Property of SCVMC

Division of Urology

(408) 885-6780

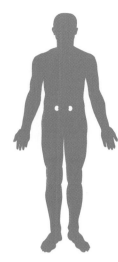

ATLAS
OF
RENAL
PATHOLOGY

ATLASES IN
DIAGNOSTIC SURGICAL PATHOLOGY

Consulting Editor

Gerald M. Bordin, M.D.
Department of Pathology
Scripps Clinic and Research Foundation

Published:

WOLD, MCLEOD, SIM, AND UNNI:
ATLAS OF ORTHOPEDIC PATHOLOGY

COLBY, LOMBARD, YOUSEM, AND KITAICHI:
ATLAS OF PULMONARY SURGICAL PATHOLOGY

WENIG:
ATLAS OF HEAD AND NECK PATHOLOGY

KANEL AND KORULA:
ATLAS OF LIVER PATHOLOGY

OWEN AND KELLY:
ATLAS OF GASTROINTESTINAL PATHOLOGY

VIRMANI:
ATLAS OF CARDIOVASCULAR PATHOLOGY

RO, GRIGNON, AMIN, AND AYALA:
**ATLAS OF SURGICAL PATHOLOGY OF
THE MALE REPRODUCTIVE TRACT**

WENIG, ADAIR, HEFESS:
ATLAS OF ENDOCRINE PATHOLOGY

FERRY AND HARRIS:
ATLAS OF LYMPHOID HYPERPLASIA AND LYMPHOMA

Forthcoming Title:

CLEMENT AND YOUNG:
ATLAS OF FEMALE GENITAL TRACT PATHOLOGY

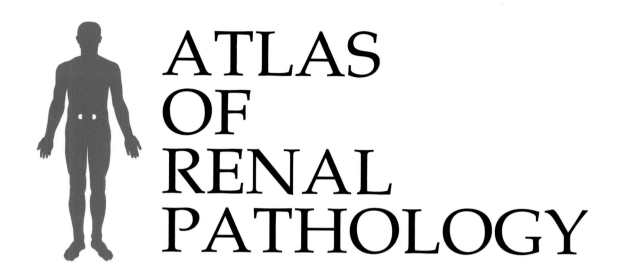

ATLAS OF RENAL PATHOLOGY

William F. Kern, MD
Assistant Professor of Pathology
Department of Pathology
University of Oklahoma College of Medicine
Oklahoma City, Oklahoma

Zoltan G. Laszik, MD, PhD
Assistant Professor of Pathology
Department of Pathology
Former Paul Kimmelstiel-Conrad Pirani Fellow in
Renal Pathology
University of Oklahoma College of Medicine
Oklahoma City, Oklahoma

Tibor Nadasdy, MD, PhD
Assistant Professor of Pathology
Department of Pathology
Johns Hopkins Hospital
Baltimore, Maryland
Former Paul Kimmelstiel-Conrad Pirani Fellow in
Renal Pathology
University of Oklahoma College of Medicine
Oklahoma City, Oklahoma

Fred G. Silva, MD
Lloyd E. Rader Professor and Chair
Department of Pathology
University of Oklahoma College of Medicine
Oklahoma City, Oklahoma

Barbara L. Bane, MD
Associate Professor of Pathology
Director, Division of Surgical Pathology
University of Oklahoma College of Medicine
Staff Pathologist
Veterans Affairs Medical Center
Oklahoma City, Oklahoma

Jan V. Pitha, MD, PhD
Professor of Pathology
University of Oklahoma College of Medicine
Chief, Pathology & Laboratory Medicine
Veterans Affairs Medical Center
Oklahoma City, Oklahoma

W. B. SAUNDERS COMPANY
A Division of Harcourt Brace & Company
Philadelphia ■ London ■ Toronto ■ Montreal ■ Sydney ■ Tokyo

W.B. SAUNDERS COMPANY
A Division of Harcourt Brace & Company

The Curtis Center
Independence Square West
Philadelphia, Pennsylvania 19106

Library of Congress Cataloging-in-Publication Data

Atlas of renal pathology / William F. Kern . . . [et al.].

p.   cm.
ISBN 0–7216–7067–9

1. Kidneys—Diseases—Atlases.   I. Kern, William
    [DNLM: 1. Kidney Diseases—pathology atlases.   2. Kidney—
pathology atlases.   WJ 17 A88171 1999]

RC903.A85   1999   616.6′107—DC21

DNLM/DLC   98–18406

ATLAS OF RENAL PATHOLOGY   ISBN 0–7216–7067–9

Printed in the United States of America.

Last digit is the print number: 9   8   7   6   5   4   3   2   1

To
Kathleen Duncan, Ph.D.
Ray Nagle, M.D., Ph.D.

Jean and Lindsay Silva
Conrad L. Pirani, M.D.

Erika, Nandi, Laura, and Aron Laszik

Robert and Alma Bane

Gyöngyi, Kriszti, and Orsi Nadasdy

To the memory of Dr. Pitha's parents, and to his family and his teachers

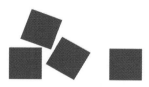

PREFACE

Renal pathology need not be difficult. Years of teaching has convinced us that the approach to the study and understanding of renal pathology can be systematic and ordered. The difficulty for neophytes in the field may relate in part to the fact that one disease can lead to many different patterns of morphologic response, and conversely that one pattern can be produced by many different etiologic agents. *Atlas of Renal Pathology* organizes the various renal patterns and diseases in a standard fashion that, we believe, is quite helpful in the approach to the study of renal diseases and their complications.

When W.B. Saunders Company approached one of us (FGS) about the development of an atlas, we were excited about the proposition of leaving to posterity the extensive renal pathology slide collection we had worked so hard to collect. For more than 20 years, a renal pathology collection of teaching slides has been assembled—what one could call the "best and brightest" of our teaching slides. These slides and the cases from which they were obtained have been collected from patient material from several institutions, including (1) The Renal Pathology Laboratory, Department of Pathology, Columbia University College of Physicians and Surgeons, formerly under the legendary direction of Dr. Conrad L. Pirani and now under the able direction of Dr. Vivette D'Agati; (2) The Southwest Pediatric Nephrology Study Group under the directorship of Dr. Ron Hogg; and (3) The University of Texas Southwestern Medical School in Dallas and The University of Oklahoma College of Medicine/The University Hospitals. If not for the renal patients, physicians, and pathologists, we would not have had the opportunity to see and collect these slides or use them for teaching a generation of interested students (at all levels).

The terminology used in the atlas is fairly consistent with that used by most North American renal pathologists. When possible, we have used the widely recognized International Nomenclature of Disease, a joint project of the Council for International Organizations of Medical Sciences and the World Health Organization. We have obviously been quite influenced over the years by our association not only with Drs. Conrad Pirani and Vivette D'Agati, but also with members of the Renal Pathology Society of North America and participants of the *Medical Diseases of the Kidney* postgraduate course held at Columbia University College of Physicians and Surgeons in New York City every year. We have tried to limit our coverage of renal patterns of disease to stable "taxonomic" groups from the large amount of published material.

A useful classification (and a subsequent approach) should be based on at least three basic requirements: (1) the classification should be *clinically significant* (for diagnosis, prognosis, and therapy), (2) it should be *easy to use and morphologically reproducible,* (3) it should be based on facts and, as far as we know, *scientifically correct.* The approach used herein allows the student to categorize the type of renal involvement, correlate it with the clinical findings, and determine the renal prognosis and, it is hoped, response to therapy.

William F. Kern, M.D.
Fred G. Silva, M.D.
Zoltan G. Laszik, M.D., Ph.D.
Barbara L. Bane, M.D.
Tibor Nadasdy, M.D., Ph.D.
Jan V. Pitha, M.D., Ph.D.

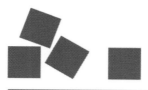

ACKNOWLEDGMENTS

We are indebted to the many various renal pathologists who over the years have contributed many of the thoughts, ideas, and dialogue that have aided in our understanding of renal diseases.

From the Department of Pathology at the University of Oklahoma College of Medicine, we are indebted to Sarah F. Johnson, M.D., Geoffrey Altshuler, M.D., and Anna Sienko, M.D., for providing pediatric pathology cases, and Mrs. Nelba Harris for secretarial assistance. From The University Hospitals in Oklahoma City, we thank Kathy Henderson, HT(ASCP), Rhonda Shuey-Drake, M.S., and Gayla Ward, HT(ASCP), for their superb job with the electron microscopy; Annie Koshy, HT(ASCP), for excellent histotechnology assistance; and Ms. Susan Heavner for secretarial assistance. From the Veterans Affairs Medical Center in Oklahoma City, our thanks go to Mrs. Jamie Yargee for secretarial assistance. We thank Sheila Lynam, M.D. (former Pathology Resident, University of Oklahoma College of Medicine), Department of Pathology, St. John's Hospital, Tulsa, Oklahoma, for providing artwork.

Many thanks go to all members of the Southwest Pediatric Nephrology Study Group (under the able direction of Ron Hogg, M.D.) for the renal biopsy material used, and to Conrad L. Pirani, M.D., for all his years of mentoring.

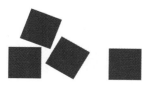

CONTENTS

■ CHAPTER 24

Tumors and Tumor-Like Conditions of the Renal Pelvis

CHAPTER 1

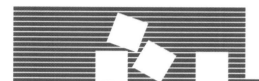

The Normal Kidney

The kidneys maintain the "internal milieu." It has been said that the body is "comprised not of what the mouth takes in, but what the kidney decides to keep." In essence, the kidney is the basis of our physiologic freedom. Its role in the filtration of plasma and secretion and reabsorption of solutes and its endocrine functions are becoming increasingly understood.

GROSS ANATOMY

- The kidneys are bean-shaped organs lying in the retroperitoneal space on each side of the vertebral column. They extend from approximately the 12th thoracic to the 3rd lumbar vertebrae; the right kidney is usually slightly caudad to the left. The left kidney lies slightly closer to the midline than the right.
- The kidneys lie in the retroperitoneum and are enclosed by the anterior and posterior layers of the renal fascia (commonly called *Gerota's fascia*).
- At full-term birth the kidneys average 6 cm in length and 26 g in weight; the adult kidney averages 11 to 12 cm in length and weighs 125 to 170 g in men and 115 to 155 g in women.
- Located on the medial surface of each kidney is the hilus, through which pass the renal artery and vein, a nerve plexus, and the ureter. The ureter originates in a cavity inside the hilus, the renal sinus, where the expanded ureter forms the renal pelvis.
- Kidneys in humans and pigs are *multipapillary*, a term referring to division of the medulla into several discrete pyramids, which range from 8 to 18 in the normal kidney. The tips of the pyramids, or *papillae*, project into extensions of the renal pelvis known as the *minor calyces.*
- Two types of papillae exist in humans: simple papillae, which are conical and drain a single lobe, and compound papillae, which drain two or more adjacent, fused lobes. Compound papillae occur primarily in the poles, especially the upper pole; simple papillae occur predominantly in the midpolar region. Simple papillae drain into the pelvis through small, often slit-like orifices; compound papillae have round or oval openings, which may be more prone to reflux of urine from the pelvis into the renal parenchyma.

- The structural unit of the kidney is the lobe, and normally each kidney has approximately 14. Each lobe is composed of a pyramid and its overlying cortex. The cortex extends downward between each pyramid to form the columns of Bertin, which flank the pyramids and receive the arterial supply of the kidney.
- The lobes contain multiple functional units called lobules that are composed of glomeruli and their related tubules, which ultimately open into the tip of the pyramid as converging collecting tubules.
- The kidney can be divided into five segments, apical, upper, middle, lower, and posterior, based on arterial blood supply. There are no anastomoses between the arteries of adjacent segments.
- There is considerable normal variation in the renal arterial supply. In the most common pattern, single renal arteries supply each side and divide into anterior and posterior branches within the extrarenal hilum. The posterior branch supplies the posterior segment of the kidney, and the anterior branch supplies the remainder of the kidney. The kidney may receive accessory arteries originating from the adrenal, superior mesenteric, or gonadal arteries. In some cases, these arteries actually represent normal segmental arteries with early origin from the aorta or main renal artery; occlusion or ligation of these "accessory" arteries results in infarction of the supplied segment.
- The renal capsule receives a dual blood supply from anastomosing intrarenal and extrarenal arteries, which allows the potential for collateral arterial supply to the kidney.
- In adults, the cortex is pale brown and averages approximately 1 cm in thickness. The medulla is darker and has a striated appearance.

MICROSCOPIC ANATOMY

For practical purposes, the kidney can be divided into four major parts: (1) *glomeruli,* (2) *tubules,* (3) the *interstitium,* and (4) *vessels.* Our approach to the morphologic diagnosis of renal diseases requires that each one of these compartments be evaluated individually and in a systematic fashion in the following order.

The Glomerulus

A normal adult kidney contains up to approximately 600,000 to 700,000 nephrons. The glomerulus was thought in the past to be a relatively inactive structure (i.e., not requiring a lot of metabolic activity) that primarily filtered renal blood flow. The glomerulus, the first part of the functional unit of the kidney, the *nephron*, is a tangle of capillaries. This capillary network is unusual in that these capillaries are the only ones in the body that are interposed between two arterioles (the afferent leading to the glomerulus and the efferent leading away from the glomerulus and supplying a large part of the renal parenchyma). The glomerulus has several important native cells and components.

Endothelium: This attenuated fenestrated endothelium has many functions, including separating blood from the glomerular basement membrane (GBM) and producing a number of vasoactive agents, adhesion molecules and growth products. Ultrastructurally, the size of the endothelial fenestrae (pores) ranges from 70 to 100 nm in diameter.

Mesangial Cells: The mesangial cell, which sits deep to the endothelium and between the capillary loops, is the reticuloendothelial system or mononuclear phagocytic system of the glomerulus. It also has major muscle-like phenotypic properties (actin and myosin positivity) and anchors the capillaries to the underlying intercapillary (mesangial) regions; it can contract under certain circumstances.

Glomerular Basement Membrane: The GBM is an acellular membrane composed of type IV collagen and heparan sulfate. Heparan sulfate gives the basement membrane a fixed anionic (negative) charge that repels negatively charged proteins such as albumin and other molecules. Ultrastructurally, the GBM is composed of a dense central layer, the lamina densa, and more electron-lucent inner and outer layers, the lamina rara interna and lamina rara externa. In healthy adults, the mean thickness of the GBM is approximately 300 nm.

Visceral Epithelial Cells (Podocytes): These complex interdigitating cells sit on top of the GBM. Like the endothelial cells, podocytes contribute to production and maintenance of the GBM. Ultrastructurally, podocytes have long cytoplasmic processes that further divide into interdigitating foot processes that come into direct contact with the lamina rara externa of the basement membrane. The distance between adjacent foot processes near the basement membrane is 25 to 60 nm in the normal glomerulus; this compartment is often referred to as a filtration slit or slit pore. In most diseases associated with proteinuria, the foot processes are replaced by a continuous cytoplasmic band, a process often referred to as *foot process effacement* or *fusion*. The cytoplasm of podocytes contains large numbers of microtubules, microfilaments, and intermediate filaments.

Parietal Epithelial Cells: Parietal epithelial cells line the inside of Bowman's capsule and form the outer limit of Bowman's space.

Together, the endothelium, mesangium, visceral epithelium, and GBM provide the permselective filter that under normal circumstances restricts passage of proteins the size of albumin and larger from crossing the glomerular capillary wall.

Tubules

What the glomerulus filters, the tubules modify through secretion and/or absorption. Ninety percent of the renal cortex is composed of tubules, and the majority of work (oxygen need) by the kidney is due to the energy requirements of these important structures. Although the tubular system of each nephron can be divided morphologically and functionally into at least 16 different segments, classically and simply the nephron is divided into the proximal tubules (convoluted and straight portions), the limb of Henle, the thick ascending limb of Henle (with its macula densa), the rest of the distal tubules, and the cortical and medullary collecting ducts (tubules).

The two segments of the proximal tubules most often identified are the proximal convoluted portion (pars convoluta), which occupies the cortical labyrinth, and the straight portion (pars recta) in the medullary rays of the cortex and outer medulla. Another classification divides the proximal tubules into three segments, P_1, P_2, and P_3 or S_1, S_2, and S_3. The lumen of the proximal tubule is patent in life but disappears if blood supply is interrupted, as seen in renal biopsy specimens. In the P_1 and P_2 portions, the proximal tubular epithelial cells have an elaborate cell shape, abundant acidophilic cytoplasm, and a well-developed periodic acid–Schiff–positive microvillous border (brush border). The P_3 pars recta cells are lower in height and have a less elaborate shape. Electron microscopy reveals an atypical junctional complex between the proximal tubular epithelial cells. Each finger-shaped microvillus has a core of microfilaments that extend into the apical cytoplasm and connect there to the cytoskeleton.

The thin descending limb of the loop of Henle originates from the proximal tubule at the boundary between the outer and the inner stripes of the outer medulla. Long-looped nephrons originating from the juxtamedullary glomeruli have a long descending thin limb followed by a long ascending thin limb that continues into the thick ascending limb. The transition from the thin to the thick ascending limb is at the border of the outer and inner medulla. The descending thin limb of the loop of Henle is lined by flat noninterdigitating epithelium with a few microvilli. The ascending thin limb has flat, interdigitating epithelium with tight junctions.

The distal tubule is composed of three segments: the thick ascending limb of the loop of Henle (pars recta), the macula densa, and the distal convoluted tubule (pars convoluta). The macula densa is a specialized region of the thick ascending limb of Henle and is part of the juxtaglomerular complex. The cells of the distal convoluted tubule resemble those of the thick ascending limb but are taller.

The collecting duct system includes the cortical and medullary collecting ducts. The collecting ducts are lined by two types of cells: collecting duct (principal) cells and intercalated (dark) cells. In the cortex the lining cells have a cuboidal shape; the morphology of the epithelial cells lining the collecting ducts gradually changes as they descend toward the papilla. They increase in cell height and have more complex tight junctions.

The Interstitium

Very little interstitial space is observable by light microscopy in the normal kidney. The interstitium provides structural support for the major elements of the kidney (tubules, blood vessels, and glomeruli), and the tubular and interstitial areas are so intimately associated with each other in the normal state that many investigators like to consider them one functional unit.

It is primarily the condition of the interstitium and tubules in disease that best correlates with altered renal function such as serum creatinine, blood urea nitrogen, or creatinine clearance.

Blood Vessels

With approximately 20% to 25% of the cardiac output of the heart coming through the kidney, the kidney is one of the most vascular tissues in the body. In essence, the kidney is nourished and sustained by the blood vessels, and most diseases of the kidney eventually alter this component. Each renal artery takes off from the aorta and divides into segmental renal arteries and then interlobar and arcuate arteries (the latter coursing between the renal cortex and the medullary areas), which then divide into the interlobular arteries and finally the afferent arterioles (which go into the glomeruli). It is important to note that these arteries and arterioles are end arteries and arterioles, which means that if they are occluded, the tissues they supply downstream will be rendered ischemic, injured, or necrotic.

All four components of the kidney (glomeruli, tubules, interstitium, and vessels) work together to excrete metabolic products or compounds that are not needed and reabsorb those that are required for maintenance of homeostasis (the "internal milieu"). Diseases of the kidney may initially involve only one of these four components individually. However, as the course of a renal disease progresses, two, three, or all of the other components of the kidneys will eventually be involved and compromised.

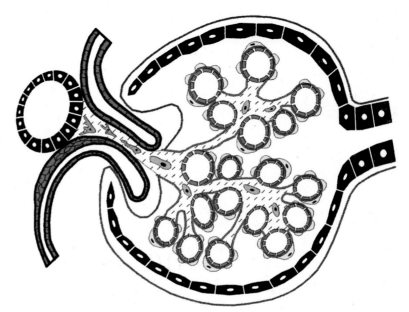

Figure 1-1. Normal glomerulus. This schematic drawing of the glomerulus illustrates a capillary network interposed between two arterioles *(red).* The capillaries are surrounded by Bowman's capsule. The basement membrane *(blue)* encircles the capillaries, the mesangial matrix *(crosshatching),* the mesangial cells *(gold),* and the lacis cells *(gold)* in the triangle between the afferent arteriole, efferent arteriole, and the tubule *(orange).* The capillary lumina are lined by endothelial cells *(red).* The visceral epithelial cells are *light yellow.* (Courtesy of Dr. Sheila Lynam, Pathology Laboratory Associates, Tulsa, Oklahoma.)

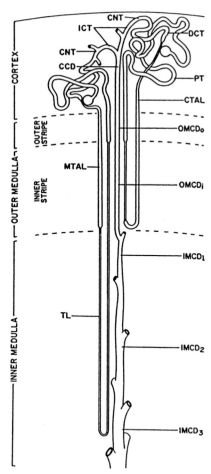

Figure 1–2. Normal nephron. The figure reveals the structure of the superficial and juxtamedullary nephrons of the kidney. Nephrons represent the functional units of the kidney. PT, proximal tubule; TL, thin limb of loop of Henle; MTAL, medullary thick ascending limb; CTAL, cortical thick ascending limb; DCT, distal convoluted tubule; CNT, connecting segment; CCD, cortical collecting duct; $OMCD_o$, collecting duct in outer stripe of outer medulla; $OMCD_i$, collecting duct in inner stripe of outer medulla; $IMCD_{1-3}$, inner medullary collecting ducts. (From Madsen KM, Tisher CC: Structural-functional relationships along the distal nephron. Am J Physiol 250:F1–F15, 1986, with permission.)

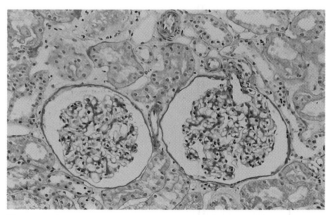

Figure 1–4. Normal renal cortex. Glomeruli, proximal and distal tubules, interstitial capillaries, and arterioles are seen. The proximal tubular epithelial brush border is periodic acid–Schiff (PAS) positive (PAS reaction).

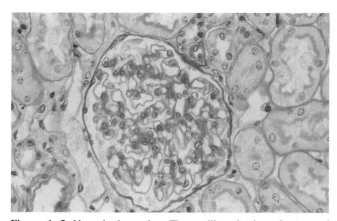

Figure 1–5. Normal glomerulus. The capillary lumina of a normal glomerulus are patent; the nuclei of the endothelial cells inside the capillary lumina are clearly visible. The basement membranes appear thin and delicate. The mesangium has as many as two to three cells per area away from the vascular pole in this thin 2- to 3-μm section. The scattered visceral epithelial cells are closely attached to the external surface of the glomerular capillary basement membranes. Bowman's capsule surrounds the glomerular capillary network (tangle of capillaries). The basement membranes, the mesangium, and Bowman's capsule are periodic acid–Schiff (PAS) positive (PAS reaction).

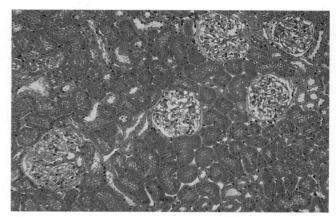

Figure 1–3. Normal renal cortex. The glomeruli occupy a small portion of the renal cortex and are separated by the tubulointerstitium, which contains tubules, delicate and quite sparse interstitial connective tissue, and vessels.

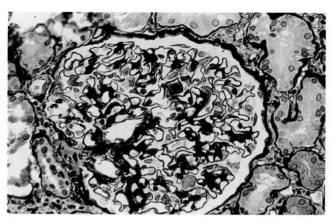

Figure 1–6. Normal glomerulus. Methenamine silver staining depicts the glomerular capillary basement membranes and the mesangium, both of which are silver positive. The basement membrane surrounds both the capillaries and the mesangium. The mesangium is a fine network of matrix and mesangial cells to which the glomerular capillaries are attached.

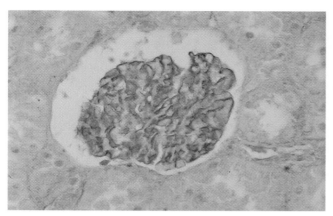

Figure 1-7. Normal glomerulus. The negatively charged fixed anionic glomerular capillary basement membranes are labeled with cationized colloidal iron.

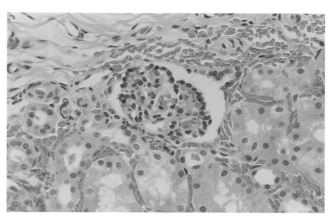

Figure 1-9. Normal glomerulus in a newborn. Prominent cuboidal visceral epithelial cells cover the capillary network of the small glomerular tuft.

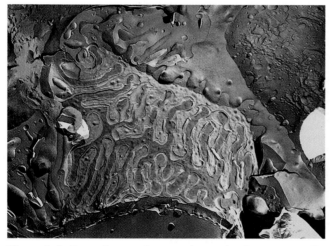

Figure 1-8. Freeze-fracture electron micrograph of a segment of a glomerular tuft. The uncolored structure at the *bottom* is the glomerular basement membrane and its fenestrated endothelium. In the *middle* above the basement membrane are three differently colored *(blue, red, yellow)* separate visceral epithelial cells. Note the complex interdigitations between the different visceral epithelial cells. (Courtesy of Dr. Vernon Schultz, Dallas.)

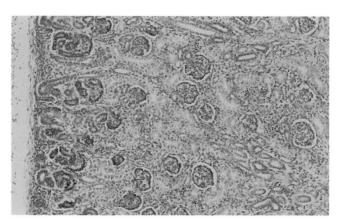

Figure 1-10. Fetal kidney. The subcapsular nephrogenic zone on the *left* contains immature glomeruli; toward the deeper portions of the cortex, small mature glomeruli are seen.

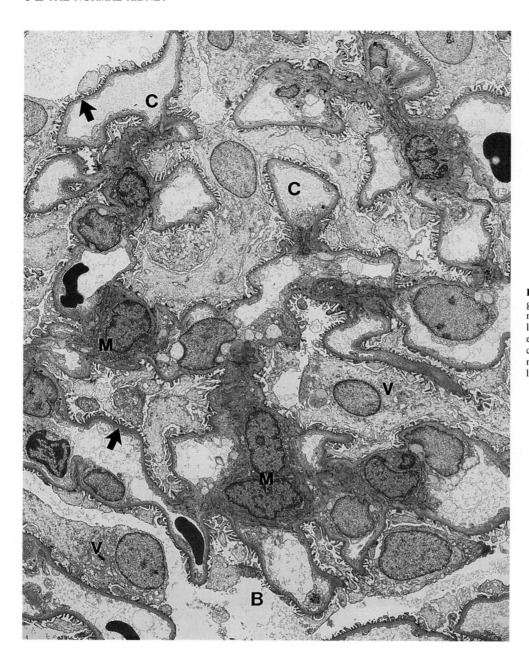

Figure 1–11. Electron microphotograph of a portion of a normal glomerulus. C, patent glomerular capillary lumina lined by fenestrated endothelial cells; *arrow,* glomerular capillary basement membranes; M, mesangial cells; V, visceral epithelial cells; B, Bowman's space.

References

Beckwith JB: Pediatric kidney. In: Sternberg SS (ed): Histology for Pathologists. New York, Raven Press, 1992, p 669.

Clapp WL: Adult kidney. In: Sternberg SS (ed): Histology for Pathologists. New York, Raven Press, 1992, p 667.

Clapp WL, Abrahamson DR: Development and gross anatomy of the kidney. In: Tisher CC, Brenner BM (eds): Renal Pathology: With Clinical and Functional Correlations, 2nd ed. Philadelphia, JB Lippincott, 1994, p 1.

Petersen RO (ed): Kidney: Normal structure. In: Urologic Pathology, 2nd ed. Philadelphia, JB Lippincott, 1992, p 1.

CHAPTER 2

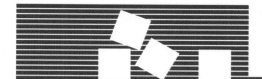

Classification of Renal Diseases and Mechanisms of Renal Injury

CLASSIFICATION OF RENAL DISEASES

Renal diseases can be classified in several ways, that is, clinically, morphologically, etiologically, or immunopathologically; combining the data of these various classifications provides a comprehensive database that allows clinicians, pathologists, and researchers to further analyze renal diseases, better understand the nature of the diseases, and ideally improve the treatment of patients with these diseases. The immunopathologic classification and electron microscopy are discussed in Chapter 3.

- The *clinical classification* defines major categories such as the *nephrotic syndrome* (proteinuria of 3.5 g or more per 24 hours, together with generalized edema, hyperlipidemia, and hyperlipiduria), the *nephritic syndrome* (hematuria, proteinuria, sodium and fluid retention, hypertension, and sometimes oliguria), and acute or chronic renal failure. Each of these clinical syndromes or symptoms may be associated with a number of renal diseases or patterns; for example, the nephrotic syndrome can be seen with focal segmental glomerulosclerosis, membranous glomerulonephropathy, membranoproliferative glomerulonephritis, and a variety of others. In addition, a specific renal disease may be associated with a variety of clinical signs and symptoms (e.g., patients who have IgA glomerulonephritis may have nephrotic syndrome, nephritic syndrome, or microscopic or macroscopic hematuria). This diverse manifestation of renal disease is often a major obstacle to making a specific diagnosis on the basis of clinical signs and symptoms alone.
- *Morphologic classification* is based on recognition of *patterns of renal injury*; however, most of the morphologic patterns do not correspond to a single specific disease entity. Therefore, in addition to the morphologic (light microscopic) findings, clinical data, immunofluorescence, and electron microscopy all are very important in attempting to classify specific renal diseases (i.e., to subclassify the pattern and type of injury).

- *Etiologic classification* requires a combination of clinical history, morphologic pattern, laboratory data, and sometimes imaging studies (radiographic or ultrasonographic). In some cases a specific etiologic diagnosis can be made; for example, *poststreptococcal acute glomerulonephritis* when the clinical history and laboratory studies indicate recent streptococcal infection in a patient with acute proliferative glomerulonephritis. In many cases, however, a specific etiology is not apparent and the pathologist can only provide a list of differential diagnoses based on the morphologic pattern.

Approach to Morphologic Classification

Light microscopic examination should be carried out in a systematic way and should deal with each of the four compartments of the kidney sequentially (glomeruli, tubules, interstitium, and vessels). The starting point is to decide which component of the kidney is the most severely affected; the component with the most severe changes defines the "primary" disease (e.g., glomerulonephritis, interstitial nephritis, vascular disease). If, however, the "primary" disease is very advanced or severe, most or all of the renal compartments are severely affected and a determination of primary versus secondary involvement may not be possible. For example, in patients who have hypertension with severe vascular disease (arteriosclerosis), advanced interstitial fibrosis and prominent interstitial inflammatory cell infiltrate, and advanced global or focal segmental glomerulosclerosis, it may not be possible to pinpoint the primary cause of the renal disease.

Glomeruli

- Glomerular lesions (if present) should be characterized next and are defined by glomerular cellularity, patency of the glomerular capillary lumina, changes in basement membranes and the mesangium, and so forth. If glomerular changes are present, one should determine whether the process is *diffuse* (i.e., a majority of the glomeruli have lesions on light microscopy) or *focal* (limited to a lesser proportion of the glomeruli).

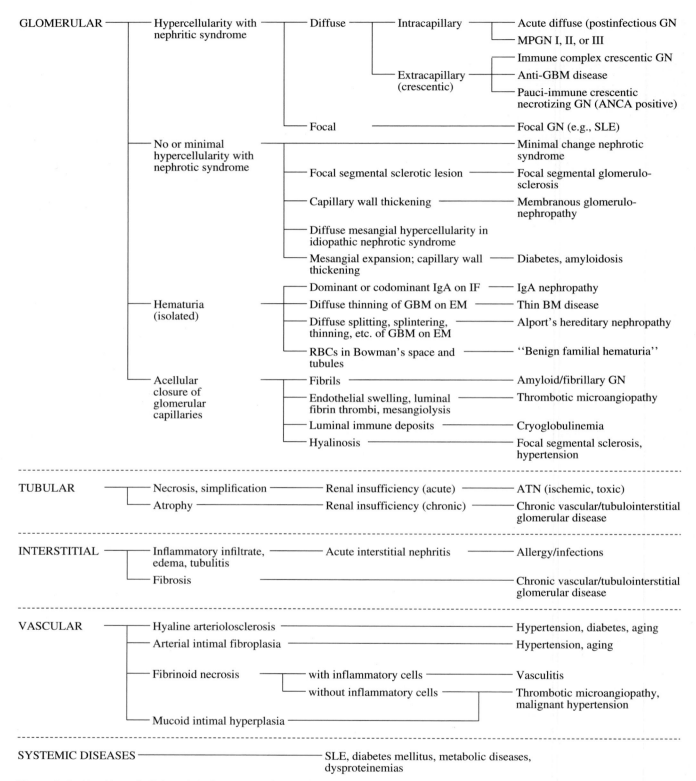

Figure 2–1. Algorithm of clinicopathologic patterns of glomerular, tubular, interstitial, and vascular diseases. GN, glomerulonephritis; MPGN, membranoproliferative glomerulonephritis; GBM, glomerular basement membrane; ANCA, antineutrophil cytoplasmic antibody; SLE, systemic lupus erythematosus; IF, immunofluorescence; EM, electron microscopy; BM, basement membrane; ATN, acute tubular necrosis.

- Mesangial hypercellularity is defined by the World Health Organization (WHO) as three or more cells in an individual mesangial region in thin 2- to 3-μm sections away from the vascular pole. The definition of intracapillary hypercellularity refers to hypercellularity *inside the glomerular capillary tuft*. Severe hypercellularity usually leads to closure of the glomerular capillary loops, which is considered by many renal pathologists to be the criterion for the diagnosis of *intracapillary proliferative glomerulonephritis*.
- The cells inside the glomerular capillary tufts in intracapillary proliferative glomerulonephritis are thought to be derived from the proliferating resident glomerular cells (e.g., mesangial and endothelial cells) and from the circulating blood. Large numbers of acute inflammatory cells (polymorphonuclear leukocytes) in the glomerular capillary loops are suggestive of either postinfectious or membranoproliferative glomerulonephritis. Accumulation of large numbers of mononuclear leukocytes (monocytes) in the glomerular capillary loops may point to cryoglobulinemic glomerulonephritis.
- Glomerular hypercellularity can also be present outside the glomerular capillary tuft in Bowman's space (i.e., *extracapillary proliferation*), in which case the mass of cells is generally described as forming a *crescent*. If a significant proportion of the glomeruli are affected by crescent formation (the WHO definition requires more than 80% of the glomeruli to be affected; however, many renal pathologists use different figures varying between 50% and 100%), the diagnosis will be *crescentic glomerulonephritis*.
- *Acellular closure* (as opposed to hypercellular closure) of the glomerular capillary lumina may result from collapse of the glomerular capillary tuft and is most often seen in focal segmental glomerulosclerosis, collapsing glomerulopathy, and glomerular ischemia. Another form of acellular closure of the glomerular capillary tuft is seen in thrombotic microangiopathies; in this case the closure is caused by swelling of endothelial cells and accumulation of subendothelial acellular material.

Tubules and Interstitium

- Changes in tubules and the interstitium (sometimes referred to as tubulointerstitial changes), such as inflammatory cell infiltrates, acute tubular necrosis, and tubular atrophy, are often secondary to changes in other compartments of the kidney such as the glomeruli or the vasculature. The presence of changes in other compartments of the kidney, the composition of the cellular infiltrate, immunofluorescence and electron microscopic findings, and clinical data are important regardless of whether we are dealing with a primary or secondary process.
- Precise dissection of the tubulointerstitial processes (i.e., tubular versus interstitial) is not always possible. For example, acute tubular epithelial injury (acute tubular necrosis) may be associated with reactive interstitial inflammatory cellular infiltrates, and interstitial nephritis may cause tubular epithelial cell injury reminiscent of changes seen in acute tubular necrosis.

Vessels

- *Arterial and arteriolar changes* are common, especially in older patients, and some degree of arteriosclerosis is considered to be part of the normal aging process. Frequently, interstitial fibrosis and/or features of glomerular ischemia are associated with the vascular changes. Arteriosclerosis (intimal fibroplasia) is most often seen in the interlobular, arcuate, and subarcuate arteries, especially in patients who have hypertension. Hyaline arteriolosclerosis is a common finding in patients who have hypertension and/or diabetes.
- Vascular changes such as mucoid intimal hyperplasia, fibrinoid necrosis, and thrombus formation are suggestive of thrombotic microangiopathy; however, fibrinoid necrosis with or without thrombus formation is also a prominent feature of vasculitis.

Although the classification herein used is widely accepted, this classification, like any other classification in medicine, is neither perfect nor absolute; it is continuously evolving, and the future—as it can be foreseen—will not leave it untouched.

MECHANISMS OF RENAL INJURY

Glomerulus

The glomerulus is a self-cleansing renewable filter; it is amazingly resistant to the numerous injuries that besiege it. However, a number of injuries can lead to glomerular disease.

Most primary glomerular diseases are immunologic in nature. Most of these immunologic glomerular diseases result from the formation of immune complexes (defined as complexes of antigens with their corresponding antibodies, sometimes including complement components). These immune complexes can be formed in the peripheral circulation and are termed circulating immune complexes (CICs), or the antigen can be localized (either planted or intrinsic [native]) and the antigen-antibody reaction occurs within the glomerulus itself (in situ immune complex formation).

In CIC diseases, antibody is generally formed in response to some antigenic determinant (immunogen) in the antigen (which is often bacterial, viral, etc.); the glomerulus acts as an "innocent bystander" that filters the large amount of blood coming to it, and for a variety of reasons (see later) the CICs impact and damage the glomerulus. Classic prototypes of this type of CIC disease are acute postinfectious glomerulonephritis and systemic lupus erythematosus; the immunofluorescence pattern is generally granular or "lumpy bumpy."

In the second type of immune complex process, termed in situ immune complex formation, the antigen is either a normal, native intrinsic antigen of the normal glomerulus or an antigen that by itself has been planted within the glomerulus. An antibody response is generated, with the antibody circulating alone in the blood until it finds its "match" (i.e., antigen) in the glomerulus. Two types of immunofluorescent patterns can be seen: (1) linear staining, as in anti–glomerular basement membrane antibody–induced glomerulonephritis, and (2) granular staining, as noted in membranous glomerulonephritis. The difference in staining patterns is related to the equal distribution of antigen in the first compared to the unequal, larger complex formation in the latter.

Factors Influencing the Glomerular Deposition of Immune Complexes

A large number of factors influence the glomerular deposition of immune complexes, including the size of the immune complex, electrical charge, and others.

Size of the Immune Complex: Larger immune complexes formed in antibody excess produce large interlinking lattice-like networks that are generally deposited in the reticuloendothelial system (RES; e.g., the spleen, liver); if they make it past these RES regions, they may be found in the glomerular subendothelial and mesangial regions. Smaller immune complexes (composed of antigen excess, the smallest immune complex being two antigens and one antibody i.e., Ag2Ab1) may make it part of the way past the inner glomerular filter and end up in the glomerular subepithelial region (although this probably requires major physicochemical alteration of the complex and the glomerulus).

Electrical Charge: In response to the existing negative electrical charge of the glomerular capillary wall, that is, the fixed glomerular polyanionic charge, immune complexes will preferentially be deposited in certain regions, depending on their own charge. For example, if the complex is strongly positively charged (cationic), it may end up in the glomerular subepithelial region. However, if the complex has a fairly weak negative electrical charge (anionic), it will be found in the subendothelial and mesangial regions. If it is very strongly negatively charged, it may not be found at all in the glomerulus.

Other Factors: Other factors influencing glomerular deposition of immune complexes include hemodynamic factors, the class and subclass of the antibodies (not well studied as yet), and the avidity and valency of the antibody-antigen association.

Mediators of Glomerular Injury

Immune complexes, once deposited in the glomerulus, are often not pathogenetic in themselves. They generally create damage by activating a cascade of inflammatory and injurious events. The list of recognized immune mediators of glomerular injury keeps growing but includes the following:

Complement (classic or alternative pathway)
Neutrophils and their products
Lymphocytes (T; sensitized) and their products
Monocytes/macrophages
Platelets
Native glomerular cells themselves
Growth factors (e.g., cytokines)

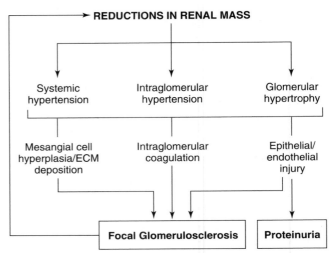

Figure 2–2. Renal ablation glomerulosclerosis. ECM, extracellular matrix. (From Cotran RS, Kumar V, Robbins SL [eds]; Robbins Pathologic Basis of Disease, 5th ed. Philadelphia, WB Saunders, 1994, p 945, with permission.)

Nonimmunologic Mechanisms of Glomerular Injury

Hemodynamic Factors

Hemodynamic factors have been demonstrated to contribute to glomerular injury in animal models of partial total nephrectomy (surgical kidney removal). In the remaining glomeruli subjected to compensatory hyperfiltration, there is an increased glomerular plasma flow rate and increased pressure. Proteinuria, polyuria, and mild arterial hypertension develop in these animals 1 week after surgery.

The increased glomerular capillary pressure could lead to direct mechanical injury to endothelial or visceral epithelial cells. Alternatively but not mutually exclusive is the possibility that increased glomerular blood flow leading to increased circulation of macromolecules is indirectly responsible for mesangial matrix increase and cellular proliferation, perhaps on the basis of growth factors.

This mode of glomerular injury is particularly important in diabetic nephropathy in humans, but it is also involved in any renal disease that results in the loss of a critical number of nephrons. Blood pressure control has been shown to reduce the rate of progression of loss of renal function.

Coagulation

Endothelial damage secondary either to direct mechanical damage, as mentioned before, or to circulating factors (bacterial endotoxin, tumor necrosis factor, and so forth) promotes platelet adhesion and the formation of fibrin thrombi. Thrombus formation and platelet activation, in turn, lead to the production of growth factors, which may either activate cellular proliferation, promote inflammation, or promote the formation of extracellular matrix, the global effect being that of eventual glomerulosclerosis and interstitial fibrosis.

Dietary Factors

The exact mechanism by which dietary protein may contribute to glomerular injury has not been determined. However, in models of renal ablation in animals, a measurable reduction in glomerular capillary pressure has been found after a low-protein diet. (It has been hypothesized that a high protein load leads to increased serum levels of prostaglandins [prostaglandin E_2], which in turn is responsible for the increased glomerular filtration rate. On the other hand, a low-protein diet is associated with an overall reduction in calorie intake. It has not been excluded that the latter is the important factor.)

Regardless of the underlying mechanism, it is important to recognize that a low-protein diet has been shown to reduce the progression of glomerular injury both in renal ablation animal models and in human glomerular diseases in which hyperfiltration has been identified as a promoter of glomerular injury, for example, diabetic nephropathy.

Studies are now under way to determine the exact role of other dietary constituents such as lipids, carbohydrates, sodium, and phosphate.

Hypertrophy

Hypertrophy as a mechanism of glomerular injury has been determined to be particularly important in early diabetes mellitus, where one of the earlier structural alterations is glomerular hypertrophy—that is, an increase in glomerular size and the caliber of glomerular capillary loops. This mechanism of glomerular injury probably also plays a role in minimal change nephrotic syndrome (nil disease) and focal segmental glomerulosclerosis. The overall detrimental effect of glomerular hypertrophy has been linked to increased glomerular capillary pressure (see earlier).

References

Schrier RW, Gottschalk CW (eds): Diseases of the Kidney, 6th ed. Boston, Little, Brown, 1996.
Silva FG, D'Agati VD, Nadasdy T (eds): Renal Biopsy Interpretation. New York, Churchill Livingstone, 1996.

CHAPTER 3

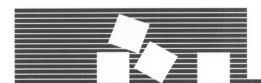

Tissue Sampling, Preparation, and Interpretation

INTRODUCTION

In many of the lesions to be described, the ability of the pathologist to provide an accurate diagnosis and estimate of severity will be determined in large part by the adequacy of the renal tissue that is obtained. This tissue is usually obtained by percutaneous or open renal biopsy or by nephrectomy. The biopsy sample is divided for light microscopy (LM), immunofluorescence (IF), and electron microscopy (EM).

LIGHT MICROSCOPY

For diagnosis of medical diseases of the kidney, slides are routinely stained for LM with hematoxylin and eosin, periodic acid–Schiff (PAS), methenamine silver, and trichrome stains. Periodic acid–Schiff and methenamine silver stains are very helpful in examining the basement membranes of the glomerular capillaries and tubules. Trichrome stain shows the severity of interstitial fibrosis or glomerular sclerosis. Fibrinogen deposition can also be seen, and in addition, glomerular immune complex deposits, if present, can be visualized (as fuchsinophilic dots) by trichrome stain.

The biopsy specimen must be examined at multiple levels to detect lesions that involve only a portion of the tissue; usually two to four slides are stained with each stain, and multiple cuts are present on each slide. It is extremely important that the histologic sections be cut as thinly as possible (2 to 3 μm). Special stains, such as Congo red for amyloid, may be useful in specific cases.

IMMUNOFLUORESCENCE

- Tissue snap-frozen for direct IF examination should be cut as thinly as possible (2 to 4 μm) and stained with antisera known to be relatively monospecific for IgG, IgM, IgA, C3, C1q (or C4), properdin, fibrin(ogen)-related antigen (FRA), and either albumin or transferrin. Other antisera such as antibodies to κ or λ light chains should be routinely applied. The following IF

characteristics should be evaluated in every renal biopsy specimen:

- What *class* of immunoglobulin and fraction of complement are being deposited? Are both types of light chains (κ and λ) positive or just one?
- Is the deposition of purported immune material (immunoglobulins or complement components) associated with *nonimmunologic* material such as albumin or transferrin? In areas of plasmatic insudation, all plasma proteins flow into the damaged region—not only immunoglobulins and complement but also albumin, transferrin, and FRA. If all these are found, one is less certain of a primary immunologic phenomenon.
- What *region* of the glomerulus is staining: capillary wall, mesangium, or Bowman's capsule? Does the staining occur in an area of segmental sclerosis? If so, this finding would again raise the possibility of nonspecific nonimmunologic trapping, especially if one found only IgM, C3, and FRA.
- Is the deposition *granular* (probably immune complex) or *linear* (classically anti–glomerular basement membrane [anti-GBM] antibodies)? It should, however, be noted that linear staining is neither sufficient nor necessary for the definitive diagnosis of anti-GBM–induced glomerulonephritis (GN).
- What is the intensity of the fluorescence? Assessment of intensity may be quite subjective, but a skilled eye can distinguish a mild, moderate, and strong reaction. Such assessment is important in certain diseases such as IgA nephropathy where, for example, an IgA predominance or codominance in glomerular deposits is a requirement for the diagnosis.

The class of immunoglobulin is important to determine because IgA can be seen, for example, in systemic lupus erythematosus (SLE) and is often associated with a "full house" of immunoglobulins, whereas IgA alone might suggest either Berger's disease (IgA nephropathy) or anaphylactoid purpura (Henoch-Schönlein purpura [HSP]). Finding C3 without C1q would suggest that the alternative complement pathway is involved, which might be detected with properdin.

Determining whether the staining is in mesangial regions or along the glomerular capillary walls may be important in determining the prognosis in such diseases as SLE, HSP, and IgA nephropathy. Examination of the extraglomerular structure (tubules, interstitium, vessels) is also quite important.

Although these IF studies give some indication of the immunologic warfare that has occurred (and allows a more crisp diagnosis), it is also obvious that the complexity of the system or systems involved is usually underestimated.

ELECTRON MICROSCOPY

Electron microscopy is especially useful in the diagnosis of medical diseases of the kidney; indeed, one of the first uses of EM in medicine was in renal disease. Tissue should be properly fixed for possible EM in all biopsy samples of native (nontransplant) kidneys. The role of routine use of EM in transplant biopsy tissue is somewhat debated. However, most renal pathologists and nephrologists agree that if significant proteinuria develops in a transplant patient several months after transplantation, it is certainly reasonable to save material for EM examination.

Material submitted for EM should be cut into small pieces ($1 \times 1 \times 1$ mm) for proper fixation and fixed in glutaraldehyde or EM-grade formalin. "Semithin" or "thick" sections (1 μm) are examined under LM to choose the proper area for ultrastructural studies.

The most important role of EM in a diseased glomerulus is the search for discrete electron-dense "immune-type" deposits. In immune-mediated glomerular disease, EM is useful for determining the presence and the exact site of the deposits, which is often difficult to determine by IF, especially if deposits are along the glomerular capillary wall (subendothelial versus subepithelial).

In certain diseases such as SLE, the presence of glomerular subendothelial deposits (especially large deposits in the peripheral glomerular capillary walls) indicates a more severe disease.

Differentiation of glomerular electron-dense "immune-type" deposits from hyalin (plasma protein) deposits may be difficult. In general, hyalin deposits are less electron dense and more homogeneous than immune-type deposits and are usually found in areas of severe sclerosis.

Glomerular mesangial deposits are present in a number of diseases such as SLE, IgA nephropathy (Berger's disease), C1q nephropathy, and others.

Occasionally it is possible to make a specific diagnosis by EM, as in Alport's hereditary nephropathy with characteristic diffuse splitting, splintering, rarefaction, and thinning of the GBMs.

GENERALIZATIONS ABOUT GLOMERULAR DISEASES

The following points are important in understanding glomerular diseases:

■ *A variety of renal morphologic patterns can lead to the same clinical syndromes;* for example, nephritic syndrome and hematuria can be caused by hereditary nephropathy, membranoproliferative GN, Berger's disease (mesangial IgA nephropathy), or acute proliferative GN. Nephrotic syndrome can be caused by minimal change nephrotic syndrome, focal sclerosis, membranous glomerulonephropathy, diabetic nephropathy, or amyloid.
■ *One disease may produce different patterns of renal injury;* for example, SLE may lead to many different patterns of injury, each with a different prognosis.
■ *One distinctive type of pathologic pattern or process may be produced or associated with many different diseases:* membranoproliferative GN (a pattern) can be seen in SLE, hepatitis B antigenemia, and various infections and can be associated with carcinomas.
■ *Renal biopsy is specific and diagnostic in only a few select conditions,* for example, Alport's hereditary nephropathy. Thus diagnostic renal pathology is an integrated "gestalt" process in which one must analyze and collate all the clinical, LM, EM, and IF studies to arrive at the best overall diagnosis.
■ *One renal syndrome may be associated with different diseases yet have common pathogenetic mechanisms that initiate it.* An example is crescentic GN, which can be seen in a variety of diseases such as SLE, anaphylactoid purpura, and acute GN; in all conditions, the crescents are probably related to FRAs that reach Bowman's space through breaks or "gaps" in the GBM.

Reference

Silva FG, D'Agati VD, Nadasdy T (eds): Renal Biopsy Interpretation. New York, Churchill Livingstone, 1996.

CHAPTER 4

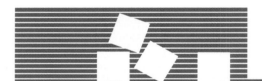

The True (Hypercellular or "Proliferative") Glomerulonephritides
Diseases Associated With the Nephritic Syndrome

INTRODUCTION

- The true glomerulonephritides include a variety of diseases with diverse etiologies and variable morphologic appearances, all of which feature an increase in cellularity in the glomerular capillary tuft with closure of capillary loops. In some cases, the renal involvement may be the primary or sole manifestation of the disease process; in others, the renal disease is secondary to a systemic process such as vasculitis or systemic lupus erythematosus (SLE). Complete pathologic evaluation of a renal biopsy performed for or demonstrating a glomerulonephritis requires a combination of clinical history, laboratory studies, light microscopy, immunofluorescence microscopy, and electron microscopy (EM). A final pathologic diagnosis should include a morphologic diagnosis and, when possible, an etiologic diagnosis (e.g., "acute diffuse proliferative [exudative] glomerulonephritis consistent with poststreptococcal glomerulonephritis").

- The clinical features of the true glomerulonephritides can be extremely variable both in signs and symptoms and in temporal evolution. Frequent manifestations include hematuria, proteinuria, renal insufficiency, or any combination thereof. Hematuria can be gross or microscopic; proteinuria can vary from minimal to nephrotic range. The *nephritic syndrome* characteristically includes hematuria, casts on urinalysis (usually red cell casts, occasionally white cell casts), fluid overload with hypertension, and variable degrees of renal insufficiency with oliguria or anuria; the onset is frequently abrupt. The term *rapidly progressive glomerulonephritis* (RPGN) indicates 50% or greater loss of renal function within 3 months as measured by creatinine clearance.

- Immunologic mechanisms underlie most cases of glomerulonephritis. Immune components (immunoglobulins, complement, or both) are present within glomeruli in the majority of cases of glomerulonephritis, and evidence of immunologic disturbances is present in many patients even when immune deposits are not found on renal biopsy; for example, antineutrophil cytoplasmic antibodies (ANCAs) are found in most cases of pauci-immune crescentic glomerulonephritis.

- The initial step in the histologic evaluation of glomerulonephritis is categorization of the process in terms of the number of glomeruli involved (i.e., whether the disease is focal and involves only some glomeruli or diffuse and involves most or all glomeruli), whether glomerular involvement is partial (segmental) or complete (global), which compartments of the glomerulus are involved, whether there is necrosis, and whether neutrophils are present (exudative). Abnormalities may involve the mesangium, mesangium plus capillary walls (mesangiocapillary or membranoproliferative), capillary lumina (intracapillary or endocapillary), or areas outside the capillary tuft in Bowman's space (extracapillary). Histologic categories of glomerulonephritis, together with common examples, are listed in Table 4–1.

- It is important to recognize that these morphologic patterns are not specific and each can be due to various causes and occur in a variety of diseases. For example, membranoproliferative (mesangiocapillary) glomerulonephritis (MPGN) can result from hepatitis B or C virus infection or can be a manifestation of SLE; the striking finding of glomerular crescents (extracapillary proliferation) occurs in a variety of diseases. A specific disease, for example, SLE, may have many histologic manifestations. There may also be transformation from one appearance to another; for instance, a resolving diffuse intracapillary proliferative (poststreptococcal) glomerulonephritis may pass through a phase characterized primarily by mesangial proliferation, which could be histologically indistinguishable from mesangial proliferative glomerulonephritis from a variety of causes.

- The prognosis of patients with histologically similar lesions may vary, depending on the primary cause; mesangial proliferative glomerulonephritis caused by IgA nephropathy, resolving poststreptococcal acute proliferative glomerulonephritis, or systemic lupus may be histologically similar but vary greatly in prognosis.

Table 4–1
HISTOLOGIC CATEGORIES OF ACUTE
HYPERCELLULAR GLOMERULONEPHRITIS

Histologic Pattern	Causes
Diffuse intracapillary proliferative (exudative) GN (with neutrophils)	Usually postinfectious Occasionally related to SLE or vasculitis
Diffuse proliferative GN (without neutrophils)	Postinfectious GN SLE
Diffuse extracapillary proliferative (crescentic) GN	Anti-GBM antibody disease Vasculitis, usually ANCA associated Immune complex GN
Membranoproliferative (mesangiocapillary) GN	Idiopathic Cryoglobulinemia SLE
Mesangial proliferative GN	Resolving postinfectious GN IgA nephropathy Common nonspecific pattern
Focal GN	Postinfectious GN Acute infectious GN (endocarditis, deep-seated visceral abscess) SLE

GN, glomerulonephritis; SLE, systemic lupus erythematosus; GBM, glomerular basement membrane; ANCA, antineutrophil cytoplasmic antibody.

■ There has been disagreement among renal pathologists whether the term *proliferative,* which implies replication of *endogenous* glomerular cells, is accurate in describing these conditions because many of the cells present appear to be recruited from the circulation or other nonglomerular sources. Accurate or not, the term *proliferative* is firmly entrenched in both clinical use and the renal pathology literature, and thus we shall use it here. Recognizing the presence of hypercellularity is critical; determining the origin of cells within the glomeruli in individual cases may be difficult and is usually unnecessary.

MESANGIAL PROLIFERATIVE GLOMERULONEPHRITIS

Synonyms and Related Terms: Mesangiopathic glomerulonephritis; diffuse mesangial proliferation; diffuse mesangial hypercellularity.

Biology of Disease

■ The term *mesangial proliferative glomerulonephritis* is defined by the World Health Organization Committee on Classification of Renal Disease as "an essentially uniform increase in mesangial cells (with clusters of four or more per mesangial area) in all or nearly all glomeruli. Cell proliferation may be accompanied by an increase in mesangial matrix." Included in this definition is the specification that *capillary lumina are patent*; patency distinguishes mesangial proliferative glomerulonephritis from conditions with endocapillary proliferation.
■ Use of the term *proliferative* in "mesangial proliferative glomerulonephritis" has been criticized for reasons discussed earlier, and therefore several synonyms have been proposed.

■ Mesangial hypercellularity is seen in a variety of conditions; thus, "mesangial proliferative glomerulonephritis" represents a heterogeneous group of conditions rather than a single disease. Therefore, although a characteristic light microscopic appearance can be described, it is not possible to describe a typical manifestation or clinical course. The findings on immunofluorescence microscopy and EM are also highly variable.
■ Diffuse mesangial hypercellularity can be seen both in primary glomerular diseases and as part of various systemic conditions; it can also be seen as a phase of a process that has a different histologic appearance, such as a resolving postinfectious glomerulonephritis. Some of the conditions that may feature diffuse mesangial hypercellularity are listed in Table 4–2. Many of these conditions are discussed and illustrated elsewhere and will not be described separately here; a few conditions characterized by diffuse mesangial hypercellularity are described later.
■ In many but not all cases, the histologic picture of diffuse mesangial hypercellularity is associated with deposits of immunoglobulins, complement components, or both that are limited to the mesangium. Extension of the deposits into the glomerular capillary loops initiates a more intense cellular response that results in closure of capillary loops.

Light Microscopy

■ Changes are generally limited to the glomeruli; other compartments usually show few changes or changes related to other diseases such as hypertension or diabetes mellitus.
■ Most or all glomeruli have four or more cells in each mesangial space, with a variable increase in mesangial area.
■ Glomerular capillaries are patent, and capillary walls are thin and delicate.
■ There is no necrosis within glomeruli and no extracapillary proliferation (crescents; proliferation in Bowman's space).

Table 4–2
CONDITIONS ASSOCIATED WITH MESANGIAL
PROLIFERATIVE GLOMERULONEPHRITIS (DIFFUSE
MESANGIAL HYPERCELLULARITY)

Primary forms of glomerulonephritis
    Resolving postinfectious glomerulonephritis
    IgA nephropahty
    IgM nephritis
    With C3 alone or with C3 and IgG
    With no immunoglobulins or complement
Accompanying systemic disease
    Systemic lupus erythematosus
    Infective endocarditis
    Henoch-Schönlein purpura
    Mixed connective tissue disease

Histologic Variants

Mesangial Proliferative Glomerulonephritis With Mesangial C3 or With C3 and IgG

- Diffuse mesangial hypercellularity associated with granular mesangial deposits of C3 on immunofluorescence microscopy has been described in patients with either gross or microscopic hematuria. In some cases, upper respiratory tract infections appear to precipitate episodes of hematuria.
- Electron microscopy usually demonstrates electron-dense granular deposits limited to the mesangium.
- In general, the outlook for patients with diffuse mesangial hypercellularity associated with mesangial C3 deposits is favorable. The presence of deposits involving glomerular capillary loops suggests another process and raises concern for a less favorable course.
- Diffuse mesangial hypercellularity with mesangial deposits of IgG and C3, without other immunoglobulins or complement components, is found in a very heterogeneous group of patients with no distinct clinicopathologic characteristics.

Mesangial Proliferative Glomerulonephritis Without Immunoglobulins or Complement

- Diffuse mesangial hypercellularity without significant immunoglobulin or complement components on immunofluorescence microscopy can be seen in patients with a broad spectrum of clinical findings. Manifestations may range from hematuria, which may be either gross or microscopic, to proteinuria or even the nephrotic syndrome.
- Light microscopy usually shows only a mild increase in cellularity in the mesangial regions, but occasionally moderate or even marked hypercellularity is present.
- The etiology of diffuse mesangial hypercellularity in the absence of significant immunoreactants is unclear. This condition probably includes a heterogeneous group of patients, and a variety of different mechanisms are likely to be involved in different cases.

ACUTE DIFFUSE INTRACAPILLARY PROLIFERATIVE GLOMERULONEPHRITIS (USUALLY POSTINFECTIOUS)

Synonyms and Related Terms: Acute proliferative (exudative) glomerulonephritis; diffuse intracapillary glomerulonephritis; diffuse endocapillary glomerulonephritis; acute poststreptococcal glomerulonephritis; acute postinfectious glomerulonephritis.

Biology of Disease

- Diffuse proliferative glomerulonephritis can occur with a variety of disorders, including infections, SLE, IgA nephropathy, and others. Glomerulonephritis related to

infections will be discussed in this section; other disorders will be discussed separately.
- The terms *acute proliferative* or *exudative* glomerulonephritis indicate diffuse proliferation with numerous neutrophils within the capillary tufts; this finding is most often related to infections, the most common infectious agent being group A β-hemolytic streptococci (*Streptococcus pyogenes*). It is commonly termed *postinfectious,* although in some examples glomerulonephritis occurs concurrently with the infection.
- Poststreptococcal glomerulonephritis may result from either pharyngitis or skin infections. Specific *Streptococcus* strains (12, 4, 1) are most frequently associated with glomerulonephritis; however, the incidence of glomerulonephritis varies widely even with the nephritogenic strains; individual predisposing factors, possibly genetic, appear to play an important role in the occurrence of renal disease.
- Acute glomerulonephritis may also occur with other bacterial infections, including infective endocarditis, deep-seated visceral abscesses, infected ventriculoatrial shunts, and others.
- Other bacteria associated with acute glomerulonephritis include *Streptococcus pneumoniae* (pneumococcus), staphylococci (both coagulase positive and coagulase negative), gram-negative bacilli, syphilis, and others.
- Infections with other organisms, including viruses (adenovirus, measles, coxsackievirus, and others), rickettsiae, mycobacteria, and parasites (malaria), may be associated with glomerulonephritis; the histopathologic appearance may vary from mesangial proliferative glomerulonephropathy to focal proliferative to diffuse proliferative to membranoproliferative glomerulonephritis.
- Occasional cases of typical acute proliferative glomerulonephritis without evidence of infection occur; such cases may represent postinfectious glomerulonephritis when appropriate laboratory studies are not performed or are performed too late for detection of the immunologic response.
- The fundamental pathogenic mechanism is believed to be deposition of immune complexes within glomerular capillary tufts, with activation of the complement sequence and other inflammatory mediators and recruitment of neutrophils and other inflammatory cells.

Clinical Features

Poststreptococcal acute glomerulonephritis is discussed as the prototypic and most common example of glomerulonephritis related to infection.

- Children and young adults are most often affected, although disease occurs at all ages.
- Males are affected approximately twice as often as females.
- There is a latent period between the streptococcal infection and the clinical onset of glomerulonephritis that averages 1 to 2 weeks after pharyngitis but 3 to 6 weeks after skin infections.
- The onset of symptoms is usually abrupt; "smoky" urine and edema are common initial manifestations.

Edema is frequently periorbital as well as peripheral; it may be more pronounced on getting up in the morning.

■ Hypertension is common and occurs in half or more of cases, but it is usually transient.

■ Transient oliguria may occur; anuria is less common.

Laboratory Values

■ Serum antibodies against streptolysin O, DNase-B, and hyaluronidase are increased; a twofold to threefold rise in titer between acute and convalescent sera is considered diagnostic.

■ Serum complement levels (C3) are usually low ($\geq$75% of cases).

■ Circulating immune complexes are present in up to 60% of cases.

■ Elevations of serum urea nitrogen and creatinine are common in the acute phase but usually resolve spontaneously.

■ Urinalysis demonstrates hematuria with "dysmorphic" or distorted erythrocytes, frequently with red and white cell casts.

■ Proteinuria is common, but usually low grade; nephrotic-range proteinuria occurs in 5% to 10% of cases.

Treatment and Clinical Course

■ The majority of children with poststreptococcal acute glomerulonephritis have spontaneous resolution within a few weeks and full recovery of renal function; the long-term prognosis is good.

■ The prognosis of adults with poststreptococcal glomerulonephritis is thought by many to be less favorable, especially in older adults. Persistent renal abnormalities are present in up to a third of patients over 60 years old.

■ Oliguria, nephrotic-range proteinuria, or numerous glomerular crescents on biopsy are unfavorable prognostic indicators, particularly in adults.

Gross Appearance

Gross examination of kidneys in acute poststreptococcal glomerulonephritis is now (fortunately) rarely performed.

■ Kidneys are enlarged, usually by 25% to 50%.

■ The surface is soft and pale, with scattered petechiae.

■ On section, the cortex is thickened and appears pale.

Light Microscopy

The histologic appearance varies both with the stage of disease and between cases. Children with typical poststreptococcal acute glomerulonephritis do not usually undergo biopsy now; biopsy is reserved for cases with atypical features such as nephrotic-range proteinuria, an unusually prolonged course, or persistent renal abnormalities after apparent resolution of the acute disease.

Glomeruli

■ All glomerular capillary tufts are hypercellular; involvement is global and usually uniform.

■ Capillary tufts are enlarged, with decreased urinary space; there may be exaggerated lobularity of tufts.

■ Capillary lumina may be occluded.

■ Capillary walls (when they can be visualized) are not thickened; capillary basement membranes appear thin on periodic acid–Schiff (PAS) and silver stains.

■ Neutrophils are frequent in the acute phase (*exudative glomerulonephritis*) but are absent or sparse in biopsies performed later in the disease. Mesangial cells and monocytes are also increased in number. Eosinophils may be seen occasionally; they may be more common in tropical cases.

■ Biopsies performed after the acute phase characteristically demonstrate primarily mesangial hypercellularity with patent capillary loops. Mesangial hypercellularity may persist for months after apparent resolution of the disease.

■ Crescents (extracapillary proliferation) may be present in a variable proportion of cases, depending on the criteria used to decide which patients should undergo biopsy, but they are usually present in only a minority of glomeruli; in rare cases, crescents involve a majority of the glomeruli, thereby justifying the term *crescentic glomerulonephritis*.

■ Fine, fuchsinophilic (red) deposits may sometimes be seen on the outer side of glomerular basement membranes (GBMs) on Masson's trichrome stain, particularly with oil immersion.

Tubules

■ Tubules are usually relatively uninvolved.

■ Protein resorption droplets may be present in proximal convoluted tubular epithelial cells.

■ Erythrocytes may be present in tubular lumina, sometimes mixed with eosinophilic cast-like material.

■ Neutrophils may be present in tubular lumina; rarely, neutrophils infiltrate into tubular epithelium.

Vessels

■ Vessels are usually not involved or show minimal change.

■ Smudgy eosinophilic material may be present within the walls of arterioles (commonly but inaccurately termed *fibrinoid necrosis*), usually associated with hypertension.

■ Very rare cases of necrotizing vasculitis associated with poststreptococcal glomerulonephritis have been reported.

Interstitium

■ Interstitial changes are usually minor; interstitial edema and scattered inflammatory cells may be present.

Immunofluorescence Microscopy

■ During the first few weeks, coarse granular ("lumpy bumpy") staining for IgG and C3 is found in glomerular capillary walls; IgM is found less frequently, and IgA and early complement components (C1q or C4) are usually absent.

- Later, staining for C3 may predominate, with scant to absent staining for IgG.
- Three patterns of immunofluorescence staining have been described by Sorger and colleagues:
  - "Garland": densely packed, sometimes confluent capillary wall deposits occurring in all stages of the disease; this finding is often seen in patients with extracapillary proliferation (crescents) and nephrotic-range proteinuria and has been suggested as having an adverse prognosis.
  - "Starry sky": fine, granular deposits, usually IgG and C3, in both capillary walls and mesangium; this finding appears to be more common in early phases of the disease.
  - "Mesangial": granular deposits, predominantly mesangial with relative sparing of capillary loops; C3 usually predominates, with IgG less common. This finding appears to be more common in resolving stages of disease.
- Combinations or transitional forms of these patterns may occur.

Electron Microscopy

- Endothelial and mesangial cells are swollen, with closure of glomerular capillary loops.
- Large, electron-dense "immune-type" deposits are present on the subepithelial (external) surface of the glomerular capillary basement membranes and are classically described as "humps." These are most common during the first few weeks of the illness and usually disappear by 6 weeks after the clinical onset of disease.
- Subendothethial, mesangial, and intramembranous deposits may be present, but they are usually sparse and small.
- Glomerular capillary basement membranes are generally normal in contour and thickness; occasional patchy thickening may be present.
- The glomerular capillary endothelium may be partially disrupted, with neutrophils directly adjacent or adherent to the denuded basement membrane.

Histologic Variants

Glomerulonephritis associated with infections may have a variety of histologic appearances other than acute proliferative glomerulonephritis.

- Diffuse proliferative glomerulonephritis with numerous glomerular crescents (crescentic glomerulonephritis): an uncommon form of postinfectious glomerulonephritis; the clinical course is often aggressive, with a significant incidence of subsequent chronic renal insufficiency. However, the presence of glomerular crescents does not preclude the possibility of recovery.
- Diffuse proliferative glomerulonephritis without neutrophils: most common appearance of glomerulonephritis associated with infective endocarditis.
- Focal segmental glomerulonephritis: another common appearance of glomerulonephritis associated with infective endocarditis that may occasionally be seen in resolving stages of postinfectious glomerulonephritis.

- Membranoproliferative (mesangiocapillary) glomerulonephritis: most common histologic appearance of glomerulonephritis associated with infected ventriculo-atrial shunts. On EM, this finding is usually associated with subendothelial and mesangial deposits, rather than subepithelial deposits; IgM is the most common immunoglobulin detected by immunofluorescence and is associated with C3 and sometimes C1q.
- Mesangial proliferative glomerulonephritis: may be seen in resolving diffuse intracapillary glomerulonephritis (as well as a large number of other conditions).

Differential Diagnosis

- The clinical differential diagnosis of postinfectious glomerulonephritis includes all the conditions listed earlier, including streptococcal infection, infective endocarditis, deep-seated visceral abscess, ventriculoatrial shunt infection, and a variety of noninfectious diseases.
- The most common noninfectious glomerulonephritis to clinically mimic poststreptococcal or postinfectious glomerulonephritis in children is idiopathic MPGN, types I and III. A clinical history of a preceding pharyngitis or skin infection, laboratory evidence of a recent streptococcal infection, or evidence of another infectious process would suggest a postinfectious process.
- The diffuse proliferative variant of SLE can resemble postinfectious glomerulonephritis; other clinical manifestations of lupus, or serologic evidence for SLE, would assist in the differential. Immunofluorescence findings of "full house" immunoglobulins (IgG, IgM, and IgA), together with the presence of C1q or C4 in addition to C3, would favor lupus nephritis over postinfectious glomerulonephritis. Predominant subendothelial deposits or the finding of numerous tubuloreticular structures on EM would also favor lupus.

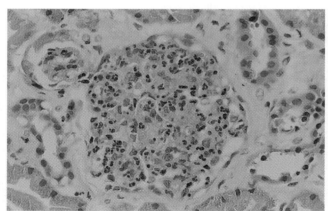

Figure 4–1. Acute diffuse intracapillary proliferative (postinfectious) glomerulonephritis. The glomeruli show diffuse and global intracapillary hypercellularity with accentuation of the lobular structure and closure of the capillaries. Note the large number of polymorphonuclear leukocytes in the glomerular capillary lumina.

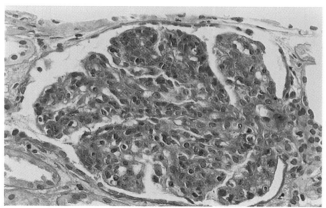

Figure 4–2. Acute diffuse intracapillary proliferative (postinfectious) glomerulonephritis. The intracapillary hypercellularity is due to proliferation of the resident glomerular endothelial and mesangial cells and accumulation of blood-borne acute inflammatory cells (including polymorphonuclear leukocytes) in the glomerular capillary lumina (periodic acid–Schiff reaction).

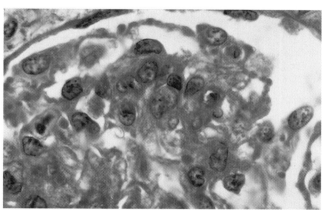

Figure 4–5. Acute diffuse intracapillary proliferative (postinfectious) glomerulonephritis. Large fuchsinophilic dots are seen along the external aspects of the glomerular capillary basement membranes. These dots represent subepithelial immune deposits (so-called humps) (Masson's trichrome stain).

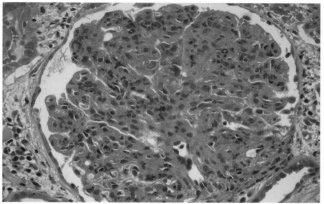

Figure 4–3. Acute diffuse intracapillary proliferative (postinfectious) glomerulonephritis. The picture shows global intracapillary hypercellularity with closure of the glomerular capillary lumina in a drug-addicted patient with acute staphylococcal endocarditis.

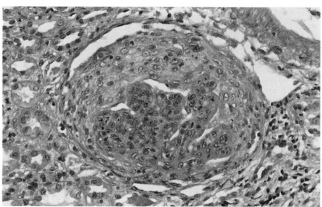

Figure 4–6. Acute diffuse intracapillary proliferative (postinfectious) glomerulonephritis with crescents. The compressed and hypercellular glomerular capillary tufts are surrounded by a cellular crescent.

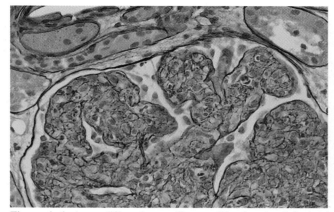

Figure 4–4. Acute diffuse intracapillary proliferative (postinfectious) glomerulonephritis. Prominent glomerular intracapillary hypercellularity is seen on a silver-stained section (i.e., all the cellularity is endorsed by the glomerular basement membranes). Note the closure of the glomerular capillary lumina (methenamine silver stain.)

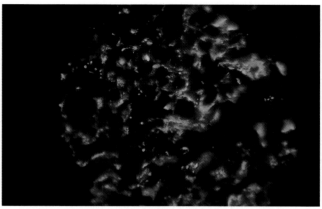

Figure 4–7. Acute diffuse intracapillary proliferative (postinfectious) glomerulonephritis. Immunofluorescence shows coarsely granular "lumpy bumpy" deposits of C3 along the glomerular capillary walls and in some mesangial regions.

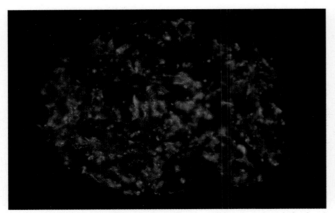

Figure 4–8. Acute diffuse intracapillary proliferative (postinfectious) glomerulonephritis. Weak granular IgG deposits are seen along the periphery of the glomerular capillary walls and in some mesangial regions.

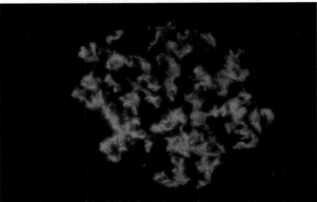

Figure 4–9. Acute diffuse intracapillary proliferative (postinfectious) glomerulonephritis. Immunofluorescence reveals strong C3 staining mostly in the mesangial regions and also along the periphery of some of the glomerular capillary walls.

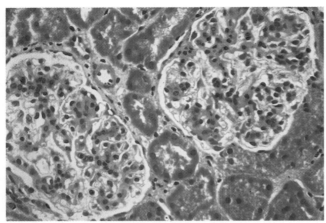

Figure 4–10. Resolving phase of acute diffuse intracapillary proliferative (postinfectious) glomerulonephritis (GN) (or so-called chronic latent GN). There is prominent mesangial widening with cellular proliferation (mesangial proliferative GN). The capillary lumina are patent and the glomerular capillary walls appear normal in thickness.

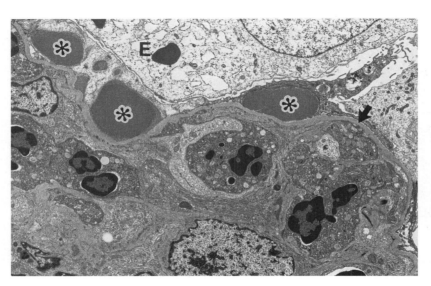

Figure 4–11. Electron micrograph of acute diffuse intracapillary proliferative postinfectious (poststreptococcal) glomerulonephritis. Hump-like discrete electron-dense subepithelial immune-type deposits (asterisks) are seen with marked intracapillary hypercellularity including polymorphonuclear leukocytes. The arrow shows glomerular capillary basement membrane. E, visceral epithelial cell. (From Laszik Z, Lajoie G, Nadasdy T, Silva FG: Medical diseases of the kidney. In: Silverberg SG, DeLellis RA, Frable WJ (eds): Principles and Practice of Surgical Pathology and Cytopathology, 3rd ed. New York, Churchill Livingstone, 1997, p 2079, with permission.)

MEMBRANOPROLIFERATIVE (MESANGIOCAPILLARY) GLOMERULONEPHRITIS

Synonyms and Related Terms: Mesangiocapillary glomerulonephritis; membranoproliferative glomerulonephritis types I, II, and III; lobular glomerulonephritis; hypocomplementemic glomerulonephritis; dense deposit disease; dense intramembranous deposit disease.

Biology of Disease

- The term *membranoproliferative glomerulonephritis* includes at least two (possibly three) distinct morphologic patterns or conditions. All are associated with activation of the complement system and have varied clinical findings and often a slowly progressive clinical course.
- Type I MPGN, the most common variant, is characterized by subendothelial electron-dense deposits and interposition of mesangial cells and matrix into the capillary wall between the basement membrane and endothelium. Type II, or dense deposit disease, is a unique variant characterized by linear, electron-dense deposits within the lamina densa of the glomerular capillary basement membrane. Two variants have each been described as type III MPGN (described in Histologic Variants later).
- Type I MPGN is associated with activation of the classic pathway of the complement system. The morphologic picture of type I MPGN can be secondary to a variety of systemic diseases, or type I MPGN can occur as an idiopathic form (Table 4–3). Mixed cryoglobulinemia associated with chronic hepatitis C virus infection has recently been implicated in a substantial number of cases of glomerulonephritis with the picture of type I MPGN.
- The cause of dense deposit disease (type II MPGN) is unknown. Many cases are associated with a serum immunoglobulin, *C3 nephritic factor*, that binds to and prevents the inactivation of C3 convertase (C3bBb), thereby resulting in persistent activation of the alternative pathway of complement activation.
- Dense deposit disease is occasionally associated with partial lipodystrophy, which is characterized by thinning of the subcutaneous fat layer of the upper extremities and trunk.
- Patients with dense deposit disease may have similar deposits to those seen in the kidney in the choroidal blood vessels, Bruch's membrane of the eye, and the spleen.
- A variety of conditions can mimic MPGN on light microscopy; the term *membranoproliferative glomerulonephritis* should be reserved for those cases with immune complex deposition in glomeruli.

Clinical Features

- All types of MPGN are most common in older children and young adults, although all can occur over a wide age range; the incidence in males and females is approximately equal.

Table 4–3
DISORDERS ASSOCIATED WITH THE MORPHOLOGIC PICTURE OF MEMBRANOPROLIFERATIVE GLOMERULONEPHRITIS TYPE I

Class of Disorder	Example
Systemic immune complex diseases	Mixed cryoglobulinemia
	Systemic lupus erythematosus
	Sjögren's syndrome
	Hereditary deficiencies of complement components
Infectious diseases	Bacterial: infected ventriculoatrial shunts, endocarditis
	Viral: hepatitis B and C, human immunodeficiency virus
	Protozoal: malaria, schistosomiasis
	Other: *Mycoplasma,* mycobacteria
Neoplasms	Leukemias and lymphomas
	Carcinomas
	Light-chain disease and plasma cell dyscrasias
	Other: Wilms tumor, melanoma
Chronic liver disease	Chronic hepatitis
	Cirrhosis
Miscellaneous	Lobular idiopathic glomerulonephritis
	Diabetes mellitus
	Amyloidosis
	α_1-Antitrypsin deficiency
	Drug abuse
	Sarcoidosis
	Sickle cell disease
	Pregnancy
	Renal artery dysplasia
	Renal vein thrombosis
	Celiac sprue

- The clinical features of the various types of MPGN are similar; the different types cannot be distinguished on the basis of clinical findings.
- The most common manifestation is the nephrotic syndrome, which occurs in half or more of patients; proteinuria is almost universal.
- Other initial signs or symptoms include recurrent episodes of gross hematuria, persistent microscopic hematuria, and an acute nephritic syndrome.
- Occasionally, renal disease may occur after an infection, usually one involving the upper respiratory tract.

Laboratory Values

- Low serum levels of the third component of the complement system (C3) are common in both type I and type II MPGN at diagnosis or at some point in the course of the disease. C3 levels are most persistently decreased in MPGN type II; in the other variants the decrease may be either transient or persistent.
- In MPGN type I, components of the classic pathway of complement activation (C1, C2, and C4), properdin, and factor B levels may also be decreased. In dense deposit disease, levels of the classic complement pathway components are usually normal.
- C3 nephritic factor, an IgG autoantibody that results in persistent activity of the alternative pathway of complement activation, is found in the serum of up to 70% of patients with MPGN type II and in approximately 20% to 30% of patients with MPGN type I; it is found in a

variable proportion of patients with MPGN associated with mixed cryoglobulinemia, SLE, and shunt nephritis.
- Urinalysis shows proteinuria and hematuria.
- Serum creatinine and urea nitrogen are increased at diagnosis in approximately one fourth of patients.

Treatment and Clinical Course

- The clinical course is generally one of slowly progressive renal insufficiency; chronic renal failure eventually develops in the majority of patients. Apparent clinical remissions occur in many patients; however, disease continues in most.
- The prognosis of dense deposit disease is poor; the majority of patients reach end-stage renal failure.
- The presence of nephrotic syndrome at diagnosis, numerous glomerular crescents (>20%), and tubular atrophy and interstitial fibrosis has been associated with higher risk of end-stage renal failure.
- No therapy has been found to be consistently effective in any of the forms of MPGN. Alternate-day therapy with corticosteroids, with or without immunosuppressive agents such as cyclophosphamide, has appeared to be effective in preventing or slowing disease progression in some cases, but benefit has not been shown in controlled clinical trials.
- Antiplatelet agents such as dipyridamole have been tried, but again benefit has not been shown in controlled clinical trials.
- Recurrence of all types of MPGN after renal transplantation is well known. Essentially all patients with dense deposit disease have recurrence after transplantation; surprisingly, recurrence does not inevitably lead to graft failure.

Gross Appearance

- Both kidneys are involved equally.
- At autopsy after death from renal failure or at nephrectomy before renal transplantation, the kidneys are small and firm and have a granular surface.

The pathology of type I and type II MPGN will be described separately.

Membranoproliferative Glomerulonephritis Type I

Light Microscopy

Glomeruli

- Cellularity within glomerular tufts is globally increased; in most cases, the increase in cellularity is predominantly in the mesangial region.
- Leukocytes, including monocytes and neutrophils, may be numerous in cases associated with mixed cryoglobulinemia.
- The lobularity of glomerular tufts is exaggerated because of increased mesangial area; capillary loops stand out individually, with distinct space between them.
- Capillary walls are thickened, with a decrease in diameter of patent capillary lumina.

- On PAS or silver stains, the capillary basement membranes appear to be doubled (two distinct layers) within many loops. This finding is described as *tram-tracking*, *splitting*, or *reduplication* of the GBM.
- Fuchsinophilic deposits may be seen in a subendothelial location in some capillary loops on trichrome stain.
- With disease progression, cellularity within the capillary tufts decreases; the mesangial space becomes progressively expanded and solidified (*mesangial sclerosis*). Centrilobular acellular nodules may be present in late stages.
- Glomerular crescents are present in approximately 10% of cases; the number may vary from occasional glomeruli to the majority of glomeruli.
- The presence of refractile eosinophilic hyalin globules in capillary lumina suggests mixed cryoglobulinemia and should be carefully sought.

Tubules

- Tubular changes generally reflect the status of glomerular disease. Tubules may appear relatively intact early in the disease course; with progressive glomerular disease, atrophic changes appear and parallel the glomerular changes in severity.
- Protein resorption droplets are commonly present in proximal convoluted tubular epithelial cells.

Interstitium

- Interstitial changes reflect the status of glomeruli. Mild fibrosis may be present on biopsy tissue early in the disease course; fibrosis becomes progressively more severe with disease progression.

Vessels

- Vascular changes usually reflect the status of glomerular disease.
- Vasculitis affecting small and medium-sized renal arteries is present in approximately one third of cases associated with mixed cryoglobulinemia.

Immunofluorescence Microscopy

- Two common patterns are described. The most common pattern is diffuse, broad, often interrupted granular staining for C3 and often immunoglobulins in glomerular capillary loops and the mesangium.
- The second pattern is mesangial staining for C3, with lesser capillary wall staining.
- Staining for C3 is present in all cases; immunoglobulins (usually IgG and IgM) are present in the majority of cases, and early complement components (C1q or C4) and properdin are also frequently present.

Electron Microscopy

- The characteristic finding is interposition of mesangial cells and matrix between the glomerular capillary basement membrane and the capillary endothelium, with layers of basement membrane–like material under the endothelium forming a new basement membrane. This interposition accounts for the characteristic splitting or "tram-track" appearance by light microscopy.

- Granular electron-dense deposits are present in the subendothelial space, under the inner side of the original basement membrane. The deposits are usually small to intermediate in size; occasionally they may be large.
- Granular deposits may be present in the mesangium, particularly in biopsy specimens harvested early in the disease. Mesangial deposits are usually small.
- Occasional, small subepithelial deposits ("humps") may be present in one half to two thirds of cases.

Dense Deposit Disease (Membranoproliferative Glomerulonephritis Type II)

Light Microscopy

Glomeruli

- Glomerular changes in dense deposit disease are variable; no single appearance is characteristic.
- Morphologic patterns that can be seen include minimal microscopic changes, pure mesangial hypercellularity, changes resembling membranous glomerulonephropathy, lobular glomerulonephritis resembling MPGN type I, focal and segmental necrotizing glomerulonephritis, and crescentic glomerulonephritis.
- The characteristic feature is the presence of elongated, irregular, brightly eosinophilic, variably refractile deposits within the GBM.
- The deposits may be continuous and ribbon-like or periodically interrupted; the latter appearance has been likened to a "string of sausages."
- The deposits stain intensely with PAS, are fuchsinophilic with trichrome stain, and are dark blue with toluidine blue.
- The deposits appear light brown with silver stains and stain less intensely than the GBM; a pale-appearing deposit bordered on each side by the thin, silver-positive GBM may give a double-contour appearance resembling that of MPGN type I.
- The deposits may stain with the fluorescent dye thioflavine T; however, such staining may also be seen in other variants of MPGN.
- Similar deposits may be seen within Bowman's capsule.
- In some cases, particularly those with the appearance of focal and segmental necrotizing glomerulonephritis, the deposits may be difficult or impossible to see by light microscopy; in such cases EM is required for diagnosis.

Tubules

- In type II MPGN, deposits similar to those in glomerular capillaries may be seen focally in tubular basement membranes; these deposits are generally small.

Interstitium and Vessels

- Changes resemble those in MPGN type I.

Immunofluorescence Microscopy

- Staining for C3 is present in glomerular capillary walls and the mesangium; staining for immunoglobulins is less frequent. Early complement components are usually absent.
- Capillary wall staining may be linear, smooth, granular, or nodular. At high magnification, capillary wall staining may demonstrate a double line or "railroad track" pattern representing C3 deposition on either side of the dense deposits.
- Mesangial staining is usually granular; under high magnification the staining may be visualized as rings.
- IgM is the most common immunoglobulin present, followed by IgG and rarely IgA. Staining for immunoglobulins is often segmental.

Electron Microscopy

- The key feature is a layer of highly electron-dense material within the lamina densa of the glomerular capillary basement membrane that splits it into two layers.
- In most cases the dense deposit layer is periodically interrupted by strands of normal-appearing basement membrane; occasionally the deposits may appear continuous.
- The dense deposit layer may be widespread within glomerular capillary loops, or it may be limited to paramesangial segments of the capillary loops.
- Granular deposits of similar dense material are usually present in the mesangium.
- Similar deposits of electron-dense material are present in Bowman's capsule.
- Electron-dense deposits are frequently found within tubular basement membranes, but they are usually smaller and less frequent than GBM deposits.

Histologic Variants

- Two distinct variants have been described, each of which has been designated MPGN type III.
- In 1970 Burkholder and colleagues described (as "mixed membranous and proliferative glomerulonephritis") a variant that had some features similar to those seen in MPGN type I, such as double contours of the GBM and subendothelial deposits, together with widespread subepithelial deposits similar to those seen in membranous glomerulonephropathy. The clinical features and course of this group of patients were similar to those of patients with MPGN type I, and the importance of making the distinction between this variant (sometimes called type III—Burkholder) and typical MPGN type I is unclear. Occasional subepithelial deposits can be seen in many cases of otherwise typical MPGN type I, as noted earlier; the difference lies in the widespread nature of the deposits in the cases described by Burkholder and associates.
- A second variant described by Strife and colleagues (sometimes called MPGN type III—Strife) has been

more widely accepted than that described by Burkholder and associates. This variant is also characterized by both subepithelial and subendothelial deposits; the deposits are large and often extend through the lamina densa of the GBM. There may be multilayering of the basement membrane material and complex disruption of the lamina densa. Subepithelial deposition with GBM spike formation is present, but these deposits are less extensive than those seen in type III—Burkholder. Histologically, hypercellularity is often less prominent than in MPGN type I. Clinical expression of this variant is generally similar to that of MPGN type I, although it may be more frequent in patients with asymptomatic hematuria and proteinuria, thus suggesting that the onset may be more insidious. The clinical course generally parallels that of MPGN type I. Identification of this variant may require silver impregnation techniques for EM because the deposits may be less electron dense with routine EM staining.

■ Cases of MPGN type I associated with mixed cryoglobulinemia differ from other cases of MPGN type I in several ways, at least in the acute phases. Eosinophilic, refractile deposits ("intraluminal thrombi") may be present within glomerular capillaries. Endocapillary proliferation is often marked, with many monocytes. Thickening and "tram-tracking" of the GBM are widespread, often with monocytes (rather than mesangial cells) interposing themselves in the capillary wall. Finally, vasculitis involving small and medium-sized arteries is seen in approximately one third of cases.

Differential Diagnosis

■ The differential diagnosis includes all of the conditions listed in Table 4–3.
■ Double contouring of the GBM on silver stains can be seen in one or a few capillary loops in a wide variety of conditions such as ischemic injury, hemolytic-uremic syndrome, radiation nephritis, and transplant glomerulopathy. In these conditions the GBM reduplication and mesangial interposition tend to be less extensive and involve only a portion of the glomerular capillary loop as opposed to the circumferential involvement in MPGN. Large, discrete electron-dense (immune complex–type) subendothelial deposits are not present in these conditions.
■ Membranoproliferative glomerulonephritis with marked cellular proliferation, especially leukocytic infiltration, may be difficult to distinguish from postinfectious acute proliferative glomerulonephritis by light microscopy; the characteristic GBM "tram-tracking" may be difficult to demonstrate. A coarse granular ("lumpy bumpy") immunofluorescence staining pattern would favor postinfectious acute glomerulonephritis; EM may be required for definitive diagnosis.
■ IgA nephropathy (Berger's disease) may have a similar clinical and light microscopic appearance as MPGN; the finding of dominant or codominant mesangial IgA deposits on immunofluorescence would indicate IgA nephropathy.

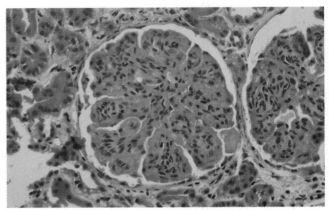

Figure 4–12. Membranoproliferative glomerulonephritis (MPGN) type I. Glomerular intracapillary hypercellularity, prominent lobularity, closure of the glomerular capillary lumina, marked thickening of the glomerular capillary walls, and occasional acute inflammatory cells within the capillaries are typical features of MPGN type I.

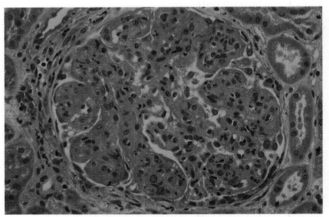

Figure 4–13. Membranoproliferative glomerulonephritis type I. Marked intracapillary hypercellularity with numerous acute inflammatory cells ("exudation") gives rise to accentuated segmentation (lobulation) of the glomerulus. Thickening of the capillary walls with large subendothelial homogeneous eosinophilic deposits is quite prominent between the 8- and 9-o'clock position.

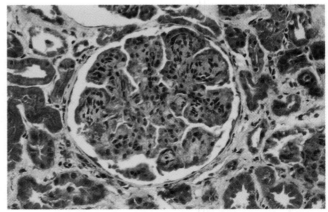

Figure 4–14. Membranoproliferative glomerulonephritis type I. Mesangial sclerosis (blue) is seen with enhanced lobulation of the tuft (Masson's trichrome stain).

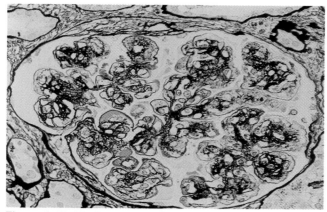

Figure 4–15. Membranoproliferative glomerulonephritis type I. The glomerulus displays extensive reduplication of the glomerular capillary walls, mesangial sclerosis, lobulation, and large subendothelial deposits in scattered capillary loops (methenamine silver stain). (From Laszik Z, Lajoie G, Nadasdy T, Silva FG: Medical diseases of the kidney. In: Silverberg SG, DeLellis RA, Frable WJ (eds): Principles and Practice of Surgical Pathology and Cytopathology, 3rd ed. New York, Churchill Livingstone, 1997, p 2079, with permission.)

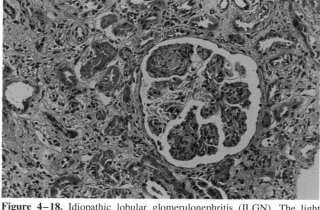

Figure 4–18. Idiopathic lobular glomerulonephritis (ILGN). The light microscopic appearance of the glomerulus in ILGN is highly reminiscent of that in membranoproliferative glomerulonephritis (MPGN) type I. However, unlike MPGN, ILGN is negative with immunofluorescence and no subendothelial deposits are seen by electron microscopy (Masson's trichrome stain).

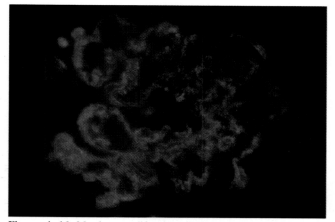

Figure 4–16. Membranoproliferative glomerulonephritis type I. The photograph shows C3 deposition mostly at the periphery of the capillary loops and also in the mesangial areas (immunofluorescence, C3).

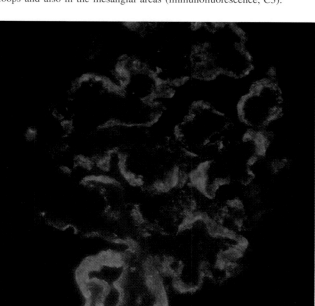

Figure 4–17. Membranoproliferative glomerulonephritis type I. Immunofluorescence microscopy reveals extensive granular peripheral/subendothelial capillary wall deposition of C3.

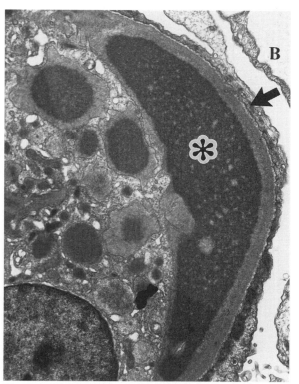

Figure 4–19. Electron micrograph of membranoproliferative glomerulonephritis type I showing a large discrete electron-dense subendothelial deposit *(asterisk)*. The foot processes of the visceral epithelial cells show effacement ("fusion") *(arrow)*. B, Bowman's space.

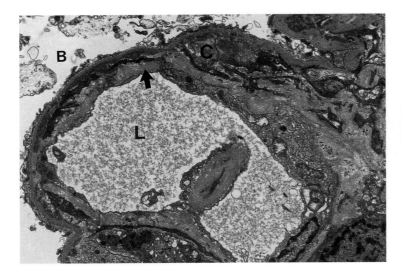

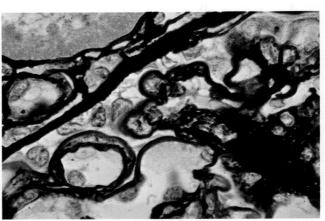

Figure 4–20. Electron micrograph of membranoproliferative glomerulonephritis type I showing glomerular capillary wall reduplication. There is circumferential mesangial cell interposition *(C)* between the newly formed *(arrow)* and the native "old" outer basement membrane. B, Bowman's space; L, glomerular capillary lumen.

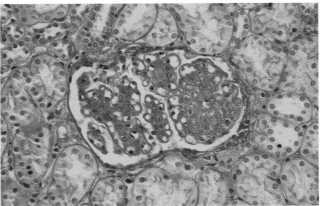

Figure 4–21. Membranoproliferative glomerulonephritis type II (dense deposit disease). The glomerulus shows moderate, segmentally accentuated intracapillary hypercellularity. Most of the glomerular capillary lumina are patent.

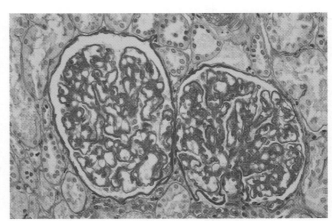

Figure 4–23. Membranoproliferative glomerulonephritis type II (dense deposit disease). Splitting of the glomerular capillary wall is seen. The nonargyrophilic intramembranous dense deposit is flanked by thin layers of the native argyrophilic basement membrane, which gives the characteristic "splitting" staining pattern (methenamine silver stain).

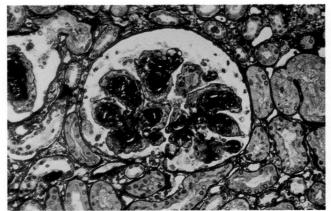

Figure 4–22. Membranoproliferative glomerulonephritis type II (dense deposit disease). Severe mesangial sclerosis with increased lobulation of the glomerular tufts is apparent (methenamine silver stain).

Figure 4–24. Membranoproliferative glomerulonephritis type II (dense deposit disease). Glomeruli reveal widespread periodic acid–Schiff (PAS)-positive thickening of the capillary walls (PAS reaction).

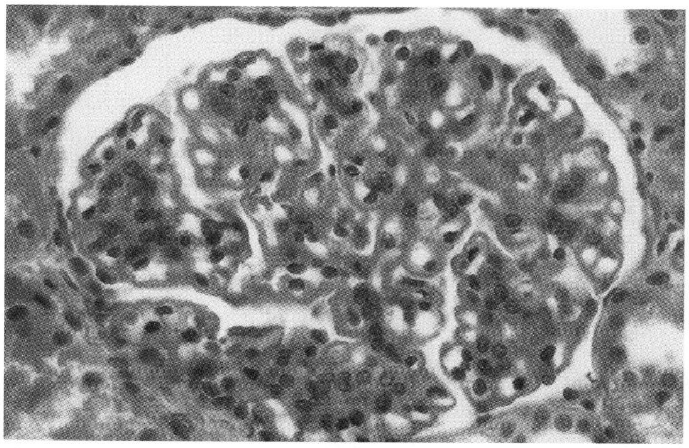

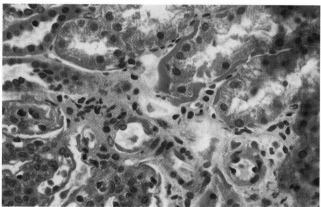

Figure 4–25. Membranoproliferative glomerulonephritis type II (dense deposit disease). There is diffuse fuchsinophilic ribbon-like staining along the glomerular capillary walls with trichrome stain because of intramembranous "dense deposits." Moderate mesangial hypercellularity is also seen (Masson's trichrome stain).

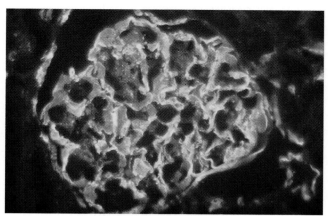

Figure 4–27. Membranoproliferative glomerulonephritis type II (dense deposit disease), immunofluorescence. Strong C3 positivity is shown along the glomerular capillary walls and also in the mesangial regions.

Figure 4–26. Membranoproliferative glomerulonephritis type II (dense deposit disease). Ribbon-like staining because of intramembranous "dense deposits" is seen in the tubular basement membranes (Masson's trichrome stain).

Figure 4–28. Electron micrograph of membranoproliferative glomerulonephritis type II (dense deposit disease). Electron-dense transformation of the glomerular lamina densa of the glomerular capillary basement membrane ("dense deposits") and mesangial deposits *(arrow)* are seen. L, glomerular capillary lumen; E, visceral epithelial cell; B, Bowman's space.

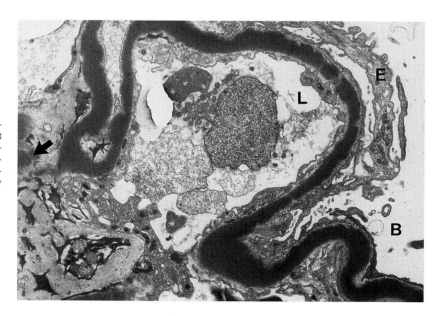

DIFFUSE EXTRACAPILLARY PROLIFERATIVE (CRESCENTIC) GLOMERULONEPHRITIS

Synonyms and Related Terms: Crescentic glomerulonephritis; rapidly progressive glomerulonephritis (RPGN); necrotizing and crescentic glomerulonephritis.

Biology of Disease

- Diffuse extracapillary proliferative or crescentic glomerulonephritis includes a variety of conditions characterized by an accumulation of cells in the extracapillary portion of the glomerulus (the urinary or Bowman's space) that form a layer at least three cells thick with the appearance of a crescent (Table 4–4).
- Glomerular crescents may be seen in occasional cases of postinfectious glomerulonephritis, lupus nephritis, IgA nephropathy, and others; however, in most of these diseases crescents are usually found in only a small proportion of the glomeruli. The terms *diffuse extracapillary proliferative glomerulonephritis* or *crescentic glomerulonephritis* should be reserved for cases in which the majority of glomeruli are affected.
- There is no universally accepted definition of crescentic glomerulonephritis in terms of the proportion of glomeruli that must have crescents; some pathologists require crescents in at least 30% of the glomeruli; others require crescents in at least 50%.
- "Rapidly progressive glomerulonephritis" is defined as glomerulonephritis causing 50% or greater loss of renal function within 3 months; the term is sometimes used synonymously with crescentic glomerulonephritis. Crescentic glomerulonephritis is the most common histologic pattern associated with the clinical syndrome of RPGN; however, the same clinical picture can occur with a variety of other histologic appearances and diseases.
- Crescentic glomerulonephritis can be divided into three immunologic types based on the results of immunofluorescence microscopy:
  - *Anti-GBM antibody disease:* 2% to 20% of cases; characterized by intense linear staining of GBMs for IgG and usually C3. Some cases are associated with

alveolar hemorrhage and hemoptysis ("Goodpasture's syndrome").
  - *Immune complex disease:* 15% to 40%; characterized by granular deposits of immunoglobulins and complement. This type comprises a heterogeneous group that includes severe cases of postinfectious glomerulonephritis, lupus nephritis, IgA nephropathy, and others.
  - *Pauci-immune crescentic glomerulonephritis:* 40% to 80%; characterized by absent to scant deposits of immunoglobulins and complement. The majority of cases in this group are associated with serum ANCAs (antineutrophil cytoplasmic antibodies), and many are associated with systemic vasculitides such as Wegener's granulomatosis or polyarteritis nodosa; however, some have no evidence of systemic disease and are considered idiopathic crescentic glomerulonephritis.
- Leakage of fibrinogen and other plasma proteins into Bowman's space is believed to stimulate proliferation of the parietal epithelial cells of Bowman's capsule and recruitment of inflammatory cells; in some cases, disruption of glomerular capillary basement membranes can be seen on PAS or silver stains.
- Necrosis of portions of the glomerular capillary tuft is present in many cases, thus justifying the term *necrotizing and crescentic glomerulonephritis.*

Clinical Features

- Two age peaks occur: adolescents to young adults, predominantly males, and middle-aged to older adults with an equal incidence in men and women.
- The clinical onset of disease is usually abrupt but may be insidious.
- Severe oliguria or anuria is common at the initial examination.
- The course is aggressive; without treatment, progression to chronic renal failure occurs within a few weeks or months.
- Some patients have evidence of systemic diseases; several syndromes occur:
  - "Pulmonary-renal syndromes": a heterogeneous group of diseases characterized by glomerulonephritis in combination with pulmonary hemorrhage. A subset of this group has anti-GBM antibodies; however, pulmonary hemorrhage can be seen with any of the immunologic types of crescentic glomerulonephritis and also other types of glomerulonephritis.
  - Glomerulonephritis associated with systemic vasculitis, such as Wegener's granulomatosis or polyarteritis nodosa.
- *"Goodpasture's syndrome"*: the original syndrome described by Goodpasture included hemoptysis associated with hematuria and rapidly progressive renal insufficiency. The term is used inconsistently; some clinicians use the term *Goodpasture's syndrome* to describe any form of pulmonary-renal syndrome with hemoptysis and use the term *Goodpasture's disease* to describe patients who have the clinical syndrome associated with strong linear staining of GBMs on immunofluorescence, with or without serum anti-GBM antibodies. Others limit the use of "Goodpasture's syndrome" to cases with evidence of anti-GBM antibodies. Not all patients

Table 4–4
CAUSES OF DIFFUSE EXTRACAPILLARY (CRESCENTIC) GLOMERULONEPHRITIS

Diseases With Crescents in Majority of Cases	Diseases With Crescents in Minority of Cases
Anti-GBM antibody disease	Postinfectious GN
With pulmonary hemorrhage	Systemic lupus erythematosus
(Goodpasture's syndrome)	IgA nephropathy (Berger's disease)
Without pulmonary hemorrhage	Henoch-Schönlein purpura
ANCA-associated GN	Mixed cryoglobulinemia
Wegener's granulomatosis	Membranoproliferative GN
Polyarteritis nodosa	
Hypersensitivity vasculitis	
Idiopathic crescentic GN	

GBM, glomerular basement membrane; GN, glomerulonephritis.

with anti-GBM antibody disease have the full clinical syndrome; glomerulonephritis occurs in the absence of hemoptysis in approximately 20% of cases of anti-GBM antibody disease. Unlike glomerular capillaries, pulmonary capillary endothelium is normally unfenestrated; thus, the antibodies may not have access to the capillary basement membrane unless the endothelium is damaged. Smoking tobacco and inhalant exposure to hydrocarbons predispose to alveolar hemorrhage in patients with anti-GBM antibodies, possibly by damaging pulmonary capillary endothelium and thus allowing the anti-GBM antibodies access to the pulmonary capillary basement membrane.

Laboratory Values

- Serum urea nitrogen and creatinine levels are elevated.
- Urinalysis discloses hematuria with dysmorphic red cells, often with erythrocyte casts; proteinuria is common but usually modest in amount.
- Anti-GBM antibodies are present in 2% to 20% of cases and should be tested for in all cases of crescentic glomerulonephritis, with or without pulmonary hemorrhage.
- Antineutrophil cytoplasmic antibodies are found in 40% to 80% of cases and again should be part of the evaluation of all cases of crescentic glomerulonephritis. Two variants of ANCAs are seen:
  - C-ANCA: cytoplasmic staining on immunofluorescence of alcohol-fixed neutrophils; most commonly seen in Wegener's granulomatosis but also seen in cases of idiopathic crescentic glomerulonephritis. Specificity for a serine protease (Pr 3) is noted.
  - P-ANCA: perinuclear staining on immunofluorescence of alcohol-fixed neutrophils; most frequent in idiopathic crescentic glomerulonephritis without evidence of systemic vasculitis. Specificity for myeloperoxidase is noted.
- Low serum complement levels suggest postinfectious glomerulonephritis, SLE, cryoglobulinemic glomerulonephritis, or MPGN.
- Antinuclear antibodies or other serologic evidence of connective tissue diseases may be present in a subset of patients but is absent in most patients with idiopathic crescentic glomerulonephritis.

Treatment and Clinical Course

- The prognosis depends in part on the primary disease; historically, cases associated with infection had a slightly less unfavorable prognosis than other cases, which almost universally progressed to complete renal failure.
- Immunosuppressive therapy, usually combining corticosteroids in relatively high doses with cytotoxic agents such as cyclophosphamide, have had a beneficial effect in a substantial number of cases when started early in the disease.
- Plasmapheresis combined with immunosuppressive therapy has been found to have a beneficial effect in cases of anti-GBM antibody disease, particularly when started early in the disease. Plasmapheresis may have a greater effect on relieving pulmonary hemorrhage and hemoptysis than on preserving renal function.

Gross Appearance

- Kidneys are enlarged and have a smooth, usually pale cortical surface.
- On section, the cortex is normal or expanded in width and appears pale; the medulla is often dark.
- Glomeruli are often visible within the cortex as gray, translucent dots.

Light Microscopy

Glomeruli

- In the acute phase, cellular crescents at least three cells in thickness are found in Bowman's space in at least 50% of glomeruli, often compressing or obliterating the glomerular capillary tuft.
- At later stages, fibrous crescents replace the cellular crescents.
- The cellular crescents are composed of Bowman's capsule parietal epithelial cells, monocytes, and other leukocytes. The presence or proportion of each type may depend on the initiating cause and also the timing of the biopsy relative to the course of the disease (early versus late).
- Glomerular capillary tufts may be very difficult to visualize on hematoxylin and eosin (H & E) staining; PAS and especially silver stains are very useful in delineating the capillary basement membranes.
- Capillary tufts are usually normocellular except in cases associated with immune complex deposition, in which event there may be diffuse intracapillary proliferation. The capillary walls are usually normal in thickness.
- Necrosis may be present within capillary tufts, as indicated by karyorrhectic nuclear debris and aggregates of material that stain strongly eosinophilic on H & E stain and fuchsinophilic on Masson's trichrome; this finding is described as "fibrinoid necrosis."
- Aggregates of eosinophilic fibrinoid material may be present within Bowman's space and consist of fibrin/fibrinogen and other plasma proteins.
- Disruptions of the GBM may sometimes be seen on PAS and silver stains.
- In some cases, disruptions of Bowman's capsule basement membrane are present; often this disruption is associated with an intense inflammatory reaction surrounding the glomeruli and extending into the interstitium, sometimes with multinucleated giant cells or eosinophils. These findings are sometimes described as "granulomatous glomerulonephritis."

Tubules

- Protein resorption droplets may be present in proximal tubular epithelial cells.
- Scattered atrophic tubules or tubular dropout may be present.
- Erythrocytes, leukocytes, or casts are present within tubule lumina.

- Necrosis of tubular epithelium, with disruption of the tubular basement membrane on silver stains, is present in occasional cases; such necrosis is most frequently seen in anti-GBM antibody disease with coexisting anti–tubular basement membrane antibodies. This condition may be associated with an interstitial inflammatory reaction, often with multinucleated giant cells.

Interstitium

- Interstitial widening and interstitial inflammation, predominantly lymphocytes and plasma cells, are frequent.
- The most severe inflammation is frequently found in the vicinity of sclerotic glomeruli.

Vessels

- Thickening of arterial and arteriolar walls may be present, especially in older patients.
- Vasculitis is occasionally seen in cases caused by polyarteritis nodosa or Wegener's granulomatosis, but is unusual.

Immunofluorescence Microscopy

- All cases: staining for fibrin/fibrinogen is frequently present within crescents and may be present within capillary tufts in foci of necrosis. Staining for fibrin/fibrinogen may persist for a long time within crescents.
- Anti-GBM antibody disease: moderate to intense linear GBM staining for IgG is present in all glomeruli; staining for C3, either linear or granular, is present in approximately two thirds of cases. Other immunoglobulins and complement components are usually absent. Linear tubular basement membrane staining for IgG, with or without C3, is present occasionally.
- Immune complex diseases: immunofluorescence findings are variable, depending on the specific disease; the immunofluorescence patterns associated with the various diseases are described in the sections relating to those entities. For example, cases associated with infections characteristically demonstrate coarse granular capillary wall staining for C3 with or without IgG; cases associated with SLE demonstrate granular capillary wall and mesangial staining for IgG, IgM, and IgA together with C3 and C1q (or C4); and cases of IgA nephropathy or Henoch-Schönlein purpura demonstrate dominant or codominant IgA staining.
- Pauci-immune crescentic glomerulonephritis: glomeruli are either negative by immunofluorescence or demonstrate weak and variable staining for immunoglobulins (usually IgM), complement components (most often C3), and other proteins (albumin).

Electron Microscopy

- In all variants, capillary loops may be collapsed, with wrinkling of the GBM. Visceral epithelial cell foot processes may demonstrate areas of simplification.
- Polymerized fibrin ("fibrin tactoids") is frequently present within the urinary space.

- Disruptions of the glomerular capillary basement membrane may be seen.
- The presence or absence of electron-dense, immune complex–type deposits depends on the immunologic type:
  - Anti-GBM antibody disease: no immune complex–type deposits are present.
  - Immune complex diseases: electron-dense, immune complex–type deposits will be present; the pattern, size, and location of deposits will vary, depending on the primary disease.
  - Pauci-immune crescentic glomerulonephritis: immune complex–type deposits are usually absent.

Histologic Variants

- Antineutrophil cytoplasmic antibody–associated glomerulonephritis and vasculitis: glomerulonephritis occurs in patients with serum ANCAs either alone (idiopathic crescentic glomerulonephritis) or in association with systemic vasculitis, usually either polyarteritis nodosa or Wegener's granulomatosis. The appearance of the glomeruli is the same in cases with and without systemic vasculitis.
- Anti-GBM antibody disease with ANCAs: ANCAs have been found concurrently with anti-GBM antibodies in up to 32% of patients with anti-GBM antibodies. The prognostic significance of the association is not clear.

Differential Diagnosis

- The clinical differential diagnosis of acute renal failure includes prerenal causes (i.e., inadequate renal perfusion), intrinsic renal diseases of various types, including both glomerular and nonglomerular diseases, and postrenal causes (urinary tract obstruction).
- The differential diagnosis of crescentic glomerulonephritis includes all the entities included in Table 4–4.

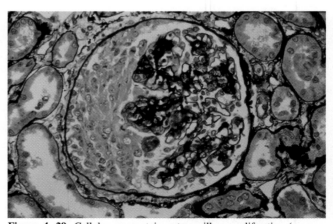

Figure 4–29. Cellular crescent in extracapillary proliferative (crescentic) glomerulonephritis. The cellular crescent is seen in Bowman's space between the 6- and 12-o'clock position on the left side of the partially compressed glomerular capillary loops. Bowman's capsule is intact (methenamine silver stain).

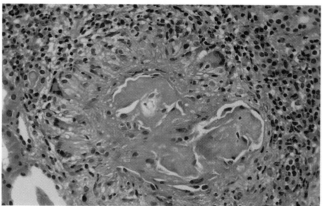

Figure 4–30. Diffuse intracapillary and extracapillary proliferative (crescentic) glomerulonephritis (GN). Cellular crescent (extracapillary hypercellularity) and slight intracapillary hypercellularity are seen in a glomerulus from a patient with postinfectious GN (trichrome stain).

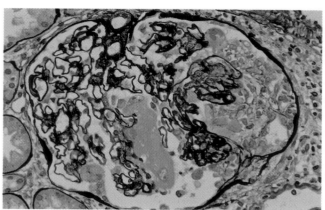

Figure 4–33. Extracapillary proliferative (crescentic) and necrotizing glomerulonephritis. Compressed capillary loops on the *right* side of the glomerulus are surrounded by cellular crescent and fibrin. The *left* part of the glomerulus is histologically unremarkable (methenamine silver stain).

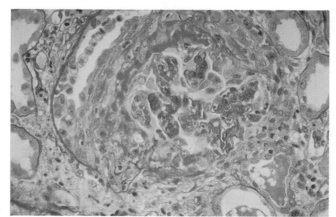

Figure 4–31. Extracapillary proliferative (crescentic) and necrotizing glomerulonephritis. The picture shows granulomatous inflammatory reaction with giant cells around the necrotic glomerulus, which has lost its Bowman's capsule. This condition is also called "granulomatous glomerulonephritis."

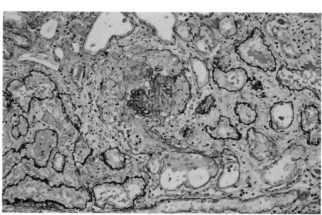

Figure 4–34. Extracapillary proliferative (crescentic) and necrotizing glomerulonephritis. Rupture of the glomerular capillary basement membranes and dissolution of Bowman's capsule are seen with reactive inflammatory cell infiltrate (methenamine silver stain).

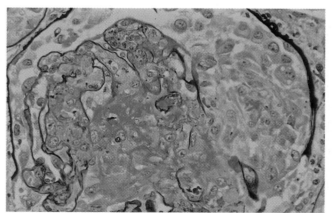

Figure 4–32. Extracapillary proliferative (crescentic) and necrotizing glomerulonephritis. The glomerular capillary loops are collapsed/compressed and fibrin is seen between the cells in the crescent (Lendrum's stain).

Figure 4–35. Extracapillary proliferative (crescentic) and necrotizing glomerulonephritis. Intracapillary and extracapillary cellular proliferation is shown with rupture of the glomerular capillary basement membranes, extravasation of fibrin, and dissolution of Bowman's capsule (*lower right;* methenamine silver stain).

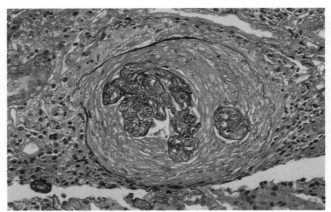

Figure 4–36. Extracapillary proliferative (crescentic) glomerulonephritis, advancing. Fibrocellular crescent is seen in a glomerulus. Bowman's capsule is partly ruptured, and the glomerular capillary tufts are collapsed (methenamine silver stain).

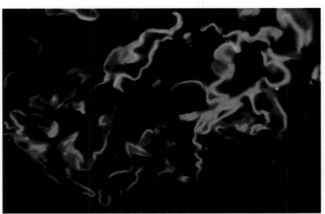

Figure 4–39. Anti–glomerular basement membrane antibody–mediated crescentic glomerulonephritis with strong linear IgG immunostaining in a segment of a glomerulus.

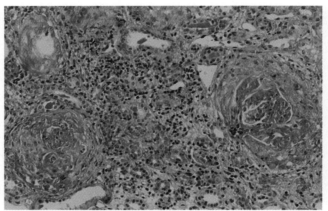

Figure 4–37. Extracapillary proliferative (crescentic) and necrotizing glomerulonephritis (GN). Marked interstitial inflammation is shown in a patient with pauci-immune crescentic GN (periodic acid–Schiff reaction).

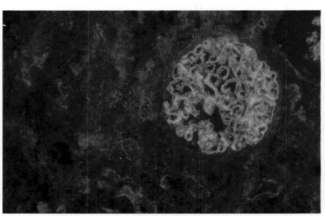

Figure 4–40. Immune complex–mediated extracapillary proliferative (crescentic) glomerulonephritis. Intense granular IgG staining is shown along the glomerular capillary walls and also in the mesangial areas. Light microscopy revealed crescents in most of the glomeruli.

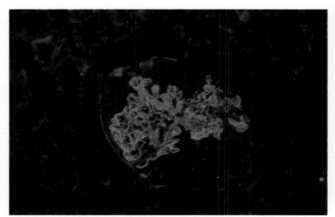

Figure 4–38. Anti–glomerular basement membrane antibody–mediated crescentic glomerulonephritis. Intense linear IgG staining is seen along the glomerular capillary basement membranes. The crescent is barely visible between Bowman's capsule and the compressed capillary loops.

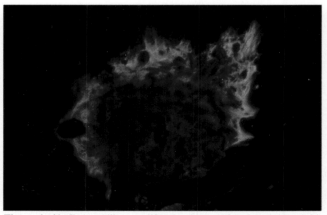

Figure 4–41. Extracapillary proliferative (crescentic) glomerulonephritis (GN). Fibrin(ogen) deposition is seen in the crescent and adjacent interstitium surrounding the glomerulus. Bowman's capsule has been destroyed in this "granulomatous" GN (see Fig. 4–31) (immunofluorescence, fibrinogen).

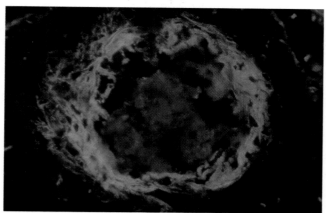

Figure 4–42. Fibrin(ogen) immunostaining in a patient with extracapillary proliferative (crescentic) glomerulonephritis. Fibrinogen staining is strongly positive in the crescent in Bowman's space.

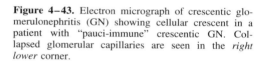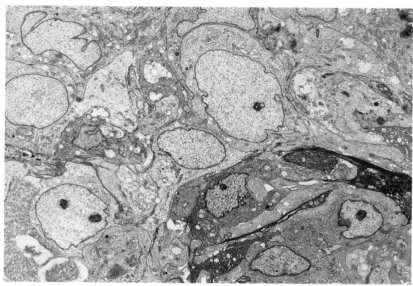

Figure 4–43. Electron micrograph of crescentic glomerulonephritis (GN) showing cellular crescent in a patient with "pauci-immune" crescentic GN. Collapsed glomerular capillaries are seen in the *right lower* corner.

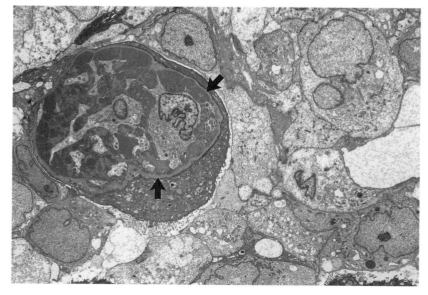

Figure 4–44. Electron micrograph of crescentic glomerulonephritis showing a cellular crescent in a patient with lupus glomerulonephritis class IV. A single glomerular capillary loop with massive discrete immune-type electron-dense subendothelial deposits is surrounded by the glomerular basement membrane *(arrows)* and a cellular crescent.

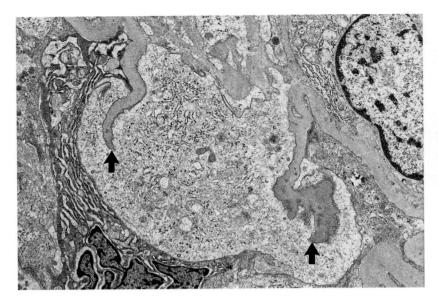

Figure 4–45. Electron micrograph of crescentic glomerulonephritis (GN). Rupture of the glomerular capillary basement membrane is shown. The site of the rupture is marked by *arrows*. The patient had anti–glomerular basement membrane antibody–mediated crescentic GN.

FOCAL GLOMERULONEPHRITIS

Synonyms and Related Terms: Focal proliferative glomerulonephritis; focal mesangiopathic glomerulonephritis; focal segmental necrotizing glomerulonephritis.

Biology of Disease

- Focal glomerulonephritis is defined as glomerulonephritis in which, by *light microscopy*, only a proportion of the glomeruli are involved; the other glomeruli have a normal appearance.
- According to the World Health Organization definition, the term *focal* is applied if fewer than 75% to 80% of the glomeruli are involved; other series restrict the term to cases in which fewer than 50% of glomeruli show microscopic evidence of involvement.
- We distinguish focal glomerulonephritis from a pure mesangial proliferative glomerulonephritis by requiring, in the former, *closure of glomerular capillary loops.* Closure of capillary loops may be caused by hypercellularity, necrosis, sclerosis, or any combination of these.
- In many cases, immunofluorescence microscopy or EM demonstrates abnormalities (complement and/or immunoglobulin deposits by immunofluorescence microscopy or electron-dense deposits by EM) in *all* glomeruli, even when only a proportion show abnormalities by light microscopy. Some of these cases are probably at an early stage in the disease process; it is possible that biopsies performed later might show diffuse involvement by light microscopy.

- *Focal* glomerulonephritis is often also *segmental*; in other words, only a portion of the glomerular tuft is involved.
- Focal glomerulonephritis lacking abnormalities by immunofluorescence or EM is often caused by polyarteritis nodosa (microscopic variant) or Wegener's granulomatosis; many patients have circulating ANCAs.
- The morphologic pattern of focal glomerulonephritis can be seen in a variety of systemic conditions, including rheumatologic diseases such as SLE, Behçet's syndrome, and relapsing polychondritis; vasculitides; infectious diseases such as endocarditis; anti-GBM antibody disease; Henoch-Schönlein purpura; sarcoidosis; and a variety of others.
- Focal glomerulonephritis may also be seen in primary renal diseases such as IgA nephropathy (Berger's disease). In some cases, focal glomerulonephritis is seen in association with mesangial C3 with or without IgM or IgG.
- Segmental necrosis is sometimes present, frequently associated with extracapillary proliferation (crescents); this pattern is common in cases associated with ANCAs and early cases of anti-GBM antibody disease.

Clinical Features

- Isolated hematuria (hematuria not accompanied by other significant abnormalities on urinalysis) is the most common manifestation of primary focal glomerulonephritis.
- The clinical features of cases associated with systemic diseases or associated with specific renal disorders such

as IgA nephropathy are discussed in the sections devoted to those diseases.

Treatment and Clinical Course

- The clinical course of focal glomerulonephritis is highly variable and depends on the disease process. No specific clinical course can be described.
- Focal necrotizing glomerulonephritis may show an aggressive course with rapid deterioration in renal function unless treated with immunosuppressive agents.
- Treatment depends on the specific disease process.

Light Microscopy

Glomeruli

- By definition, significant changes are found in only some glomeruli. The proportion involved may vary from occasional glomeruli up to 80% of the glomeruli (50% according to some pathologists); the remaining glomeruli show minimal or no change.
- The changes are frequently segmental and involve only a portion of the glomerular capillary tuft.
- Cellularity may vary from minimally to markedly increased; in some cases, neutrophils may be present.
- The mesangial space is expanded on PAS and silver stains, often segmentally.
- Segmental necrosis may be present and is often accompanied by extracapillary proliferation (crescents).
- In late stages, segmental sclerosis replaces the active cellular lesions; adhesions (synechiae) between the capillary tuft and Bowman's capsule may be present.

Tubules, Interstitium, and Blood Vessels

- Tubular, interstitial, and vascular changes are highly variable and may be absent.
- Interstitial inflammation and tubular damage may be present.
- Occasionally, vasculitis involving arteries or arterioles, often leukocytoclastic (with neutrophil nuclear debris), is present in focal necrotizing glomerulonephritis.

Immunofluorescence Microscopy

- Immunoglobulin and complement deposits are often found in all glomeruli despite the focal pattern of changes on light microscopy.
- Deposits usually have a predominantly mesangial ("pruned tree") distribution; occasionally, deposits will be present in short capillary wall segments.
- The pattern of immunoreactants present is variable, depending on the disease process. Cases corresponding to IgA nephropathy contain predominantly IgA, with or without C3 and other immunoglobulins; in other cases, C3 may predominate, with or without IgG or IgM.
- Linear GBM staining for IgG may be present and corresponds to anti-GBM antibody disease.
- In many cases, no or only minimal immunoreactants are present; cases with minimal staining on immunoflu-

orescence often demonstrate segmental necrosis on light microscopy.

Electron Microscopy

- There are no specific ultrastructural changes; discrete immune-type deposits may be present or absent. When present, they are found predominantly in the mesangium.

Differential Diagnosis

- The clinical differential diagnosis includes all the conditions mentioned in Biology of Disease (see earlier).
- IgA nephropathy is the most common renal disorder associated with the morphologic pattern of focal proliferative glomerulonephritis; the presence of dominant mesangial IgA deposits on immunofluorescence microscopy will establish the diagnosis.
- Focal necrotizing glomerulonephritis may represent the microscopic variant of polyarteritis nodosa, renal involvement by Wegener's granulomatosis, or early anti-GBM antibody disease; immunofluorescence microscopy will demonstrate no or minimal deposits in the first two conditions and intense linear GBM staining with IgG in the latter. Assay for serum ANCAs should be recommended when few or no immunoreactants are found in association with focal glomerulonephritis, especially if necrosis is present.
- Focal segmental glomerulosclerosis (FSGS) enters into the differential diagnosis of healing or healed focal glomerulonephritis when there is a predominance of sclerosis and little proliferation; distinction can be difficult, sometimes impossible. Focal glomerulonephritis should be favored when significant immunoreactants are present; the presence of prominent glomerular hyalin favors FSGS but can be seen in focal glomerulonephritis.
- The presence of fibrous crescents or disruption of Bowman's capsule on PAS or silver stains favors focal glomerulonephritis but may also be found in late stages of FSGS.

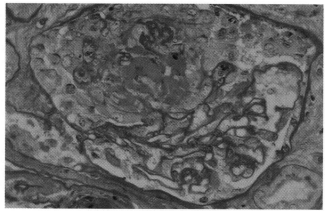

Figure 4–46. Focal segmental glomerulonephritis. Segmental necrosis of the glomerular capillary loops admixed with fibrin is seen; the rest of the glomerulus appears histologically normal and has patent capillary lumina.

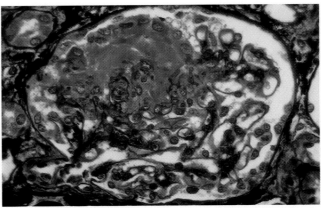

Figure 4–47. Focal segmental necrotizing glomerulonephritis. The glomerulus has segmental necrosis of the capillary loops with fibrin deposition (methenamine silver stain).

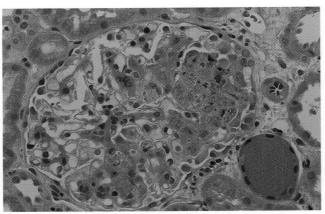

Figure 4–49. Focal segmental proliferative and necrotizing glomerulonephritis in a patient with lupus (focal proliferative lupus nephritis class III). Segmental glomerular intracapillary hypercellularity with closure of some lumina and necrosis is seen. The uninvolved part of the glomerulus appears normal by light microscopy.

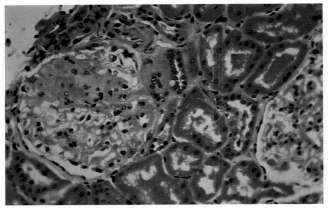

Figure 4–48. Healed focal glomerulonephritis versus focal segmental glomerulosclerosis. A segmental sclerotic lesion is seen in a glomerulus. The differential diagnosis of this lesion involves healed focal glomerulonephritis and focal segmental glomerulosclerosis; differentiation is often impossible by light microscopy. The patient had polyarteritis nodosa treated with steroids and immunosuppressive therapy.

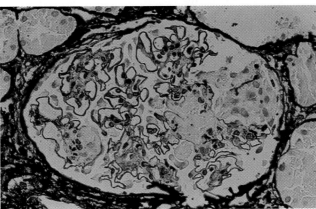

Figure 4–50. Focal segmental proliferative glomerulonephritis with crescents in a patient with lupus (focal proliferative lupus nephritis class III). Except for slight mesangial widening, large portions of the glomerulus appear normal by light microscopy. On the *right*, the glomerular capillary basement membranes are disrupted and a small crescent has formed (methenamine silver stain).

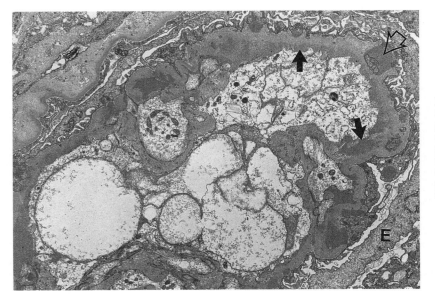

Figure 4–51. Electron micrograph of focal glomerulonephritis (GN) showing immune complex–mediated glomerular disease in a patient with bacterial endocarditis. Note the discrete glomerular subendothelial *(solid arrows)* and subepithelial *(empty arrow)* electron-dense "immune-type" deposits. Light microscopy showed focal proliferative GN. Immunofluorescence and electron microscopy revealed immune deposition in all glomeruli. E, visceral epithelial cell.

References

General

Heptinstall RH: Classification of glomerulonephritis; focal, and mesangial proliferative forms of glomerulonephritis; recurrent hematuria. In: Heptinstall RH (ed): Pathology of the Kidney, 4th ed. Boston, Little, Brown, 1992, p 261.

Jennette JC, Falk RJ: Nephritic syndrome and glomerulonephritis. In: Silva FG, D'Agati VD, Nadasdy T (eds): Renal Biopsy Interpretation. New York, Churchill Livingstone, 1996, p 71.

Acute Diffuse Intracapillary Proliferative Glomerulonephritis (Usually Postinfectious)

Edelstein CL, Bates WD: Subtypes of acute postinfectious glomerulonephritis: A clinico-pathological correlation. Clin Nephrol 38:311, 1992.

Lewy JE, Salinas-Madrigal L, Herdson PB, et al: Clinico-pathologic correlations in acute poststreptococcal glomerulonephritis: A correlation between renal functions, morphologic damage and clinical course of 46 children with acute poststreptococcal glomerulonephritis. Medicine (Baltimore) 50:453, 1971.

Pankewycz OG, Sturgill BC, Bolton WK: Proliferative glomerulonephritis: postinfectious, noninfectious, and crescentic forms. In: Tisher CC, Brenner BM (eds): Renal Pathology: With Clinical and Functional Correlations, 2nd Ed. Philadelphia, JB Lippincott, 1994, p 222.

Silva FG: Acute postinfectious glomerulonephritis and glomerulonephritis complicating persistent bacterial infection. In: Jennette JC, Olson JL, Schwartz MM, Silva FG (eds): Heptinstall's Pathology of the Kidney, 5th ed. Philadelphia, Lippincott-Raven, 1998, p 389.

Sorger K, Gessler U, Hübner FK, et al: Subtypes of acute postinfectious glomerulonephritis. Synopsis of clinical and pathological features. Clin Nephrol 17:114, 1982.

Membranoproliferative (Mesangiocapillary) Glomerulonephritis

Burkholder PM, Marchand A, Krueger RP: Mixed membranous and proliferative glomerulonephritis: A correlative light, immunofluorescence, and electron microscopic study. Lab Invest 23:459, 1970.

D'Amico G, Fornasieri A: Cryoglobulinemic glomerulonephritis: A membranoproliferative glomerulonephritis induced by hepatitis C virus. Am J Kidney Dis 25:361, 1995.

Donadio JV, Slack TK, Holley KE, et al: Idiopathic membranoproliferative (mesangiocapillary) glomerulonephritis: A clinicopathologic study. Mayo Clin Proc 54:141, 1979.

Habib R, Gubler M-C, Loirat C, et al: Dense deposit disease: A variant of membranoproliferative glomerulonephritis. Kidney Int 7:204, 1975.

Holley KE, Donadio JV: Membranoproliferative glomerulonephritis. In: Tisher CC, Brenner BM (eds): Renal Pathology: With Clinical and Functional Correlations, 2nd Ed. Philadelphia, JB Lippincott, 1994, p 294.

Sibley RK, Kim Y: Dense intramembranous deposit disease: New pathologic features. Kidney Int 25:660, 1984.

Silva FG: Membranoproliferative glomerulonephritis. In: Jennette JC, Olson JL, Schwartz MM, Silva FG (eds): Heptinstall's Pathology of the Kidney, 5th ed. Philadelphia, Lippincott-Raven, 1998, p 309.

Southwest Pediatric Nephrology Study Group: Dense deposit disease in children: Prognostic value of clinical and pathologic indicators. Am J Kidney Dis 6:161, 1985.

Strife CF, McEnery PT, McAdams AJ, et al: Membranoproliferative glomerulonephritis with disruption of the glomerular basement membrane. Clin Nephrol 7:65, 1977.

West CD: Idiopathic membranoproliferative glomerulonephritis in childhood. Pediatr Nephrol 6:96, 1992.

Zamurovic D, Churg J: Idiopathic and secondary mesangiocapillary glomerulonephritis. Nephron 38:145, 1984.

Diffuse Extracapillary Proliferative (Crescentic) Glomerulonephritis

Couser WG: Rapidly progressive glomerulonephritis: Classification, pathogenetic mechanisms, and therapy. Am J Kidney Dis 9:449, 1988.

Falk RJ, Jennette JC: Anti-neutrophil cytoplasmic autoantibodies with specificity for myeloperoxidase in patients with systemic vasculitis and idiopathic necrotizing and crescentic glomerulonephritis. N Engl J Med 318:1651, 1988.

Heaf JG, Jørgensen F, Nielsen LP: Treatment and prognosis of extracapillary glomerulonephritis. Nephron 35:217, 1983.

Jennette JC: Crescentic glomerulonephritis. In: Jennette JC, Olson JL, Schwartz MM, Silva FG (eds): Heptinstall's Pathology of the Kidney, 5th ed. Philadelphia, Lippincott-Raven, 1998, p 625.

Jennette JC, Falk RJ: Diagnosis and management of glomerulonephritis and vasculitis presenting as acute renal failure. Med Clin North Am 74:893, 1990.

Kallenberg CGM, Brouwer E, Weening JJ, et al: Anti-neutrophil cytoplasmic antibodies: Current diagnostic and pathophysiological potential. Kidney Int 46:1, 1994.

McLeish KR, Yum MN, Luft FC: Rapidly progressive glomerulonephritis in adults: Clinical and histologic correlations. Clin Nephrol 10:43, 1978.

Focal Proliferative Glomerulonephritis

Furlong TJ, Ibels LS, Eckstein RP: The clinical spectrum of necrotizing glomerulonephritis. Medicine (Baltimore) 66:192, 1987.

Germuth FG, Rodriguez E: Focal mesangiopathic glomerulonephritis: Prevalence and pathogenesis. Kidney Int 7:216, 1975.

Grishman E, Churg J: Focal segmental lupus nephritis. Clin Nephrol 17: 5, 1982.

Morel-Maroger L, Leathem A, Richet G: Glomerular abnormalities in nonsystemic diseases. Relationship between findings by light microscopy and immunofluorescence in 433 renal biopsy specimens. Am J Med 53:170, 1972.

Vernier RL, Resnick JS, Mauer SM: Recurrent hematuria and focal glomerulonephritis. Kidney Int 7:224, 1975.

Weiss MA, Crissman JD: Segmental necrotizing glomerulonephritis: Diagnostic, prognostic, and therapeutic significance. Am J Kidney Dis 6:199, 1985.

Whitworth JA, Turner DR, Leibowitz S, et al: Focal segmental sclerosis or scarred focal proliferative glomerulonephritis? Clin Nephrol 9:229, 1978.

CHAPTER 5

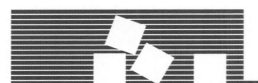

The Nonglomerulonephritic Glomerulonephropathies
Diseases Manifested as Severe Proteinuria or Idiopathic Nephrotic Syndrome

INTRODUCTION

- Proteinuria is a common manifestation of many renal diseases; however, proteinuria exceeding 1.0 g per 24 hours almost always indicates a glomerular disorder. A variety of diseases, both primary renal and systemic, may cause severe proteinuria or the nephrotic syndrome (Table 5–1). Primary renal diseases manifested predominantly with proteinuria will be discussed in this chapter; the various systemic diseases that cause severe proteinuria, such as diabetic nephropathy and amyloidosis, will be discussed separately.

- These conditions are classified on the basis of morphologic pattern determined by routine light microscopy, immunofluorescence microscopy, and electron microscopy. However, as is so often the case in renal pathology, each of these morphologic patterns may be caused by different disease processes. Therefore, the prognosis and treatment of different patients, with similar or even identical morphologic pictures, may be greatly different.

- These diseases may be associated with varying levels of proteinuria, with or without the full nephrotic syndrome. Nephrotic syndrome is defined as proteinuria of 3.5 g or greater per 24 hours in adults ($\geq$40 mg/m²/hr in a timed overnight collection in children) in association with hypoalbuminemia, edema, hypercholesterolemia, and hypercholesteroluria. However, patients may have nephrotic-range proteinuria without manifesting the full nephrotic syndrome.

- The causes of idiopathic nephrotic syndrome are numerous; fortunately, the majority of cases are associated with only three morphologic patterns: minimal change nephrotic syndrome (MCNS), focal segmental glomerulosclerosis (FSGS), and membranous glomerulonephropathy (MGN). The most common causes differ in pediatric and adult patients; MCNS is by far the most common cause in childhood, whereas MGN and other glomerulonephritides are the most common causes of idiopathic nephrotic syndrome in adults.

- The usual pathophysiologic basis of proteinuria lies in loss of the normal negative charge of the glomerular capillary wall, which is predominantly an effect of the proteoglycan heparan sulfate. This negative charge restricts the passage of negatively charged proteins across the glomerular basement membrane (GBM) by electrostatic repulsion; there is also a size-selective mechanism that primarily restricts the passage of larger molecules. In some conditions such as MCNS in childhood, the size-selective function is preserved and the proteinuria consists largely of smaller molecules such as albumin (*selective proteinuria*). In other conditions, the size-selective function is lost, and both smaller and larger proteins are excreted (*nonselective proteinuria*).

- Certain morphologic changes occur in glomeruli with proteinuria of any cause. These include effacement of the visceral epithelial cell foot processes, microvillous transformation, and the appearance of vacuoles and protein resorption droplets in epithelial cells.

- Nephrotic-range proteinuria of any cause can be associated with a variety of complications, including malnutrition caused by protein loss, impaired humoral and cellular immunity, accelerated atherosclerosis secondary to hyperlipidemia, and a hypercoagulable state that is believed to be due to increased hepatic synthesis of fibrinogen and other clotting factors, together with urinary loss of antithrombin III and other coagulation inhibitors. Complications of the hypercoagulable state include renal vein thrombosis (formerly believed to be a cause of nephrotic syndrome but now instead believed to be a complication thereof) and pulmonary thromboembolism.

Table 5–1
CONDITIONS ASSOCIATED WITH THE NEPHROTIC SYNDROME

Primary Renal Diseases	Other Causes
Minimal change nephrotic syndrome	Medications
Focal segmental glomeru-losclerosis	Mercury
	Organic gold compounds
Membranous glomerulo-nephropathy	Penicillamine
	Probenecid
Mesangial proliferative glomerulonephritis	Captopril
	NSAIDs
Membranoproliferative glomerulonephritis	Lithium
	Interferon-α
Diffuse mesangial sclero-sis	Allergens, venoms, immunizations
	Infections
Endocapillary or prolifer-ative glomerulonephri-tis	Bacterial: endocarditis, shunt nephri-tis, others
	Viral: hepatitis, CMV, EBV, HIV-1
Fibrillary and immunotac-toid glomerulonephritis	Protozoal: malaria, toxoplasmosis
	Helminthic: schistosomiasis
	Neoplasms
	Carcinoma: lung, colon, stomach, other
	Leukemia and lymphoma: Hodgkin's disease, CLL, plasma cell dyscra-sias
	Multisystem diseases
	Systemic lupus erythematosus
	Amyloidosis
	Henoch-Schönlein purpura
	Metabolic diseases
	Diabetes mellitus
	Miscellaneous
	Pregnancy (preeclampsia)
	Chronic renal allograft failure

NSAIDs, nonsteroidal anti-inflammatory drugs; CMV, cytomegalovirus; EBV, Epstein-Barr virus; HIV-1, human immunodeficiency virus type 1; CLL, chronic lymphocytic leukemia.

MINIMAL CHANGE NEPHROTIC SYNDROME

Synonyms: Minimal change disease; minimal change nephropathy; lipoid nephrosis; nil disease; visceral epithelial foot process disease.

Biology of Disease

■ Minimal change nephrotic syndrome occurs in primary (idiopathic) or secondary forms. The cause or causes of primary MCNS are unknown; abnormalities of cell-mediated immunity occur and may be of pathophysiologic significance. Secondary forms of MCNS most often occur in adults and are associated with lymphoproliferative disorders (i.e., lymphomas) or the use of nonsteroidal anti-inflammatory drugs (NSAIDs) or other medications.

■ In older series, MCNS was found on biopsy in approximately 65% to 75% of cases of idiopathic nephrotic syndrome in children; the current frequency of MCNS in pediatric biopsies is probably lower because many children are treated empirically and do not undergo biopsy unless resistant to corticosteroids. In adults, MCNS accounts for approximately 10% to 22% of

cases of idiopathic nephrotic syndrome. During childhood, the median age at diagnosis is 3 to 4 years, with 80% of patients younger than 6 years of age. In children, MCNS is approximately twice as common in males as in females; in adults, the incidence in men and women is equal.

■ The proteinuria of primary MCNS usually responds to corticosteroids with reversal of the ultrastructural changes; the overall prognosis is good.

Clinical Features

■ The most common features are proteinuria and periorbital edema, with or without the other manifestations of nephrotic syndrome. Onset may follow an upper respiratory tract infection.

Laboratory Values

■ The proteinuria is usually *selective* and consists of albumin and other low-molecular-weight proteins; the presence of higher-molecular-weight proteins (*nonselective proteinuria*) suggests another diagnosis.

■ Microscopic hematuria may occur (10% to 30%); gross hematuria is rare.

■ Renal excretory function, as measured by serum urea nitrogen (BUN) and creatinine, is usually normal.

■ Serum complement levels are normal and serologic tests for autoimmune ("collagen vascular" or "connective tissue") diseases are usually negative.

Treatment and Clinical Course

■ Idiopathic MCNS usually responds to corticosteroids (up to 90% of children; 60% to 90% of adults), although relapses may occur. Cytotoxic immunosuppressive agents such as cyclophosphamide (Cytoxan) are often used in steroid-resistant cases.

■ The long-term prognosis for overall and renal survival in idiopathic MCNS is good; the majority of patients maintain normal or nearly normal renal function.

■ The prognosis of secondary forms of MCNS depends on the condition with which the MCNS is associated. Minimal change nephrotic syndrome associated with NSAIDs has a good prognosis; complete resolution of proteinuria can be expected, provided that treatment with the drug is discontinued.

Gross Pathology

■ Today, few kidneys involved by MCNS are examined grossly. Historical reports of kidneys involved by MCNS describe enlarged, pale kidneys with yellow discoloration of the cortex because of lipid accumulation within tubules, which may be focal; the medulla is usually spared.

Light Microscopy

The defining overall characteristic is that *the light microscopic appearance shows no or only minimal histologic changes.*

Glomeruli

- Glomerular cellularity is usually normal.
- Capillaries may appear slightly dilated; capillary walls are thin and capillary basement membranes are thin and delicate on periodic acid–Schiff (PAS) and Jones (silver) stains.
- Visceral epithelial cells appear prominent and may contain cytoplasmic protein resorption droplets.
- Occasional globally obsolescent glomeruli may be present (fewer than 6% to 10%, depending on the age of the patient), but *glomeruli with segmental sclerotic lesions must be absent.*

Tubules

- Proximal convoluted tubular epithelial cells may contain PAS-positive resorption droplets; occasional tubules may contain hyaline casts.
- Adult patients may have focal areas of tubular atrophy. Tubules are otherwise unremarkable.

Vessels

- Vessels are characteristically unremarkable; adult patients may have arterial and arteriolar sclerosis related to preexisting hypertension.

Interstitium

- The interstitium is characteristically not expanded, and no interstitial inflammation is present.
- Interstitial nephritis or tubular injury is occasionally present, possibly related to medications (NSAIDs, diuretics, or antibiotics).
- Interstitial nephritis is present in half or more of patients with MCNS caused by NSAIDs; however, interstitial inflammation can be completely absent.

Fluorescence Microscopy

- No immunofluorescent staining is seen within the glomerular mesangium or capillary walls in typical cases; staining may be seen within visceral epithelial cells and represents reabsorbed serum proteins.
- Granular staining, primarily for albumin and C3, may be seen within proximal convoluted tubular cells and represents lysosomes with reabsorbed protein.
- Glomerular mesangial staining for IgM may be seen in some cases (see IgM Nephropathy later).

Electron Microscopy

- Glomerular basement membranes are not thickened. No basement membrane spikes are present, and no electron-dense deposits are present within the glomerular mesangium or within capillary walls.
- Visceral epithelial cell foot processes (podocytes) are diffusely broadened and simplified, with effacement of the normal architecture; this finding is commonly but inaccurately described as "fusion."

- Visceral epithelial cells may contain vacuoles or protein resorption droplets and have numerous long, narrow projections extending from their surface ("microvillous transformation").

Histologic Variants

Diffuse Mesangial Hypercellularity in Idiopathic Nephrotic Syndrome

- Some patients with clinical and pathologic features otherwise consistent with MCNS have a diffuse increase in mesangial cellularity, defined as three or more cells in a single mesangial area on thin (2- to 3-μm) sections away from the vascular pole.
- A proportion of cases demonstrate mesangial staining for IgM, with or without C3, and occasionally other immunoglobulins; thus there may be overlap with the entity of IgM nephropathy (see later).
- The significance of this change is controversial. Some series have suggested a worse prognosis; however, in the series of the International Study of Kidney Disease in Children and the Southwest Pediatric Nephrology Study Group, the incidence of initial resistance to corticosteroid therapy was higher in patients with mesangial hypercellularity, but the final response to therapy and the overall outcome were not significantly different.

IgM Nephropathy

- The presence of mesangial staining for IgM, sometimes with C3, in biopsy tissue, which would otherwise be considered minimal change disease, was first described in the late 1970s and is sometimes designated IgM nephropathy. At present, IgM nephropathy as an entity remains controversial; some believe that it may represent a variant or early form of FSGS. The clinical features, pathologic findings, and response to therapy are heterogeneous, and the prognostic implications are unclear.
- One possibly confounding variable is the presence or absence of mesangial hypercellularity. In many series, no distinction is made between cases with or without diffuse mesangial hypercellularity; patients with hypercellularity could represent a distinct group with a different prognosis and probability of response to therapy.
- Electron-dense mesangial deposits are found by electron microscopy in approximately half of cases.
- The etiology of IgM nephropathy is unknown; it is possible, perhaps probable, that there are heterogeneous causes.
- The majority of patients have proteinuria or the nephrotic syndrome. A proportion of patients have hematuria, either recurrent gross hematuria or persistent microhematuria.
- The clinical course is heterogeneous; there is a tendency for proteinuria to be resistant to corticosteroids. It has been suggested that the prognosis of patients with nephrotic syndrome may be worse than that of patients with hematuria alone.

Differential Diagnosis

- Focal segmental glomerulosclerosis is a difficult diagnostic problem, particularly if the biopsy specimen is small. There is no widely accepted minimum number of glomeruli required for an adequate biopsy sample; one author has recommended that biopsies containing fewer than 10 glomeruli be considered inadequate. The diagnosis of FSGS can never be totally excluded, even in specimens with a generous number of glomeruli, because of the focal nature of the defining lesion.

- The presence of numerous sclerotic glomeruli (more than 10%), significant interstitial fibrosis or tubular atrophy, or vascular disease out of proportion to the degree of glomerular sclerosis raises a concern for FSGS in a patient with proteinuria, particularly a young patient. In such a case, examination of the biopsy tissue at multiple levels is recommended to reduce the possibility of a missed diagnosis of FSGS.

- The possibility of a secondary form of MCNS should always be considered in adults; in particular, the possibility of MCNS from NSAIDs should be excluded.

- Prominent interstitial nephritis suggests MCNS associated with NSAIDs; however, MCNS secondary to NSAIDs can occur without interstitial nephritis.

- Early MGN can be indistinguishable from MCNS on light microscopy; the presence of granular glomerular capillary wall staining on immunofluorescence and electron-dense subepithelial deposits on electron microscopy distinguish MGN from MCNS.

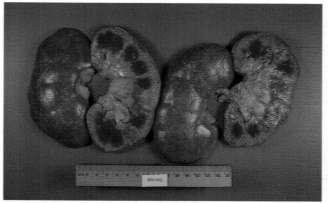

Figure 5–1. Minimal change nephrotic syndrome (synonym, lipoid nephrosis). A gross photograph of an autopsied kidney reveals a *dotted yellow* cortical cut surface and deep-dark medulla. The old term "lipoid nephrosis" was given because of the deposition of fat (lipid) in the renal tubules in these patients with nephrotic syndrome. (Courtesy of Dr. Alex Miller, Downers Grove, IL.)

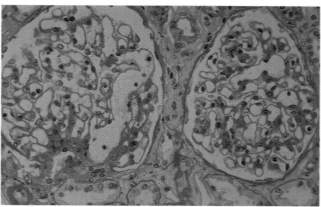

Figure 5–3. Minimal change nephrotic syndrome. Histologically normal-appearing glomeruli are seen in a renal biopsy specimen from a patient with nephrotic syndrome (periodic acid–Schiff reaction).

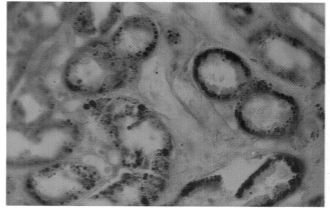

Figure 5–2. Minimal change nephrotic syndrome ("lipoid nephrosis"). Sudan black stain shows extensive lipid accumulation in the tubular epithelial cells of the proximal convoluted tubules. Originally, lipoid nephrosis was thought to be a tubular metabolic disorder with fat deposition in the tubules. Now, with the advent of electron microscopy and other studies, we know that the primary change is glomerular.

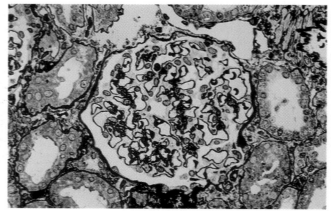

Figure 5–4. Minimal change nephrotic syndrome. A silver-stained section shows patent glomerular capillary lumina. No glomerular hypercellularity is noted (methenamine silver stain).

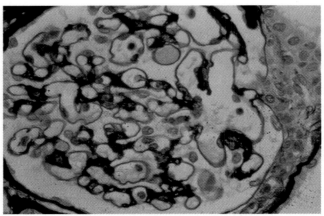

Figure 5–5. Minimal change nephrotic syndrome. The glomerular capillary basement membranes appear delicate; a few capillary loops are slightly ectatic. A few visceral epithelial cells are enlarged (methenamine silver stain).

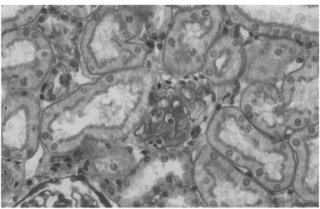

Figure 5–6. Minimal change nephrotic syndrome (MCNS), globally sclerotic glomeruli. Occasional globally sclerotic glomeruli can be seen in patients with MCNS. However, glomeruli with segmental sclerosis must be absent to make the diagnosis of MCNS. The presence of globally sclerotic glomeruli is considered to be abnormal if the ratio of the globally sclerotic glomeruli exceeds 6% to 10% of all glomeruli in a patient under 40 years of age.

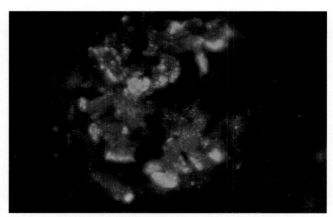

Figure 5–7. Minimal change nephrotic syndrome (MCNS). In typical cases of MCNS, no immunofluorescent staining is seen in the glomeruli. However, deposition of IgM in the mesangial areas may sometimes be seen (see so-called IgM nephropathy in the text).

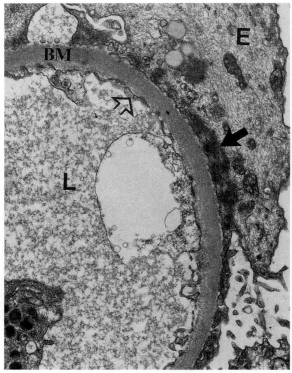

Figure 5–8. Electron micrograph of minimal change nephrotic syndrome. Note the effacement (so-called fusion) of the foot processes of visceral epithelial cells. Condensation of the microfilaments in the cytoplasm *(arrow)* can be confused with subepithelial deposits by trichrome staining on light microscopy. The *empty arrow* points to the glomerular capillary endothelial cell. BM, glomerular capillary basement membrane; E, visceral epithelial cell; L, glomerular capillary lumen. (From Laszik Z, Lajoie G, Nadasdy T, Silva FG: Medical diseases of the kidney. In: Silverberg SG, DeLellis RA, Frable WJ [eds]: Principles and Practice of Surgical Pathology and Cytopathology, 3rd ed. New York, Churchill Livingstone, 1997, p 2079, with permission.)

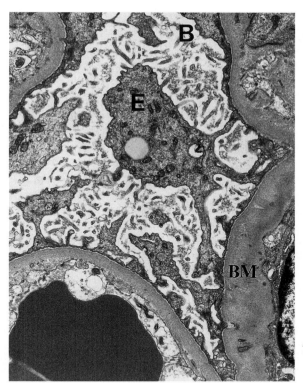

Figure 5–9. Electron micrograph of minimal change nephrotic syndrome (MCNS). Microvillous transformation of the visceral epithelial cells *(E)* is a frequent nonspecific finding in MCNS (and in any cause of a "leaky" glomerulus and subsequent nephrotic syndrome). B, Bowman's space; BM, glomerular capillary basement membrane.

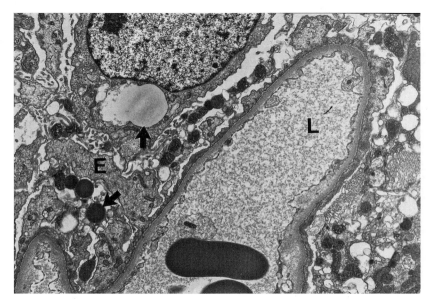

Figure 5–10. Electron micrograph of minimal change nephrotic syndrome (MCNS) with protein and lipid droplets in the visceral epithelial cells. Intracytoplasmic protein and/or lipid droplets *(arrows)* are frequently seen in patients with proteinuria, including MCNS and focal segmental glomerulosclerosis. Note the effacement of the visceral epithelial cell foot processes and the mild microvillous transformation. E, visceral epithelial cell; L, glomerular capillary lumen.

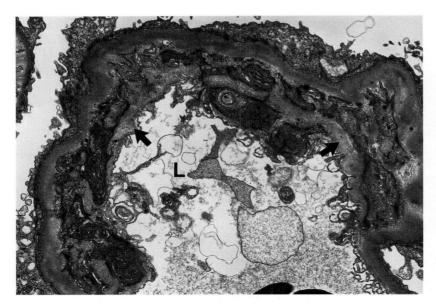

Figure 5–11. Electron micrograph of reduplication of the glomerular capillary wall with circumferential mesangial cell interposition in a single capillary loop in a patient with minimal change nephrotic syndrome (MCNS); the remainder of the capillary loops revealed only foot process effacement. Severe widespread basement membrane reduplication is a typical finding in membranoproliferative glomerulonephritis; it is also somewhat common in advanced glomerular diseases but occasionally occurs focally in various glomerular diseases as well, including even MCNS. The new basement membrane is marked by *arrows.* L, glomerular capillary lumen.

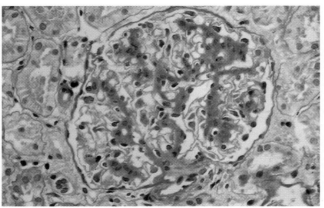

Figure 5–12. Diffuse mesangial hypercellularity with idiopathic nephrotic syndrome. Slight mesangial widening with mesangial hypercellularity is shown. The capillaries are still patent.

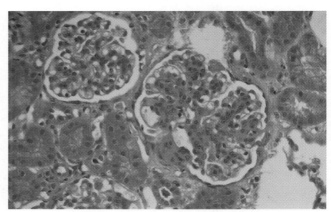

Figure 5–13. Moderate diffuse mesangial hypercellularity with idiopathic nephrotic syndrome (MCNS). Diffuse mesangial hypercellularity in MCNS is associated with an increased incidence of hematuria and may have a less favorable initial response to steroid therapy without affecting the long-term good prognosis.

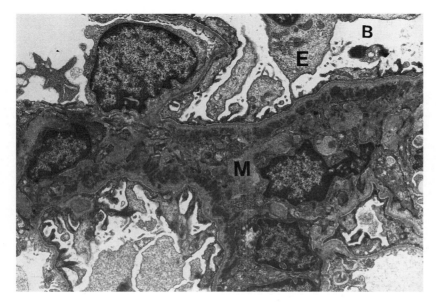

Figure 5–14. Electron micrograph of minimal change nephrotic syndrome with discrete mesangial electron-dense "immune-type" deposits. The widened mesangium shows slight hypercellularity. The deposits are just under the glomerular basement membrane, overlying the mesangial regions. These types of deposits can be seen in so-called IgM nephropathy. B, Bowman's space; E, visceral epithelial cell; M, mesangium.

FOCAL SEGMENTAL GLOMERULOSCLEROSIS

Synonyms: Focal and segmental glomerulosclerosis; focal sclerosis; focal sclerosis with hyalinosis.

Biology of Disease

- Focal segmental glomerulosclerosis (FSGS) is a histologic pattern associated with a variety of renal and nonrenal diseases (Table 5–2). Like MCNS, there are primary (idiopathic) and secondary forms; also like MCNS, the cause or causes of FSGS are unknown. Historically, FSGS was identified in a group of children with idiopathic nephrotic syndrome that exhibited resistance to corticosteroids and a higher incidence of progression to chronic renal insufficiency; the histologic lesion has subsequently been associated with reflux nephropathy, congenital unilateral kidney, partial nephrectomy (in laboratory animals), intravenous drug abuse, and a variety of other conditions.
- A variety of possible causes of FSGS have been proposed, including circulating systemic factors, hyperfiltration, abnormalities of the humoral or cellular immune systems, localized coagulation disorders, persistent proteinuria per se, and a variety of other causes or mechanisms; no explanation is completely satisfactory, and multiple factors or mechanisms are most likely involved.
- Focal segmental glomerulosclerosis is found in 7% to 15% of cases of idiopathic nephrotic syndrome in children and in 10% to 20% of adult cases.

Clinical Features

- The most common manifestation of FSGS is severe proteinuria or the nephrotic syndrome. Unlike MCNS, the proteinuria is usually nonselective and includes both smaller and larger proteins.
- Hematuria is common (25% to 75%) and usually microscopic.
- Hypertension is more common than in MCNS (30% to 50%).
- A male preponderance is noted in most series.
- There is a higher incidence of FSGS in African-Americans and other persons of African descent.

Laboratory Values

- Elevated serum urea nitrogen (BUN) and creatinine are present in 20% to 30% at diagnosis.
- Serum complement levels are usually normal, and serologic tests for collagen vascular disorders are negative.

Table 5–2
CONDITIONS ASSOCIATED WITH FOCAL
SEGMENTAL GLOMERULOSCLEROSIS

Primary (idiopathic) focal segmental glomerulosclerosis
Congenital or acquired reduction of renal parenchyma
Human immunodeficiency virus–associated nephropathy
Reflux nephropathy

Treatment and Clinical Course

- There is no widely accepted treatment for FSGS; corticosteroids have been of apparent benefit in a subset of patients (10% to 15%) in some series, although the majority of patients are resistant.
- The overall outlook for patients with FSGS is not favorable; approximately 25% to 40% of patients die or chronic renal insufficiency develops over 10 to 15 years of follow-up.
- The presence of interstitial fibrosis or numerous globally sclerotic glomeruli on biopsy at the initial diagnosis may be an unfavorable histologic indicator.
- Recurrence of FSGS occurs in approximately 20% to 30% of patients after renal transplantation; the recurrence rate may be higher in patients with a rapid decline in renal function originally (progression to renal failure in 3 years or less). However, recurrence does not necessarily indicate inevitable early graft failure.

Gross Pathology

- Early: kidneys may be swollen and pale; yellow streaks may be present in the cortex because of lipid within tubular epithelial cells.
- Late: kidneys may be small and have finely granular surfaces.

Light Microscopy

Glomeruli

- The key histologic feature is segmental sclerosis of some glomerular tufts, with expansion of the mesangium and collapse of capillary lumina. In advanced disease the glomeruli become globally obsolescent, indistinguishable from obsolescent glomeruli secondary to any chronic renal disease. The sclerosis is said to be more pronounced at the vascular pole of the tuft, especially near the afferent arteriole.
- The sclerotic areas stain positively with PAS and silver stains.
- Juxtamedullary glomeruli are said by some pathologists to be preferentially involved early in the disease, with later involvement of superficial cortical glomeruli.
- Uninvolved glomeruli may appear large and hypertrophic.
- Glomerular cellularity usually appears normal, although there may be segmental or diffuse mesangial hypercellularity.
- Visceral epithelial cells overlying the sclerotic loop may be enlarged and hyperplastic, with hyperchromatic nuclei, basophilic cytoplasm, and PAS-positive resorption droplets. This appearance is known as a "cap" or "cellular" lesion.
- Intracapillary cells within sclerotic tufts may have cytoplasmic vacuolization, described as a "foam cell" appearance. This appearance may be more common during the early phases of the disease.
- "Glomerular tip lesion": adhesion of the glomerular tuft to Bowman's capsule adjacent to the origin of the proximal convoluted tubule is seen in association with

obstruction of capillaries and proliferation of the parietal epithelial cells of Bowman's capsule. The tip lesion is most often present in FSGS but can be seen in other conditions.

■ "Hyalinosis": homogeneous, eosinophilic material may be present at the glomerular hilum, at the periphery of sclerotic foci, or within the capillary subendothelial space, probably representing leakage ("insudation") of plasma proteins into the capillary wall. It stains positively with PAS and fuchsinophilic with trichrome stains but does not stain with silver stains.

Tubules

■ Tubular epithelial cells may contain PAS-positive resorption droplets.
■ Focal tubular atrophy with hyaline casts and thickening of tubular basement membranes may be present at the initial diagnosis; tubular atrophy is common in biopsy specimens harvested later in the disease course.

Vessels

■ Arterial wall hyperplasia and hyaline arteriolosclerosis are frequent, particularly in adults.

Interstitium

■ Focal interstitial fibrosis may be present. Interstitial inflammation is usually absent or minimal.

Fluorescence Microscopy

■ Glomeruli are either negative or demonstrate staining for IgM and C3 in sclerotic areas; staining, when present, is believed to represent entrapment of plasma proteins rather than true immune complexes and often corresponds to areas of hyalinosis. Staining for albumin, immunoglobulins, C3, and other proteins may be seen in visceral epithelial cells and represents protein absorption; it can sometimes be difficult to distinguish this staining from capillary wall staining.
■ Tubules may demonstrate staining of lysosomes for albumin and other proteins, and this finding probably represents protein reabsorption.

Electron Microscopy

■ Visceral epithelial foot processes are effaced, focally or diffusely; microvillous transformation is common.
■ Sclerotic regions contain increased mesangial matrix and basement membrane–like material.
■ Cells containing cytoplasmic lipid vacuoles may be present within capillary lumina and represent the "foam cells" seen by light microscopy.
■ Visceral epithelial cells may become detached from the glomerular basement membrane (GBM); a laminated appearance of the GBM may develop at the site of detachment because of new basement membrane synthesis. This change is most commonly seen in FSGS but is not specific.

Histologic Variants

Focal Segmental Glomerulosclerosis With Mesangial Hypercellularity

■ The presence of diffuse mesangial hypercellularity is said by some to indicate more aggressive disease. In the Southwest Pediatric Nephrology Study Group series, the outcome of patients with mesangial hypercellularity was not significantly different from that of patients lacking this feature.

Collapsing Glomerulopathy

■ Collapsing glomerulopathy is a recently described variant of FSGS with an aggressive course. Clinically, it is characterized by a strong predilection for African-Americans, massive proteinuria (frequently exceeding 10 g/day), and a high incidence of renal insufficiency at diagnosis. Pathologically, it is characterized by extensive segmental or global collapse of the glomerular tuft with less mesangial matrix expansion and adhesion formation, more striking visceral epithelial cell hypertrophy, and more extensive tubulointerstitial changes than seen in typical FSGS. The clinical course is aggressive, with a majority of patients in renal failure within 1 to 2 years (often much less). Many patients with this variant are infected with human immunodeficiency virus (HIV); however, collapsing glomerulopathy has been described in patients with no evidence of HIV infection; the etiology in this group is unclear.

Differential Diagnosis

■ Differentiation of FSGS from MCNS is critical because of the lower probability of response to corticosteroid therapy and worse long-term prognosis of FSGS. Unfortunately, this distinction can be difficult or, at times, impossible. The presence of numerous obsolescent glomeruli in biopsy tissue from a patient with nephrotic syndrome should raise a concern for FSGS rather than MCNS, as should interstitial fibrosis or vascular disease out of proportion to the glomerular changes. Careful scrutiny of glomeruli for segmental changes at multiple levels is required, and sectioning through the biopsy specimen should be done in an attempt to exclude segmental sclerosis. When in doubt, it may be most appropriate to give a descriptive diagnosis with a comment that the biopsy findings are consistent with MCNS and a description of any features that raise concern for FSGS.
■ Segmental glomerular scarring caused by previous proliferative glomerulonephritis may be confused with FSGS; the clinical history is helpful in this differential. The presence of hyalinosis within sclerotic areas is said to be a clue to FSGS rather than segmental scarring from other causes, but hyalinosis is frequently absent.
■ Nephropathy associated with intravenous drug use (heroin-associated nephropathy) is histologically somewhat similar to idiopathic FSGS; African-Americans appear to be predisposed to both.

■ Nephropathy associated with HIV (HIV-associated nephropathy [HIV-AN]) also resembles FSGS by light microscopy; the presence of numerous tubuloreticular structures within glomerular capillary endothelial cells on electron microscopy and the presence of microcystic tubules should suggest HIV-AN.

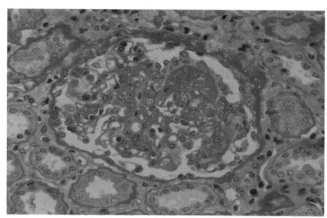

Figure 5–17. Focal segmental glomerulosclerosis (focal sclerosis). There is prominent visceral epithelial cell hyperplasia overlying the segmental sclerotic lesion between the 12- and 3-o'clock position. The nonsclerotic segments of the glomerulus reveal some moderate mesangial widening with hypercellularity. The significance of mesangial hypercellularity in focal segmental glomerulosclerosis is uncertain.

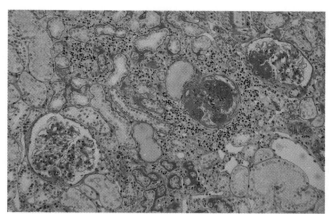

Figure 5–15. Focal segmental glomerulosclerosis (focal sclerosis). The characteristic lesion of this disease is the focal segmental sclerotic lesion seen in the glomerulus on the *upper right*; the glomerulus in the *middle* is globally sclerotic, whereas the one on the *left* appears histologically normal. Note the tubular atrophy and chronic inflammatory cell infiltrate in the tubulointerstitium. Light microscopy usually does not differentiate between primary (idiopathic) and secondary (known causes) focal segmental glomerulosclerosis (periodic acid–Schiff reaction).

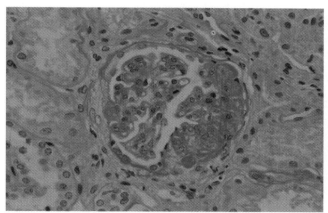

Figure 5–18. Focal segmental glomerulosclerosis (focal sclerosis). The segmental sclerosis involves approximately half of the glomerulus on the *right* side; a few sclerotic loops are attached to Bowman's capsule at the 9-o'clock position.

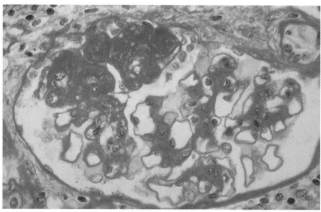

Figure 5–16. Focal segmental glomerulosclerosis (focal sclerosis). The sclerotic glomerular segment between the 10- and 12-o'clock position shows collapsed capillary loops, accumulation of basement membrane–mesangial matrix–like material, and fibrous attachment (synechiae) to Bowman's capsule. The mesangial areas of the nonsclerotic segments appear slightly widened. The typical site of a segmental sclerotic lesion within the glomerulus is near the vascular pole (especially near the afferent arteriole) (periodic acid–Schiff reaction).

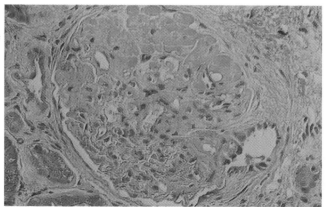

Figure 5–19. Focal segmental glomerulosclerosis (focal sclerosis). Intracapillary hyalin deposits are shown in the sclerotic glomerular segment. The presence of hyalinosis (plasmatic insudation) accounts for the term *focal sclerosis and hyalinosis* (Masson's trichrome stain).

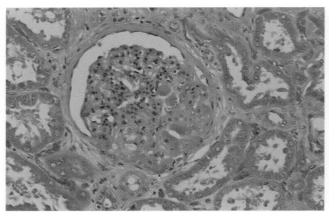

Figure 5–20. Focal segmental glomerulosclerosis (focal sclerosis). There is fibrous adhesion between the segmental sclerotic lesion that involves more than half of the glomerulus and Bowman's capsule. Foam cells and hyalinosis are also seen within the sclerotic glomerular segment.

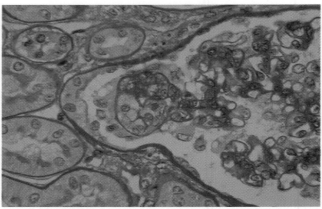

Figure 5–22. Focal segmental glomerulosclerosis (focal sclerosis), "tip" lesion. The lesion consists of a few effaced (or closed) capillary loops at the glomerular "tip" with intracapillary foam cells and hypertrophy and vacuolization of podocytes. Adhesions between the glomerular capillary loops and Bowman's capsule—a common feature of the tip lesion—are not present in this particular lesion. This type of glomerular injury has also been described in various other glomerular diseases.

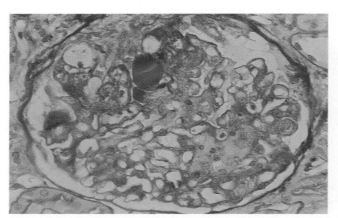

Figure 5–21. Focal segmental glomerulosclerosis (focal sclerosis). The glomerulus displays a segmental sclerotic lesion *(left upper glomerular quadrant)* with collapse of the capillary loops, intracapillary hyalinization and foam cells, accumulation of mesangial matrix, and adhesion between the sclerotic loops and Bowman's capsule (periodic acid–Schiff reaction).

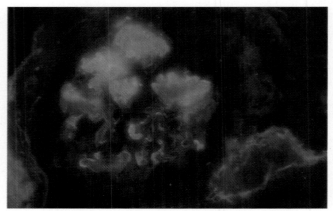

Figure 5–23. IgM immunofluorescence in focal segmental glomerulosclerosis (focal sclerosis). The staining is restricted to the sclerotic segments, glomerular mesangial regions and capillary loops; the positivity is possibly related to nonimmune absorption of IgM in the damaged sclerotic areas. A positive staining is also seen in a small artery.

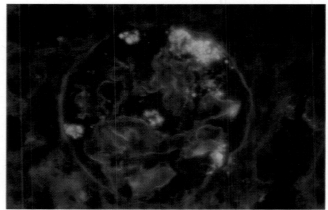

Figure 5–24. Focal segmental glomerulosclerosis (focal sclerosis), immunofluorescence, albumin staining. A few visceral epithelial cells are loaded with protein resorption droplets.

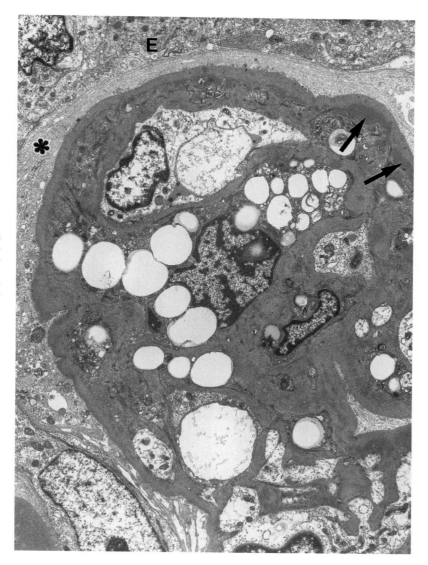

Figure 5–25. Electron micrograph of focal segmental glomerulosclerosis (focal sclerosis). An effaced glomerular capillary loop shows amorphous subendothelial hyalin deposits *(arrows)* and intracapillary foam cells. Note the lifting/separation of the visceral epithelial cells from the underlying glomerular basement membrane (GBM) with loose lamination between the GBM and the visceral epithelial cell *(asterisk).* E, visceral epithelial cell.

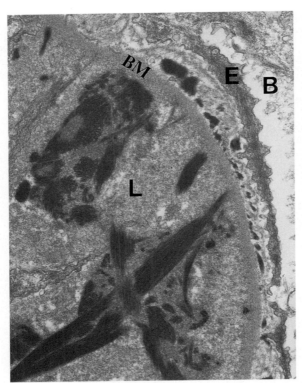

Figure 5–26. Electron micrograph of focal segmental glomerulosclerosis (FSGS). Glomerular intracapillary, intraluminal, subendothelial, and subepithelial fibrin deposits are present. Fibrin is not uncommon in FSGS. Subepithelial fibrin deposition, however, is uncommon. BM, glomerular capillary basement membrane; E, visceral epithelial cell; B, Bowman's space; L, glomerular capillary lumen.

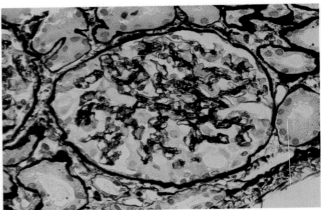

Figure 5–27. Focal segmental glomerulosclerosis (focal sclerosis), collapsing glomerulopathy. Most of the glomeruli from biopsy tissue of a 24-year-old African-American female showed global collapse of the glomerular capillary loops and hypertrophic visceral epithelial cells. Note the lack of silver-positive matrix accumulation within the collapsed glomerulus (methenamine silver stain).

MEMBRANOUS GLOMERULONEPHROPATHY

Synonyms: Membranous glomerulonephritis; membranous nephropathy; epimembranous or extramembranous nephropathy.

Biology of Disease

■ Membranous glomerulonephropathy is the most common cause of idiopathic nephrotic syndrome in adults and may rarely lead to idiopathic nephrotic syndrome in childhood.

■ The etiology in the majority of cases is unknown (*idiopathic* or *primary MGN*); MGN can also be secondary to or associated with a variety of conditions, including systemic lupus erythematosus and other autoimmune disorders, chronic infections such as with hepatitis B virus, drugs such as penicillamine, and malignant neoplasms (Table 5–3). Thus like MCNS and FSGS, MGN represents a morphologic appearance with numerous causes rather than a homogeneous disease entity.

■ The characteristic finding in MGN is the presence of diffuse, discrete, granular glomerular capillary wall staining for immunoglobulins and complement on immunofluorescence and subepithelial electron-dense deposits on electron microscopy. It has generally been thought that the deposits are derived from circulating immune complexes that become trapped within glomerular capillary walls; more recently it has been suggested that in many cases the immune complexes may form in situ, with circulating antibodies recognizing either native renal antigens or foreign antigens previ-

Table 5–3

CONDITIONS ASSOCIATED WITH MEMBRANOUS GLOMERULONEPHROPATHY

Primary (idiopathic) membranous glomerulonephropathy
Infections: hepatitis B, syphilis
Drugs: gold, D-penicillamine, mercury, captopril
Systemic diseases: systemic lupus, rheumatoid arthritis
Malignant neoplasms: carcinomas (lung, colorectal, gastric, breast, kidney), leukemia, and lymphomas (Hodgkin's and non-Hodgkin's)

ously localized in glomerular capillaries near the sub-epithelial space.

Clinical Features

- The most common finding is proteinuria, with or without the full nephrotic syndrome.
- The peak incidence is in the fourth to fifth decades, although MGN is seen at all ages.
- There is a male preponderance in most series.

Laboratory Values

- The proteinuria is usually nonselective (both high- and low-molecular-weight proteins).
- Microscopic hematuria is present in 25% to 85% of patients; gross hematuria is uncommon.
- Elevations in serum creatinine and urea nitrogen are present in approximately half of the patients, but the degree of elevation is usually mild.

Treatment and Clinical Course

- The clinical course in the majority of patients appears to be indolent, although some series have suggested a higher incidence of progression to end-stage renal failure. Spontaneous remissions of proteinuria occur in approximately one quarter of patients; approximately half will have stable renal function, with or without continued proteinuria.
- A minority of patients will demonstrate slow decline in renal function, and a few will have rapid decline leading to renal failure or death.
- Treatment of MGN is controversial. Controlled trials of corticosteroids with or without cytotoxic agents have had variable results.

Gross Pathology

- Kidneys with MGN are seldom examined grossly. Historical reports of patients dying of acute nephrotic syndrome describe enlarged, pale kidneys with smooth surfaces.

Light Microscopy

The characteristic changes of MGN involve glomerular capillary walls; changes in the other compartments are secondary and usually minor until the late stages of disease.

Glomeruli

- In early or mild cases of the disease, glomeruli may appear remarkably normal and the diagnosis may be missed without immunofluorescence and electron microscopy. Capillary loops may appear round and rigid; the GBM may appear slightly amphophilic on hematoxylin and eosin stain.
- The earliest sign by light microscopy is a mottled or "moth-eaten" appearance of the GBM in *en face* orientation on silver stains.

- Linear projections or "spikes" that protrude from the outer surface of the GBM into Bowman's space are seen on silver stains; initially these may be focal and fine and require careful examination under high magnification for detection. With disease progression they become widespread and larger, and club-shaped ends may develop.
- Fine, fuchsinophilic speckles may be distributed along the outer surface of the GBM on trichrome stain.
- With disease progression, capillary walls and the GBM become progressively thickened.
- Glomerular cellularity is frequently normal.

Tubules

- Proximal convoluted tubular epithelial cells may contain PAS-positive resorption droplets.
- With disease progression, tubular atrophy may occur.

Vessels

- Vessels may appear unremarkable; thickening of arterial and arteriolar walls may be present.

Interstitium

- Interstitial widening with fibrosis may be present, particularly in disease of longer duration.

Fluorescence Microscopy

- The characteristic immunofluorescence picture of MGN is granular glomerular capillary wall staining for immunoglobulins and complement that varies from fine to coarse.
- IgG is present in virtually all cases, C3 is present in approximately three quarters, IgM and IgA are present in a minority of cases, and other complement components are usually absent.
- Mesangial deposits are usually absent; the presence of prominent mesangial deposits suggests MGN associated with systemic lupus erythematosus.
- Granular staining for albumin and possibly other reactants will be present in proximal convoluted tubules.

Electron Microscopy

- Electron-dense deposits are present on the epithelial side of glomerular capillary loops, between the GBM and the visceral epithelial cells; this location is described as *subepithelial* or *epimembranous*. Deposits are usually diffusely distributed over all capillary loops, but they may be irregular or segmental in distribution.
- Irregular projections of the GBM may be present between the deposits and correspond to the GBM spikes seen on silver stains by light microscopy.
- With disease progression, the GBM spikes become longer and thicker; deposits may become surrounded by GBM material and incorporated within a thickened GBM.

- Deposits may become rarefied and lose their electron density.
- Visceral epithelial foot processes are variably effaced.

Ehrenreich and Churg Staging System for Membranous Glomerulonephropathy

Stage I: The GBM is normal in thickness, with no or only minimal spike formation.

Stage II: GBM spikes are present and extend between deposits; broadening of the ends of spikes may be present.

Stage III: Electron-dense deposits are fully enclosed by GBM material and incorporated within a thickened GBM.

Stage IV: Deposits are incorporated within the GBM and become rarefied.

Differential Diagnosis

- Early MGN can be difficult or impossible to distinguish from MCNS by light microscopy; the presence of characteristic granular capillary wall staining on immunofluorescence microscopy or subepithelial electron-dense deposits on electron microscopy will distinguish MGN from MCNS.
- Membranous nephropathy may be the initial manifestation of systemic lupus erythematosus, with other non-renal manifestations of lupus developing months or years later. The presence of "full house" immunoglobulins (IgG, IgM, and IgA) plus C4 or C1q in addition to C3 on immunofluorescent staining or the presence of numerous tubuloreticular structures on electron microscopy suggests MGN associated with systemic lupus erythematosus.

- Secondary cases of MGN cannot be distinguished from idiopathic MGN by morphologic findings alone. It has been suggested that the electron-dense deposits tend to be more variable in size and more irregular in distribution in secondary MGN; however, this distinction is not always reliable. The presence of mesangial deposits suggests MGN associated with systemic lupus but mesangial deposits can be seen in non-SLE cases of MGN.
- Membranoproliferative (mesangiocapillary) glomerulonephritis (MPGN) may show capillary wall thickening suggestive of MGN by light microscopy; the presence of mesangial expansion and hypercellularity in MPGN distinguishes it from MGN. On electron microscopy, the presence of subendothelial rather than subepithelial deposits, mesangial cell interposition, and synthesis of new GBM-like material distinguishes MPGN from MGN.
- Very fine granular capillary wall deposits may be mistaken for linear GBM staining on immunofluorescence and suggest anti-GBM antibody disease. The histologic appearance will differ; anti-GBM is usually associated with focal necrosis of the glomerular capillary tuft and crescents in Bowman's space, which are rare in MGN. Anti-GBM disease will also lack the characteristic electron-dense subepithelial deposits seen in MGN.

Histologic Variants

Membranous Glomerulonephropathy Associated With Crescents

- Rare cases with the typical subepithelial deposits of MGN but with the added feature of cellular crescents have been reported. The clinical course is usually one of rapid decline in renal function ending in renal failure. Anti-GBM antibodies are present in some cases but not all.

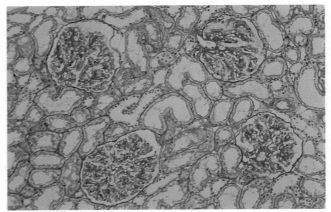

Figure 5–28. Membranous glomerulonephropathy, mild stage. This low-magnification photograph shows normal-appearing glomeruli with widely patent glomerular capillary lumina. In a case like this, electron or immunofluorescence microscopy may be necessary to make the diagnosis (periodic acid–Schiff reaction).

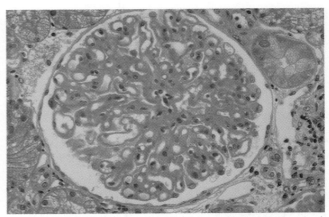

Figure 5–29. Membranous glomerulonephropathy. Beside the prominent uniform thickening of the glomerular capillary walls (basement membranes) slight sclerotic lesions are also seen (case of systemic lupus erythematosus).

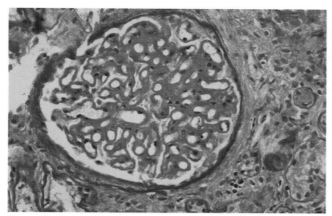

Figure 5–30. Membranous glomerulonephropathy. The glomerular capillary walls show diffuse uniform thickening; the capillary lumina are patent. No glomerular hypercellularity is noted (periodic acid–Schiff reaction).

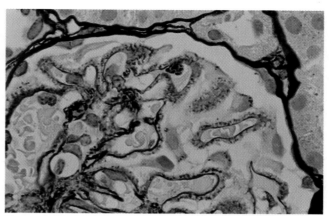

Figure 5–33. Membranous glomerulonephropathy. Numerous silver-positive spikes are seen protruding from the outer aspects of the glomerular capillary basement membranes into Bowman's space (methenamine silver stain).

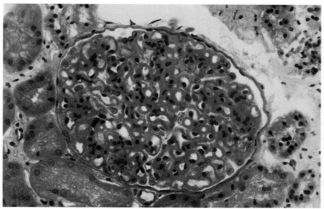

Figure 5–31. Membranous glomerulonephropathy. Masson's trichrome stain demonstrates uniform marked thickening of the glomerular capillary basement membranes; slight sclerotic changes of the glomerulus are also seen.

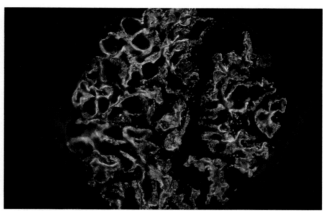

Figure 5–34. Membranous glomerulonephropathy (MGN). Widespread granular IgG immunostaining along the glomerular capillary basement membranes is shown. This pattern is highly characteristic for MGN.

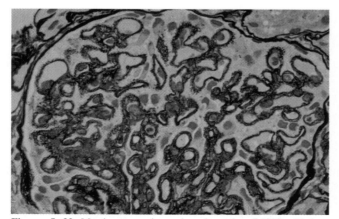

Figure 5–32. Membranous glomerulonephropathy (MGN). Methenamine silver stain shows "spikes" protruding from the glomerular capillary basement membranes. This patient had MGN associated with hepatitis B virus infection.

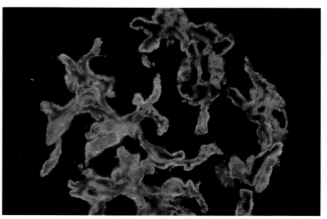

Figure 5–35. Membranous glomerulonephropathy (MGN). Finely granular/pseudolinear immunostaining with antibodies against IgG is shown on this photograph. This staining pattern is typical for mild/early stages of MGN.

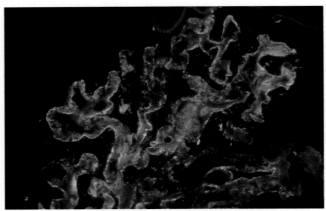

Figure 5–36. Membranous glomerulonephropathy with higher magnification of anti-IgG staining showing granular capillary wall staining.

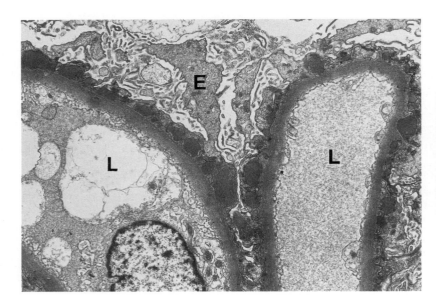

Figure 5–37. Electron micrograph of idiopathic membranous glomerulonephropathy, stage I to II. Discrete granular subepithelial electron-dense immune-type deposits are seen along the external aspects of the glomerular basement membranes (GBMs); the outline of the GBM is smooth; however, a few small basement membrane–like protrusions between some of the deposits are already seen. The foot processes of the visceral epithelial cells show effacement; microvillous transformation is also seen. E, visceral epithelial cell; L, glomerular capillary lumen.

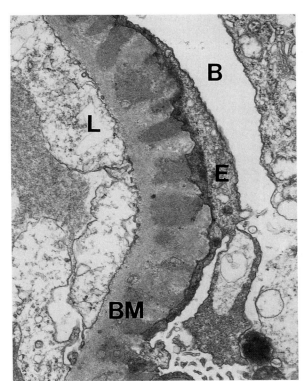

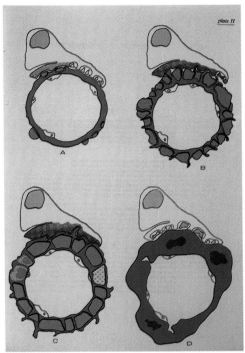

Figure 5–38. Electron micrograph of idiopathic membranous glomerulonephropathy, stage II to III: segment of glomerular capillary. Basement membrane–like "spikes" protrude from the glomerular basement membrane (GBM) between the discrete electron-dense immune-type deposits toward Bowman's space; some of the deposits are already embedded in the thickened GBM. L, glomerular capillary lumen; B, Bowman's space; E, visceral epithelial cell; BM, glomerular capillary basement membrane.

Figure 5–39. Membranous glomerulonephropathy, schematic illustration of various stages of the disease. Stage I *(A):* a few deposits *(red)* are on the top of the basement membrane. Stage II *(B):* there is spike formation of the glomerular basement membrane between the deposits. Stage III *(C):* the deposits are incorporated-embedded in the thickened basement membrane. Stage IV *(D):* the glomerular capillary basement membrane shows irregular thickening with complete replacement of the deposits. (Courtesy of Drs. Ehrenreich and Churg, from Somers S [ed]: Kidney Pathology Decennial 1966–1975. Paramus, NJ, Prentice-Hall, 1975, with permission.)

References

General

Glassock RJ, Cohen AH, Adler SG: Primary glomerular diseases. In: Brenner BM (ed): Brenner & Rector's The Kidney, 5th ed. Philadelphia, WB Saunders, 1996, p 1797.

Mallick NP: Epidemiology and natural course of idiopathic nephrotic syndrome. Clin Nephrol 35(suppl 1):3, 1991.

Olson JL, Schwartz MM: The nephrotic syndrome: Minimal change disease, focal segmental glomerulosclerosis, and miscellaneous causes. In: Jennette JC, Olson JL, Schwartz MM, Silva FG (eds): Heptinstall's Pathology of the Kidney, 5th ed. Philadelphia, Lippincott-Raven, 1998, p 187.

Schwartz MM: Nephrotic syndrome and proteinuria. In: Silva FG, D'Agati VD, Nadasdy T (eds): Renal Biopsy Interpretation. New York, Churchill Livingstone, 1996, p 115.

Zech P, Colon S, Pointet PH, et al: The nephrotic syndrome in adults aged over 60: Etiology, evolution and treatment of 76 cases. Clin Nephrol 18:232, 1982.

Minimal Change Nephrotic Syndrome

Churg J, Habib R, White RHR: Pathology of the nephrotic syndrome in children: A report for the International Study of Kidney Disease in Children. Lancet 1:1299, 1970.

Corwin HL, Schwartz MM, Lewis EJ: The importance of sample size in the interpretation of the renal biopsy. Am J Nephrol 8:85, 1988.

International Study of Kidney Disease in Children: Primary nephrotic syndrome in children: Clinical significance of histopathologic variants of minimal change and of diffuse mesangial hypercellularity. Kidney Int 20:765, 1981.

Nadasdy T, Silva FG, Hogg RJ: Minimal change nephrotic syndrome–

focal sclerosis complex (including IgM nephropathy and diffuse mesangial hypercellularity). In: Tisher CC, Brenner BM (eds): Renal Pathology: With Clinical and Functional Correlations, 2nd ed. Philadelphia, JB Lippincott, 1994, p 389.

Southwest Pediatric Nephrology Study Group: Childhood nephrotic syndrome associated with diffuse mesangial hypercellularity. Kidney Int 23:87, 1983.

Waldherr R, Gubler MC, Levy M, et al: The significance of pure diffuse mesangial proliferation in idiopathic nephrotic syndrome. Clin Nephrol 10:171, 1978.

White RHR, Glascow EF, Mills RJ: Clinicopathologic study of nephrotic syndrome in childhood. Lancet 1:1353, 1970.

Focal Segmental Glomerulosclerosis

Cameron JS, Turner DR: The long-term prognosis of patients with focal segmental glomerulosclerosis. Clin Nephrol 10:213, 1978.

Detwiler RK, Falk RJ, Hogan SL, et al: Collapsing glomerulopathy: A clinically and pathologically distinct variant of focal segmental glomerulosclerosis. Kidney Int 45:1416, 1994.

Magil AB: Focal and segmental glomerulosclerosis. Mod Pathol 4:383, 1991.

Nadasdy T, Silva FG, Hogg RJ: Minimal change nephrotic syndrome–focal sclerosis complex (including IgM nephropathy and diffuse mesangial hypercellularity). In: Tisher CC, Brenner BM (eds): Renal Pathology: With Clinical and Functional Correlations, 2nd ed. Philadelphia, JB Lippincott, 1994, p 330.

Schoeneman MJ, Bennett B, Greifer I: The natural history of focal segmental glomerulosclerosis with and without mesangial hypercellularity in children. Clin Nephrol 9:45, 1978.

Southwest Pediatric Nephrology Study Group: Focal segmental glomerulosclerosis in children with idiopathic nephrotic syndrome. Kidney Int 27:442, 1985.

Velosa JA, Donadio JV, Holley KE: Focal sclerosing glomerulonephropathy: A clinicopathologic study. Mayo Clin Proc 50:121, 1975.

Whitworth JA, Turner DR, Leibowitz S, et al: Focal segmental sclerosis or scarred focal proliferative glomerulonephritis? Clin Nephrol 9:229, 1978.

Membranous Glomerulonephropathy

Falk RJ, Hogan SL, Muller KE, et al: Treatment of progressive membranous glomerulopathy. A randomized trial comparing cyclophosphamide and corticosteroids with corticosteroids alone. Ann Intern Med 116:438, 1992.

Jennette JC, Iskandar SS, Dalldorf FG: Pathologic differentiation between lupus and nonlupus membranous glomerulopathy. Kidney Int 24:377, 1983.

Murphy BF, Fairley KF, Kincaid-Smith PS: Idiopathic membranous glomerulonephritis: Long-term follow-up in 139 cases. Clin Nephrol 30:175, 1988.

Rosen S, Tornroth T, Bernard DB: Membranous glomerulonephritis. In: Tisher CC, Brenner BM (eds): Renal Pathology: With Clinical and Functional Correlations, 2nd ed. Philadelphia, JB Lippincott, 1994, p 258.

Schieppati A, Mosconi L, Perna A, Mecca G, et al: Prognosis of untreated patients with idiopathic membranous nephropathy. N Engl J Med 329:85, 1993.

Schwartz MM: Membranous glomerulonephritis. In: Jennette JC, Olson JL, Schwartz MM, Silva FG (eds): Heptinstall's Pathology of the Kidney, 5th ed. Philadelphia, Lippincott-Raven, 1998, p 259.

CHAPTER 6

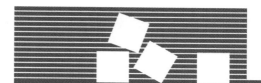

Conditions With Isolated or Predominant Hematuria
IgA Nephropathy, Henoch-Schönlein Purpura, and Loin Pain–Hematuria Syndrome

CONDITIONS WITH ISOLATED HEMATURIA

- The main conditions discussed in this chapter, IgA nephropathy (IgAN) and Henoch-Schönlein purpura (HSP), are associated with isolated or predominant hematuria. Other conditions typically manifested as predominant hematuria include Alport's syndrome, thin-basement-membrane disease, and nail-patella syndrome, which are discussed in Chapter 11.
- Although hematuria is usually the *predominant* manifestation of renal disease in this group of conditions, proteinuria of a variable degree is often present. The clinical features of these conditions can overlap with those of the glomerulonephritides, as well as disorders associated with proteinuria or the nephrotic syndrome, and these disorders must be considered in the pathologic differential diagnosis.
- Hematuria can be the initial manifestation of a wide variety of conditions, both renal and extrarenal (Table 6–1). The most important initial differential is between hematuria of renal parenchymal or urinary tract (pelvis, ureter, bladder, urethra, and prostate) origin. An important consideration in the evaluation of any patient with hematuria, particularly adults, is the detection or exclusion of a urologic malignancy.
- The presence of red blood cell casts or significant proteinuria on urinalysis strongly suggests a glomerular origin for the hematuria; however, these findings may be absent. In the absence of these abnormalities, distinguishing renal parenchymal from urinary tract origin can be difficult. The presence of dysmorphic erythrocytes on urinalysis, best seen on phase-contrast microscopy, has been reported to be a reliable indicator of renal origin. However, the detection of dysmorphic erythrocytes can be challenging, and the reliability of this test in the routine office setting is uncertain.
- An important question is whether the hematuria is microscopic or gross. In adults, gross hematuria raises a strong concern for urologic cancer; malignancies are found in one fifth to one quarter of adults seen with gross hematuria, with transitional cell carcinoma of the urinary bladder accounting for approximately three fourths. In contrast, malignancies are found in only 5% of adults with microhematuria. No source is found in approximately 40% of cases of microhematuria; on the other hand, a source is found in up to 90% of cases of gross hematuria.
- Evaluation of a renal biopsy specimen for hematuria requires careful examination by three modalities: light, immunofluorescence, and electron microscopy. In particular, the diagnoses of IgAN or HSP cannot be made without immunofluorescence, and Alport's syndrome or thin-basement-membrane nephropathy cannot be diagnosed without electron microscopy.
- An important question on light microscopy is whether erythrocytes are seen in Bowman's space or tubular lumina. In a percutaneous needle biopsy, the presence of erythrocytes within Bowman's space and/or tubular lumina is generally considered strong evidence for a renal origin of the hematuria; the significance of this same finding on an *open* biopsy of the kidney is less clear. An additional question is whether "foam" cells are present in the interstitium; in nonnephrotic patients, the presence of foam cells suggests Alport's syndrome (progressive hereditary nephritis).
- On immunofluorescence microscopy, are there significant glomerular deposits of immunoglobulins and/or complement? The presence of dominant or codominant IgA suggests IgAN (Berger's disease). Mesangial deposits of IgG and/or IgM (without IgA) suggest IgG-IgM mesangial nephropathy and, generally, a good prognosis for renal function. Alternatively, immunofluorescence may suggest another immune complex glomerular disease such as systemic lupus erythematosus.
- On electron microscopy, is the glomerular basement

Table 6–1
CONDITIONS WITH ISOLATED OR PREDOMINANT HEMATURIA

Renal Parenchymal Origin	Non–Renal Parenchymal Origin
Glomerular lesions with immune complex deposition	Transitional cell carcinoma
IgA nephropathy (Berger's disease)	Urinary bladder
	Ureter
IgG and/or IgM mesangial deposition	Renal pelvis
	Nephrolithiasis
Abnormalities of the glomerular basement membrane	Prostatic carcinoma
Alport's syndrome	Urinary tract infection
Nail-patella syndrome	Parasitic infection (*Schistosoma haematobium*)
Thin glomerular basement membrane	
Hematologic disorders	
Sickle cell disease	
Coagulopathy	
Viral illness	
Physical exercise or trauma	

Table 6–2
CONDITIONS ASSOCIATED WITH GLOMERULAR IgA DEPOSITS

Rheumatologic
  Behçet's syndrome
  Rheumatoid arthritis
  Ankylosing spondylitis
  Psoriatic arthritis
  Reiter's disease
  Relapsing polychondritis
  Others
Gastrointestinal
  Hepatic cirrhosis
  Portal hypertension
  Celiac disease
  Inflammatory bowel disease
  Others
Neoplastic
  Renal cell carcinoma
  Non-Hodgkin's lymphoma
  Bronchogenic carcinoma
  Others
Infectious
  Epstein-Barr virus
  Human immunodeficiency virus
  Osteomyelitis
  Mycoplasma pneumoniae
  Leprosy
  Brucella
Dermatologic
  Psoriasis
  Erythema nodosum
  Dermatitis herpetiformis
Ophthalmologic
  Uveitis
  Scleritis
Miscellaneous
  Familial Mediterranean fever
  Myasthenia
  Hemochromatosis
  Sarcoidosis
  Others

membrane (GBM) diffusely thinned as in thin-basement-membrane nephropathy? Is there diffuse thickening, splitting, or splintering of the GBM suggestive of Alport's disease?

IGA NEPHROPATHY

Synonyms and Related Terms: Berger's disease; IgA-IgG nephropathy; IgA-IgG mesangial nephropathy.

Biology of Disease

- First described in 1968, IgAN is now recognized as the most common form of glomerulonephritis worldwide.
- Henoch-Schönlein purpura is a systemic disease characterized by small vessel vasculitis with frequent renal involvement; the renal changes of HSP are pathologically similar or identical to those of IgAN, and the two conditions are now considered to be closely related.
- The finding common to IgAN and HSP is the presence of dominant (or codominant) mesangial deposits of IgA on immunofluorescence microscopy, frequently with C3 and sometimes with IgG or IgM.
- The cause or causes of IgAN are unknown. The proposed mechanisms include deposition of circulating immune complexes or macromolecular IgA, abnormal regulation of the immune response, abnormal IgA molecules, and an autoimmune response to normal or planted mesangial antigens; none of the mechanisms have been found to apply to all cases. These mechanisms are not mutually exclusive, and each may be involved alone or in combination in different cases. In the individual patient, it is usually idiopathic.
- Mesangial deposits of IgA may also be found in association with other systemic conditions, including cirrhosis and other hepatic diseases, a variety of rheumatologic disorders, various gastrointestinal diseases, infections, neoplasms, dermatologic and hematologic diseases, and others (Table 6–2). Overt renal disease is unusual in some of these conditions despite the presence of glo-

merular immune deposits. The mechanism(s) of the renal deposition of IgA in these disorders is unknown.
- The incidence of IgAN varies widely in different regions; IgAN appears to have the highest incidence in the Far East, it is less common in Europe and North America, and it is uncommon in Africa. Much of the apparent variation may reflect differences in clinical practice and in common indications for renal biopsy. Many countries with the highest incidence, such as Japan, conduct screening of children for urinary abnormalities; renal biopsy is often performed on children with asymptomatic microhematuria in Japan, whereas many similar patients in the United States would probably not undergo biopsy.
- The incidence of IgAN also varies between different ethnic groups; it appears low in African-Americans and relatively high in Native Americans.

Clinical Features

- IgA nephropathy occurs in all ages but is most common during the second and third decades. There is a male preponderance, the male-to-female ratio being 2 : 1 in Japan and higher in Europe and the United States.

- Renal manifestations of IgAN vary widely from asymptomatic microhematuria to rapidly progressive renal failure. The two most common findings are episodes of macrohematuria on the one hand and microscopic hematuria and proteinuria on the other.
- Episodes of macroscopic hematuria sometimes follow infections, most often infections involving the upper respiratory tract. The period between the infection and the appearance of macrohematuria is frequently short; hematuria may last for a few hours to several days and may be accompanied by flank or loin pain. Occasionally, oliguric renal failure may accompany the hematuria, possibly because of obstruction of tubules by red cell casts or as a result of tubular necrosis; spontaneous recovery is usual.
- Patients with microscopic hematuria and proteinuria are often asymptomatic, the condition being discovered only on urinalysis performed for a routine physical examination. The microhematuria may be either intermittent or persistent; the degree of proteinuria is variable but may include the nephrotic syndrome.
- Approximately 5% to 15% of patients with IgAN have the nephrotic syndrome.
- Hypertension, impairment of renal function, or both are present in a significant number of patients at initial evaluation, particularly in adults. Hypertension may be present in the absence of renal function impairment or may develop during the course of the illness, even in the absence of impaired renal function.

Laboratory Values

- Serum IgA levels are elevated in up to 50% to 70% of patients with IgAN or active HSP; in some series, higher IgA levels were associated with a worse prognosis, but other studies found no correlation. Serum levels of polymeric IgA have also been found to be elevated by some researchers.
- Circulating immune complexes containing IgA have been found in one third to one half of patients in some series; IgA rheumatoid factors have also been found in some patients.
- Serum complement levels are usually normal; however, some researchers have found evidence of increased activation of the alternative pathway of complement activation with sensitive tests for breakdown products of C3.
- Urinalysis demonstrates erythrocytes and proteinuria in most cases; proteinuria may reach nephrotic levels.
- Renal function as measured by serum creatinine is normal in most cases at initial diagnosis.

Light Microscopy

Glomeruli

- The appearance of the glomeruli in IgAN includes a broad spectrum of histologic changes; no single appearance can be considered characteristic. In part, this variability may reflect differences in stage of the disease at the time the biopsy is performed.

- The most common histologic appearance, approximately 60% of the total, is mesangiopathic glomerulonephritis; the second most common appearance is focal segmental glomerulonephritis. Other patterns include normal or nearly normal glomeruli, diffuse endocapillary proliferation (with closure of glomerular capillary loops), crescentic glomerulonephritis, membranoproliferative glomerulonephritis, and a variety of other less common patterns.
- The mesangiopathic pattern includes variable degrees of mesangial proliferation and increased mesangial matrix; capillary loops remain patent. The changes may involve only some or all glomeruli (i.e., may be focal or diffuse); the relative proportion of proliferation versus increase in mesangial matrix may vary between glomeruli. The increase in mesangial space is best visualized with periodic acid–Schiff stain.
- The focal segmental pattern involves only a proportion of the glomeruli (varying from a few to a majority); the involved glomeruli show segmental changes, which may include necrosis, proliferation with closure of capillary loops, sclerosis, or any combination of these changes.
- Segmental capillary tuft necrosis may be seen in all variants, sometimes with crescents in Bowman's space.
- Synechiae, segmental areas of scarring and adhesion between the capillary tuft and Bowman's capsule, are frequently present; hyperplasia of the parietal cells of Bowman's capsule may be present in scarred areas.
- Fuchsinophilic deposits may be visible in the mesangium on trichrome stain; occasionally such deposits may be seen in a subendothelial capillary wall location.
- Global sclerosis of some glomeruli is frequently seen on initial biopsy but is more frequent on subsequent biopsies.

Tubules

- The most common change seen in tubules is the presence of erythrocytes or erythrocyte casts within tubular lumina.
- Degenerative changes of tubular cells such as desquamation, loss of the microvillous brush border, and cytoplasmic vacuolization may be present.
- Atrophic tubules may be present on initial biopsy, and with increased disease duration they become progressively more frequent .

Interstitium

- Interstitial fibrosis may be present on initial biopsy and becomes more frequent and extensive with increased disease duration.

Vessels

- Arterial wall hyperplasia and hyaline arteriosclerosis may be present on initial biopsy and become more severe on later biopsies.

Immunofluorescence Microscopy

- By definition, staining for IgA is present in glomeruli in all cases and is predominant or codominant in intensity of staining.
- IgA is the sole immunoglobulin present in approximately one quarter of cases; IgG is found along with IgA in approximately one third, IgM is found in approximately 10%, and all three are found in one quarter.
- C3 is present in most cases (approximately 95%); properdin or factor B is also present when staining for them is performed. Components of the classic pathway of complement activation (C1 and C4) are usually absent.
- Staining is usually present in a mesangial location; the pattern has been described as resembling a "pruned bush." Staining may be present in short segments of glomerular capillary walls in more severe cases.
- Tubular or vascular staining for immunoglobulins or complement components is unusual.

Electron Microscopy

- Electron-dense deposits are present in the glomerular mesangium, frequently below the basement membrane where it overlies the mesangium (the paramesangium). Occasionally, large deposits may be present deeper in the mesangium; this finding may indicate more advanced disease.
- In some but not all series, deposits may be present in glomerular capillaries. Subendothelial deposits have been described in approximately 10% to 20% of cases in some series; usually they are present in only a few capillary loops. Subepithelial and intramembranous deposits are sometimes present.
- Mesangial cells are increased in size and number. The mesangial matrix may be expanded and appear fibrillar; collagen fibrils may be present.
- Glomerular capillary basement membranes may appear thinned or have a laminated appearance; occasionally breaks are present in the GBM.
- Tubular injury may be present
- Collagen fibrils may be present within the interstitium.

Differential Diagnosis

- IgA nephropathy may resemble virtually any form of glomerulonephritis by light microscopy. The presence of diffuse, dominant, or codominant IgA within the glomerular mesangium strongly suggests IgAN but can be seen in hepatic disease and nephritis associated with systemic lupus erythematosus. Clinical correlation may help exclude these entities.
- The distinction between IgAN and HSP depends primarily on the clinical features and cannot be made on renal biopsy alone.
- Trace amounts of IgA may be found within the glomerular mesangium in cases that are otherwise clinically and histologically typical of minimal change nephrotic syndrome. The presence of trace (or even moderate) amounts of immunofluorescence staining for IgA does not appear to affect the clinical course or prognosis, and such cases should be diagnosed as minimal change nephrotic syndrome rather than IgAN.
- The presence of mesangial IgA deposits alone is not diagnostic of IgAN or HSP; IgA may be found on renal biopsy in patients with hepatic cirrhosis or other chronic liver disease, celiac sprue, and other conditions. These patients usually have little or no clinical evidence of renal disease. The reason for the discrepancy between the presence of deposits and the absence of overt renal disease is unclear.

Treatment and Clinical Course

- When first described, IgAN was considered benign; it is now clear that chronic renal failure develops in a proportion of patients, and IgAN is now considered to be responsible for a significant fraction of end-stage renal disease.
- The incidence of chronic renal failure in patients with IgAN appears to be approximately 10% to 15% after 5 years, 15% to 25% after 10 years, and 20% to 45% after 15 years. A small proportion of patients (approximately 5%) progress rapidly to end-stage renal failure.
- Heavy proteinuria (>1 g/day) or the nephrotic syndrome appear, in general, to be adverse clinical prognostic indicators. However, those cases with heavy proteinuria that have minimal morphologic changes (the morphologic picture of minimal change nephrotic syndrome with mesangial IgA deposits) have a good prognosis.
- Histologic indicators of poor outcome include a high proportion of glomeruli with extracapillary proliferation (crescents), numerous sclerotic glomeruli, interstitial fibrosis and tubular atrophy, and extension of IgA deposits into the peripheral glomerular capillary walls.
- Several histologic classifications of IgA nephropathy have been proposed in an effort to predict the clinical outcome based on the histologic appearance. A recently proposed system is outlined in Table 6–3. In a clinicopathologic study, this system defined three groups of IgAN patients with significantly different outcomes in terms of survival of renal function: an excellent-prognosis group (subclasses I and II), an intermediate-prognosis group (subclass III), and a poor-prognosis group (subclasses IV and V).
- No treatment has been shown to be effective at preventing progression to chronic renal failure in prospective, controlled trials. Anecdotal reports suggest that corticosteroids or immunosuppressive agents, alone or in combination, may be of value in some patients.
- Immunofluorescence staining for IgA is found on biopsy in approximately half of the patients who receive transplants for end-stage renal failure caused by IgAN; however, overt clinical recurrence of IgAN is uncommon after renal transplantation. The reason for the discrepancy between deposition of IgA and clinical recurrence is unknown.

Table 6–3
HISTOLOGIC SUBCLASSES OF IgA NEPHROPATHY

Subclass	Definition
I: Minimal histologic lesion	Glomeruli show no more than a minimal increase in mesangial cellularity, without segmental sclerosis or crescents.
II: Focal segmental glomerulosclerosis–like	Glomeruli show focal segmental sclerosis in a pattern resembling primary focal segmental glomerulosclerosis, with at most a minimal increase in mesangial cellularity and no crescents.
III: Focal proliferative glomerulonephritis	Fifty percent or fewer of glomeruli are hypercellular. The increase in cellularity may be limited to mesangial areas, or there may be obstruction of glomerular capillaries by proliferated endocapillary cells. Crescents may be present. Although the great majority of subclass III lesions show segmental glomerular hypercellularity, this is not a requisite for assigning a biopsy specimen to this subclass.
IV: Diffuse proliferative glomerulonephritis	More than 50% of glomeruli are hypercellular. The hypercellularity may be segmental or global, and crescents may be present.
V: Advanced chronic glomerulonephritis	Forty percent or more of glomeruli are globally sclerotic, and/or there is 40% or greater tubular atrophy or loss in the cortex as estimated from periodic acid–Schiff–stained sections. If these features are present, the biopsy specimen is assigned to subclass V regardless of other histologic features.

From Haas M: Histologic subclassification of IgA nephropathy: A clinicopathologic study of 244 cases. Am J Kidney Dis 29:829, 1997, with permission.

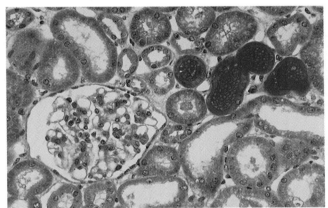

Figure 6–1. IgA nephropathy. An essentially normal-appearing glomerulus is shown. A few tubules contain red blood cells. The presence of erythrocytes in the tubules in a percutaneous renal biopsy specimen in a patient with hematuria is a strong indication that the hematuria is of glomerular origin (trichrome stain).

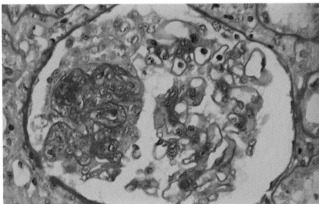

Figure 6–3. IgA nephropathy with focal segmental glomerulonephritis. Segmental intracapillary cellular proliferation and sclerosis are seen involving approximately half of the glomerulus. The other half of the glomerulus appears histologically normal (periodic acid–Schiff reaction).

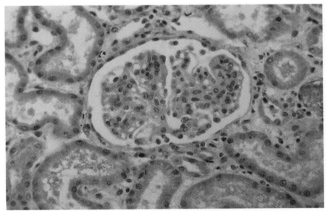

Figure 6–2. IgA nephropathy. The mesangial hypercellularity shown represents one of the most typical light microscopic manifestations of IgA nephropathy.

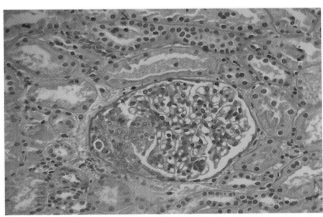

Figure 6–4. IgA nephropathy. Extracapillary cellular proliferation (crescent) is seen in a glomerulus with patent capillary loops and normal cellularity. If present, crescents can be focal and involve only a few glomeruli or be diffuse and involve the majority of the glomeruli.

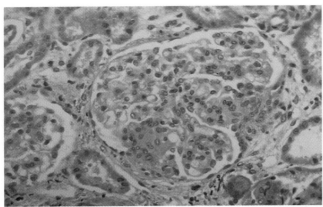

Figure 6–5. IgA nephropathy with focal glomerulonephritis. Synechiae (adhesions) between the glomerular capillary loops and Bowman's capsule as seen here at the 7-o'clock position are a common histologic feature of IgA nephropathy.

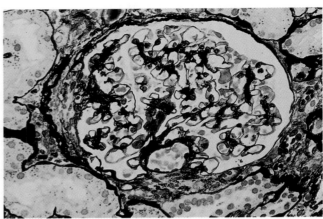

Figure 6–8. IgA nephropathy. There is an adhesion (synechia) seen between the glomerular capillary loops and the Bowman's capsule in a glomerulus, which shows only slight mesangial widening. Adhesions (synechiae) are often seen, even at the early stages of the disease, but they are not pathognomonic for IgA nephropathy.

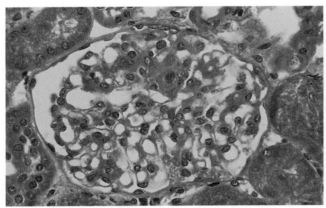

Figure 6–6. IgA nephropathy with focal glomerulonephritis. A focal segmental lesion with some intracapillary proliferation and necrosis is present. Some would interpret this as an intraluminal thrombus (trichrome stain).

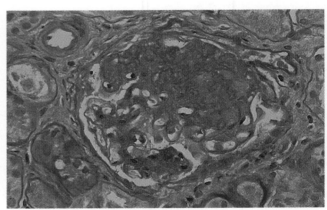

Figure 6–9. IgA nephropathy with focal sclerosing glomerulonephropathy. Advanced sclerosis is seen in a glomerulus with closure of most of the capillary lumina. No significant hypercellularity is noted.

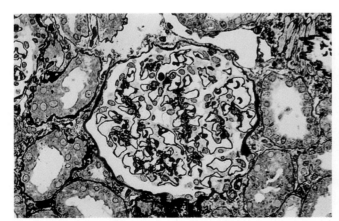

Figure 6–7. IgA nephropathy in a patient with nephrotic syndrome. The glomerulus appears normal and has thin glomerular capillary basement membranes and patent capillary lumina. This patient responded to steroid therapy and did well (methenamine silver stain).

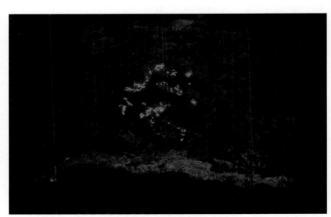

Figure 6–10. IgA nephropathy. Immunofluorescence shows glomerular mesangial IgA staining.

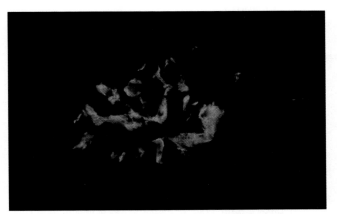

Figure 6–11. IgA nephropathy. Mesangial IgA positivity is shown.

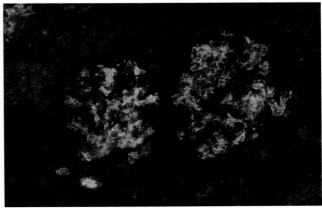

Figure 6–13. IgA nephropathy. IgA positivity is seen both in the mesangial regions and along the glomerular capillary walls.

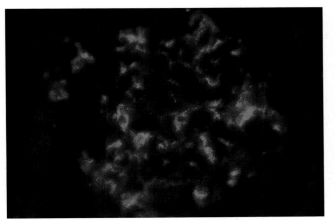

Figure 6–12. IgA nephropathy. A high-magnification immunofluorescence photograph shows IgA positivity limited to the mesangial regions.

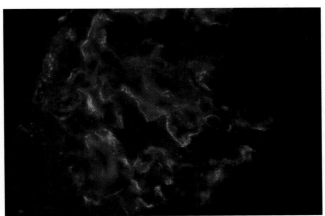

Figure 6–14. IgA nephropathy. High-magnification immunofluorescence shows what was initially interpreted as linear staining but really represents staining in the paramesangial regions just under the overlying glomerular basement membranes.

Figure 6–15. Electron micrograph of IgA nephropathy (Berger's disease). Discrete electron-dense immune-type deposits are present in the mesangium. The deposits are most prominent in the paramesangial areas between the mesangial cells and the anchoring glomerular basement membranes *(arrows)*. Although no deposits are seen along the capillary loops, peripheral deposits are not uncommon in IgA nephropathy. Immunofluorescence revealed predominant mesangial IgA staining (L, glomerular capillary lumen).

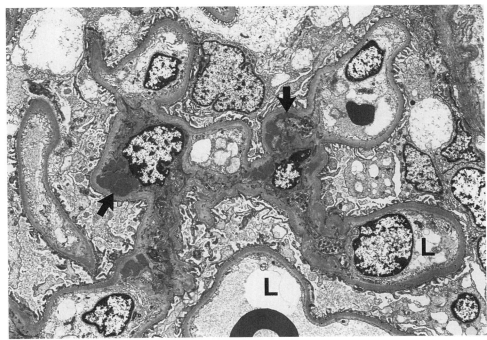

HENOCH-SCHÖNLEIN PURPURA

Synonyms and Related Terms: Schönlein-Henoch purpura; anaphylactoid purpura.

Biology of Disease

■ Henoch-Schönlein purpura (HSP), also known as anaphylactoid purpura, is a systemic, small vessel vasculitis; histologically, it is characterized as a leukocytoclastic vasculitis. The clinical syndrome of HSP includes purpuric skin lesions, gastrointestinal symptoms, arthritis, and (in a minority of cases) renal lesions.

■ The cause of HSP is unknown. Many of the same pathogenetic mechanisms that appear to be involved in IgAN may also be involved in HSP. There appears to be an increased incidence of upper respiratory tract infections preceding the onset of HSP, thus suggesting the possibility of an aberrant immune response to viral or bacterial antigens.

■ The morphologic, immunofluorescence microscopic, and electron microscopic changes in the kidney in HSP closely resemble those in IgAN. Therefore, the pathologic features of HSP will be summarized with an emphasis on features that might differ from those of IgAN.

Clinical Features

■ HSP occurs predominantly in children and adolescents between the ages of 3 and 15 years; it also occurs in adults, although the incidence is much lower. There is a male preponderance, with a male-to-female ratio of approximately 1.5:1 to 2:1.

■ The incidence of HSP varies with the season, with a higher incidence noted during the winter months.

■ Overall, clinical evidence of renal involvement occurs in approximately 10% to 25% of cases of HSP. The incidence varies in different countries, with a lower incidence (10% to 20%) in Italy, France, and Israel; the incidence appears higher in the United States, with renal disease occurring in approximately 40% to 50% of cases. Interestingly, the incidence of renal involvement appears to have little or no relationship to the severity of extrarenal manifestations.

■ The most common manifestation of renal involvement is asymptomatic hematuria, either microscopic or gross; proteinuria is also common and may range up to nephrotic levels. Transient renal insufficiency may occur but usually resolves spontaneously. Renal manifestations usually occur during the first few weeks after the onset of purpura but may occasionally be the initial manifestation.

■ Extrarenal manifestations of HSP most commonly involve the skin, gastrointestinal tract, and joints. Purpura of the skin is usually the initial manifestation, followed within a few days by gastrointestinal symptoms and joint pain. The skin lesions are usually symmetrical and are most frequently located on the lower extremities, particularly on the malleoli and buttocks; the elbows are also a common site of involvement. Biopsies of the purpura demonstrate small vessel vasculitis, usually leukocytoclastic (with perivascular leukocytes and nuclear debris); immunofluorescence microscopy demonstrates deposits of IgA within the walls of involved vessels.

■ Joint involvement occurs in approximately two thirds of cases and is usually manifested by arthralgias. The knees and ankles are most commonly involved, followed by the wrists and small joints of the hands. The joints usually appear unremarkable on examination, but there may be joint swelling; joint destruction does not occur.

■ Gastrointestinal manifestations may be mild, with colicky abdominal pain and vomiting, or severe, with intussusception, bowel necrosis, or perforation.

■ Fever and weight loss are also common. Other extrarenal manifestations can include bleeding around arteritic lesions in various parts of the body, including muscle, testes, lungs, pancreas, central nervous system, and occasionally the peripheral nervous system.

Laboratory Values

■ Laboratory values are similar to those in IgAN.

Light Microscopy

Glomeruli

■ The morphologic changes in HSP resemble those in IgAN. However, biopsy is more often performed during the acute phase in HSP; in IgAN, biopsies are performed at much more variable times during the course of the illness.

■ The key features in HSP are the degree of glomerular hypercellularity and the number of glomeruli that have extracapillary crescents (crescents in Bowman's space).

■ The glomerular appearance in HSP can be divided into four main categories:

• *Mesangiopathic glomerulonephritis:* normal or nearly normal glomeruli with widening of mesangial stalks are noted.

• *Focal segmental glomerulonephritis:* a variable number of glomeruli have segments with increased mesangial matrix and cellularity superimposed on a mesangiopathic pattern with closure of capillaries. Necrosis may be present in some segments. Small crescents or synechiae often overlie segments with hypercellularity or necrosis.

• *Diffuse proliferative endocapillary glomerulonephritis:* the mesangium is hypercellular, with increased mesangial matrix; capillary walls are thickened, with occlusion of capillary loops. Capillaries may have a double-contour appearance resembling membranoproliferative glomerulonephritis.

• *Endocapillary and extracapillary glomerulonephritis:* glomeruli are diffusely and globally hypercellular, with occlusion of capillary loops; a variable proportion of extracapillary crescents are present. In contrast to the focal segmental glomerulonephritis pattern, extracapillary crescents are more common and tend to be larger. In a small proportion of patients, the majority of glomeruli have large, cellular crescents.

- Biopsies performed later in the disease course will show variable numbers of glomeruli with segmental or global sclerosis; crescents, if present, will be fibrous rather than cellular.

Tubules, Interstitium, and Vessels

- In biopsies performed during the early stages of the illness, these compartments show minor changes that resemble those in IgAN. In biopsies performed later, there may be tubular atrophy and interstitial fibrosis, generally proportional to the degree of glomerulosclerosis.

Immunofluorescence Microscopy

- The findings on immunofluorescence microscopy resemble those of IgAN.

Electron Microscopy

- The ultrastructural features in HSP resemble those in IgAN.

Treatment and Clinical Course

- The prognosis of HSP is considered to be good; the majority of patients recover completely, although the disease may recur. However, HSP has been reported to be a significant cause of progression to chronic renal failure in childhood in Europe.
- The proportion of patients who progress to chronic renal failure is unknown; the majority of series come from referral centers and are probably biased toward severe disease with unfavorable outcomes.
- In general, the prognosis tends to be better for children than for adults.
- Heavy proteinuria at diagnosis appears to be generally an adverse prognostic indicator.
- The presence of numerous glomerular crescents on biopsy (more than 50%) appears to be predictive of a poor outcome.
- Anecdotal reports suggest that corticosteroids or immunosuppressive agents, alone or in combination, may be of value in some patients. However, no treatment has been shown to be effective at preventing progression to chronic renal failure in prospective, controlled trials.

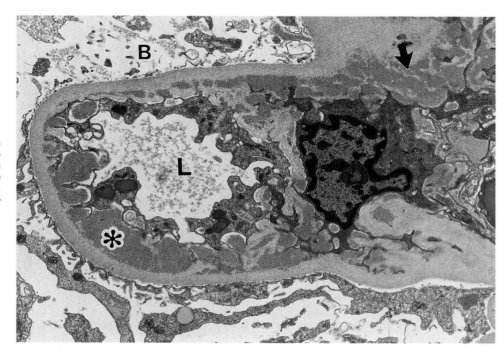

Figure 6–16. Electron micrograph of Henoch-Schönlein (anaphylactoid) purpura. Large discrete electron-dense glomerular subendothelial *(asterisk)* and mesangial *(arrow)* immune complex deposits are seen (L, glomerular capillary lumen; B, Bowman's space).

LOIN PAIN-HEMATURIA SYNDROME

Biology of Disease

- Loin pain-hematuria syndrome (LPHS) is an uncommon, poorly understood condition that includes intermittent episodes of flank (loin) pain associated with variable amounts of hematuria.

- First described in young women taking oral contraceptives, LPHS was initially believed to be limited to that population. It is now clear that it occurs in both males and females, although there is a marked female preponderance (nearly 10 : 1). The usual age of onset is in the mid-20s, although onset may occur over a wide age range. The initial association with oral contraceptives has not been confirmed in later studies; the majority of patients have no known predisposing factors.

- The cause of LPHS is unknown. Some evidence suggests that abnormalities in the coagulation system may be important, possibly by causing intrarenal coagulation. However, the findings in different studies are inconsistent, and the importance of the coagulation system in LPHS is unclear.

- Vascular abnormalities on renal angiography have been described in patients with LPHS and may be important in the pathogenesis. The most common abnormalities include widened bifurcations of the interlobar and interlobular arteries, tortuosity and abrupt termination of the smaller arteries, and irregularities of the renal outline on angiography. However, these abnormalities are not found in all patients with LPHS; in addition, they are not specific for LPHS. Similar abnormalities are found in older patients with no evidence of accompanying renal disease; in addition, renal angiography itself can induce similar changes. However, the prevalence of these abnormalities appears to be higher in patients with LPHS, and they tend to be present at younger ages in patients with LPHS.

- There is no specific diagnostic test for LPHS. The physical findings are minimal, all laboratory studies are normal in most patients, imaging studies are unrevealing, and the morphologic changes are mild and nonspecific. The diagnosis becomes one of exclusion, with few objective findings to explain patients' symptoms.

- Patients with LPHS appear to experience severe, often intolerable pain. A significant psychological overlay may develop, and patients have often been described as "neurotic" and have been accused of exaggerating their pain and faking the hematuria and proteinuria. It has been suggested that a significant component of this behavior is due to frustration from continuing symptoms and attempts to get adequate pain relief from physicians who have become both frustrated at their lack of success in treating these patients and suspicious that the victims are faking symptoms in order to obtain narcotics.

Clinical Features

- Episodes of pain and hematuria occur at variable intervals ranging from several per week to a few per year.

They may last a few hours or persist for weeks. The attacks do not seem to be associated with exertion, infection, menstruation, or medications.

- The pain is described as constant, severe, or incapacitating. It is most intense in the flank and may radiate to the abdomen, groin, or medial aspect of the thigh. The pain is usually unilateral initially but eventually becomes bilateral in the majority of patients. Patients often have low-grade fever during episodes and sometimes urinary frequency and dysuria.

- The hematuria may be gross or microscopic; it may be constant or intermittent and associated with exacerbations of pain. In most cases, both hematuria and loin pain are present during the initial episodes of symptoms; in occasional cases one manifestation may precede the other, sometimes by several years. Rare cases of recurrent loin pain without hematuria have been described.

- Patients frequently have low-grade fever and costovertebral angle tenderness; physical examination is otherwise unremarkable.

Laboratory Values

- Proteinuria of modest degree, not exceeding 1.5 g per 24 hours, may be present during episodes.

- Serum urea nitrogen and creatinine are normal, as are electrolytes, calcium, phosphate, and other serum values. The hematologic profile, including routine coagulation studies, is also normal.

- Serum complement levels are normal; serologic studies for autoimmune disorders (antinuclear antibodies, anti-DNA antibodies, etc.) are negative.

- Urine cultures are negative; when positive cultures are present, they are not temporally associated with exacerbations of symptoms.

- Excretory urography (intravenous pyelography) and other renal imaging studies are normal, with the exception of renal angiography in some patients as described earlier.

Light Microscopy

- Changes on light microscopy are variable, nonspecific, and generally mild.

- Occasional sclerotic glomeruli, slight periglomerular fibrosis, and rare capsular adhesions may be present. There may be mild to moderate mesangial hypercellularity.

- Scattered areas of interstitial fibrosis and occasional atrophic tubules may be present.

- There may be intimal fibrosis or hyalinosis in arterioles; larger vessels may show intimal fibrin deposition or focal disruptions of the internal elastic lamina. When these changes are present, they are usually mild.

Immunofluorescence Microscopy

- The most consistent abnormality seen on biopsies of patients with LPHS is deposition of C3 in the walls of arterioles. The frequency of this finding is variable; some investigators have found it in all or nearly all

cases, but others have found it in only occasional cases. It has been totally absent in some series. The significance of this finding is unclear; in our experience, C3 deposition (in the absence of immunoglobulins) in the walls of arterioles is common in all types of biopsies, and we interpret it as nonspecific evidence of injury.
- Staining for immunoglobulins and other complement components is negative.

Electron Microscopy

- In general, there are no significant changes on electron microscopy. Occasional wrinkling of glomerular capsular basement membranes may be present; this finding is common, but its significance is unclear.
- No electron-dense, immune complex–type deposits are present.

Differential Diagnosis

- The most common causes of the combination of loin pain and hematuria are pyelonephritis and obstruction of a ureter (by a renal stone, blood clot, or tissue). Less common causes include a ruptured renal cyst, renal or ureteral neoplasms, and renal infarction.
- Loin pain and hematuria may be a manifestation of IgAN and occasionally IgM nephropathy. In some cases, patients with the sole morphologic abnormality of thin glomerular capillary basement membranes have a history of both hematuria and loin pain.
- Rare renal vascular disorders may mimic LPHS, including arteriovenous fistulas, aortic–left renal vein fistula resulting from an abdominal aortic aneurysm, entrapment of the left renal vein between the superior mesenteric artery and the aorta, acute renal vein thrombosis, and acute renal artery occlusion.
- Factitious hematuria or the Munchausen syndrome must be considered.

Treatment and Clinical Course

- The prognosis for renal function is excellent. Renal function is normal at diagnosis and remains normal over prolonged follow-up.
- Up to one third of patients will have spontaneous resolution of symptoms after a median of approximately 3 to 4 years. Resolution of symptoms has been reported in a few patients after pregnancies. The experience of the remaining patients is often unfortunate, with recurring episodes of severe or unrelenting pain, disruption of work and family relationships, and even suicide attempts.
- A variety of treatments have been tried, including long-term antibiotic therapy, anticoagulation, splanchnic nerve blockade, longitudinal excision of the renal capsule, and surgical stripping of the renal capsule to denervate the kidney. Despite case reports of apparent success with these therapies, none have proved successful in a substantial proportion of patients over prolonged follow-up. Unilateral nephrectomy was performed on a few patients, but a strong tendency for symptoms to recur on the opposite side led to the abandonment of this procedure.
- Renal autotransplantation involving nephrectomy with resection of the ureter and renal blood vessels, followed by implantation of the kidney in the iliac fossa as performed for renal allografts, has been performed in a few patients. It appears to be successful in relieving pain in a high proportion of patients, probably because of complete denervation of the kidney. Interestingly, hematuria persists despite relief of pain. Unfortunately, up to 10% of patients have recurrence of pain localized to the transplanted kidney, usually after approximately 1 year and presumably as a result of reinnervation of the kidney from the iliac vessels.

References

Introduction

Sutton JM: Evaluation of hematuria in adults. JAMA 263:2475, 1990.

IgA Nephropathy and Henoch-Schönlein Purpura

Alamartine E, Sabatier JC, Berthoux FC: Comparison of pathological lesions on repeated renal biopsies in 73 patients with primary IgA glomerulonephritis: Value of quantitative scoring and approach to final prognosis. Clin Nephrol 34:45, 1990.

Emancipator SN: IgA nephropathy and Henoch-Schönlein syndrome. In: Jennette JC, Olson JL, Schwartz MM, Silva FG (eds): Heptinstall's Pathology of the Kidney, 5th ed. Philadelphia Lippincott-Raven, 1998, p 479.

Fogazzi GB, Pasquali S, Moriggi M, et al: Long-term outcome of Schönlein-Henoch nephritis in the adult. Clin Nephrol 31:60, 1989.

Haas M: Histologic subclassification of IgA nephropathy: A clinicopathologic study of 244 cases. Am J Kidney Dis 29:829, 1997.

Habib R, Niaudet P, Levy M: Schönlein-Henoch purpura nephritis and IgA nephropathy. In: Tisher CC, Brenner BM (eds): Renal Pathology: With Clinical and Functional Correlations, 2nd ed. Philadelphia, JB Lippincott, 1994, p 472.

Hogg RJ: Usual and unusual presentations of IgA nephropathy in children. Contrib Nephrol 104:14, 1993.

Ibels LS, Györy AZ: IgA nephropathy: Analysis of the natural history, important factors in the progression of renal disease, and a review of the literature. Medicine (Baltimore) 73:79, 1994.

Lee SMK: Prognostic indicators of progressive renal disease in IgA nephropathy: Emergence of a new histologic grading system. Am J Kidney Dis 29:953, 1997.

Sinniah R, Feng PH, Chen BTM: Henoch-Schoenlein syndrome: A clinical and morphological study of renal biopsies. Clin Nephrol 9:219, 1978.

van Es LA: Pathogenesis of IgA nephropathy. Kidney Int 41:1720, 1992.

Loin Pain–Hematuria Syndrome

Weisberg LS, Bloom PB, Simmons RL, et al: Loin pain hematuria syndrome. Am J Nephrol 13:229, 1993.

CHAPTER 7

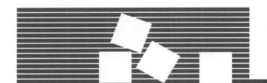

Diseases Associated With Acellular Closure of Glomerular Capillaries
The Thrombotic Microangiopathies

HEMOLYTIC-UREMIC SYNDROME AND THROMBOTIC THROMBOCYTOPENIC PURPURA

Synonyms and Related Terms: Thrombotic microangiopathy; primary malignant nephrosclerosis.

Introduction

- Hemolytic-uremic syndrome (HUS) and thrombotic thrombocytopenic purpura (TTP) are closely related clinical syndromes/diseases with virtually identical renal morphologic pictures. The clinical features of HUS and TTP may show a significant overlap, and it may not always be possible to distinguish the two conditions. Therefore some investigators prefer the term HUS-TTP.
- Hemolytic-uremic syndrome and TTP, along with a number of related conditions such as preeclampsia/eclampsia, postpartum renal failure, malignant hypertension, scleroderma renal crisis, humoral allograft rejection, and cyclosporine nephrotoxicity, can be grouped together under the generic term *thrombotic microangiopathy*. The first part of this chapter considers HUS and TTP, and the second part deals with preeclampsia/eclampsia.

Biology of Disease

- Endothelial injury is a key player in the pathogenesis of HUS and TTP and probably in other thrombotic microangiopathies as well. Factors initiating endothelial damage include verotoxins and Shiga toxin, neuraminidase, lytic anti–endothelial cell antibodies, apoptosis-inducing factor, cyclosporine, mitomycin, and so forth. Additional factors such as endotoxin, proinflammatory cytokines, and activated polymorphonuclear leukocytes may also contribute to endothelial damage.
- Features such as altered endothelial cell procoagulant-

anticoagulant properties, unusually large circulating von Willebrand factor multimers, hypercoagulable plasma, and platelet activation may cause microthrombosis and/or intimal proliferation in glomeruli, arteries, and arterioles.

- The minimum diagnostic criteria for HUS-TTP are microangiopathic hemolytic anemia and thrombocytopenia (the diagnostic "diad") without another apparent cause. Additional features, such as fever, renal manifestations, neurologic involvement, and clinical history may help establish the diagnosis. Renal biopsy is not required to make the diagnosis of either HUS or TTP.
- The renal manifestations of HUS are usually more severe than those of TTP. Acute renal failure with oliguria or anuria, hematuria, hemoglobinuria, proteinuria, various types of casts in the urine, hyperkalemia, and elevated blood urea nitrogen (BUN) and serum creatinine levels is common in HUS.
- In TTP, renal involvement with hematuria, proteinuria, pyuria, urinary casts, and elevation of BUN and serum creatinine levels is frequently seen; however, severe renal damage is uncommon.
- Extrarenal organs can also be affected in HUS, and involvement of extrarenal organs is commonly seen in TTP; microthrombi are most frequent in the brain, heart, adrenals, pancreatic islets, intestinal tract, and spleen.
- In general, the kidney is the most severely affected organ in HUS, whereas in TTP, central nervous system involvement is more severe than the nephropathy. However, there may be a significant overlap when groups of cases are compared.
- *Escherichia coli, Shigella dysenteriae* I, *Streptococcus pneumoniae, Salmonella typhi,* and viruses are the most frequent infectious agents to cause or precipitate HUS-TTP. The most common form of HUS is associated with the 0157:H7 strain of verotoxin-producing *E. coli* infection.
- Hereditary forms of HUS also exist, and there are cases seen in association with abnormalities in the comple-

ment system and with systemic diseases such as systemic sclerosis (scleroderma), systemic lupus erythematosus, and malignant hypertension.

- Additional "miscellaneous" forms of HUS are related to pregnancy, the use of oral contraceptives, bone marrow transplantation, irradiation of the kidney, use of cyclosporine or FK 506, transplant humoral rejection, and the use of antineoplastic drugs such as mitomycin.
- Most cases of TTP are considered to be *idiopathic*.

Clinical Features

Classic Form of Hemolytic-Uremic Syndrome (D+ [Diarrhea Positive] or Epidemic)

- The classic form occurs mainly in young children, accounts for most cases seen, and develops in isolated cases or as outbreaks mostly in the summer.
- In most cases, classic HUS is associated with prodromal diarrhea, followed by various combinations of acute renal failure (oliguria, proteinuria, hematuria, elevated BUN and serum creatinine levels), anemia, thrombocytopenia, central nervous system disturbances, and cardiovascular changes.
- Most of these cases are associated with infection from verotoxin-producing strains of *E. coli* (especially 0157 : H7).
- Thrombotic microangiopathy is most often confined to the glomeruli.

Atypical Form of Hemolytic-Uremic Syndrome (D− [Diarrhea Negative] or Sporadic)

- The atypical form occurs without prodromal diarrhea in both children and adults and accounts for approximately 5% to 12% of all cases.
- Severe renal failure with marked proteinuria and hypertension is a characteristic feature.
- Most patients with diarrhea-negative HUS have an unknown etiology. Cases may be associated with neuraminidase-producing *S. pneumoniae*, hypocomplementemia, chemotherapy, bone marrow transplantation, and others. They may also be familial and may follow a relapsing or progressive course.
- Renal arteriolar involvement is more frequent in this group.

Thrombotic Thrombocytopenic Purpura

- Thrombotic thrombocytopenic purpura occurs mainly in adults, with a peak incidence in the third decade of life.
- The classic pentad of symptoms includes fever, hemolytic anemia, thrombocytopenia, neurologic involvement, and renal manifestations. However, the "classic pentad" is present in only one third of patients.
- Clinical features indicating renal involvement are frequent; however, severe renal damage is uncommon.

Laboratory Findings

- Thrombocytopenia and Coombs-negative microangiopathic hemolytic anemia with abnormal erythrocytes (helmet cells, burr cells, red cell fragments or schistocytes) are characteristic findings in both HUS and TTP. Mechanical forces (i.e., shearing of red blood cells by coagulation-induced fibrin strands in the vessel wall and lumen), neuraminidase, altered lipid peroxidation, etc., could be contributing factors to the red blood cell damage.

Treatment and Clinical Course

- Children with classic diarrhea-positive HUS have a better prognosis/renal outcome than those with diarrhea-negative HUS. The overall mortality rate is approximately 12% in cases of HUS and only 4% with classic HUS. In over 90% of cases, the renal damage spontaneously resolves in HUS.
- Adult HUS is less common and more heterogeneous than childhood HUS, with up to 30% overall mortality. Adults with diarrhea-associated HUS seem to have a better prognosis than those without diarrhea.
- Better management of acute renal failure during the acute phase significantly decreases the mortality of HUS. Better outcome is also related to better recognition of milder forms of the disease.
- The survival rate for patients with TTP is up to 80%, which reflects a significant improvement from a survival rate of 10% only a few decades ago. The improved survival rate is due to earlier detection, recognition of milder forms, and also the introduction of more effective forms of therapy.
- There has been an approximately 2.5-fold increase in TTP-associated mortality rates during the period from 1968 to 1991; the increase in the mortality rate despite significant improvement in survival rates suggests an increasing incidence of more severe forms and/or better recognition of the disease.
- Plasma exchange is the single most important treatment modality in both TTP and HUS. Glucocorticoids and antiplatelet agents may be beneficial. Treatment includes supportive measures and management of the acute renal failure.
- Age at onset, diarrheal episode in the prodromal phase, the duration of anuria, the severity of hypertension, and occurrence in summer months are the most reliable clinical prognostic factors in HUS.
- The severity of gastrointestinal tract symptoms and the presence of peripheral leukocytosis at diagnosis predict a poor prognosis for renal function in diarrhea-positive HUS.
- The better outcome of HUS in infants is thought to be related to the high incidence of the atypical subset (diarrhea negative) of HUS in children over 3 years, a subset that is very uncommon in infants and carries a worse prognosis.
- Long-term renal outcome studies in childhood HUS indicate residual nephropathy in up to 39% of patients.
- The presence and severity of renal arterial changes in HUS-TTP correlate with the severity of renal damage.

The prognosis is also related to the extent of renal cortical necrosis. However, the extent of renal cortical necrosis cannot be evaluated on biopsy specimens.

■ Extensive glomerular changes in themselves do not signify a poor prognosis in patients with HUS-TTP as long as the changes are confined to the glomeruli.

Gross Appearance

■ Renal cortical necrosis is frequently seen in patients who die of HUS. The necrosis is usually patchy and the swollen kidney has a reddish, mottled appearance. If patients survive for a longer period, calcification may be present in the previously necrotic areas.

■ Petechial hemorrhages can be seen beneath the capsule and in the renal parenchyma.

■ The kidneys can be reduced in size, particularly if there has been severe arterial narrowing because of HUS-TTP; arterial narrowing related to dialysis may also play a role.

Light Microscopy

Glomeruli

■ The morphology varies according to the severity and duration of the disease and whether arterial changes are present.

Early (Acute) Phase

■ Thickening of the glomerular capillary walls is present because of subendothelial (lamina rara interna) swelling. The endothelial cells can also be swollen. Severe subendothelial/endothelial swelling with associated mesangial cell interposition may cause occlusion of capillary lumina ("bloodless" glomeruli).

■ The glomerular capillary walls may have a double-contour appearance. This double contour is due to (1) separation of the endothelium from the underlying basement membrane and (2) production of a new basement membrane–like material by endothelial and/or interposed mesangial cells.

■ Fragmented red blood cells, fibrin, and platelet thrombi/aggregates can be seen in the glomerular capillary lumina or even within the glomerular capillary wall. Fibrin and fragmented red blood cells can also be present in the mesangium.

■ The glomeruli may be congested (so-called "glomerular paralysis"), especially in cases with severe vascular involvement. This congestion is a typical change in the early stages of patients with cortical necrosis; frank global glomerular necrosis usually develops later.

■ Accumulation of polymorphonuclear leukocytes in the glomerular capillaries can occur.

■ Small crescents may occasionally be present.

■ The glomerular mesangium often displays a fibrillar appearance, the reason for which is not obvious; mesangial edema may be a contributing factor. The fibrillar appearance is most striking in patients with severe vascular involvement.

■ Mesangial cells are often swollen and hypertrophic. Mesangial hypercellularity is uncommon; if present, it is usually slight, focal, and segmental.

■ Mesangiolysis can be seen. The term *mesangiolysis* refers to partial or complete dissolution of the mesangial matrix and cells. Mesangiolysis is particularly severe in HUS after bone marrow transplantation or mitomycin therapy. "Healing" of mesangiolysis may lead to proliferating and/or sclerosing glomerular changes.

■ Ischemic-type glomerular injury (collapse of the glomerular capillary tuft and thickening and wrinkling of the capillary basement membranes) during the acute stage of HUS usually indicates severe vascular lesions.

Advanced Stages

■ Mesangial widening is present along with matrix accumulation (mesangial sclerosis), thick capillary walls with occasional double contours, and chronic ischemic glomerular injury.

■ Double contours of the glomerular capillary walls may persist for several months or years. Double contours with mesangial sclerosis and occasional mild hypercellularity may be somewhat reminiscent of a membranoproliferative glomerular pattern.

■ Double contours of the glomerular capillary walls in advanced HUS are usually sparse, and no or only minor mesangial hypercellularity is present; these features distinguish HUS from membranoproliferative glomerulonephritis type I. In addition, electron microscopy does not disclose discrete electron-dense immune-type deposits in HUS, only an electron-lucent "fluff" in the lamina rara interna of the glomerular capillary basement membrane.

■ Glomerular hypercellularity is seen in patients who have HUS superimposed on a proliferative glomerulonephritis such as lupus nephritis.

Tubules

■ Hyaline casts and red blood cells are often seen in tubules; tubular necrosis and tubular atrophy may be present.

■ Small patchy infarcts or larger necrotic areas are seen in patients who have cortical necrosis.

■ Focal calcifications in the cortex can be present (these calcifications are usually a sequela of cortical necrosis).

Interstitium

■ The interstitium may be widened because of edema or fibrosis; a slight mononuclear cellular infiltrate can occasionally be seen.

■ Interstitial hemorrhage is associated with cortical necrosis.

Vessels

■ The renal arteries and arterioles may be normal; if affected, the *early stages* are characterized by swelling of the endothelial cells and widening of the subendothelial space. The arteriolar lumen may be severely narrowed, and sometimes fragmented red blood cells are seen in the thickened arteriolar wall.

- Infiltration of the arteriolar wall by fibrin may occur (*fibrinoid necrosis*). Unlike in true leukocytoclastic vasculitis, acute inflammatory cell infiltrate (polymorphonuclear leukocyte infiltrate) is rarely seen in fibrinoid necrosis with HUS.
- Fibrin thrombi can be seen in the afferent arterioles; the thrombi often continue into the glomerular capillary tuft.
- Aneurysmal dilatation of arterioles can sometimes be seen, particularly in the hilar region of the glomerulus; this finding is most frequent in patients with TTP.
- "Glomeruloid structures" somewhat resembling the glomeruli are formed when thrombosis in dilated segments of the arterioles is followed by organization and cellular proliferation. The origin of the proliferating cells is unknown. This feature is most common in TTP.
- Swelling of the intima accompanied by infiltration of red blood cells and/or fibrin is a common feature of the interlobular and arcuate arteries. Fibrin may extensively permeate the wall (fibrinoid necrosis).
- The intimal swelling may cause severe narrowing of the lumen.
- Cells in the thickened intima (myointimal cells) are thought to be of medial muscle cell origin. Proliferation of the myointimal cells is believed to be a sign of organization of the intimal edema. Proliferating myointimal cells may form concentric, ring-like layers admixed with delicate connective tissue fibrils ("onionskin" lesion).
- The arterial changes may result in severe narrowing or occlusion of the vascular lumen with a consequent reduction in blood flow.
- Fibrous replacement of the thickened intima is a later change in the arteries.
- In patients with preexisting chronic hypertension, the acute vascular lesions of HUS may be superimposed on chronic vascular changes such as intimal fibroplasia, medial hypertrophy, or arteriolar/arterial hyalinosis.

Immunofluorescence Microscopy

- In the *glomeruli,* the most typical finding is fibrinogen/fibrin staining along the capillary walls in a continuous, broken linear, or granular pattern. Intracapillary thrombi also contain fibrinogen/fibrin. Fibrinogen/fibrin is found less frequently in the mesangium.
- Deposition of fibrinogen/fibrin in the glomerular capillary walls (and also in the arteriolar/arterial walls—see later) is thought to be related to abnormal intravascular coagulation.
- The glomerular capillary walls may also display IgM, C3, IgG, and rarely IgA positivity. Glomerular factor VIII positivity has also been described.
- *Arterioles* and *small arteries* often exhibit fibrinogen/fibrin in their walls, usually in a subendothelial position. Fibrin II has also been described in the arterial and arteriolar walls.
- IgM positivity can be seen in arterial/arteriolar walls;

C3, C1q, IgG, IgA, and factor VIII staining is present less often.
- When present, intravascular thrombi show positive fluorescence for fibrinogen/fibrin.

Electron Microscopy

Early (Acute) Stages

- The glomerular capillary walls are thickened because of widening of the subendothelial space (lamina rara interna of the glomerular capillary basement membrane), swelling of endothelial cells, and occasional mesangial interposition.
- The subendothelial "fluff" is acellular, pale, and rarefied and contains irregular collections of electron-dense material with an occasional fibrillar or beaded appearance; it usually lacks the periodicity and electron density of fully developed fibrin.
- The exact nature of the subendothelial material is unknown; it is thought to represent the breakdown products of intravascular coagulation and/or cell debris organized into the capillary wall. Fibronectin has been found in it.
- Additional signs of glomerular capillary endothelial cell damage are commonly seen and include localized areas of detachment of the endothelial cytoplasm from the basement membrane and cytolysis.
- Glomerular intracapillary thrombi are composed of amorphous osmiophilic material admixed with platelets and deformed red blood cells. Remnants of platelets are occasionally seen within the lamina densa of the glomerular capillary basement membrane.
- Electron-dense fibrin wisps and tactoids are sometimes seen in glomerular capillary lumina and the subendothelial space.
- The swollen mesangial matrix appears as a meshwork filled with electron-dense, finely granular or fibrillar material similar to the subendothelial changes.
- Mesangiolysis may be seen, and this progressive disintegration results in capillary ectasia. There is frequent visceral epithelial foot process effacement, especially with membranoproliferative-type glomerular lesions and proteinuria.
- In older lesions, wrinkling, thickening, and collapse of glomerular basement membranes may occur as a result of severe accompanying renal artery/arteriolar lesions and lead to ischemia.
- Multiple layers of basement membrane–like material are often seen in the glomerular capillary wall with cellular (mesangial) interposition.
- Arterioles and arteries show changes in endothelial cells similar to those seen in the glomeruli. There is swelling, cytolysis, and detachment of the endothelium from the underlying structures, as well as widening of the intima.
- The intima has a lucent appearance with strands or granules of greater electron density.
- Structures consistent with fibrin are found at various depths of the vessel wall; luminal thrombi made up of platelets, fibrin, and electron-dense material may be present.

Later Stages

■ Elongated myointimal cells abound in the thickened intima.

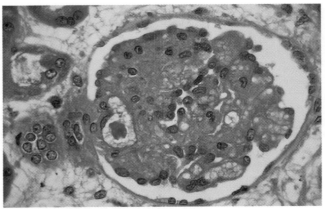

Figure 7-1. Thrombotic microangiopathy (TMA), "bloodless glomerulus." The glomerular capillary lumina are closed and the glomerulus appears hypocellular. This is one of the most typical patterns seen in TMA. The patient had hemolytic-uremic syndrome.

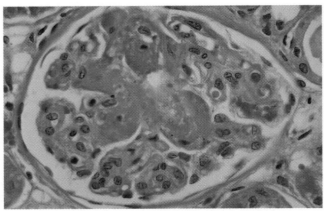

Figure 7-2. Thrombotic microangiopathy, intraluminal thrombi versus fibrinoid necrosis. Some of the glomerular capillary lumina/tufts show insudation by eosinophil acellular material (i.e., fibrin).

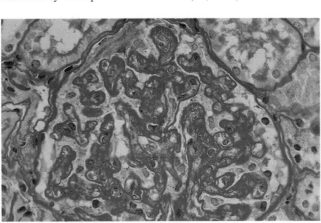

Figure 7-3. Thrombotic microangiopathy. Marked endothelial cell swelling is present along with narrowing of the glomerular capillary lumina. There is also focal thickening of the glomerular capillary walls and mild reduplication of the glomerular capillary basement membranes. This specimen is from a patient with eclampsia/preeclampsia (periodic acid–Schiff reaction).

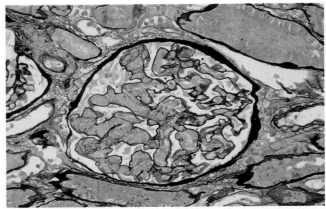

Figure 7-4. Thrombotic microangiopathy. Swelling of the endothelial cells resulted in closure of the glomerular capillary lumina in this patient (same patient as in Fig. 7–3) with eclampsia/preeclampsia (methenamine silver stain).

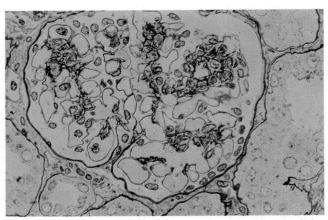

Figure 7-5. Thrombotic microangiopathy. Mesangiolysis (dissolution of mesangial matrix/anchor with dilated capillary lumina) is seen affecting a segment of the glomerulus in a case of Epstein-Barr virus–related glomerular disorder (methenamine silver stain).

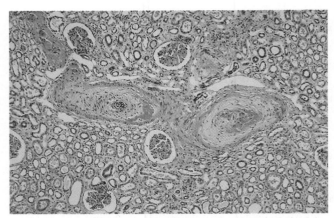

Figure 7-6. Thrombotic microangiopathy. Severe mucoid intimal hyperplasia with segmental fibrin insudation is seen in an arcuate artery. The lumen of the artery is severely narrowed. The patient had acute scleroderma.

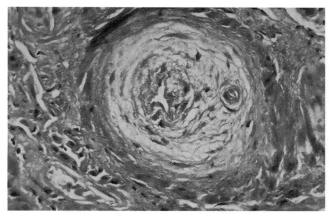

Figure 7–7. Thrombotic microangiopathy, mucoid intimal hyperplasia. The edematous widened intima with a mucoid appearance has only a few scattered cellular elements. The lumen is severely compromised. The patient had acute scleroderma (Masson's trichrome stain).

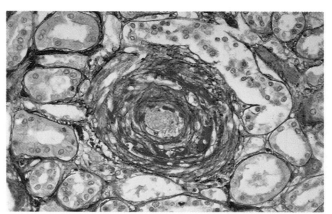

Figure 7–10. Thrombotic microangiopathy. Massive fibrin deposition in the thickened wall of a renal small artery is seen along with luminal narrowing in a case of acute scleroderma (Lendrum's stain).

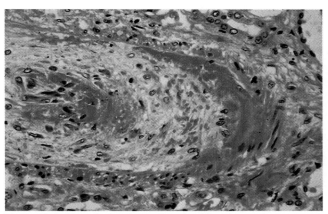

Figure 7–8. Thrombotic microangiopathy. The picture shows a complex lesion in a renal artery with severe mucoid swelling of the intima, detachment of the endothelial cells, and fibrin deposition both in the lumen and in the widened intima. Fragmented red blood cells are also seen in the intima. The patient had scleroderma renal crisis.

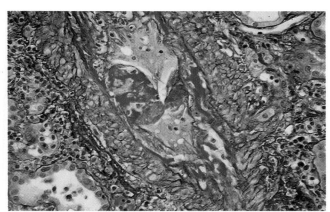

Figure 7–11. Thrombotic microangiopathy. Swelling and partial detachment of the endothelial cells from the underlying basement membranes and subendothelial fibrin deposition are seen in an artery from a patient with humoral transplant (allograft) rejection (Lendrum's stain).

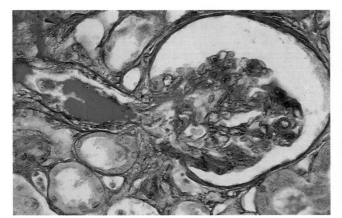

Figure 7–9. Thrombotic microangiopathy. There is arteriolar fibrin deposition in the afferent arteriole with signs of severe ischemia in the glomerulus in a patient with acute scleroderma (Lendrum's stain).

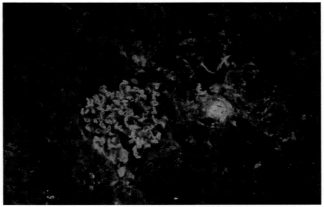

Figure 7–12. Thrombotic microangiopathy. There is strong fibrinogen staining in the glomerulus and also in an arteriole in a patient with scleroderma renal crisis.

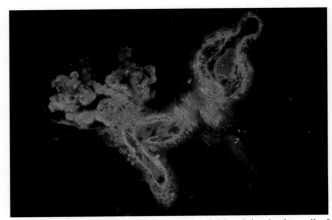

Figure 7–13. Thrombotic microangiopathy. IgM staining in the wall of a small renal interlobular artery is seen in a patient with renal humoral transplant (allograft) rejection.

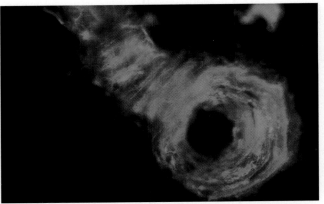

Figure 7–14. Thrombotic microangiopathy. IgM deposition is seen in the entire thickness of a subarcuate artery in a patient with acute scleroderma.

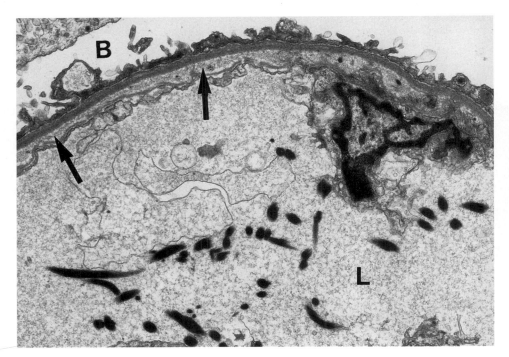

Figure 7–15. Electron micrograph of thrombotic microangiopathy. Electron-dense fibrin wisps are seen in a glomerular capillary lumen, as well as widening of the lamina rara interna *(arrows)* by subendothelial electron-lucent fluffy material (signs of abnormal coagulation). Signs of intravascular coagulation are seen not only in the thrombotic microangiopathies but also in other glomerular diseases such as focal segmental glomerulosclerosis (L, glomerular capillary lumen; B, Bowman's space).

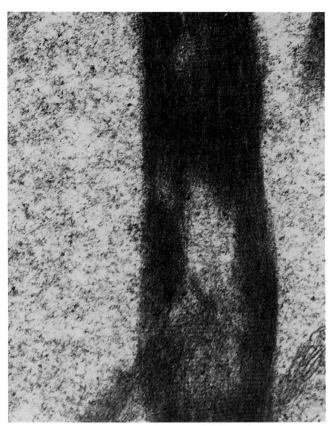

Figure 7–16. Electron micrograph of thrombotic microangiopathy. A high-magnification photograph of an electron-dense intracapillary fibrin wisp shows characteristic cross-striations.

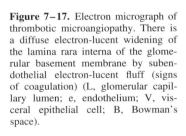

Figure 7–17. Electron micrograph of thrombotic microangiopathy. There is a diffuse electron-lucent widening of the lamina rara interna of the glomerular basement membrane by subendothelial electron-lucent fluff (signs of coagulation) (L, glomerular capillary lumen; e, endothelium; V, visceral epithelial cell; B, Bowman's space).

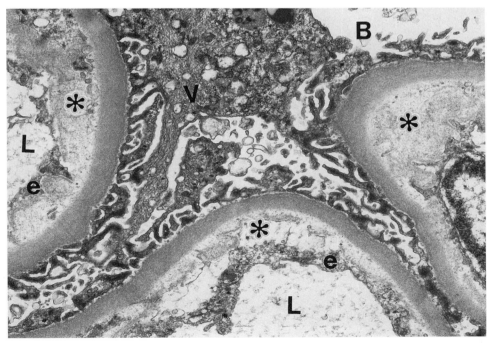

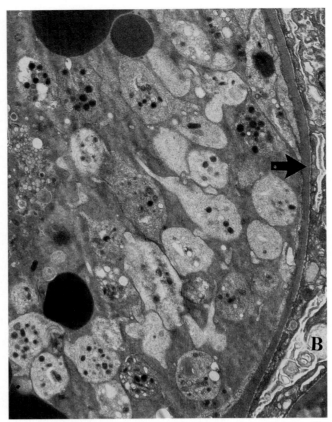

Figure 7–18. Electron micrograph of thrombotic microangiopathy. The glomerular capillary lumen is occluded by numerous small platelets. The glomerular capillary basement membrane is seen on the right *(arrow)* (B, Bowman's space).

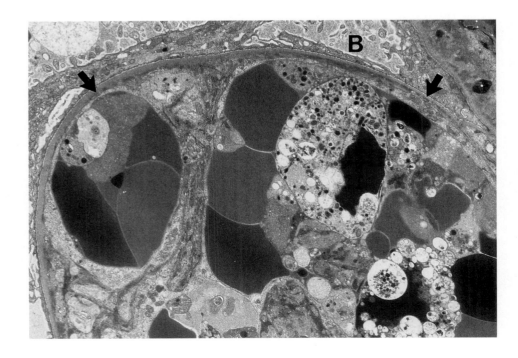

Figure 7–19. Electron micrograph of thrombotic microangiopathy. The glomerular capillary lumen contains red blood cells, inflammatory cells, platelet fragments, fibrin, and what appears to be necrotic inflammatory cells. The glomerular capillary basement membrane is marked by arrows (B, Bowman's space).

PREECLAMPSIA AND ECLAMPSIA

- Preeclampsia is characterized by hypertension, proteinuria (usually below the nephrotic range), and edema in the third trimester of pregnancy (almost always occurring in the first pregnancy and then often the subsequent pregnancies). Eclampsia is defined as the occurrence of convulsions in association with the signs of preeclampsia. The eclampsia may be life threatening.
- Placental abnormalities with placental hypoperfusion caused by vascular injury may be underlying factors for preeclampsia/eclampsia.
- The prognosis of patients with preeclampsia/eclampsia is good; signs and symptoms of preeclampsia and eclampsia resolve with cessation of pregnancy, usually within 24 hours of delivery. In near-term patients, preeclampsia is best treated by induction of labor. Magnesium sulfate is used for treating impending eclampsia.
- The clinical features of preeclampsia in pregnancy (hypertension, proteinuria, and edema) are nonspecific and can be related to various underlying renal and/or nonrenal disorders that are accentuated by the physiologic changes occurring in the pregnant woman.
- A definitive diagnosis of preeclampsia can be established only by renal biopsy, although this view is not generally shared by practicing obstetricians. Renal biopsy is almost never performed at this time.
- The kidneys of women with preeclampsia/eclampsia do not show distinctive gross features.
- The changes of preeclampsia/eclampsia are mostly confined to the glomeruli and are similar to those seen in HUS and TTP. The most typical glomerular change of preeclampsia/eclampsia is marked swelling and hypertrophy of the endothelial cells (so-called capillary endotheliosis). Capillary endotheliosis is, however, not a specific feature of preeclampsia/eclampsia; patients with abruptio placentae may show similar changes.
- Mesangial and endothelial cell vacuolization, increase in the mesangial matrix, slight mesangial hypercellularity, and mesangial interposition with double contours may also be seen in preeclampsia/eclampsia. Mesangial interposition is more prominent in severe disease and in the healing phase.
- Additional glomerular changes include vacuolization of the endothelial cells and protein and lipid droplets in the visceral epithelial cells; electron microscopy discloses focal foot process effacement.
- Glomerular capillary thrombosis is a rare feature in preeclampsia/eclampsia.
- The relatively frequent finding of focal segmental glomerulosclerosis in preeclamptic patients does not necessarily imply a poor prognosis.
- Protein resorption droplets are frequently seen in the tubular epithelial cells in preeclampsia/eclampsia.
- If present, arterial/arteriolar changes of preeclampsia/eclampsia are usually nonspecific. The changes include hyalinization of the vessel wall, medial hyperplasia, and intimal fibroplasia.
- Vascular changes in preeclampsia/eclampsia similar to those of acute stages of HUS and TTP are rare; if present, they are most often associated with antiphospholipid antibody positivity in plasma.
- The immunofluorescence findings of preeclampsia/eclampsia are similar to those seen in HUS and TTP; most cases show glomerular and arteriolar wall fibrinogen/fibrin and IgM staining.

References

Bell BP, Goldoft M, Griffin PM, et al: A multistate outbreak of *Escherichia coli* 0157:H7–associated bloody diarrhea and hemolytic uremic syndrome from hamburgers. The Washington experience. JAMA 272:1349, 1994.

Boyce TG, Swerdlow DL, Griffin PM: *Escherichia coli* O157:H7 and the hemolytic-uremic syndrome. N Engl J Med 333:364, 1995.

Gaber LW, Spargo BH, Lindheimer MD: Renal pathology in preeclampsia. Clin Obstet Gynecol 1:971, 1987.

Griffin PM, Tauxe RV: The epidemiology of infections caused by *Escherichia coli* O157:H7, other enterohemorrhagic *E. coli*, and the associated hemolytic uremic syndrome. Epidemiol Rev 13:60, 1991.

Laszik Z, Silva FG: Hemolytic-uremic syndrome, thrombotic thrombocytopenic purpura, and systemic sclerosis (systemic scleroderma). In: Jennette JC, Olson JL, Schwartz MM, Silva FG (eds): Heptinstall's Pathology of the Kidney, 5th ed. Philadelphia, Lippincott-Raven, Philadelphia, 1998, p 1003.

Lindheimer MD, Katz AL: Preeclampsia: Pathophysiology, diagnosis, and management. Annu Rev Med 40:223, 1989.

Morita T, Churg J: Mesangiolysis. Kidney Int 24:1, 1983.

Remuzzi G, Ruggenenti P: The hemolytic uremic syndrome. Kidney Int 47:2, 1995.

Roberts JM, Redman CWG: Pre-eclampsia: More than pregnancy-induced hypertension. Lancet 341:1447, 1993.

Török TJ, Holman RC, Chorba TL: Increasing mortality from thrombotic thrombocytopenic purpura in the United States—analysis of national mortality data. 1968–1991. Am J Hematol 50:84, 1995.

CHAPTER 8

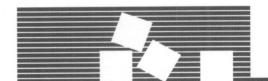

The Nephropathies of Systemic Lupus Erythematosus and Other Rheumatologic Disorders

INTRODUCTION

- The rheumatologic disorders, otherwise known as the "connective tissue" or "collagen vascular" diseases, are a heterogeneous group of diseases characterized by autoimmune reactions of various types.
- Renal disease is common in systemic lupus erythematosus (SLE), and the kidneys may also be involved in many of the other rheumatologic disorders; however, in most, the frequency of renal disease is lower than that in SLE, and the severity tends to be less.
- Renal involvement may be a prominent component of progressive systemic sclerosis (scleroderma); the usual acute manifestation is a thrombotic microangiopathy resembling that seen in hemolytic-uremic syndrome (HUS) and other thrombotic microangiopathies.
- The vasculitides (Wegener's granulomatosis, polyarteritis nodosa, and others) are discussed in Chapter 15 and in the section on crescentic (extracapillary) glomerulonephritis.

SYSTEMIC LUPUS ERYTHEMATOSUS

Biology of Disease

- Systemic lupus erythematosus is a multisystem disorder associated with faulty regulation of the immune system along with production of autoantibodies and resulting immune complex reactions.
- A wide range of autoantibodies are found in patients with SLE, and these antibodies are believed to be important in the pathogenesis of the disease. Many of these autoantibodies are directed against nuclear components (antinuclear antibodies [ANAs]), including RNA and DNA, nuclear proteins such as histones, and others. Other antibodies may be directed against cytoplasmic or cell membrane antigens. Antibodies against the so-called Smith antigen and double-stranded DNA

(anti-Sm and anti-dsDNA) are considered relatively specific for SLE.
- Complexes of these autoantibodies and their respective antigens are deposited or form in tissues; here they initiate complement activation and other inflammatory systems, which results in tissue injury.
- The diagnosis of SLE requires correlation of clinical and laboratory features. The revised diagnostic criteria published in 1982 consist of 11 criteria; for the purpose of identifying patients with SLE for clinical trials, any 4 or more criteria must be present serially or simultaneously during any interval of observation (Table 8–1).
- Renal involvement is frequent in SLE, with clinical evidence of renal disease in approximately two thirds of patients (up to 90% in some series).
- The presence of immune complex deposits within the subendothelial space of glomerular capillary loops appears to be critical to the induction of severe glomerular injury in SLE; the degree of intracapillary proliferation and necrosis generally correlates with the number of subendothelial deposits.
- Renal disease was formerly one of the most common causes of death in patients with SLE; despite advances in therapy and maintenance hemodialysis, renal disease (or treatment for renal disease) remains a significant cause of morbidity and mortality in lupus patients.
- Other systems commonly involved in SLE include the joints, skin, blood, central nervous system, heart, lungs, and others; in essence, any system or organ in the body can be affected.
- The cause or causes of SLE are unknown. Genetic predispositions appear to exist, possibly an inherited predisposition to autoimmune reactions; some triggering event, possibly a viral infection, appears to be required to initiate the clinical onset of disease. Some cases are associated with inherited deficiencies in components of the complement system. Interactions with other factors are also important, possibly including hormones and environmental factors.

Table 8–1
REVISED CRITERIA FOR THE CLASSIFICATION OF
SYSTEMIC LUPUS ERYTHEMATOSUS

Criterion*	Definition
Malar rash	
Discoid rash	
Photosensitivity	
Oral ulcers	
Arthritis	
Serositis	Pleuritis *or* pericarditis
Renal disorder	Persistent proteinuria >0.5 g/day *or* cellular casts (red cell, hemoglobin, granular, tubular, or mixed)
Neurologic disorder	Seizures *or* psychoses
Hematologic disorder	Hemolytic anemia, leukopenia, lymphopenia, *or* thrombocytopenia
Immunologic disorder	Positive LE cell preparation, anti-DNA, anti-Sm antibodies, *or* false-positive serologic test for syphilis

*For the purpose of identifying patients in clinical studies, a person shall be said to have SLE if any 4 or more of the 11 criteria are present serially or simultaneously during any interval of observation.

Modified from Tan EM, Cohen AS, Fries JF, et al: The 1982 revised criteria for the classification of systemic lupus erythematosus (SLE). Arthritis Rheum 25:1271, 1982, with permission.)

- Some cases of SLE appear to be induced by drugs (procainamide and others); renal involvement appears to be less frequent in drug-induced SLE.
- Clinical and laboratory criteria for the diagnosis of SLE were established by the American Rheumatism Association; definitive diagnosis requires the presence of a sufficient number of clinical and/or laboratory criteria and cannot be based on renal biopsy alone.

Clinical Features

- Systemic lupus erythematosus is more common in women than men by a substantial margin (approximately 9:1); the incidence is higher in African-Americans than in whites.
- Onset at young ages is frequent, although SLE occurs over a wide range of ages.
- Renal manifestations of SLE, like other manifestations of the disease, are highly variable. Clinical findings may include asymptomatic proteinuria or hematuria, the nephrotic syndrome, tubulointerstitial nephritis, or a syndrome of rapidly progressive glomerulonephritis.
- The nephrotic syndrome is common in SLE and occurs in up to two thirds of those with clinical renal disease; SLE may be responsible for 6% to 10% of all cases of nephrotic syndrome.
- Renal insufficiency is not uncommon at diagnosis of renal involvement. This insufficiency may be due to glomerulonephritis or acute tubulointerstitial nephritis; the latter may be due to deposition of immune complexes within the interstitium or at the tubular basement membrane or a reaction to nonsteroidal anti-inflammatory drugs (NSAIDs) or other medications.
- Most patients have other manifestations of SLE at the discovery of renal disease. However, renal disease, particularly the nephrotic syndrome, may be the initial

manifestation of SLE; other manifestations may not appear until several years later.
- Clinical evidence of renal disease (based on urinalysis and serum measures of renal function) may not correlate well with pathologic evidence of disease activity; renal biopsy may show significant renal disease, including diffuse proliferative glomerulonephritis, with little or no clinical evidence of renal involvement.

Laboratory Values

- Serum urea nitrogen and creatinine levels may be normal or elevated.
- Urinalysis usually shows proteinuria, with or without hematuria; leukocytes and casts may be present.
- A variety of autoantibodies may be present in the serum, including ANAs, anti-dsDNA, anti-Sm, and others.
- Serum complement levels (C3, C4, and total hemolytic complement [CH_{50}]) are often decreased in association with active renal disease; in some patients, complement levels correlate with activity of renal disease.
- Antibodies directed against DNA may correlate with renal disease activity; such antibodies are believed to be important in the pathogenesis of active lupus glomerulonephritis.

Treatment and Clinical Course

- Treatment generally includes corticosteroids (prednisone or equivalent) given either on a daily basis at low or moderate doses or as intermittent pulse therapy at higher doses.
- Cytotoxic agents such as cyclophosphamide (Cytoxan) are frequently used in combination with corticosteroids, again either on a continuous daily basis or as intermittent pulse therapy.
- Renal disease was formerly one of the main causes of death in systemic lupus; with improvements in therapy, overall survival has improved and renal function has been preserved in a majority of patients.
- Patients with SLE in whom end-stage renal disease develops tolerate hemodialysis as well as patients with renal failure from other causes; other manifestations of SLE frequently decrease in severity in patients undergoing hemodialysis.
- Recurrence of lupus nephritis after renal transplantation is uncommon, and survival of transplants in patients with SLE is similar to that in other patients. Again, other manifestations of lupus frequently decrease in severity after renal transplantation. The immunosuppression required for transplantation may be responsible, at least in part, for the amelioration of disease in transplant patients.
- Adverse clinical prognostic factors in lupus nephritis include the nephrotic syndrome, elevated serum urea nitrogen and creatinine levels at clinical onset of disease, and failure to respond to therapy.
- Adverse histologic prognostic indicators include tubular atrophy and interstitial fibrosis on renal biopsy.
- Necrotizing arteritis or arteriolitis is not commonly seen in biopsies, but these conditions are associated with a poor prognosis.

■ Various activity and chronicity indices have been proposed for lupus nephritis (Table 8–2). The activity index is reported to correspond best to a likelihood of response to therapy, whereas long-term likelihood of renal survival is reported to correlate best with the chronicity index.

■ The utility of these indices has been questioned because of lack of pathologic reproducibility; in addition, they may only apply to diffuse proliferative variants of lupus nephritis. However, they may be useful in providing clinicians with a more objective (although semiquantitative) estimate of disease activity and the degree of underlying renal injury.

World Health Organization Histologic Classification of Lupus Nephritis (Modified)

■ A World Health Organization (WHO) classification system for lupus nephritis was published in 1982; a modified version was published in 1995 and is described in Table 8–3.

■ Transitions from one WHO class to another occur; for example, class II or III may progress to class IV, or class IV may transform to class III or II with therapy. Similarly, transitions may occur from class V to class IV and vice versa.

■ The inclusion of biopsy specimens with deposits by immunofluorescence microscopy (IF) or electron microscopy (EM) within class I disease (normal by light microscopy) represents a significant change from the original WHO classification, which included such cases within class II. Patients with class I disease generally have a benign clinical course.

■ The majority of patients with class II disease (pure mesangiopathy) *who have not been treated* also have a benign course; however, approximately 20% will progress to diffuse glomerulonephritis, which has a more guarded prognosis. Patients whose biopsy tissue shows pure mesangial proliferation *after therapy* may show clinical and histologic relapse despite continued therapy.

■ Class III lupus nephritis should be limited to cases with focal segmental necrosis and/or sclerosis but without significant proliferation or extensive subendothelial immune complex deposits; cases with significant proliferation and closure of capillary loops should be included with class IV, diffuse glomerulonephritis. The distinction between class III and class IV no longer rests on the proportion of glomeruli involved as it did in the original WHO classification. Thus defined, class III disease has a much better prognosis than class IV. (Not all pathologists or nephrologists accept this new definition of class III.)

■ Diffuse glomerulonephritis (class IV) includes all cases with severe mesangial, endocapillary, or mesangiocapillary proliferation *or* those cases with extensive subendothelial deposits with or without the proliferative changes. Cases that would previously have been called class V with diffuse proliferation are now included in class IV, as are cases with the proliferative changes present in fewer than half of the glomeruli.

■ Class V, or membranous lupus nephritis, is defined more strictly in the new WHO classification than in the old; cases with diffuse intracapillary proliferation superimposed on diffuse membranous change are now included within class IV. This new classification recognizes that the prognosis of membranous disease with diffuse intracapillary (endocapillary) proliferation more closely resembles that of class IV than membranous disease without proliferation; cases of pure membranous disease have a much more favorable prognosis.

■ *Results of published series using the initial WHO classification may not be directly applicable to cases classified according to the modified WHO classification.* Pathologists should therefore specify which WHO classification they are using, and it might be advisable to include the category according to the older system as well as the modified system.

Gross Appearance

■ There is no characteristic gross appearance of lupus nephritis.

■ The kidneys may be moderately reduced in size, with fine granularity of the surface and thinning of the cortex on section.

■ The surface may be pale, particularly in patients with nephrotic syndrome.

Light Microscopy

Glomeruli

■ The general categories of glomerular appearance in lupus nephritis correspond to the WHO classification of lupus nephritis (Table 8–3).

■ Glomerular appearance is highly variable: from minimal abnormalities to diffuse and global intracapillary proliferation with necrosis and extracapillary proliferation (crescents).

Table 8–2
ACTIVITY AND CHRONICITY INDICES IN LUPUS NEPHRITIS*

Activity Index	Chronicity Index
Glomerular Abnormalities	*Glomerular Abnormalities*
Cellular proliferation	Glomerular sclerosis
Fibrinoid necrosis,† karyorrhexis	Fibrous crescents
Cellular crescents†	
Hyaline thrombi, wire loops	
Leukocyte infiltration	
Tubulointerstitial Abnormalities	*Tubulointerstitial Abnormalities*
Mononuclear cell infiltration	Interstitial fibrosis
	Tubular atrophy

*Each factor is semiquantitatively graded on a scale of 0, 1, 2, or 3 (absent, mild, moderate, and severe, respectively), and the sum of all factors is calculated as the total activity and chronicity scores. The maximum activity index is 24; the maximum chronicity index is 12.

†Fibrinoid necrosis and cellular crescents are multiplied by a factor of 2.

From Austin HA, Muenz LR, Joyce KM, et al: Prognostic factors in lupus nephritis: Contribution of renal histologic data. Am J Med 75:382, 1983, with permission.

Table 8–3
WORLD HEALTH ORGANIZATION CLASSIFICATION OF LUPUS GLOMERULONEPHRITIS

Original WHO Classification	Modified WHO Classification
Class I: Normal	
Class II: Mesangial Alterations	**Class I: Normal Glomeruli**
IIa: Normal by light microscopy but mesangial deposits by electron or immunofluorescence microscopy	A. Nil by all techniques
IIb: Mesangial expansion with or without hypercellularity	B. Normal by light microscopy but deposits seen by electron or immunofluorescence microscopy
Class III: Focal Segmental Glomerulonephritis	**Class II: Pure Mesangial Alterations (Mesangiopathy)**
(<50%)	A. Mesangial widening and/or mild hypercellularity (+)
Class IV: Diffuse Proliferative Glomerulonephritis	B. Moderate hypercellularity (++)
(≥50%)	**Class III: Focal Segmental Glomerulonephritis**
Class V: Membranous Glomerulonephritis	A. Active necrotizing lesions
Va: Pure membranous	B. Active and sclerosing lesions
Vb: Mesangial widening	C. Sclerosing lesions
Vc: Segmental proliferation	**Class IV: Diffuse Glomerulonephritis**
Vd: Diffuse proliferation	A. Without segmental lesions
	B. With active necrotizing lesions
	C. With active and sclerosing lesions
	D. With sclerosing lesions
	Class V: Diffuse Membranous Glomerulonephritis
	A. Pure membranous glomerulonephritis
	B. Associated with lesions of category II (A or B)
	Class VI: Advanced Sclerosing Glomerulonephritis

- The most common glomerular lesions in lupus nephritis are immune deposits in the mesangium and/or capillary walls, mesangial increase and hypercellularity, intracapillary proliferation, thickening of capillary walls, intracapillary hyaline thrombi, and glomerular sclerosis.
- A variety of histologic lesions are described in lupus nephritis, including "wire loops" and "hyaline thrombi"; however, the only lesion that is probably *pathognomonic* for lupus nephritis is the *hematoxylin body*. Hematoxylin bodies are smudgy inclusions, pale blue or lilac on hematoxylin and eosin stain, with indistinct margins and variable size; they probably represent degenerated nuclei and correspond to the inclusions seen in lupus erythematosus (LE) cells.
- *Normal glomeruli (modified WHO class I):*
  - By definition, no abnormalities are present by light microscopy (deposits may be present within the mesangium on IF or EM).

Table 8–4
DEFINITION OF ACTIVE AND SCLEROTIC LESIONS IN THE MODIFIED WORLD HEALTH ORGANIZATION CLASSIFICATION

Active Lesions	Sclerosing Lesions
Glomerular	Glomerular sclerosis
Capillary proliferation	1. Segmental
Disruption of capillary walls	2. Mesangial
Polymorphs and karyorrhexis	3. Global
Hematoxylin bodies	Fibrous crescents
Crescents, cellular or fibrocellular	Tubular atrophy
"Wire loops" (light microscopy)	Interstitial fibrosis
Fibrin thrombi	Vascular sclerosis
Hyaline thrombi	
Segmental fibrin deposition	
Vascular	
Hyaline (immune complex) deposits	
Necrotizing arteritis	
Tubular degeneration and necrosis	
Interstitial inflammation, active	

- *Pure mesangial alterations (mesangiopathy; modified WHO class II):*
  - The mesangial space is widened; mesangial cellularity may be normal to mildly increased (IIA), or moderate hypercellularity may be present (IIB).
  - Capillary loops appear unremarkable.
  - Mesangial deposits are not usually visible by light microscopy; no capillary wall deposits are present.
  - Necrosis, neutrophils, and extracapillary proliferation (crescents) are absent.
- *Focal segmental glomerulonephritis (modified WHO class III):*
  - Foci of necrosis may be present (IIIA).
  - Segmental areas of sclerosis may be present, with (IIIB) or without (IIIC) changes of active disease (see Table 8–4 for a definition of active changes).
  - Mild or moderate mesangial alterations (expansion and/or hypercellularity) are usually present.
  - Mesangial deposits may be visible as fuchsinophilic specks on trichrome stain; extensive subendothelial deposits are not present.
- *Diffuse glomerulonephritis (modified WHO class IV):*
  - Many or all glomeruli show changes such as severe mesangial, endocapillary, or mesangiocapillary proliferation and/or extensive subendothelial deposits.
  - Segmental capillary loop lesions may be absent (IVA), or there may be segmental necrosis (IVB), active and sclerosing lesions (IVC), or segmental sclerosis without active lesions (IVD).
  - Necrosis, if present, is usually segmental; evidence of necrosis includes eosinophilic fibrinoid material (fuchsinophilic on trichrome stain), karyorrhectic nuclear debris, and dissolution of capillary basement membranes on periodic acid–Schiff (PAS) or Jones stains.
  - Neutrophils may be present within capillary loops, usually segmentally and frequently associated with necrosis.
  - Some capillary loops may be markedly thickened and

have a rigid, refractile appearance—the characteristic *"wire loop"* lesion of lupus nephritis. This appearance is due to dense, confluent subendothelial deposits.
  • Mesangial deposits (fuchsinophilic on trichrome stain) are invariably present. Subendothelial capillary loop deposits are usually present and may be extensive; subepithelial deposits are often present and may be numerous.
  • Capillary loops may appear occluded by eosinophilic material, so-called *hyaline thrombi.* In some cases this occlusion is due to large, dense subendothelial deposits; in others, true intracapillary thrombi are present in capillary loops.
  • Cellular crescents may be present in Bowman's space, usually in association with necrosis of capillary loops.
  • Some capillary loops may show mesangial interposition, with "tram-track" changes of the glomerular basement membrane (GBM) on PAS or Jones stains resembling membranoproliferative (mesangiocapillary) glomerulonephritis (MPGN).
■ *Diffuse membranous glomerulonephritis (modified WHO class V):*
  • Capillary walls are diffusely and evenly thickened; the basement membranes appear diffusely thickened on PAS and Jones stains, and GBM spikes may be seen.
  • Subepithelial deposits may be seen as fuchsinophilic specks on trichrome stain.
  • Occasional cases are indistinguishable from idiopathic membranous glomerulopathy (class VA); however, in many or most cases superimposed mesangial changes are present (class VB).
  • The diagnosis of membranous lupus glomerulonephritis should be restricted to cases with predominantly subepithelial deposits. A few subendothelial deposits may be present; however, cases with extensive subendothelial deposits should be classified as diffuse glomerulonephritis (class IV).
  • Similarly, cases with significant degrees of proliferation should be classified as diffuse glomerulonephritis.

Tubules

■ Proximal convoluted tubules frequently show protein resorption droplets; epithelial cells may have vacuolated cytoplasm in patients with marked proteinuria or nephrotic syndrome.
■ Variable degrees of tubular atrophy may be present; in general, the degree of tubular atrophy correlates with the severity of glomerular injury but may vary depending on the duration of disease.
■ In severe cases, inflammatory cells (usually lymphocytes) may be seen infiltrating into tubular epithelium; this infiltration is associated with epithelial flattening and necrosis or sloughing of epithelial cells.
■ Erythrocytes, leukocytes, and/or casts may be present within tubular lumina.
■ Immune complexes may occasionally be seen within tubular basement membranes on trichrome stain, most

commonly with severe diffuse proliferative lupus nephritis.

Interstitium

■ The interstitium may appear unremarkable, or there may be variable degrees of interstitial fibrosis and/or inflammation. The degree of interstitial inflammation generally correlates with the severity of glomerular changes.
■ Inflammation, when present, generally consists predominantly of lymphocytes; neutrophils and eosinophils may be present, but the presence of *numerous* neutrophils should raise the question of infection.

Vessels

■ Arteritis or arteriolitis with fibrinoid necrosis is rarely seen in lupus nephritis; they are usually seen in association with severe, necrotizing glomerulonephritis or malignant hypertension.
■ There may be PAS-positive hyaline material within the intima of arterioles.
■ Fibromyxoid material within the intima of arteries or arterioles suggests the presence of a thrombotic microangiopathy.

Immunofluorescence Microscopy

■ Staining for IgG is almost invariably present (90% of cases or more); IgM and IgA are found slightly less often (60% to 70% each).
■ C3 is the most common complement component found (approximately 80% of cases). C1q is almost as common, and often staining is intense; C4 is less common and often stains less intensely. Staining for properdin may be present when looked for.
■ The presence of "full house" immunoglobulins (IgG, IgM, and IgA) together with both C3 and C1q (or C4) is characteristic of lupus nephritis and rarely seen in other conditions.
■ Granular deposits of immunoglobulin and complement may be seen within tubular basement membranes, most often in association with diffuse proliferative glomerulonephritis (class IV). Occasionally, linear tubular basement membrane staining may be present.
■ Subendothelial staining for immunoglobulins and complement may be present in small arteries and arterioles, again most commonly with class IV.
■ *Normal glomeruli (modified WHO class I):*
  • IA: No staining is present.
  • IB: Mesangial staining for immunoglobulins and complement is present.
■ *Pure mesangial alterations (modified WHO class II):*
  • Mesangial staining for IgG and complement is present; IgM and IgA may also be present.
  • No capillary wall staining is found.
■ *Focal segmental glomerulonephritis (modified WHO class III):*
  • Mesangial staining for IgG and C3 is present in all glomeruli; staining for IgM and IgA is also frequently noted.

- Scattered capillary wall staining for immunoglobulins and complement may be seen; however, extensive capillary wall (particularly subendothelial) deposits are not present.
- Segmental staining for fibrin/fibrinogen may be present and corresponds to segmental necrosis, sometimes associated with staining within Bowman's space.

■ *Diffuse glomerulonephritis (modified WHO class IV):*
- Mesangial and capillary wall staining for immunoglobulins and complement is invariably present.
- Capillary wall staining is usually widespread; extensive subendothelial deposits are usually present, and subepithelial deposits may also be found.
- Segmental staining for fibrin/fibrinogen is frequently present and corresponds to areas of necrosis, often accompanied by staining within Bowman's space and within crescents.

■ *Pure membranous glomerulonephritis (modified WHO class V):*
- Diffuse, granular capillary wall (subepithelial) staining for IgG and C3 is present, frequently accompanied by IgM and C1q; IgA and C4 are less frequently found.
- Small mesangial deposits are frequently present, even in cases in which the mesangium appears unremarkable by light microscopy.
- Scattered, small subendothelial deposits of immunoglobulins and complement are sometimes seen; however, extensive subendothelial deposits are not present.

Electron Microscopy

- Ultrastructural findings in lupus nephritis may vary from small mesangial deposits to large subendothelial deposits that may almost occlude glomerular capillary lumina; subepithelial deposits may be present in almost any class of lupus nephritis but are a dominant feature in class V only.
- Deposits may be found simultaneously in mesangial, subendothelial, and subepithelial locations; it is unusual to find deposits in *all* these locations in conditions other than lupus nephritis.
- Deposits in lupus nephritis may have a distinctive substructure termed the *fingerprint* pattern. The deposits consist of arrays of parallel, curved, regularly stacked linear structures that may have a whorled, intersecting pattern closely resembling fingerprints. These structures often appear to represent cryoglobulins; they may be seen in other conditions with cryoglobulins but are most often found in lupus nephritis.
- Interlacing, branching tubular structures, termed *tubuloreticular structures, tubuloreticular inclusions,* or *myxovirus-like particles,* are characteristically seen in glomerular capillary endothelial cells in lupus nephritis. These inclusions are believed to represent an effect of interferon and thus have also been termed *interferon footprints.* Originally thought to be specific for lupus nephritis, they have since been found in a wide variety of conditions, including transplant rejection, human immunodeficiency virus (HIV)-associated nephropathy, and others.
- Glomerular visceral epithelial cell foot processes are often diffusely simplified and effaced, similar to the changes seen in minimal change nephrotic syndrome and other conditions associated with proteinuria.
- *Pure mesangial alterations (modified WHO class II):*
  - Electron-dense deposits are usually small and limited to the mesangial region.
- *Focal segmental glomerulonephritis (modified WHO class III):*
  - Scattered subendothelial capillary wall deposits of varying size may be present in addition to mesangial deposits; extensive subendothelial deposits are not present.
- *Diffuse glomerulonephritis (modified WHO class IV):*
  - Subendothelial deposits are widespread and may be large; mesangial deposits are also present, and scattered subepithelial deposits are frequent.
- *Pure membranous glomerulonephritis (modified WHO class V):*
  - Subepithelial deposits are widespread and involve most or all capillary loops; the distribution and size of deposits may be variable, however.
  - Mesangial deposits are usually present; subendothelial deposits may be present but are not extensive.
- Granular electron-dense deposits may be seen in tubular basement membranes.

Histologic Variants

- A picture of thrombotic microangiopathy resembling thrombotic thrombocytopenic purpura may occur in patients with systemic lupus, usually patients with antiphospholipid antibodies (the "lupus anticoagulant"). This condition is characterized by intimal fibromyxoid changes in small arteries and arterioles, similar to changes seen in other thrombotic microangiopathies.

Differential Diagnosis

- The clinical features of lupus nephritis may mimic many other forms of renal disease from membranous glomerulonephropathy to diffuse intracapillary proliferative glomerulonephritis to crescentic glomerulonephritis; however, the presence of multisystem disease with signs or symptoms consistent with SLE would indicate lupus nephritis rather than other forms of glomerulonephritis.
- The presence of high titers of ANA, anti-Sm, or anti-dsDNA antibodies would support the diagnosis of SLE.
- Histologically, lupus nephritis may mimic virtually any form of glomerulonephritis and vice versa.
- Hematoxylin bodies (described earlier) are the only histologic feature that is probably pathognomonic for lupus nephritis; the presence of "wire loops" and hyaline thrombi would strongly suggest lupus nephritis, although structures resembling hyaline thrombi may be seen in mixed cryoglobulinemia.
- The presence of "full house" immunoglobulins (IgG, IgM, and IgA), together with the presence of early

complement components (C1q or C4) in addition to C3, also favors lupus nephritis.

- Ultrastructurally, the presence of deposits in all three locations (mesangial, subendothelial, and subepithelial), a "fingerprint" substructure in the immune deposits, or numerous tubuloreticular structures supports the diagnosis of lupus.

- Class V lupus nephritis (pure membranous) is a particular problem; membranous glomerulonephritis with nephrotic syndrome may be the initial manifestation of systemic lupus, with other manifestations not occurring

for up to several years afterward. The immunohistologic and ultrastructural features just noted would favor membranous glomerulonephritis secondary to lupus; however, the diagnosis of lupus nephritis cannot be made by renal biopsy alone. The pathologist can only raise the question of SLE and suggest that the patient be monitored for further evidence of lupus. Fortunately, in this situation, therapy for idiopathic membranous glomerulonephropathy and lupus nephritis (membranous) would probably be the same; immediate management would not change.

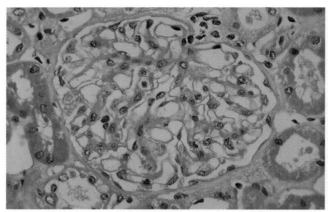

Figure 8-1. Systemic lupus erythematosus, class IIa (original WHO classification). The light microscopic appearance of the glomerulus is normal. The immunofluorescence showed mesangial deposits. In the modified WHO classification, this is class IB (normal by light microscopy but deposits seen by immunofluorescence microscopy).

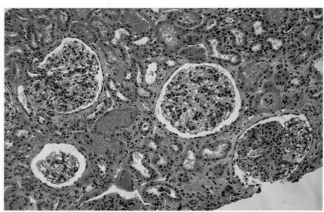

Figure 8-3. Systemic lupus erythematosus, focal glomerulonephritis, class III (original WHO classification). Focal segmental intracapillary hypercellularity with effacement of capillary lumina is seen in the glomerulus on the right. The remainder of the glomeruli show only moderate mesangial widening with hypercellularity by light microscopy. In the WHO classification, this is best classified as class IVA, mild lesion.

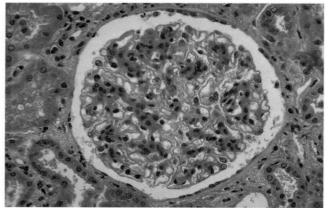

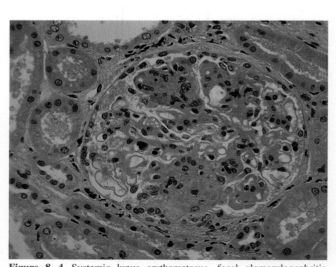

Figure 8-2. Systemic lupus erythematosus, class IIb (original WHO classification). Mesangial hypercellularity is present without closure of the glomerular capillary lumina. In the modified WHO classification, this is class IIB (moderate mesangial hypercellularity).

Figure 8-4. Systemic lupus erythematosus, focal glomerulonephritis, class III (original WHO classification). Segmental intracapillary hypercellularity with closure of the glomerular capillary lumina and some necrosis is seen. Intracapillary cellular proliferation with closure of the capillary lumina (either global or segmental) affects less than 50% of the glomeruli in class III lupus nephritis. In the modified WHO classification, this is class IVB, based on the severity of the glomerular lesion and large subendothelial deposits on immunofluorescence and electron microscopy.

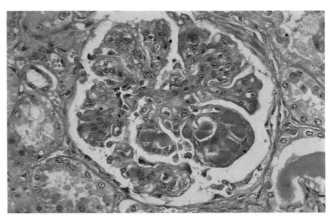

Figure 8–5. Systemic lupus erythematosus, diffuse glomerulonephritis, class IV (original WHO classification). Prominent mesangial hypercellularity and some segmental intracapillary cellular proliferation are seen in the glomerulus on the left. On the right, severe intracapillary hypercellularity gives rise to hypersegmentation (lobulation) of the capillary tufts. In the modified WHO classification, this is class IVA.

Figure 8–8. Systemic lupus erythematosus, diffuse glomerulonephritis, class IV (original WHO classification). The glomerulus displays global intracapillary cellular proliferation with scattered "hyaline intracapillary thrombi." These "thrombi" usually represent large subendothelial immune (wire loop) deposits, some of which are protruding into the capillary lumina. In the modified WHO classification, this is class IVB.

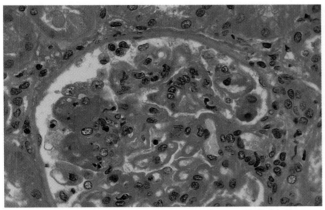

Figure 8–6. Systemic lupus erythematosus. Segmental fibrinoid necrosis is seen with nuclear dust (karyorrhexis) in a patient with class IV lupus nephritis (original WHO classification). Necrosis is common in class III and class IV lupus nephritides. In the modified WHO classification, this is class IVB.

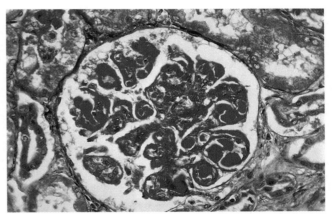

Figure 8–9. Systemic lupus erythematosus, diffuse glomerulonephritis, class IV (original WHO classification). Trichrome stain displays numerous globules occluding the capillary lumina; thickened capillary walls secondary to wire loop deposits are also seen. Wire loop deposits are large subendothelial immune deposits readily visible by light microscopy (Masson's trichrome stain). In the modified WHO classification, this is class IVB.

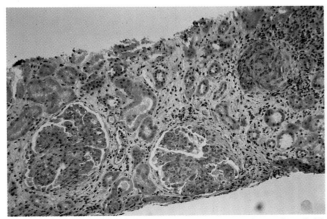

Figure 8–7. Systemic lupus erythematosus, diffuse glomerulonephritis (GN), class IV (original WHO classification). The glomerulus on the upper right displays a cellular crescent. Occasional crescents or even crescentic GN can be seen in severe cases of lupus nephritis. Also note the prominent interstitial widening caused by fibrosis and diffuse inflammatory cell infiltrate. In the modified WHO classification, this is class IVC.

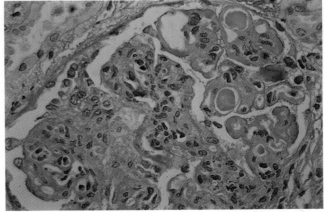

Figure 8–10. Systemic lupus erythematosus, diffuse glomerulonephritis, class IV (original WHO classification). The photograph depicts extensive "wire loop" deposits (i.e., subendothelial) along the thickened glomerular capillary walls; intracapillary "hyaline thrombi" are also present (modified Masson's trichrome stain). In the modified WHO classification, this is class IVB.

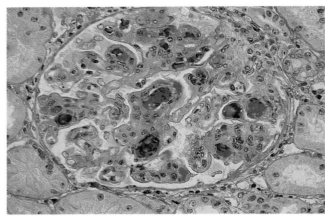

Figure 8–11. Systemic lupus erythematosus. Glomerular capillary thrombosis (thrombotic microangiopathy) is seen in a few capillary loops; the incidence of thrombotic microangiopathy seems to be higher in patients who are antiphospholipid antibody positive. There is also moderate global intracapillary cellular proliferation, thickening of the glomerular capillary walls, and closure of many of the capillary loops (Lendrum's stain). The patient had diffuse glomerulonephritis, class IV (original as well as modified WHO classification).

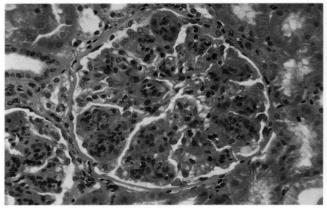

Figure 8–12. Systemic lupus erythematosus, diffuse glomerulonephritis (GN), class IV (membranoproliferative variant; original as well as modified WHO classification). Lobulation of the glomerulus is due to prominent intracapillary hypercellularity. This pattern is reminiscent of that of a primary (idiopathic) membranoproliferative GN.

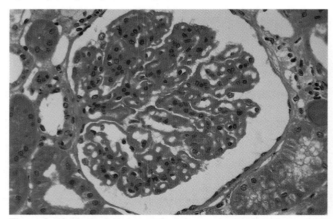

Figure 8–13. Systemic lupus erythematosus, membranous glomerulonephropathy, class V (original WHO classification). The light microscopic morphology is similar to that seen in idiopathic membranous glomerulonephropathy; there is diffuse uniform thickening of the glomerular capillary walls. A slight segmental mesangial/intracapillary hypercellularity is also seen. In the modified WHO classification, this is best classified as class VB.

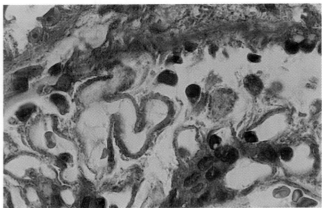

Figure 8–14. Systemic lupus erythematosus, membranous glomerulonephropathy, class V (original as well as modified WHO classification). Fuchsinophilic dots along the external aspects of the glomerular capillary basement membranes represent subepithelial deposits (Masson's trichrome stain).

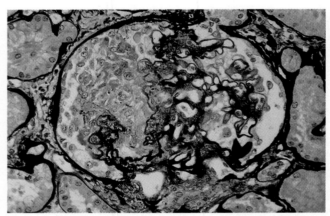

Figure 8–15. Systemic lupus erythematosus, class V plus III (original WHO classification). The photograph depicts a cellular crescent in a patient with focal proliferative lupus nephritis superimposed on membranous glomerulonephritis. Crescents are usually seen in patients who have either focal proliferative or diffuse proliferative lupus nephritis (methenamine silver stain). If electron microscopy shows not only subepithelial deposits but also large subendothelial deposits, this is class IV in the modified WHO classification.

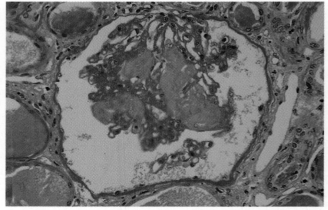

Figure 8–16. Systemic lupus erythematosus. The picture shows a glomerulus with acellular sclerotic changes ("healed lesions") in a patient with treated focal segmental lupus nephritis (class III; original as well as modified WHO classification).

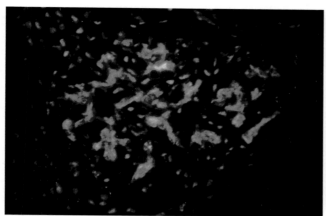

Figure 8–17. Systemic lupus erythematosus, immunofluorescence. Mesangial IgG deposition is seen in a patient with a light microscopic glomerular pattern consistent with class IIa (original WHO classification). In the modified WHO classification, this is class IB (normal by light microscopy, but deposits seen by immunofluorescence microscopy). The nuclear immunoreactivity indicates the presence of antinuclear antibodies.

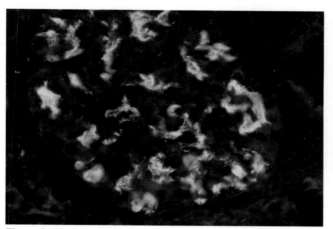

Figure 8–18. Systemic lupus erythematosus, immunofluorescence. C1q staining is clearly restricted to the mesangial regions in a patient with class IIb glomerular disease (original WHO classification). In the modified WHO classification, this is either class IIA or IIB, based on the severity of the mesangial widening/hypercellularity by light microscopy.

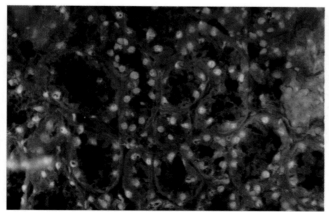

Figure 8–19. Systemic lupus erythematosus. Nuclear immunostaining with antibodies against IgG in the tubular epithelial cells depicts the presence of antinuclear antibodies.

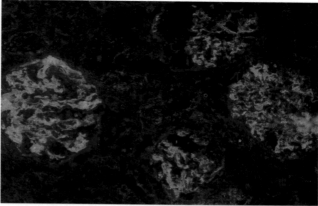

Figure 8–20. Systemic lupus erythematosus, diffuse glomerulonephritis, class IV (original as well as modified WHO classification). Immunofluorescence typical of class IV lupus nephritis shows massive strong glomerular IgG staining in the mesangial areas and also along the periphery of the capillary loops (subendothelial).

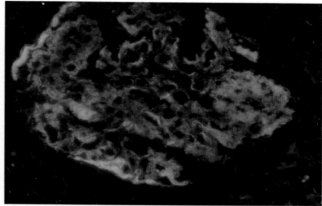

Figure 8–21. Systemic lupus erythematosus, diffuse glomerulonephritis, class IV (original as well as modified WHO classification). There is strong mesangial and peripheral glomerular capillary wall staining (subendothelial) with antibodies against IgG.

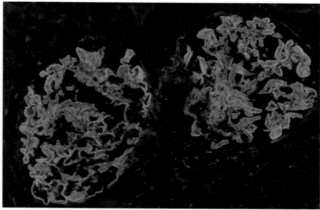

Figure 8–22. Systemic lupus erythematosus, immunofluorescence, membranous glomerulonephropathy, class V (original WHO classification). Both glomeruli show granular uniform peripheral staining along the glomerular capillary walls with antibodies against IgG. Electron microscopy disclosed discrete electron-dense immune-type deposits subepithelially along the glomerular capillary basement membranes; scattered electron-dense deposits were also seen in the mesangial areas. In the modified WHO classification, this is also class V.

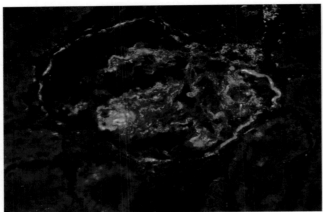

Figure 8–23. Systemic lupus erythematosus, immunofluorescence, diffuse glomerulonephritis, class IV (original as well as modified WHO classification). IgG staining is strongly positive not only in the glomerular tuft but also along Bowman's capsule.

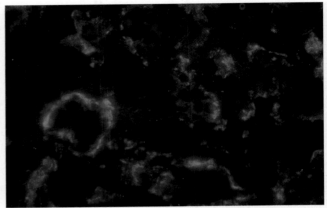

Figure 8–25. Systemic lupus erythematosus, immunofluorescence, tubular deposits. Granular κ light-chain–positive deposits are present along the tubular basement membranes. Tubular deposits are common in focal or diffuse proliferative lupus nephritis.

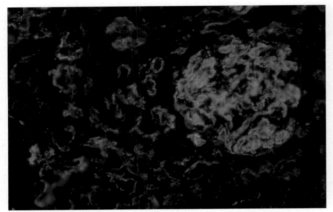

Figure 8–24. Systemic lupus erythematosus, immunofluorescence, diffuse glomerulonephritis, class IV (original as well as modified WHO classification). There is strong C3 staining in the glomerulus and along the tubular basement membranes (so-called tubulointerstitial deposits).

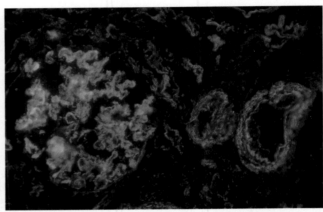

Figure 8–26. Systemic lupus erythematosus, immunofluorescence, diffuse glomerulonephritis, class IV (original as well as modified WHO classification). Strong glomerular, tubular, and arterial wall staining signals immune deposition in various compartments of the kidney (κ light-chain immunofluorescence).

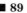

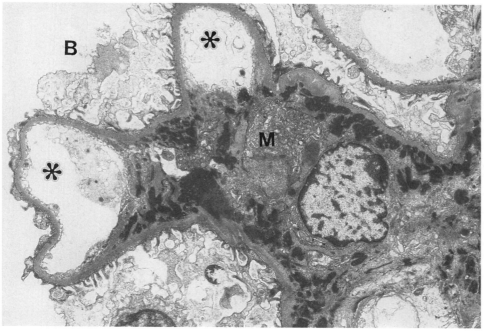
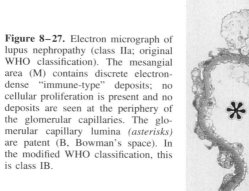

Figure 8–27. Electron micrograph of lupus nephropathy (class IIa; original WHO classification). The mesangial area (M) contains discrete electron-dense "immune-type" deposits; no cellular proliferation is present and no deposits are seen at the periphery of the glomerular capillaries. The glomerular capillary lumina *(asterisks)* are patent (B, Bowman's space). In the modified WHO classification, this is class IB.

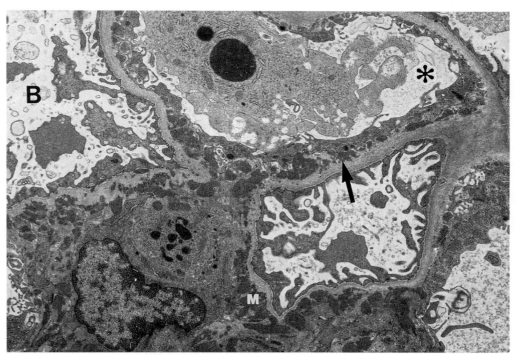

Figure 8–28. Electron micrograph of diffuse proliferative lupus nephritis, class IV (original as well as modified WHO classification). Discrete electron-dense "immune-type" mesangial (M) and adjacent numerous contiguous subendothelial deposits *(arrow)* are present (B, Bowman's space; asterisk, glomerular capillary lumen).

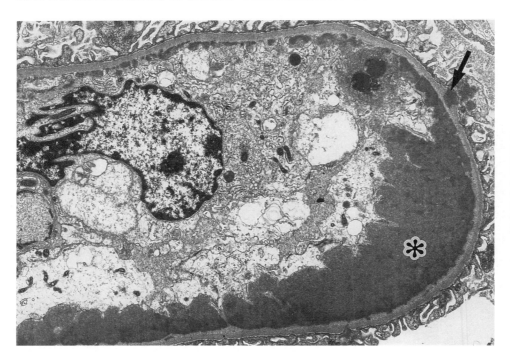

Figure 8–29. Electron micrograph of diffuse proliferative lupus glomerulonephritis, class IV (original as well as modified WHO classification). Large discrete electron-dense "immune-type" subendothelial deposits *(asterisk)* and a few smaller subepithelial deposits *(arrow)* are seen in a glomerular capillary loop.

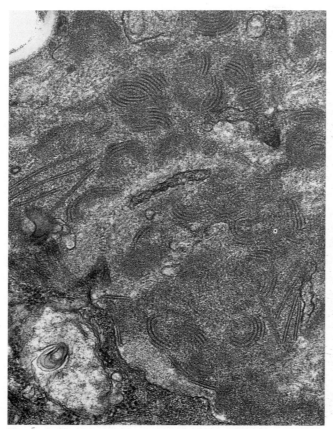

Figure 8–30. Electron micrograph of lupus nephropathy, class IV (original as well as modified WHO classification). Organized "fingerprint" deposits can be seen in the mesangium. When present, these types of deposits are thought to be quite characteristic of lupus.

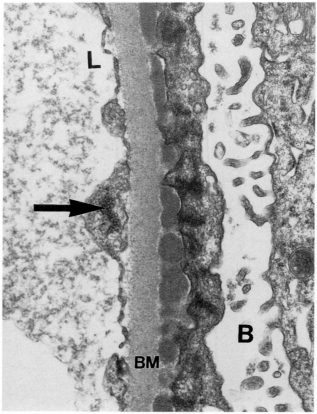

Figure 8–31. Electron micrograph of membranous lupus glomerulonephropathy, class V (original WHO classification). Discrete subepithelial electron-dense "immune-type" deposits and endothelial tubuloreticular inclusions ("myxovirus-like particles") *(arrow)* are seen. The glomerular capillary basement membrane (BM) appears normal (L, glomerular capillary lumen; B, Bowman's space).

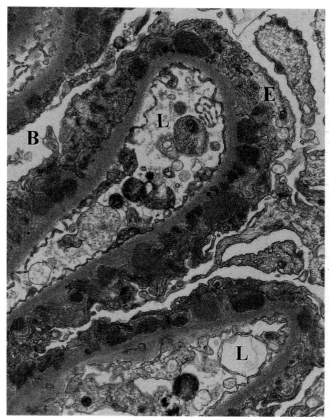

Figure 8–32. Electron micrograph of membranous lupus glomerulonephropathy, class V (original WHO classification). Numerous large discrete granular electron-dense "immune-type" subepithelial deposits are present in the glomerular capillary loops (B, Bowman's space; L, glomerular capillary lumen; E, visceral epithelial cell).

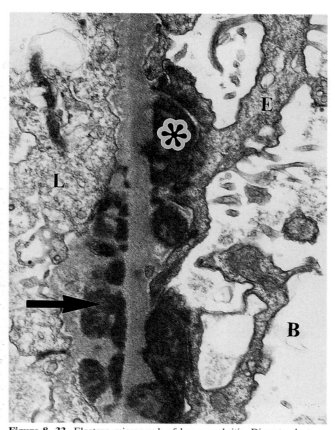

Figure 8–33. Electron micrograph of lupus nephritis. Discrete electron-dense "immune-type" deposits are present subendothelially *(arrow)* and subepithelially *(asterisk)* along the glomerular basement membranes. Subendothelial deposits are seen in focal and diffuse proliferative lupus glomerulonephritis (classes III and IV); however, a few subendothelial deposits can also occasionally be seen in mesangial proliferative lupus glomerulopathy (class II), although if common and peripheral, they may represent an impending explosion/transformation to a more active class III or IV. The subepithelial deposits may indicate a membranous glomerulonephropathy component (class V); however, scattered subepithelial deposits are frequently seen in association with either class III or class IV lupus nephritis. "Mixed" (subendothelial and subepithelial deposits) can also be seen in patients with severe/active lupus nephropathy observed (and treated) for many years (B, Bowman's space; L, glomerular capillary lumen with endothelial cell; E, visceral epithelial cell). (The WHO classes refer to the original WHO classification.)

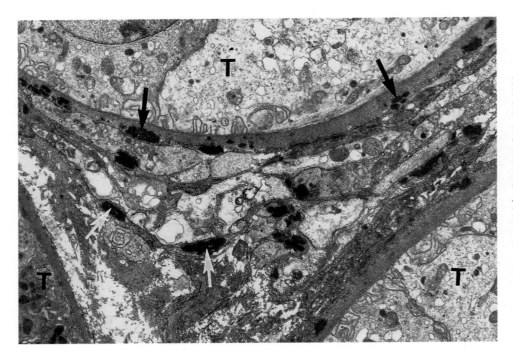

Figure 8–34. Electron micrograph of lupus nephritis. Tubulointerstitial immune deposits are present in a patient with diffuse proliferative lupus glomerulonephritis. Granular electron-dense "immune-type" deposits are present along the tubular basement membranes *(black arrows)* and in the interstitium *(white arrow)* (T, tubular epithelial cells). (From Laszik Z, Lajoie G, Nadasdy T, Silva GS: Medical diseases of the kidney. In: Silverberg SG, DeLellis RA, Frable WJ, [eds]: Principles and Practice of Surgical Pathology and Cytopathology, 3rd ed. New York, Churchill Livingstone, 1997, p 2079, with permission.)

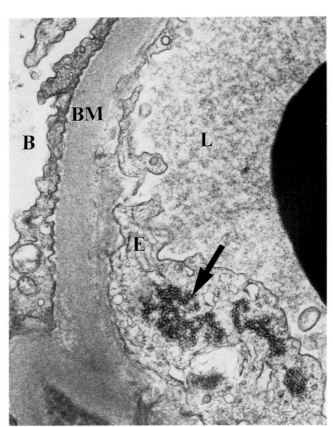

Figure 8–35. Electron micrograph of lupus nephritis. Endothelial tubuloreticular inclusions (myxovirus-like particles) *(arrow)* are present in a patient with diffuse proliferative lupus nephritis. Although tubuloreticular inclusions are seen in virtually all patients with systemic lupus erythematosus, the inclusions are not specific for lupus. They represent "interferon footprints" (B, Bowman's space; BM, glomerular capillary basement membrane; L, glomerular capillary lumen; E, endothelium).

RHEUMATOID ARTHRITIS

- Clinical evidence of renal involvement in rheumatoid arthritis (RA) is relatively uncommon; more often, renal involvement is related to complications of therapy rather than the disease itself.
- The most common forms of primary renal disease in RA are membranous glomerulonephropathy and a pure mesangial proliferative glomerulonephritis; rare patterns of renal involvement include MPGN, rheumatoid nodules in the kidney (necrosis with palisading epithelioid histiocytes), tubulointerstitial nephritis, and necrotizing vasculitis.
- In most cases of membranous and mesangial proliferative glomerulonephritis associated with RA, the histologic, IF, and EM features are similar to those of the same conditions not associated with RA and will not be discussed here.
- Necrotizing vasculitis occurs in severe cases of RA; however, renal involvement is rare.
- Amyloidosis may occur and involve the kidneys in RA; the amyloid protein is the AA type and related to serum amyloid-associated protein. The histologic and ultrastructural features of amyloidosis associated with RA are similar to those of amyloidosis associated with other conditions.
- Treatment of RA with gold salts and penicillamine may be associated with membranous glomerulonephropathy and the nephrotic syndrome; proteinuria develops in approximately 1% to 10% of patients treated with these medications.
- Less common complications of gold or penicillamine therapy include proliferative glomerulonephritis with hematuria, focal glomerulosclerosis, and tubulointerstitial nephritis.
- Therapy with NSAIDs may be associated with tubulointerstitial nephritis, manifested as impaired renal function; minimal change nephrotic syndrome ("nil disease") may also complicate NSAID use.

MIXED CONNECTIVE TISSUE DISEASE

- The term *mixed connective tissue disease* (MCTD) describes a group of patients whose illness has some features of SLE, scleroderma, polymyositis, and RA but does not completely fulfill the criteria for any one of these disorders.
- Serum from patients frequently contains antibodies to extractable nuclear antigen; they usually lack autoantibodies characteristic of SLE such as anti-Sm or anti-dsDNA.
- The original description of MCTD suggested that renal disease was uncommon and usually less severe than in SLE; it now appears that clinical evidence of renal disease occurs in approximately 50% of cases.
- Two common patterns of renal disease in MCTD are described: the most frequent is immune complex–mediated glomerulonephritis, which can resemble the various patterns of lupus nephritis; less frequently there is vascular sclerosis resembling renal involvement in scleroderma.
- The most common pattern of glomerulonephritis related to MCTD is pure mesangial proliferative glomerulonephritis resembling class II lupus nephritis; a membranous glomerulonephropathy occurs, often with mesangial proliferation, that resembles class V lupus nephritis. A diffuse proliferative glomerulonephritis with subendothelial immune complex deposits can also occur, and rare cases resemble MPGN.
- The histologic, IF, and ultrastructural features of the various types of glomerulonephritis in MCTD resemble those in the corresponding types of lupus nephritis.
- The vascular disease seen in MCTD consists of vascular proliferation and sclerosis similar to that in scleroderma; medial and intimal thickening occurs in both small and large arteries, frequently associated with hypertension.

PROGRESSIVE SYSTEMIC SCLEROSIS (SYSTEMIC SCLERODERMA)

Synonyms and Related Terms: Systemic sclerosis; CREST syndrome.

Biology of Disease

- Progressive systemic sclerosis (PSS), or systemic scleroderma, is characterized by symmetrical collagenous thickening and hardening of the skin, most marked on the distal extremities with later involvement of the face; vascular abnormalities, particularly those involving digital arteries; fibrosis of the gastrointestinal tract with motility abnormalities; pulmonary fibrosis; cardiovascular abnormalities; and occasional involvement of a wide variety of other systems.
- The kidneys are frequently involved in PSS; acute renal failure, frequently associated with severe hypertension *(scleroderma renal crisis),* occurs in approximately 15% to 20% of patients with the systemic disease. A lesser degree of renal involvement, such as proteinuria without renal failure, occurs in a substantial number of patients.
- A related but more limited disease can occur, called the *CREST syndrome* (*c*alcinosis, *R*aynaud's phenomenon, *e*sophageal dysmotility, *s*clerodactyly, and *t*elangiectasias); renal involvement is unusual in patients with this variant.
- Localized cutaneous forms of scleroderma occur; renal involvement seldom occurs in patients with disease limited to the skin.
- The cause of scleroderma is unknown. A variety of autoantibodies occur in patients with PSS, thus suggesting an autoimmune basis.
- Renal disease in patients with scleroderma usually takes one of two forms: an acute form with vascular changes resembling those of HUS, which is seen with scleroderma renal crisis, and a chronic form characterized by arterial sclerosis. The cause or causes of these changes in systemic sclerosis are unknown.

- Injury to the endothelium may be involved in the initiation of the process; however, the mechanism or mechanisms of such injury are unknown.

Clinical Features

- Systemic scleroderma is more common in women, with a female-to-male ratio of approximately 3:1.
- Onset is most frequent between the ages of 30 and 50 years.
- The diffuse form, which has more extensive skin and visceral involvement, makes up about 40% of cases (excluding the localized cutaneous variants); the remainder consist of patients with the CREST syndrome and other limited systemic forms.
- The initial symptom is thickening and tightening of the skin of the fingers, sometimes preceded by Raynaud's phenomenon. The cutaneous changes spread to the forearms and upper part of the arms, chest, abdomen, thighs, and eventually the face. The skin becomes reddened, shiny, firm, and adherent to the underlying subcutaneous tissue. Telangiectasias develop in small vessels in the fingers.
- Scleroderma renal crisis usually occurs in patients with diffuse cutaneous involvement; frequently they have had PSS for a relatively short time, with a mean of approximately 2.4 years.
- Symptoms of acute renal crisis include headaches, blurred vision, dyspnea, and sometimes convulsions.
- Severe elevation of blood pressure is common in the acute crisis, often reaching "malignant" hypertension levels. However, in some patients hypertension never develops, and in others the blood pressure is only mildly elevated.
- Oliguria is frequent.

Laboratory Values

- A variety of autoantibodies are seen in patients with scleroderma, including ANAs (present in up to 90%), frequently with a speckled pattern; antinucleolar antibodies may also be seen. Anticentromere antibodies occur in approximately half of patients with the CREST syndrome but in only about 12% of patients with diffuse disease. Anti-Scl (directed against DNA topoisomerase I) is found in nearly three quarters of patients with diffuse systemic disease but in fewer than half of patients with the CREST syndrome.
- Elevated serum renin levels are common in acute renal crisis.
- Proteinuria and microscopic hematuria are common.
- With onset of scleroderma renal crisis, serum urea nitrogen and creatinine levels progressively increase.

Treatment and Clinical Course

- Acute renal involvement carries the most adverse prognostic significance of all organs involved in PSS; formerly, the acute renal crisis was nearly uniformly fatal, with survival usually only a few months.
- Aggressive control of hypertension, particularly with angiotensin-converting enzyme inhibitors, has dramatically improved the outlook of patients with renal involvement; improvement in the cutaneous manifestations of the disease has also been reported.

Gross Appearance

- Kidneys examined during or shortly after acute renal crisis are usually normal or slightly enlarged in size.
- The capsular surface often shows petechial hemorrhages or pale areas representing infarcts.
- On section, wedge-shaped infarcts may be present; these infarcts are frequently smaller than typical renal infarcts due to emboli.
- The chronic form of scleroderma kidney is characterized by small kidneys with a finely granular surface.

Light Microscopy

Light microscopic changes in the acute form generally resemble those seen in HUS, thrombotic thrombocytopenic purpura, and other thrombotic microangiopathies with renal involvement.

Glomeruli

- Glomerular appearance in the acute form is variable and may range from little change to diffuse congestion or infarction.
- Glomeruli may appear swollen and "bloodless," with swelling of capillary endothelial cells and thickened capillary walls; capillary walls may have a double-contour appearance on silver stains.
- Glomerular cellularity is usually normal or only slightly increased; significant leukocytic infiltration is uncommon.
- Afferent arterioles and capillaries may be occluded by hyaline material with the staining qualities of fibrin; in some cases fragmented erythrocytes may be present.
- Larger areas of hyaline material may be present within capillary tufts and suggest fibrinoid necrosis.
- The juxtaglomerular apparatus may appear prominent.

Tubules

- Tubular atrophy is frequently present; occasionally, necrotic tubules are found in infarcted areas.

Interstitium

- The interstitium frequently shows few changes in the acute form; fibrosis may be present.
- Variable degrees of interstitial fibrosis are present in chronic renal involvement in scleroderma.

Vessels

- The most striking changes involve vessels, usually the subarcuate and interlobular arteries and arterioles. Larger arteries are frequently spared or show fibrous intimal thickening.
- There is intimal thickening in the subarcuate and interlobular arteries, with narrowing of the lumina. The in-

tima appears myxoid, mucinous, or loosely fibrous and may contain fibrin. Red blood cells or fragments may be seen within vessel walls. Small thrombi may be found within the lumina of small arteries.

- The walls of arterioles are thickened; fibrin may be present, sometimes having the appearance of fibrinoid necrosis.
- Arterioles with fibrinoid necrosis may contain thrombi, which may continue into the hilar region of glomeruli.

Immunofluorescence Microscopy

- Staining for fibrin/fibrinogen may be present in glomerular capillary walls. Staining for complement components may be present, but staining for immunoglobulins is usually not seen.
- Staining for fibrin/fibrinogen is present in the intima of interlobular arteries and arterioles. Staining for IgM, C3, and sometimes C1q is frequently present in the same areas; staining for IgG and IgA is less common.

Electron Microscopy

- The intima of interlobular arteries contains parallel bands of basement membrane–like material in a loose bed of finely granular material; fibrin deposits and erythrocyte fragments may be present. Myointimal cells may also be present.
- Granular deposits are found in the intima of arterioles.
- Aggregates of platelets and fibrin may be present within the lumina of arteries and arterioles.
- The subendothelial space (lamina rara interna) of glomerular capillaries is widened and contains finely granular, electron-lucent ("fluffy") material.
- There may be thickening and sometimes reduplication of glomerular capillary basement membranes. In the later stages of the disease there is wrinkling and contraction of thickened GBMs.
- Immune complex–type electron-dense deposits are not usually present.

Histologic Variants

- Most of the aforementioned pathologic changes are found in acute scleroderma renal crisis. In chronic forms of the disease, the changes are primarily limited to thickening of the walls of arteries and arterioles.

Differential Diagnosis

- The clinical diagnosis of diffuse systemic sclerosis is usually evident, although other rheumatologic disorders such as MCTD may enter into the differential.
- The pathologic findings of acute renal scleroderma crisis are essentially similar to those of malignant hypertension, HUS, thrombotic thrombocytopenic purpura, and other thrombotic microangiopathies.

SJÖGREN'S SYNDROME

- Sjögren's syndrome is a chronic disorder characterized by inflammation, fibrosis, and atrophy of the lacrimal and salivary glands that results in keratoconjunctivitis sicca and xerostomia (dry eyes and mouth; the "sicca complex").
- Sjögren's syndrome may occur in isolation or in association with other rheumatologic disorders such as SLE, RA, scleroderma, or MCTD.
- Sjögren's syndrome occurs most commonly in women (female-to-male ratio, approximately 9:1); the average age of onset is approximately 50 years.
- Autoantibodies are frequently present in the serum of patients with Sjögren's syndrome and include rheumatoid factor, ANAs, and anti-La.
- Renal disease occurs in up to one third of patients with Sjögren's syndrome; the most common type is interstitial nephritis manifested clinically as renal tubular acidosis and nephrogenic diabetes insipidus; glomerulonephritis of various histologic types may also occur.
- Both the interstitial nephritis and glomerulonephritis associated with Sjögren's syndrome have been shown to respond to corticosteroids.

Light Microscopy

- The most common histologic change is an interstitial infiltrate of inflammatory cells, predominantly lymphocytes, plasma cells, and histiocytes.
- Interstitial edema and/or fibrosis may be present.
- Tubular atrophy may be prominent.
- Calcium deposition within renal tubules may occur.
- Glomerulonephritis occurring in patients with Sjögren's syndrome may be of several types, including focal, membranous, membranoproliferative, and mesangial proliferative glomerulonephritis.

Immunofluorescence Microscopy

- In many cases, no positive staining is found by IF.
- IgG with or without C3 may be found in tubular cells and in the interstitium; interstitial staining for IgA and IgM is occasionally present.
- Glomeruli usually show no positive IF staining; occasionally, diffuse granular staining for IgG, IgM, IgA, and C3 is present.

Electron Microscopy

- Ultrastructural findings are usually nonspecific. Electron-dense deposits are sometimes present in tubular basement membranes; occasionally, glomerular subepithelial, mesangial, or subendothelial deposits are seen.

References

General

Adler SG, Cohen AH, Glassock RJ: Secondary glomerular diseases. In: Brenner BM (ed): Brenner & Rector's The Kidney, 5th ed. Philadelphia, WB Saunders, 1996, p 1498.

Systemic Lupus Erythematosus

Appel GB, Cohen DJ, Pirani CL, et al: Long-term follow-up of patients with lupus nephritis: A study based on the classification of the World Health Organization. Am J Med 83:877, 1987.

Appel GB, Silva FG, Pirani CL, et al: Renal involvement in systemic lupus erythematosus (SLE): A study of 56 patients emphasizing histologic classification. Medicine (Baltimore) 57:371, 1978.

Austin HA III, Muenz LR, Joyce KM, et al: Prognostic factors in lupus nephritis: Contribution of renal histologic data. Am J Med 75:382, 1983.

Baldwin DS, Gluck MC, Lowenstein J, et al: Lupus nephritis: Clinical course as related to morphologic forms and their transitions. Am J Med 62:12, 1977.

Balow JE, Austin HA III, Muenz LR, et al: Effect of treatment on the evolution of renal abnormalities in lupus nephritis. N Engl J Med 311:491, 1984.

Churg J, Bernstein J, Glassock RJ: Lupus nephritis. In: Classification and Atlas of Glomerular Diseases, 2nd ed. New York, Igaku-Shoin, 1995, p 51.

D'Agati VD: Renal disease in systemic lupus erythematosus, mixed connective tissue disease, Sjögren's syndrome, and rheumatoid arthritis. In: Jennette JC, Olson JL, Schwartz MM, Silva FG (eds): Heptinstall's Pathology of the Kidney, 5th ed. Philadelphia, Lippincott-Raven, 1998, p 541.

Jennette JC, Iskandar SS, Dalldorf FG: Pathologic differentiation between lupus and nonlupus membranous glomerulopathy. Kidney Int 24:377, 1983.

Kashgarian M, Hayslett JP: Renal involvement in systemic lupus erythematosus. In: Tisher CG, Brenner BM (eds): Renal Pathology: With Clinical and Functional Correlations, 2nd ed. Philadelphia, JB Lippincott, 1994, p 442.

Magil AB, Ballon HS, Chan V, et al: Diffuse proliferative lupus nephritis: Determination of prognostic significance of clinical, laboratory and pathologic factors. Medicine (Baltimore) 63:210, 1984.

Schwartz MM, Shu-Ping L, Bernstein J, et al: Irreproducibility of the activity and chronicity indices limits their utility in the management of lupus nephritis. Am J Kidney Dis 21:374, 1993.

Schwartz MM, Shu-Ping L, Bonsib SM, et al: Clinical outcome of three discrete histologic patterns of injury in severe lupus glomerulonephritis. Am J Kidney Dis 13:273, 1989.

Rheumatoid Arthritis, Mixed Connective Tissue Disease, Systemic Sclerosis, and Sjögren's Syndrome

D'Agati V, Cannon PJ: Scleroderma (systemic sclerosis). In: Tisher CG, Brenner BM (eds): Renal Pathology: With Clinical and Functional Correlations, 2nd ed. Philadelphia, JB Lippincott, 1994, p 1058.

Eigenbrodt EH, Molony DA, DuBose TD: Renal involvement in hepatic disease, rheumatoid arthritis, Sjögren syndrome, and mixed connective tissue disease. In: Tisher CG, Brenner BM (eds): Renal Pathology: With Clinical and Functional Correlations, 2nd ed. Philadelphia, JB Lippincott, 1994, p 596.

Laszik Z, Silva FG: Hemolytic-uremic syndrome, thrombotic thrombocytopenic purpura, and systemic sclerosis (systemic scleroderma). In: Jennette JC, Olson JL, Schwartz MM, Silva FG (eds): Heptinstall's Pathology of the Kidney, 5th ed. Philadelphia, Lippincott-Raven, 1998, p 1003.

Sellars L, Siamopoulos K, Wilkinson R, et al: Renal biopsy appearances in rheumatoid disease. Clin Nephrol 20:114, 1983.

CHAPTER 9

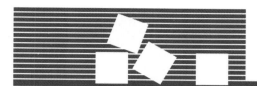

The Kidney in Metabolic Disorders
Diabetes Mellitus, Hyperuricemia, Oxalosis, Nephrocalcinosis, and Nephrolithiasis

DIABETIC NEPHROPATHY

Biology of Disease

- Diabetes mellitus, the single most common cause of end-stage renal disease (ESRD) in the United States, is responsible for one quarter to one third of patients with ESRD.
- Renal disease is associated with high morbidity and mortality in diabetic patients; much of the excess mortality in diabetics occurs in patients with diabetic nephropathy, although many of the deaths are due to cardiovascular disease rather than renal disease directly.
- Two common types of diabetes occur, both resulting in hyperglycemia and a variety of secondary metabolic abnormalities:
  - *Insulin-dependent diabetes mellitus (IDDM)* is associated with complete loss of endogenous insulin production; it occurs predominantly in younger patients, who are predisposed to episodes of diabetic ketoacidosis.
  - *Non–insulin-dependent diabetes mellitus (NIDDM)* is associated with decreased (but not absent) insulin production, resistance to insulin activity, or both. It occurs predominantly in older persons; episodes of diabetic ketoacidosis are less common. Non–insulin-dependent diabetes represents approximately 90% of cases of diabetes in the United States.
- Diabetic nephropathy occurs in both types of diabetes; renal failure occurs in approximately 25% to 35% of patients with IDDM and 15% to 25% of patients with NIDDM.
- The changes that occur in the kidney in the two common types, as well as in less common causes of diabetes such as hemochromatosis, are similar. It is believed that the pathophysiologic mechanisms underlying renal disease are similar in all types of diabetes.
- Proteinuria is the hallmark of diabetic nephropathy; diabetes is one of the most common causes of the nephrotic syndrome in adults.
- The pathogenesis of diabetic nephropathy is not com-

pletely understood. Hyperglycemia per se appears to play an important role; several studies have shown that poor control of glucose predisposes to diabetic nephropathy and the other long-term vascular complications of diabetes. However, other factors such as hemodynamic alterations (hyperfiltration) may also be involved.
- One consequence of hyperglycemia is nonenzymatic glycosylation of proteins, which occurs at a rate directly proportional to the level of blood glucose. An example is the glycosylation of hemoglobin (the level of glycosylated hemoglobin, or hemoglobin A_{1c}, is used to monitor glucose control). Other proteins are also glycosylated, including albumin, collagen, other matrix proteins, and basement membrane proteins.
- Advanced glycosylation end products (AGEs) may result from the glycosylation of proteins; some of these AGEs are capable of forming covalent bonds to amino groups on other proteins, thereby resulting in cross-linking. Advanced glycosylation end product formation on collagen and other matrix proteins may result in decreased endothelial cell adhesion and replication, mesangial cell vasoconstriction and growth, and increased lipoprotein and immune complex adhesion to monocytes and macrophages. Inhibitors of AGE formation decrease albuminuria in diabetic animal models.
- Conversion of glucose to sorbitol by the enzyme aldose reductase has been proposed as another mechanism of injury in diabetes; however, clinical trials of aldose reductase inhibitors have been disappointing, at least in part because of toxicity.
- The characteristic morphologic changes of diabetic nephropathy are expansion of the extracellular matrix, thickening of basement membranes, and intimal thickening in arteries and arterioles.
- Hemodynamic alterations are also characteristic of diabetic nephropathy. A 20% to 50% increase in the glomerular filtration rate (GFR) has been found early in the course of diabetic nephropathy, even before any clinical evidence of renal disease. The incidence of eventual renal failure appears to be increased in patients with IDDM who have higher initial GFR rates,

thus suggesting that hyperfiltration plays a direct role in the pathogenesis of diabetic nephropathy; however, the mechanism or mechanisms are unclear.

■ In the early stages of diabetes, glomeruli are characteristically enlarged; this enlargement correlates with the increased GFR. The kidneys themselves are also frequently enlarged.

■ Hyperfiltration appears to be directly related to the degree of hyperglycemia; correction of hyperglycemia with insulin leads to return of the GFR toward normal and a decrease in renal size.

■ Vascular changes similar to those in the glomerulus also occur in the retina. Diabetic nephropathy is associated with diabetic retinopathy; retinopathy is present in more than 90% of patients with IDDM and over half of patients with NIDDM and nephropathy. However, fewer than half of the patients with retinopathy have nephropathy.

■ There is evidence of a genetic predisposition for the development of renal disease in diabetics; the risk of nephropathy appears to be higher in African-Americans than in whites with diabetes. Hypertension and tobacco use also appear to increase the risk of nephropathy in diabetics.

Clinical Features

■ The initial change in diabetes is microalbuminuria, defined as urinary albumin excretion between 30 and 300 mg per 24 hours; this level of proteinuria is not detected by standard urine dipsticks. Microalbuminuria is present early after the onset of disease in many diabetic patients; control of hyperglycemia may decrease albumin excretion.

■ Microalbuminuria appears to be an early marker of renal injury; patients with early microalbuminuria have a higher incidence of the development of overt nephropathy. Overall mortality from cardiovascular disease appears to be higher in the cohort of patients with early microalbuminuria.

■ Detection of proteinuria by standard dipstick analysis, which occurs at a proteinuria level of approximately 500 mg/day, indicates the onset of overt diabetic nephropathy. Overt nephropathy rarely occurs in patients with IDDM before 10 years after diagnosis; on average, nephropathy is diagnosed 15 to 20 years after the clinical onset of diabetes. Interestingly, the risk of *new-onset* diabetic nephropathy appears to *decrease* after 20 years of diabetes, which suggests that the risk of nephropathy is limited to a subset of patients.

■ Occasional patients with new-onset or recently diagnosed NIDDM have significant pathologic evidence of diabetic nephropathy; most likely such patients actually had undiagnosed diabetes for several years before the actual diagnosis.

■ Hypertension is usually present in diabetic patients with renal disease; the degree to which hypertension contributes to the renal disease, and vice versa, is unknown or difficult to separate from each other.

Laboratory Values

■ Urinalysis shows proteinuria in virtually all patients with diabetic nephropathy; 5% to 10% have nephrotic-range proteinuria.

■ Microhematuria may be present; however, in many cases the microhematuria appears to be due to superimposed renal disorders and cannot be definitely attributed to diabetes. The incidence of microhematuria in uncomplicated diabetic nephropathy is unclear.

■ Serum urea nitrogen and creatinine levels may be normal or mildly elevated at the time nephropathy is diagnosed and then become progressively elevated over time.

■ Hyperkalemia and acidosis may appear out of proportion to the degree of uremia because of the propensity of diabetic patients for hyporeninemic hypoaldosteronism.

Gross Pathology

■ Early in the disease course the kidneys may be diffusely and symmetrically enlarged.

■ Later, kidney size may be highly variable; in part this difference in size depends on the presence or absence of superimposed diseases such as vascular disease or pyelonephritis.

■ End-stage kidneys may be small or normal in size, with granular surfaces and irregular, deep scars; diabetes is a cause of large, contracted and scarred kidneys.

■ Papillary necrosis may be present, with loss of pyramids.

Light Microscopy

Glomeruli

■ Early in the disease the glomeruli may appear hypertrophic, particularly in patients with IDDM. The mesangium may appear slightly expanded and capillary walls slightly thickened, but these changes are better appreciated by electron microscopy.

■ The most characteristic lesion of diabetic glomerulonephropathy is *nodular intercapillary glomerulosclerosis,* also known as *Kimmelstiel-Wilson nodules.* These nodules are eosinophilic and round; the center of the nodule is largely acellular, but there may be a cellular rim. They stain strongly with periodic acid–Schiff and silver stains and stain blue or green on trichrome stains; they may appear laminated on silver stains. Kimmelstiel-Wilson nodules are located in the mesangial or intercapillary regions of the glomerulus. One or more may be present in a single glomerulus; if multiple, they tend to vary in size. Occasionally they may appear to originate as microaneurysms and thickening of capillary walls. Although Kimmelstiel-Wilson nodules are virtually pathognomonic of diabetic glomerulonephropathy (except for a few mimics, discussed later), they are found in only a quarter of diabetic cases.

■ The second characteristic glomerular lesion is *diffuse intercapillary glomerulosclerosis,* which is found in all cases of diabetic glomerulonephropathy. There is diffuse and global expansion of the mesangium by material with staining properties similar to those of Kimmelstiel-Wilson nodules. Glomerular capillary basement membranes are diffusely thickened. Mesangial cellularity is usually normal but may be increased. Mesangial sclerosis progressively increases, with resulting compromise of capillary lumina. Diffuse glomerulosclerosis frequently coexists with nodular lesions.

- A third characteristic lesion of diabetic glomerulonephropathy is the *capsular drop*. This lesion is a homogeneous, eosinophilic, hyaline or "waxy"-appearing mass located within Bowman's capsule that may represent insudation of plasma proteins. Capsular drops do not stain with silver stains; they are fuchsinophilic with trichrome stains. If present, capsular drops are strongly suggestive, but not quite pathognomonic of diabetic glomerulonephropathy.
- Another characteristic lesion is the *fibrin cap,* which is an exudative lesion located between the glomerular capillary endothelial cells and the glomerular basement membrane (GBM). The appearance and staining qualities resemble those of the capsular drop. Fibrin caps may grow to occlude the capillary lumen, and adhesions may form between the fibrin cap and Bowman's capsule. Fibrin caps are not specific for diabetes; similar lesions may occur in other diseases such as focal segmental glomerulosclerosis, reflux nephropathy, arteriolosclerosis, and others.
- Microaneurysms of the glomerular capillaries may be present. Glomerular capillary loops may become dilated as a result of mesangiolysis.
- The glomerular capillary walls become diffusely and progressively thickened; the capillary lumina become progressively compromised by thick capillary walls, diffuse mesangial sclerosis, and fibrin cap lesions. Eventually, the glomeruli become globally sclerotic.

Tubules

- Tubular epithelial cells contain protein droplets; there may be vacuolization of cytoplasm because of lipid droplets.
- With disease progression, tubules become increasingly atrophic; tubular basement membranes become progressively thickened, occasionally with splitting.
- The *Armanni-Ebstein change,* or glycogen deposits within the tubular epithelial cells, is now very rare.
- The presence of inflammatory cells infiltrating into tubular epithelium or collections of neutrophils in tubular lumina suggests superimposed pyelonephritis.

Interstitium

- The most common interstitial change is fibrosis, which is usually proportional to the degree of vascular change.
- Interstitial inflammation may result from superimposed infection or be caused by chronic renal failure. In the latter circumstance, the amount of inflammation is proportional to the amount of glomerulosclerosis and interstitial fibrosis.

Vessels

- Vascular disease is common and may be striking in diabetic nephropathy.
- Intimal hyaline thickening of arterioles is the most characteristic change; the presence of marked hyaline arteriolosclerosis, especially in a young patient, should alert the pathologist to look for other changes of diabetes. If the pathologist is fortunate enough to have a glomerulus cut so that both the afferent and efferent arterioles are present, both may be involved; the presence of arteriolar hyalinosis involving *both* the afferent and efferent arterioles is virtually pathognomonic of diabetic nephropathy.
- Arteriosclerosis is usually present; however, it is difficult to separate the effects of diabetes from those of hypertension.

Immunofluorescence Microscopy

- The most characteristic finding on immunofluorescence is linear staining of glomerular capillary basement membranes for IgG and albumin and occasionally for other immunoreactants; this staining probably represents nonspecific adhesion to the GBM rather than a specific immunologic reaction. This finding is sometimes seen in other conditions but is most often seen in diabetes.
- Linear GBM staining in diabetes may suggest anti-GBM antibody disease to an inexperienced renal pathologist. The coexistence of staining for albumin and IgG suggests diabetes rather than anti-GBM antibodies; the intensity of staining is also usually less in diabetes than in true anti-GBM antibody disease. Some pathologists prefer the term *pseudolinear* staining to avoid confusion with anti-GBM antibody disease.
- Linear staining of tubular basement membranes for IgG and albumin may also be present.
- Granular cytoplasmic staining for albumin, C3, and occasionally other immunoreactants is commonly present in proximal convoluted tubular epithelial cells, probably representing lysosomes containing reabsorbed protein.
- Fibrin cap and arteriolar hyaline lesions usually demonstrate staining for IgM and C3.

Electron Microscopy

- The glomerular mesangium is expanded, primarily because of extracellular matrix material, which appears amorphous or granular. This material appears relatively electron dense, although not usually to the degree seen in immune complex deposits.
- Kimmelstiel-Wilson nodules are formed from similar amorphous or granular, relatively electron-dense material.
- Glomerular capillary basement membranes become progressively thickened. Normal GBM thickness is approximately 300 to 400 nm; in advanced diabetic nephropathy, GBMs may be up to 4,000 nm in thickness.
- The fibrillary nature of the glomerular basement membrane may appear accentuated, and it may appear laminated.

- Glomerular capillary basement membranes commonly appear wrinkled or corrugated, most likely representing ischemic changes resulting from the accompanying arteriosclerosis.
- There may be interposition of mesangial matrix and mesangial cell cytoplasmic processes into the peripheral capillary loops, between the GBM and endothelial cells, resembling the changes seen in membranoproliferative glomerulonephritis (MPGN) type I. This change is limited and localized in diabetes, in contrast to the widespread changes seen in MPGN.
- Capsule drop, fibrin cap, and arteriolar subintimal hyaline lesions are seen to be accumulations of amorphous, electron-dense material, probably plasma proteins.
- Tubular basement membranes are thickened and demonstrate changes similar to those seen in GBMs.

Differential Diagnosis

- Clinically, the differential diagnosis includes any cause of proteinuria or the nephrotic syndrome; thus minimal change nephrotic syndrome, focal segmental glomerulosclerosis, membranous glomerulonephropathy, amyloidosis, and others enter into the differential diagnosis.
- Any cause of advanced glomerulosclerosis and tubulointerstitial fibrosis may enter the histologic differential of diabetic nephropathy, including focal segmental glomerulosclerosis, hypertensive renal disease, and ischemia secondary to arteriosclerosis and arteriolosclerosis.
- Differentiation of diabetic nephropathy from hypertensive renal disease may be difficult because of the similarity of some morphologic features (e.g., thickened GBMs) and the frequent coexistence of the two diseases. Hyaline arteriolosclerosis is a common feature in both diseases; the presence of hyaline change involving both afferent *and efferent* arterioles strongly favors diabetic nephropathy but often cannot be demonstrated on needle biopsies.
- Light-chain deposition disease (LCDD) may cause nodular lesions in glomeruli that resemble Kimmelstiel-Wilson nodules. The nodules in LCDD are frequently remarkably uniform in size, both within single glomeruli and between different glomeruli in the same biopsy specimen; in contrast, true Kimmelstiel-Wilson nodules characteristically vary in size, both within single glomeruli and between glomeruli. Staining for immunoglobulin light chains may also be helpful; LCDD may stain for either κ or λ light chains (more often κ), whereas staining for both will be observed in diabetes.
- Amyloidosis may have a nodular appearance resembling Kimmelstiel-Wilson nodules. In contrast with Kimmelstiel-Wilson nodules, amyloid nodules do not stain with silver stains; they stain with Congo red and demonstrate the characteristic "apple green" birefringence of amyloid under polarized light.
- Glomeruli in advanced membranoproliferative (mesangiocapillary) glomerulonephritis may have sclerotic nodules suggesting Kimmelstiel-Wilson nodules. Increased mesangial cellularity, diffuse GBM "tram-tracking," granular glomerular staining for immunoglobulins and complement on immunofluorescence, and discrete "immune-type" electron-dense deposits on electron microscopy would favor MPGN.

Treatment and Clinical Course

- Inexorable deterioration in renal function usually follows the development of overt proteinuria; however, the rate of deterioration is highly variable. The time from overt proteinuria to ESRD averages 4 to 5 years but may vary from only months to a decade or longer. The reasons for the marked variability are unclear; some evidence suggests that control of hypertension may slow this progression; however, there is little evidence that control of hyperglycemia is beneficial after overt renal disease is present.
- There is no specific therapy for diabetic nephropathy once it has developed; prevention is therefore the long-term goal in treating diabetic patients.
- Animal models of diabetes suggest that strict control of blood glucose may prevent nephropathy. Until recently there has not been as strong evidence that strict glucose control in *humans* prevents nephropathy; in part, this lack of strong evidence may have been due to the fact that strict control of blood glucose over a period of years would be required to demonstrate an effect, and this control has been hard to achieve in a large number of patients.
- Recent studies have suggested that aggressive blood sugar control may delay or prevent the onset of microalbuminuria, thus suggesting that nephropathy might also be delayed or prevented. However, once overt nephropathy is present, control of hyperglycemia appears to have little effect on progression of the disease.
- Aggressive control of hypertension appears to slow the development of diabetic nephropathy. Angiotensin-converting enzyme inhibitors such as captopril have demonstrated renal protective effects in animal models and appear to decrease proteinuria in humans. Preliminary evidence suggests that they may also prevent or delay the onset of nephropathy.
- Dietary protein restriction has been shown to decrease urinary albumin excretion and hyperfiltration; trials in patients with IDDM and nephropathy suggest that progression of nephropathy may be slowed.
- Pancreas transplantation to replace pancreatic islet cells is now being performed to restore normal glucose metabolism; in some cases, pancreas transplantation is combined with renal transplantation.
- Maintenance dialysis and renal transplantation are the final therapeutic modalities for diabetic nephropathy. Survival rates for patients undergoing hemodialysis are lower than those for nondiabetic patients with ESRD; the leading cause of death in diabetic patients undergoing maintenance hemodialysis is cardiovascular disease.
- Renal transplantation provides improved survival for diabetics with ESRD in comparison to maintenance hemodialysis; however, graft survival and overall survival are less than in nondiabetic patients. The increase in mortality in diabetic transplant recipients is again primarily due to cardiovascular disease.
- Diabetics appear to be predisposed to severe urinary

tract infections. The spectrum of bacteria that cause urinary tract infections appears to be similar in diabetic and nondiabetic patients; diabetics appear to have a higher incidence of fungal infections, primarily *Candida* species.

Other Renal Diseases Associated With Diabetic Nephropathy

■ Diabetic nephropathy is the most common renal disease to be complicated by another form of glomerular disease. Virtually any form of glomerulonephritis may complicate diabetic nephropathy, but the most common complicating condition is membranous glomerulonephropathy.

■ Nephropathy in patients with NIDDM is more frequently complicated by second glomerular diseases; such an occurrence is less common in patients with IDDM.

■ Papillary necrosis is a serious complication of diabetic nephropathy. It usually occurs in association with nodular glomerulosclerosis or significant vascular disease combined with pyelonephritis.

■ In the past, diabetics had a high incidence of pyelonephritis. This finding no longer appears to be true, possibly because of more effective antibiotic therapy for pyelonephritis.

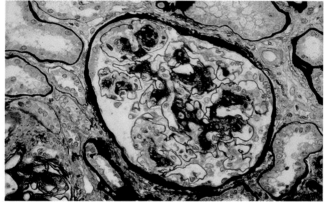

Figure 9–1. Diabetes mellitus with diffuse and nodular diabetic glomerulosclerosis. Silver staining depicts silver-positive mesangial widening with a small mesangial (intercapillary) nodule (Kimmelstiel-Wilson nodule) at the 11-o'clock position (methenamine silver stain).

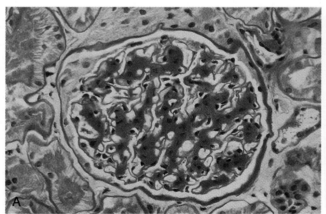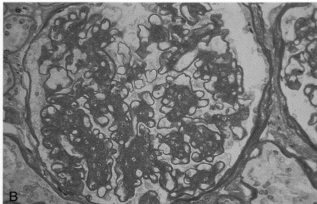

Figure 9–2. *A*, and *B*, Diabetes mellitus with diffuse diabetic glomerulosclerosis. The mesangial widening is due to periodic acid–Schiff (PAS)–positive matrix accumulation. The capillary lumina are patent although narrowed (PAS reaction). *A* shows a mild change and *B* shows a moderate to severe mesangial widening.

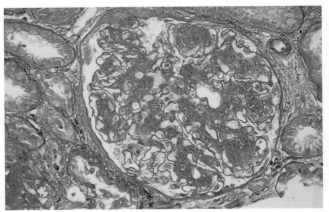

Figure 9–3. Diabetes mellitus with diffuse and nodular diabetic glomerulosclerosis, moderately advanced. Mesangial nodules (Kimmelstiel-Wilson nodules) are located in the center of the glomerular lobules; at the periphery of the nodules are patent glomerular capillaries (Masson's trichrome stain).

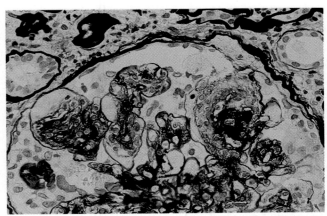

Figure 9–4. Diabetes mellitus with diffuse and nodular diabetic glomerulosclerosis, advanced. This high-magnification picture of a segment of a glomerulus depicts the lamellar nature of a Kimmelstiel-Wilson nodule (methenamine silver stain).

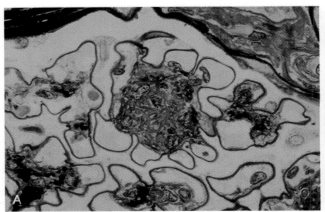
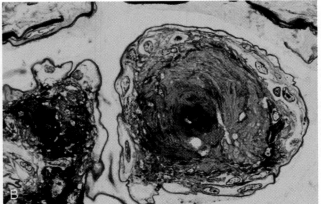

Figure 9–5. *A* and *B*, Diabetes mellitus with Kimmelstiel-Wilson nodule. The large, almost acellular mesangial (intercapillary) nodule represents the characteristic lesion of nodular diabetic glomerulosclerosis. *A* shows the mesangial localization of the nodule with widely patent capillary lumina; *B* shows a more advanced acellular nodule with lamellation and narrow capillary lumina at the periphery.

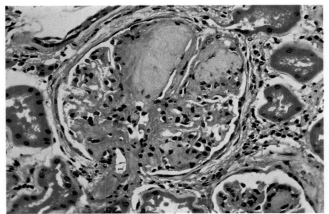

Figure 9–6. Diabetes mellitus with diffuse and nodular diabetic glomerulosclerosis, advanced. The Kimmelstiel-Wilson mesangial nodules are large and acellular. At the periphery of the nodules the capillary lumina are occluded. Arteriolar hyalinization is also seen at the vascular pole.

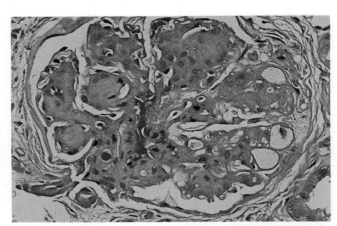

Figure 9–7. Diabetes mellitus with diffuse and nodular diabetic glomerulosclerosis. The mesangial nodules are *blue* on trichrome stain. The nodules vary in size and contain only a few cells (Masson's trichrome stain).

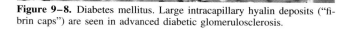

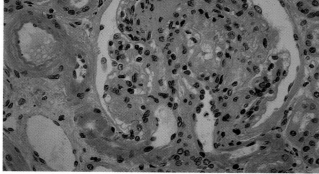

Figure 9–8. Diabetes mellitus. Large intracapillary hyalin deposits ("fibrin caps") are seen in advanced diabetic glomerulosclerosis.

Figure 9–11. Diabetes mellitus with diffuse and nodular diabetic glomerulosclerosis. The mesangial matrix accumulation is quite prominent. Both the afferent and the efferent arterioles reveal severe hyalinization (the latter quite characteristic of diabetes).

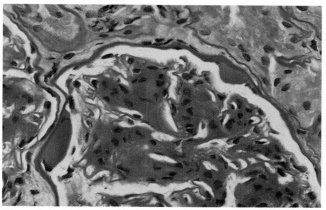

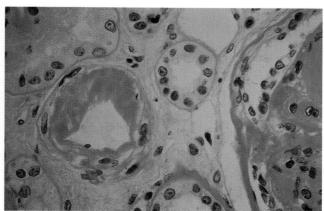

Figure 9–9. Diabetes mellitus with capsular drops. The eosinophil capsular drops are seen between Bowman's capsule and the parietal epithelium.

Figure 9–12. Diabetes mellitus with arteriolar hyalinization. Severe arteriolar hyalinization is a common feature in diabetes mellitus. Both the afferent and the efferent arterioli may be hyalinized.

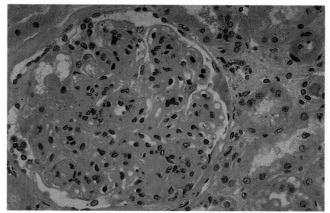

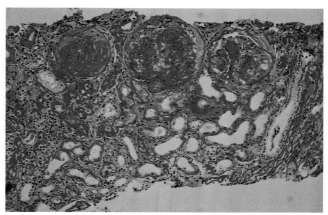

Figure 9–10. Diabetes mellitus with diffuse diabetic glomerulosclerosis. Diffuse mesangial matrix accumulation, mesangial hypercellularity, and enlargement of the glomerulus can be seen. This pattern is quite characteristic although not specific for diabetes mellitus. Note the small capsular drop at the 2-o'clock position in Bowman's capsule and the "fibrin caps" at the 10-o'clock position. Hyaline arteriolosclerosis is noted at the far upper right.

Figure 9–13. Diabetes mellitus with advanced diabetic glomerulosclerosis. The glomeruli reveal advanced sclerotic changes; unlike the situation in advanced glomerulosclerosis secondary to glomerulonephritis, the sclerotic glomeruli may retain a relatively large size in diabetes. Kimmelstiel-Wilson nodules are still apparent.

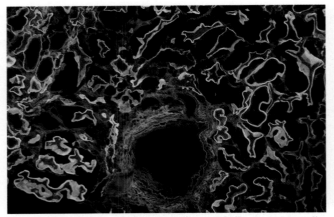

Figure 9–14. Diabetes mellitus. Immunofluorescence demonstrates linear (pseudolinear) immunostaining along the tubular basement membranes with antibodies against albumin.

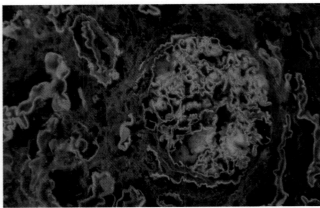

Figure 9–15. Diabetes mellitus. Immunofluorescence demonstrates linear (pseudolinear) albumin staining along the glomerular capillary and tubular basement membranes.

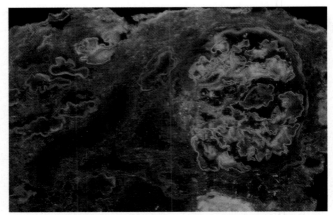

Figure 9–16. Diabetes mellitus. Immunofluorescence demonstrates linear (pseudolinear) IgG staining along the glomerular capillary basement membranes in a glomerulus with features of nodular diabetic glomerulosclerosis; there is also some linear staining along the tubular basement membranes.

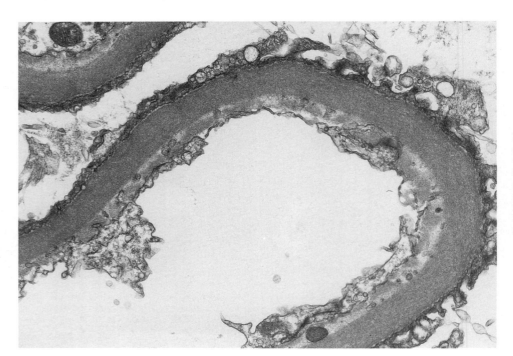

Figure 9–17. Electron micrograph of diabetic nephropathy. The glomerular capillary basement membrane reveals moderate uniform thickening (average, 730 nm) in a patient with diffuse diabetic glomerulosclerosis. The normal thickness of the glomerular capillary basement membrane is approximately 300 to 330 nm.

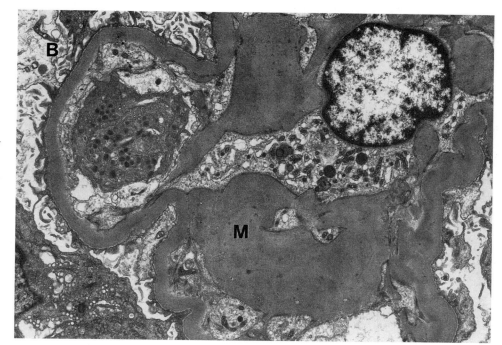

Figure 9–18. Electron micrograph of diabetic glomerulosclerosis. Note the mesangial matrix (M) accumulation and the thickening of the glomerular capillary basement membranes (B, Bowman's space).

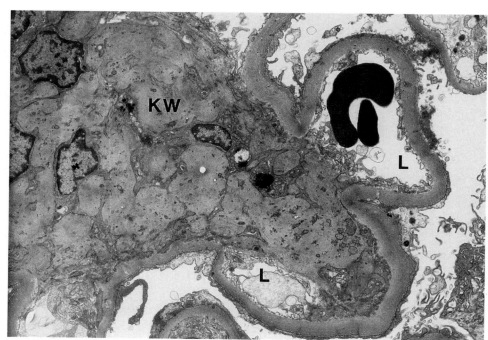

Figure 9–19. Electron micrograph of diabetic nephropathy (nodular diabetic glomerulosclerosis, moderately advanced). Patent but narrowed capillary lumens (L) are present at the periphery of the acellular mesangial (Kimmelstiel-Wilson) nodule (KW). The basement membranes have uniform thickening. (From Laszik Z, Lajoie G, Nadasdy T, Silva FG: Medical diseases of the kidney. In: Silverberg SS, DeLellis RA, Frable WJ [eds]: Principles and Practice of Surgical Pathology and Cytopathology, 3rd ed. New York, Churchill Livingstone, 1997, p 2079, with permission.)

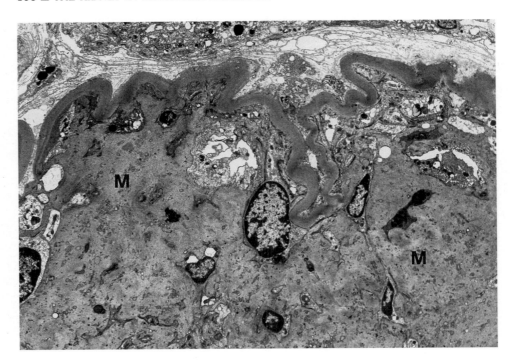

Figure 9–20. Electron micrograph of diabetic glomerulosclerosis, advanced. The mesangium (M) is expanded and sclerotic; the glomerular capillary lumina are closed/effaced.

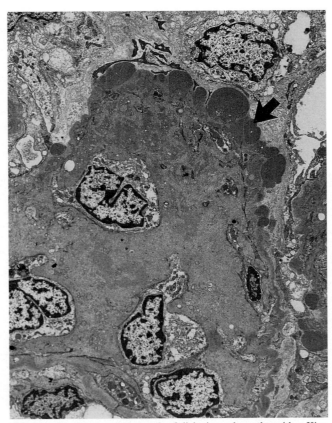

Figure 9–21. Electron micrograph of diabetic nephropathy with a Kimmelstiel-Wilson nodule, advanced. Mesangial expansion with matrix accumulation is the basis for formation of Kimmelstiel-Wilson nodules. Note the extensive electron-dense amorphous hyalin insudation or accumulation, closure of the capillary loops at the periphery of the nodule *(arrow),* and a few residual cells inside the nodule.

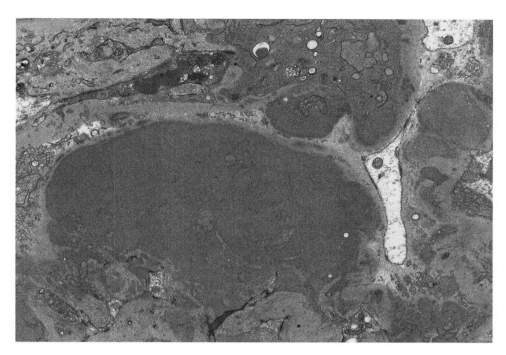

Figure 9–22. Electron micrograph of diabetic nephropathy. Intracapillary electron-dense amorphous hyalin deposits (so-called "fibrin caps") are seen in a patient with advancing diabetes mellitus. Hyalin deposits are usually finely granular and less electron dense than immune deposits.

URATE NEPHROPATHY

Synonyms and Related Terms: Gouty nephropathy; hyperuricemia.

Biology of Disease

- Hyperuricemia may involve the kidney in a variety of ways: acute hyperuricemic nephropathy, chronic urate nephropathy, and renal stones composed of uric acid.
- Acute hyperuricemia may occur as part of the tumor lysis syndrome after chemotherapy for acute leukemia or a high-grade lymphoma; this association is discussed in Chapter 18. Chronic urate nephropathy will be discussed in this section.
- Uric acid is an end product of purine metabolism. The majority of purines are endogenous, derived from cellular turnover with breakdown of DNA and RNA; a smaller amount is derived from the diet.
- At normal pH, the majority of uric acid is in the form of monosodium urate. Urate is freely filtered by the glomerulus and then undergoes both tubular reabsorption and secretion. Renal clearance of urate is a complex process influenced by a variety of factors, including urine pH, urine flow rate and volume, systemic acid-base balance, drugs, and many others.
- The normal upper limit of urate is approximately 7 mg/dL but varies with age, sex, and ethnicity. There are multiple causes of hyperuricemia, including inherited disorders of purine metabolism such as a deficiency of hypoxanthine-guanine phosphoribosyltransferase (the

Lesch-Nyhan syndrome) or glucose-6-phosphatase, increased turnover of purines in neoplasms, renal insufficiency secondary to lead poisoning, a variety of drugs including thiazide diuretics, a purine-rich diet, hypertension, preeclampsia, and others. In a majority of cases the cause is unknown.
- The most common complication of hyperuricemia is gouty arthritis, followed in frequency by renal disease.
- Increased excretion of uric acid (hyperuricuria) may occur in the absence of hyperuricemia and is an important predisposition to nephrolithiasis. Pure uric acid stones occur; in addition, urate crystals commonly form a nidus for crystallization of calcium oxalate stones.
- Chronic urate nephropathy was formerly widely accepted as an entity, but this concept is now controversial. The association among lead overload, renal insufficiency, and hyperuricemia is well established ("saturnine gout"); it is unclear whether hyperuricemia in the absence of lead poisoning or hypertension can cause renal insufficiency. Some evidence suggests that the majority of patients previously accepted as having chronic urate nephropathy actually had unsuspected lead toxicity. A description of the accepted morphologic appearance of chronic urate nephropathy will be given nonetheless.

Clinical Features

- The typical manifestation is an insidious onset of renal insufficiency, usually with hypertension.

■ There may be a history of gouty arthritis, renal stones, or both.

Gross Appearance

■ The characteristic abnormality is yellow-white streaks in the medulla or pyramids that represent deposition of urate crystals within collecting ducts.

■ Stones may be present within the pelvis.

Light Microscopy

■ Monosodium urate is soluble in water, so demonstration of the urate crystals may require fixation and processing in nonaqueous solutions such as alcohol.

■ Urate crystals deposit in tubules and collecting ducts. The crystals are usually needle shaped but may be rectangular or amorphous. They are birefringent under polarized light.

■ The crystals may disrupt the tubular lining and protrude into the interstitium, where they elicit an inflammatory response. The inflammation includes macrophages, lymphocytes, and multinucleated giant cells; interstitial fibrosis is often present.

■ Arteries and arterioles frequently show hypertensive changes, including medial hypertrophy and luminal narrowing.

■ Glomeruli may show ischemic changes and global obsolescence as a result of the accompanying vascular disease. Glomeruli are otherwise unremarkable.

Treatment and Clinical Course

■ The prognosis of patients with urate nephropathy depends primarily on the underlying disease causing the hyperuricemia. In the majority of cases the prognosis is favorable; hyperuricemia is more of a nuisance than a threat to life or kidney function.

■ Allopurinol (Zyloprim) is an inhibitor of the enzyme xanthine oxidase, which prevents the formation of uric acid from xanthine. It is effective in lowering the serum uric acid concentration.

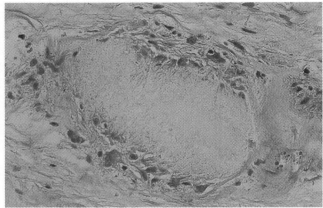

Figure 9–23. Urate tophus in gout. The trichrome-negative tophus deep in the renal medulla (i.e., close to the pelvis) is surrounded by cells, including multinucleated giant cells (Masson's trichrome stain).

OXALOSIS

Synonyms and Related Terms: Primary hyperoxaluria.

Biology of Disease

■ Oxalic acid, like uric acid, can affect the kidney in several ways. Toxicity may occur with acute hyperoxalemia and hyperoxaluria, which are predominantly due to poisoning, with chronic hyperoxalemia and consequent deposition in the renal parenchyma, and as a component of renal stones.

■ "Oxalosis" is the pathologic deposition of oxalate in tissues; deposits occur in the kidneys as well as other tissues.

■ In the normal state, oxalic acid is derived from both endogenous metabolism and the diet. The majority is derived from endogenous synthesis; the immediate precursor is glyoxylate, which is an intermediate metabolite in the synthesis of glycine. Oxalic acid is also derived from other amino acids (tryptophan, phenylalanine, and serine) and ascorbic acid.

■ Dietary sources of oxalic acid include cocoa, tea, coffee, parsley, rhubarb, spinach, pepper, and nuts.

■ Hereditary ("primary") hyperoxalemia is hyperoxalemia caused either by a genetic deficiency in an enzyme in one of the metabolic pathways that produce oxalic acid or by inherited intestinal hyperabsorption. Type I hyperoxalemia is due to a deficiency in hepatic alanine-glyoxylate aminotransferase, type II is due to a deficiency in D-glycerate dehydrogenase, and type III is due to intestinal hyperabsorption.

■ Acquired ("secondary") causes of increased absorption include excessive consumption of foods high in oxalate, excessive ascorbic acid intake, and a variety of gastrointestinal diseases resulting in hyperabsorption.

■ Gastrointestinal hyperabsorption is the most common cause of chronic hyperoxalemia. Hyperabsorption occurs in celiac sprue, ileal resection, pancreatic insufficiency, small intestinal bypass surgery, blind loop syndrome, and chronic inflammatory bowel disease. Malabsorption of bile salts is a common mechanism of increased absorption inasmuch as increased amounts of bile salts reaching the colon increase the absorption of oxalate. Dietary calcium decreases the absorption of oxalate from the gastrointestinal tract; therefore, diets low in calcium result in increased oxalate absorption.

■ Ethylene glycol poisoning results in metabolic acidosis

and acute hyperoxalemia and hyperoxaluria; acute hyperoxalemia can also be a complication of methoxyflurane anesthesia. Acute hyperoxalemia may result in acute renal failure secondary to precipitation of oxalate crystals within tubules with subsequent tubular obstruction.

- Oxalate is excreted by the kidney, and decreased renal function results in hyperoxalemia.
- Calcium oxalate, the most common compound identified in renal calculi, is present in approximately 40% to 47% of stones.
- The presence of oxalate crystals within renal tubules is not specific for hyperoxaluria; acute renal failure of any cause may result in small amounts of oxalate crystals being deposited within renal tubules.

Gross Appearance

- Kidneys of patients with chronic hyperoxaluria are usually small; they may be gritty on sectioning.
- Calculi are frequently present within the pelvis.

Light Microscopy

- Acute hyperoxalemia results in the deposition of calcium oxalate crystals in renal tubular lumina. The crystals appear irregular, laminated, or fan shaped; they are colorless under ordinary light and birefringent under polarized light.

- Chronic hyperoxalemia results in crystals in tubular lumina that penetrate through the tubular walls. This penetration of tubular walls results in an inflammatory response that includes lymphocytes, histiocytes, giant cells, and interstitial and periglomerular fibrosis.

Treatment and Clinical Course

- The prognosis and treatment of renal oxalosis depend on the underlying disease process.

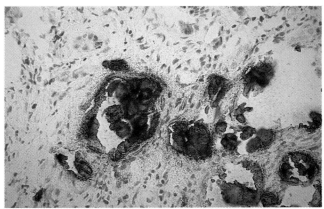

Figure 9–24. Oxalosis. Large oxalate crystals are seen with destruction of renal tubular epithelial cells.

NEPHROCALCINOSIS

Synonyms and Related Terms: Chronic calcium nephropathy; hypercalciuria.

Biology of Disease

- Hypercalcemia and consequent increased calcium excretion in the urine *(hypercalciuria)* can be associated with a variety of renal manifestations. The level of serum calcium greatly influences the clinical manifestations of hypercalcemia; an additional factor that influences the clinical and pathologic features is whether the hypercalcemia developed acutely or was chronic.
- The term *nephrocalcinosis* indicates the deposition of calcium crystals within the renal parenchyma. Calcium can also be deposited within the renal pelvis as renal stones (see Nephrolithiasis).
- Nephrocalcinosis usually occurs with chronic hypercalcemia and hypercalciuria; the most common causes of hypercalcemia are listed in Table 9–1. Nephrocalcinosis is also occasionally seen in patients with acquired immunodeficiency syndrome, often in conjunction with calcification in multiple organs; in Bartter's syndrome (metabolic alkalosis associated with hypokalemia, juxta-

glomerular apparatus hyperplasia, and hyperreninemic hyperaldosteronism, probably caused by defective tubular reabsorption of chloride ions); in occasional patients with cystic fibrosis; after acute tubular necrosis or cortical necrosis; in patients with hypochloremic alkalosis from excessive vomiting, often as a result of pyloric stenosis; and in a variety of other conditions.

- Renal calcifications also occur in many normal older people and patients with proteinuria from any cause. In addition, calcium oxalate crystals are frequently found in renal transplants. In such circumstances, the calcifications are not associated with significant functional deficits.
- Hypercalcemia itself can result in significant impairment in kidney function, even without deposition of calcium in the renal parenchyma.

Clinical Features

- The earliest manifestation of hypercalcemia is an inability to concentrate the urine, with resulting polyuria. Hypercalcemia may also result in renal tubular acidosis, both proximal and distal.
- Patients with severe, acute hypercalcemia (such as is

Table 9–1
CAUSES OF HYPERCALCEMIA

Hyperparathyroidism caused by excess production by the parathyroid
    glands
    Parathyroid adenoma
    Parathyroid hyperplasia
Malignancies
    Parathyroid hormone–related protein: squamous cell carcinoma, renal
      cell carcinoma, transitional cell carcinoma of the bladder, breast
      carcinoma
    True parathyroid hormone production: ovarian carcinoma, small cell
      lung carcinoma
    Osteolytic tumors and metastases: multiple myeloma, lymphomas and
      leukemias, carcinomas (breast, other)
Increased intestinal absorption of calcium
    Idiopathic infantile hypercalcemia (Williams syndrome)
    Vitamin D excess
    Sarcoidosis
    Milk-alkali syndrome
Increased bone turnover
    Thyrotoxicosis
    Paget's disease of bone with immobilization

---

sometimes seen in multiple myeloma) may have nausea, vomiting, extracellular volume contraction, lethargy, obtundation or other mental status changes, cardiac arrhythmias, and renal failure.
- Chronic calcium nephropathy, such as may be seen in primary hyperparathyroidism, is manifested as interstitial nephritis. Patients have polyuria with a bland urine sediment and little or no proteinuria; a variable degree of renal insufficiency may be present.

Gross Appearance

- The kidneys in chronic nephrocalcinosis will vary in size from small to normal.
- The kidneys may feel "gritty" on sectioning.
- The cut surface shows alternating areas of normal parenchyma and wedge-shaped scars.

Light Microscopy

- Occasional basophilic calcifications within tubular epithelial cells or tubular lumina may be seen in normal older individuals or patients with proteinuria. The tubular epithelium usually appears atrophic or is absent.
- Small foci of calcification are quite common in renal papillae and occur either as small round deposits, as linear streaks, or as plaque covering the tips of papillae (Randall's plaque). These foci may form a nidus for

the crystallization of renal stones, but they are otherwise of no functional significance.
- In acute hypercalcemia there is usually sparse calcium deposition within the kidney. Calcifications within tubular lumina may appear to obstruct the tubules.
- In chronic nephrocalcinosis, the most striking change is calcification in tubular basement membranes. Calcification appears most prominent in proximal convoluted tubules; however, all segments of the nephron may be involved. Calcification occurs in the tubular basement membranes of both atrophic and apparently intact tubules and in both scarred and viable areas.
- Calcification may be present in Bowman's capsule of glomeruli and in sclerotic glomeruli.
- The calcification appears as a purplish tinge or stippling on hematoxylin and eosin stains; it is emphasized by the von Kossa stain for calcium.
- Intratubular calcifications similar to those just described are often present; they are more common in scarred areas, particularly in collecting ducts.
- Calcifications may be present in the interstitium, often adjacent to tubules. Interstitial deposits may appear dense and basophilic or fine and less darkly staining.

Treatment and Clinical Course

- The prognosis of patients with nephrocalcinosis depends primarily on the underlying disease process.
- Treatment of nephrocalcinosis is directed at the primary disease process.

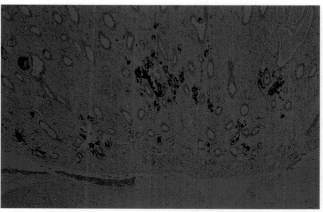

Figure 9–25. Randall's plaque. Calcification of the distal portion of the renal medullary collecting ducts (of Bellini) is seen (Randall's plaque). Randall's plaque has been described in association with nephrolithiasis.

NEPHROLITHIASIS

Synonyms and Related Terms: Kidney stones; renal calculi.

Biology of Disease

- Kidney stones affect approximately 5% to 10% of people in the United States during their lifetime. Although seldom life threatening, renal calculi are associated with substantial economic cost and cause considerable pain and suffering.
- The major types of stones, the relative frequency, and the characteristics of each type are listed in Table 9–2; the most common causes of each are listed in Table 9–3.
- The formation of renal calculi depends on a balance of factors: the concentration of the specific component in the urine, the presence of nucleating factors, and a deficiency of factors that inhibit crystallization.
- An absolute requirement for stone formation is that the urine be supersaturated for the specific solute. Many compounds are supersaturated in normal urine; for example, the concentration of calcium oxalate in normal urine is four times its solubility.
- Nucleating factors function as a surface on which crystallization can begin *(heterogeneous nucleation)*; rarely, stones form without such nucleating factors *(homogeneous nucleation)*. Possible nucleating factors in the urine include epithelial lining, cell debris, urinary casts, and other crystals (for example, uric acid crystals frequently act as nucleating factors for calcium oxalate stones).
- Several factors in normal urine inhibit stone formation. Among them are *nephrocalcin*, an acidic glycoprotein; *uropontin*; the *Tamm-Horsfall protein*; and urinary citrate, which increases the solubility of calcium oxalate. The pH of the urine also has an important effect; a pH above 6.5 increases calcium phosphate saturation.

Table 9–2
TYPES AND CHARACTERISTICS OF RENAL CALCULI

Type	Proportion of Total (%)	Characteristics
Calcium oxalate	75	Black, gray, or white; small (<1–2 cm); sharply circumscribed Radiopaque
Struvite	10–15	Yellow-tan; branching ("staghorn") Radiopaque
Uric acid	5–6	White or orange, may fill the pelvis Radiolucent
Brushite (calcium monohydrogen phosphate)	5	Similar to calcium oxalate
Cystine	1	Greenish yellow, flecked with shiny crystallites Radiopaque: "sculpted wax" or "soap" appearance
Other	10	

Table 9–3
CAUSES OF RENAL CALCULI

Type of Stone	Causes	Proportion of Total (%)
Calcium oxalate	Hypercalcemia and hypercalciuria	5
	Hypercalciuria without hypercalcemia Absorptive Renal Idiopathic	55
	Hyperuricosuria	20
	Hyperoxaluria Enteric Primary	5
	Hypocitraturia	20–50
Struvite	Renal infection	
Brushite	Renal tubular acidosis	
Uric acid	Hyperuricemia with hyperuricosuria Hyperuricosuria without hyperuricemia Low urine pH	
Cystine	Defective tubular reabsorption of cystine	

- The vast majority of renal calculi (approximately 75%) are calcium oxalate stones formed predominantly from calcium oxalate or calcium oxalate and calcium phosphate; approximately 10% to 12% also contain uric acid. Over half of renal calculi are associated with hypercalciuria without hypercalcemia, approximately one fifth are associated with hyperuricosuria, a small proportion is associated with hypercalciuria secondary to hypercalcemia, and another small proportion is linked with hyperoxaluria.
- Hypercalciuria is generally considered to be 24-hour urine calcium over 300 mg in men and over 250 mg in women. The cause in the majority of cases of hypercalciuria is unknown; a small proportion is associated with hyperparathyroidism, vitamin D excess, sarcoidosis, and other rare conditions.
- Struvite (magnesium ammonium phosphate) stones are strongly associated with infection with urea-splitting bacteria, most often *Proteus* or *Staphylococcus* species. Urease produced by bacteria splits urea to form ammonia, which alkalinizes the urine. Struvite stones can be among the largest renal calculi and may form branching structures that fill the renal pelvis and calyces ("staghorn" calculi).
- Some patients with uric acid stones have hyperuricemia and hyperuricosuria; however, the majority of patients have neither. Uric acid stones in these patients are believed to be due to a tendency to excrete urine with pH below 5.5 because the solubility of uric acid is lower in relatively acidic urine.

Clinical Features

- The syndrome of renal colic, caused by the passage of a stone from the kidney into the ureter or bladder, is well known (particularly to persons who have experienced it!). The pain begins suddenly and rapidly becomes excruciating; nausea and vomiting are frequent. Characteristically the pain passes downward from the flank, curves anteriorly, and descends toward the groin.

The pain vanishes abruptly when the stone passes into the bladder or moves in the ureter to decompress the urinary system.
- Renal calculi may also be painless if they remain in the renal pelvis; in some cases calculi may cause obstructive uropathy without causing pain.
- Hematuria is also a frequent manifestation of renal calculi.

Laboratory Values

- All renal calculi should be sent for chemical analysis to determine their composition and guide future evaluation and therapy.
- The majority of renal calculi are visible on noncontrast radiographs (approximately 85%). However, pure uric acid stones are radiolucent and are not seen without contrast.

Treatment and Clinical Course

- Renal calculi may cause a variety of complications, including renal colic and urinary tract obstruction. In general, smaller stones are more likely to cause complications because they are free to pass from the kidney into the ureter.
- Calculi also predispose to infection by causing obstruction and trauma to the pelvis or ureter.
- Stones less than 5 mm in diameter are likely to pass spontaneously; stones greater than 7 mm in size are unlikely to do so. Stones less than 2 cm can often be treated with extracorporeal shock wave lithotripsy; nephrolithotomy may be required for stones greater than 2 cm or for stones in the lower pole that exceed 1 cm in diameter. Stones lodged in the distal ureter may be managed by ureteroscopic stone removal.
- Without treatment, the majority of patients who have had one stone will experience at least one recurrence. Therefore, determination of the chemical composition

and investigation of possible predisposing factors are recommended to prevent recurrences. Prophylactive therapy is beyond the scope of this text.

References

Diabetic Nephropathy

Breyer JA: Diabetic nephropathy in insulin-dependent patients. Am J Kidney Dis 20:533, 1992.

Fioretto P, Steffes MW, Brown DM, et al: An overview of renal pathology in insulin-dependent diabetes mellitus in relationship to altered glomerular hemodynamics. Am J Kidney Dis 20:549, 1992.

Lewis EJ, Hunsicker LG, Bain RP, et al: The effect of angiotensin-converting-enzyme inhibition on diabetic nephropathy. N Engl J Med 329:1456, 1993.

Olson JL: Diabetes mellitus. In: Jennette JC, Olson JL, Schwartz MM, Silva FG (eds): Heptinstall's Pathology of the Kidney, 5th ed. Philadelphia, Lippincott-Raven, 1998, p 1247.

Parving H-H, Østerby R, Anderson PW, et al: Diabetic nephropathy. In: Brenner BM (ed): Brenner & Rector's The Kidney, 5th ed. Philadelphia, WB Saunders, 1996, p 1864.

Ritz E, Stefanski A: Diabetic nephropathy in type II diabetes. Am J Kidney Dis 27:167, 1996.

Selby JV, FitzSimmons SC, Newman JM, et al: The natural history and epidemiology of diabetic nephropathy: Implications for prevention and control. JAMA 263:1954, 1990.

Tisher CG, Hostetter TH: Diabetic nephropathy. In: Tisher CG, Brenner BM (eds): Renal Pathology: With Clinical and Functional Correlations, 2nd ed. Philadelphia, JB Lippincott, 1994, p 1387.

Venkataseshan VS, Churg J: Diabetes and other metabolic diseases. In: Silva FG, D'Agati VD, Nadasdy T (eds): Renal Biopsy Interpretation. New York, Churchill Livingstone, 1996, p 221.

Urate Nephropathy and Oxalosis

Chonko AM, Richardson WP: Urate and uric acid nephropathy, cystinosis, and oxalosis. In: Tisher CG, Brenner BM (eds): Renal Pathology: With Clinical and Functional Correlations, 2nd ed. Philadelphia, JB Lippincott, 1994, p 1413.

Nephrocalcinosis and Nephrolithiasis

Coe FL, Parks JH, Asplin JR: The pathogenesis and treatment of kidney stones. N Engl J Med 327:1141, 1992.

Hill GS: Calcium and the kidney, hydronephrosis: In: Jennette JC, Olson JL, Schwartz MM, Silva FG (eds): Heptinstall's Pathology of the Kidney, 5th ed. Philadelphia, Lippincott-Raven, 1998, p 891.

CHAPTER 10

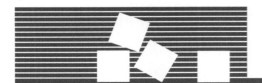

The End-Stage Kidney

INTRODUCTION

- Deterioration of renal function in a chronic progressive or acute rapidly progressive renal disease may culminate in end-stage renal disease (ESRD); at this point the glomerular filtration rate falls below 20% and the patient requires renal dialysis or transplantation to survive.
- In the United States the leading causes of ESRD are diabetes, hypertension, glomerulonephritis, cystic kidney disease, and interstitial nephritis. Diabetes and hypertension account for more than 60% of cases of ESRD.
- After beginning dialysis, the kidneys continue to atrophy and eventually all glomeruli become sclerotic. The arterial bed is obliterated by intimal thickening, and cysts frequently develop in the kidneys (see Acquired Cystic Kidney Disease in Chapter 20), in addition to renal tubular epithelial hyperplasia and epithelial neoplasms (see Chapter 22).

MORPHOLOGIC CHANGES

- Certain features may allow recognition of the cause (i.e., original disease) that led to ESRD. Sometimes, however, the disease is so advanced that the characteristic pathognomonic features of the primary underlying disease are "burned out" and microscopy reveals only nonspecific changes such as global glomerulosclerosis, interstitial fibrosis, and advanced tubular atrophy; in these cases the original disease cannot be determined morphologically.

GROSS FINDINGS

- The gross findings of ESRD depend on the original (underlying) disease and also how long the patient has been undergoing dialysis. In patients maintained on dialysis, kidneys usually undergo continuing atrophy, with some kidneys weighing only a few dozen grams (normal kidney, 150 g).
- End-stage kidneys secondary to diabetes usually retain a normal size (the so-called large contracted kidney) or

can be slightly smaller than normal. The surface is slightly granular.
- The kidneys of end-stage glomerulonephritis usually weigh significantly less than normal and the surface is granular. The granularity is usually coarser than that of vascular-induced nephrosclerosis. On cut surface, a slightly irregular thinning of the cortex is seen and differentiation from the medulla is poor.
- End-stage kidneys secondary to essential hypertension (i.e., end-stage nephrosclerosis) are smaller than normal; however, they are usually much less shrunken than in chronic glomerulonephritis or chronic pyelonephritis. The surface is more often granular or sometimes smooth. If granular, the surface is fine and regular. The consistency of the kidney is firm, but no significant capsular adhesions are usually present.
- End-stage kidneys secondary to malignant hypertension are usually normal in size or only slightly smaller than normal, especially if there was an underlying essential hypertension before the malignant hypertension. Petechial hemorrhages beneath the capsule and on the cut surface of the cortex are common.
- Differentiation of atherosclerotic (vascular) cortical scars and chronic pyelonephritis may be difficult; the scars of both atherosclerosis and chronic pyelonephritis may be large and deep. Typically, atherosclerotic scars are V shaped; scars caused by chronic pyelonephritis are broad based and U shaped with irregular borders. Deformation of the underlying renal pelvis and retraction and destruction of the renal papillae (concave rather than convex papillae) are additional features of chronic pyelonephritis. Of course, the clinical history may be of great help.
- As more and more renal cortical tissue undergoes fibrosis because of atherosclerosis or chronic pyelonephritis, the surface of the kidneys gradually flattens and the kidneys become smaller with an irregular smooth or granular surface.
- The frequent combination of various diseases such as vascular renal disease (arterial and/or arteriolar nephrosclerosis) and chronic pyelonephritis makes the gross findings more complex.
- In amyloidosis, the kidneys are usually firm, pale, and significantly enlarged; the cortex is thicker than normal

and has a waxy, gray, translucent appearance. In late stages the kidneys can still be larger than normal, the surface is usually slightly granular, and the medulla is gray. Application of Lugol's iodine to the cut surface may help disclose amyloidosis.

■ Numerous cortical and medullary cysts (acquired cystic kidney disease) will develop in approximately 20% to 35% of end-stage kidneys in patients who undergo dialysis.

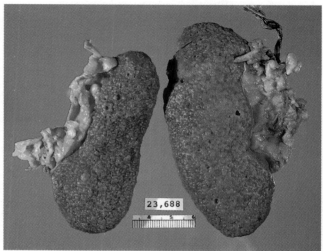

Figure 10–1. Chronic glomerulonephritis. The surface of the small shrunken kidneys is granular. The gross appearance is somewhat similar to that of arteriolar nephrosclerosis; however, kidneys with chronic glomerulonephritis are usually smaller. This morphology was quite typical for chronic glomerulonephritis before the hemodialysis era.

LIGHT MICROSCOPY

In ESRD, eventually all four components (glomeruli, tubules, interstitium, vessels) of the kidney become progressively damaged irrespective of the primary disease.

Glomeruli

■ Even in end-stage kidneys there are usually some glomeruli that are nonglobally sclerotic. The clue to the original or primary glomerular disease in an end-stage kidney often comes from examination of these relatively better preserved glomeruli. Therefore, a careful search for less affected (best preserved) glomeruli is recommended to decide what process was primary and led to the ESRD. Features of the sclerotic glomeruli (size, presence or absence of hyalinosis, mesangial nodules, etc.) may be very helpful in establishing the original disease.

■ The presence of globally sclerotic (obsolescent) glomeruli in end-stage kidneys with expansion of the glomerular tufts (i.e., the glomeruli are sclerotic without prominent collapse of the glomerular capillary tufts) usually indicates the following diseases as the underlying (primary) disorders: diabetes, glomerulonephritis, focal segmental glomerulosclerosis, or amyloidosis.

■ In end-stage diabetic glomerulosclerosis the sclerotic glomeruli are large; some glomeruli may show increased mesangial matrix and intercapillary (Kimmelstiel-Wilson) sclerotic nodules. Marked glomerular hyalinosis may be present.

■ In end-stage focal segmental glomerulosclerosis the glomerular hyalinosis is usually prominent, but no Kimmelstiel-Wilson nodules are present.

■ Glomerular hyalinosis is also common in patients who have ESRD secondary to hypertension; however, glomerular hyalinosis can also be found in chronic glomerulonephritis and chronic pyelonephritis.

■ The obsolescent glomeruli of hypertensive patients are usually smaller and contain simplified wrinkled and simplified sclerotic capillary loops. Accumulation of collagen inside Bowman's space surrounding the sclerotic/collapsed glomerular tuft is characteristic of hypertension; however, ischemic glomeruli may also occur in advanced vascular diseases (i.e., atherosclerosis without hypertension) and in any advanced process (ESRD) irrespective of etiology. Features of glomerular ischemia (simplification of the glomerular capillary tuft, thickening and wrinkling of the glomerular capillary basement membranes) are often seen in the nonglobally sclerotic glomeruli of hypertensive patients.

■ In end-stage membranoproliferative glomerulonephritis (MPGN), some of the accentuated/sclerotic glomerular lobules and other characteristic changes of MPGN may still be usually recognizable in the best preserved/mildest involved glomeruli.

■ In end-stage membranous glomerulonephropathy the marked uniform thickening of the glomerular capillary basement membranes may still be recognizable in at least some of the least involved (i.e., less sclerotic) glomeruli.

■ In end-stage kidneys secondary to amyloidosis, recognition of massive glomerular/vascular/interstitial amyloid is the clue to correct diagnosis. Special stains (Congo red and thioflavin T) are used to verify the diagnosis of amyloidosis.

- In end-stage crescentic glomerulonephritis, rupture (gaps) of Bowman's capsule on special stains (periodic acid–Schiff, silver) with remnants of fibrous crescents may help establish the diagnosis.
- In ESRD caused by chronic pyelonephritis, the relatively less affected parts of the kidney may retain glomeruli with normal-appearing tufts; some of these better preserved glomeruli may show superimposed focal segmental glomerulosclerosis. Focal segmental glomerulosclerosis can also be seen in the late stages of many other renal disease processes. Periglomerular fibrosis is commonly seen in chronic pyelonephritis.
- Globally sclerotic glomeruli can, with time, merge almost imperceptibly with the inflamed and fibrotic interstitium. Periodic acid–Schiff, trichrome, or silver stains can aid in the identification of these "disappearing" glomeruli.

Tubules, Interstitium

- Tubular atrophy, interstitial fibrosis, and interstitial chronic inflammatory cell infiltrate are the common features in ESRD.
- Atrophic tubules in end-stage kidneys (and also in less advanced renal diseases) may be seen in three different patterns. "Classic" atrophic tubules have thick, occasionally lamellated basement membranes and simplified epithelium. The "thyroidization" pattern designates uniform round tubules with flattened simplified epithelium and casts. "Endocrine"-type atrophic tubules, which are most commonly seen in ischemia, are "bunched" close together and have narrow or no lumina, clear epithelial cells, and relatively thin basement membranes.
- Large areas with thyroidization-type atrophic tubules are common in end-stage kidneys with chronic pyelonephritis.
- In end-stage kidneys with chronic pyelonephritis, the interstitial inflammatory cell infiltrate (primarily lymphocytic) is usually more prominent than in other renal diseases and is often nested near the urothelium.

Vessels

- The arteries of end-stage kidneys undergo fibrous intimal thickening, the severity of which is related to the duration of dialysis; this change affects arteries of all sizes.
- Fibrinoid arterial/arteriolar necrosis can be seen in patients with uncontrolled hypertension and associated end-stage kidney disease.
- The veins of end-stage kidneys are thickened by hypertrophic smooth muscle.

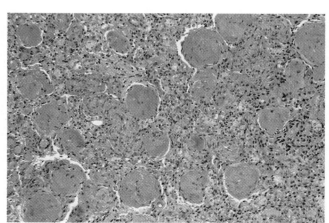

Figure 10–2. Chronic glomerulonephritis/end-stage renal disease. The globally sclerotic glomeruli appear as small sclerotic and hyaline "tombstones" situated quite close to each other because of the severe tubulointerstitial injury/loss.

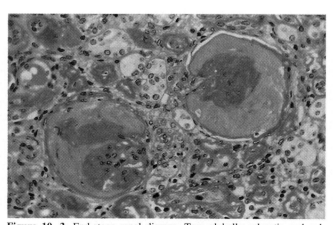

Figure 10–3. End-stage renal disease. Two globally sclerotic and collapsed glomeruli display weakly periodic acid–Schiff (PAS)–positive collagen halos in Bowman's space in an end-stage kidney. The tubules are markedly atrophic; some of the atrophic tubules have thick basement membranes, whereas others are somewhat reminiscent of the tubules of endocrine glands ("endocrine tubules"). These changes are consistent with the changes induced by vascular ischemia (PAS reaction).

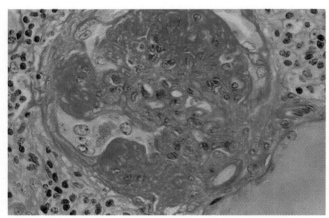

Figure 10–4. End-stage renal disease. The globally sclerotic glomerulus displays hyalinization at the 7-o'clock position. Hyalinization can be seen in globally sclerotic glomeruli irrespective of the etiology of the sclerosis. There appears to be some residual hypercellularity, but this may just be the result of the glomerular collapse and does not necessarily indicate a proliferative glomerulonephritis as the cause of the renal disease (periodic acid–Schiff reaction).

IMMUNOFLUORESCENCE MICROSCOPY

- Immunofluorescence is particularly helpful in diagnosing IgA nephropathy; also, other immune complex–mediated glomerulonephritides can occasionally be diagnosed by positive glomerular fluorescence months or even years after ESRD has developed. However, it should be remembered that globally sclerotic glomeruli (irrespective of cause) often have nonspecific staining for IgM and C3.

ELECTRON MICROSCOPY

- Electron microscopy has limited value in establishing the underlying cause in ESRD. It may be helpful in diagnosing end-stage immune complex–type glomerulonephritis (by detecting electron-dense mesangial, subendothelial, intramembranous, or subepithelial immune-type deposits) if material is not available for immunofluorescence microscopy. However, distinction of "hyalinosis" from discrete electron-dense immune-type deposits may be difficult, and the least involved (sclerotic) glomerulus needs to be studied because hyalinosis usually affects the more sclerotic areas.

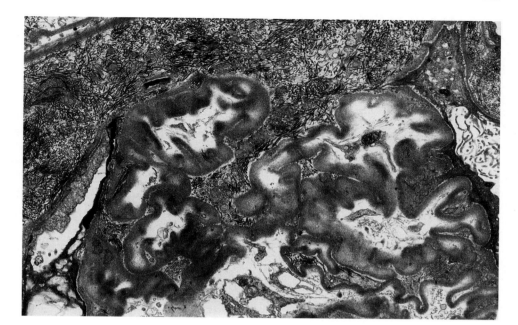

Figure 10–5. Electron micrograph of global glomerulosclerosis. Advanced glomerulosclerosis with collapsed/sclerotic capillary loops and extracapillary collagen deposition is illustrated. At this late stage, the etiology of the process is usually unclear morphologically.

CHANGES IN THE RENAL MEDULLA

- The medullae of end-stage kidneys are usually fibrotic; medullary fibrosis is, however, difficult to evaluate. In some cases the medullary interstitium of end-stage kidneys can be focally composed of smooth muscle.
- Medullary fibrosis resulting in loss of the glycosaminoglycan matrix and possibly loss of medullary interstitial cells has been associated with aging and hypertension.

OXALATE DEPOSITS

- Oxalosis has been found to be more common in the kidneys of hemodialysis patients than in control nondialysis cases and to increase in severity with the duration of dialysis.
- Oxalate crystals can be found in noncystic tubules, within the walls of renal cysts intermixed with cyst epithelium, or embedded in interstitial connective tissue.

COMPLICATIONS

- Acquired polycystic kidney disease and ESRD-associated renal tumors are considered in separate chapters (Chapters 20 and 22, respectively).

References

Hughson MD: End-stage renal disease. In: Jennette JC, Olson JL, Schwartz MM, Silva FG (eds): Heptinstall's Pathology of the Kidney, 5th ed. Philadelphia, Lippincott-Raven, 1998, p. 1371.

Hughson MD, Fox M, Garvin AJ: Pathology of the end-stage kidney after dialysis. Prog Reprod Genitourin Tract Pathol 2:157, 1991.

Meadows R: The obsolescent glomerulus and the disappearance of glomeruli from the kidney. In: Meadows R: Renal Histopathology. Oxford, Oxford University Press, 1978, p 153.

The United States Renal Data System's 1995 Annual Data Report: III. Incidence and causes of treated ESRD. Am J Kidney Dis 26(suppl 2): 39, 1995.

CHAPTER 11

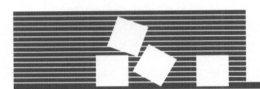

Disorders of the Glomerular Basement Membrane
Alport's Syndrome, Nail-Patella Syndrome, and Thin-Basement-Membrane Disease

ALPORT'S SYNDROME

Synonyms and Related Terms: Progressive hereditary nephritis.

Biology of Disease

- Alport's syndrome is an inherited abnormality of collagen that in its classic form consists of progressive renal insufficiency terminating in renal failure, neurosensory deafness, and various ocular disturbances. The incidence is approximately 1 in 5,000 individuals.
- The majority of cases are caused by a mutation of the gene for the $\alpha5$ chain of type IV collagen, designated *COL4A5,* which is located on the long arm of the X chromosome (Xq22). Collagen IV, the major collagen in basement membranes, makes up about 50% of the basement membrane's dry weight.
- Abnormalities in the $\alpha5$ chain result in abnormal biosynthesis, secretion, or degradation of other basement membrane constituents. However, the exact mechanisms by which abnormalities in collagen IV result in progressive nephropathy and deafness are not known.
- Inheritance is sex linked in the majority of cases (approximately 85%); a smaller number of cases with the clinical features of Alport's syndrome appear to be transmitted in either autosomal recessive or autosomal dominant fashion. Autosomal recessive variants of Alport's syndrome can arise from mutations in either the *COL4A3* or *COL4A4* gene; the genetic basis of the autosomal dominant form of Alport's syndrome is unclear.
- Interestingly, the anti–glomerular basement membrane (GBM) antibodies found in patients with Goodpasture's syndrome usually fail to react with the GBMs of patients with Alport's syndrome. After renal transplantation, anti-GBM antibody will develop in a proportion of patients with Alport's syndrome; fortunately, it is uncommon to lose the transplant because of anti-GBM antibody disease (approximately 5% of cases).

Clinical Features

- Males are usually affected more often, more severely, and earlier than females, who are usually heterozygous for the mutation and have mosaic expression of the altered gene product. End-stage renal failure develops in virtually all affected males; end-stage renal disease is rare in females but does occur. Only mild abnormalities in renal function develop in the majority of affected women, and approximately 10% to 15% of obligate carriers never have clinical evidence of renal disease.
- There may be no family history of the disease because of the occurrence of new mutations, lack of clinical disease in female carriers, and autosomal recessive variants.
- Affected males have persistent microscopic hematuria beginning within the first year of life; episodes of gross hematuria may follow upper respiratory tract infections. Women usually have intermittent microscopic hematuria.
- Proteinuria is also common in affected males. It is usually absent during the first few years but becomes progressively worse with age; the full nephrotic syndrome develops in approximately 30% to 40% of patients.
- Decreased creatinine clearance is usually demonstrable by the second decade of life in males and is associated with proteinuria and hypertension.
- Sensorineural deafness is the second most common manifestation of Alport's syndrome. Hearing is normal at birth, but high-frequency hearing loss usually begins in affected males by 15 years of age; hearing loss is uncommon in females. In its early stages the hearing deficit can be detected only by audiometry. In some families, progressive renal disease occurs without deaf-

ness; thus deafness is not required for the diagnosis of progressive hereditary nephritis.

- Ocular defects occur in 15% to 30% of patients with Alport's syndrome. A variety of abnormalities can occur, the most characteristic of which is *anterior lenticonus*, or conical protrusion of the central portion of the lens into the anterior chamber. Pigmentary changes in the retina such as whitish or yellowish granulations around the foveal area are also common.
- Other abnormalities reported in a few families with Alport's syndrome include platelet and granulocyte anomalies and diffuse leiomyomatosis of the upper gastrointestinal tract and tracheobronchial tree.

Laboratory Values

- Urinalysis shows variable degrees of hematuria and proteinuria.
- Serum creatinine and urea nitrogen values are elevated.
- The usual serologic tests for systemic lupus erythematosus and other "connective tissue" or "collagen vascular" diseases are negative, and serum complement levels are normal.

Light Microscopy

The light microscopic changes in progressive hereditary nephritis are nonspecific, and hereditary nephritis can resemble a primary glomerular, tubular, interstitial, or vascular disease by light microscopy. Electron microscopy is required to establish the diagnosis.

Glomeruli

- The earliest changes consist of mild mesangial expansion, focal mesangial hypercellularity, and thickening of Bowman's capsule.
- Later changes include segmental to global mesangial expansion and hypercellularity, capillary wall thickening, and globally sclerotic glomeruli. Capillary walls may appear split on silver stains.
- Eventually, segmental sclerosis and hyalinosis become widespread, capillary walls are diffusely thickened with GBM duplication on silver stains, and numerous obsolescent glomeruli are present.
- So-called fetal glomeruli, which are smaller and contain fewer capillary loops than do normal glomeruli, may be present on biopsy in young males; fetal glomeruli are not usually seen in older patients.

Tubules

- Tubules may have protein resorption droplets in epithelial cells and contain occasional erythrocyte casts; otherwise, they appear unremarkable on biopsy early in the course of the disease. Later biopsies show tubular atrophy.

Interstitium

- The most characteristic interstitial change is the presence of cells with vacuolated or bubbly appearing cytoplasm, designated *interstitial foam cells*. These cells may be more prominent near the corticomedullary junction.
- Interstitial foam cells were once thought to be pathognomonic of Alport's syndrome; it is now clear that foam cells can be seen in other conditions, particularly in patients with nephrotic syndrome. The presence of interstitial foam cells in *nonnephrotic* patients should alert pathologists to carefully consider hereditary nephritis in their differential diagnostic list.
- Scattered areas of interstitial fibrosis and inflammation are early biopsy findings and become progressively more generalized and severe as the disease progresses.

Vessels

- Vessels demonstrate the usual changes seen with progressive renal disease.

Immunofluorescence Microscopy

- Findings on immunofluorescence microscopy are usually minor and nonspecific; many biopsies are entirely negative.
- Granular deposits of IgM and C3 may be present within the glomerular mesangium and capillary walls. IgM and C3 are frequently present in sclerotic areas and represent leakage of plasma proteins into damaged segments of the glomeruli.

Electron Microscopy

- The typical change in males consists of diffuse, widespread irregularities in the glomerular capillary basement membranes, with variation in thickness and alterations in the appearance of the lamina densa.
- The lamina densa consists of strands of electron-dense material enclosing electron-lucent zones, which gives it a multilayered, laminated, "splintered," or "basket-weave" appearance. The lucent zones may appear clear or may contain finely granular material.
- The GBM varies in thickness, with thin and thick segments on the same or adjacent capillary loops. Basement membrane thickness may be increased threefold to fivefold over normal thickness.
- Discontinuities in the GBM that allow the outer surface of capillary endothelial cells and inner surface of visceral epithelial cells to become contiguous are often present.
- The GBMs in women and young boys often show diffuse thinning, without the thickening and basket-weave appearance seen in men. This difference suggests that diffuse attenuation of the GBM may be the initial change in Alport's syndrome, with thickening and multilayering occurring later.
- Simplification and effacement of visceral epithelial cell foot processes may be present.
- The mesangium initially appears unremarkable; later, mesangial expansion and increased mesangial cellularity are seen.
- Tubular basement membranes (TBMs) and Bowman's capsule may show thickening and multilayering similar to that seen in GBMs.

Immunohistochemistry

- Immunohistochemical analysis of type IV collagen in skin and renal basement membranes can confirm the diagnosis of Alport's syndrome when other features are equivocal and assist in determining the mode of inheritance.
- Absence of epidermal basement membrane staining for α5(IV) or absence of basement membrane staining for α3, α4, and α5(IV) in renal tubules and glomerular capillaries is diagnostic of X-linked Alport's syndrome.
- Autosomal recessive Alport's syndrome is characterized by absent GBM staining for α3, α4, and α5(IV); absent TBM and Bowman's capsule staining for α3(IV) and α4(IV); and preserved TBM and Bowman's capsule staining for α5(IV).

Differential Diagnosis

- The characteristic GBM changes in Alport's syndrome are not absolutely specific, although they tend to be much more diffuse and widespread in Alport's syndrome than in other conditions. Foci of GBM splitting may also be seen in postinfectious glomerulonephritis, focal segmental glomerulosclerosis, IgA nephropathy, and membranoproliferative glomerulonephritis associated with the nephrotic syndrome, etc. A careful family history, audiometric and ophthalmologic examinations, and follow-up for proteinuria or progressive renal insufficiency may help distinguish Alport's syndrome from these other conditions in cases in which the morphologic changes are equivocal.
- Widespread thinning of the GBM, characteristically associated with benign familial hematuria, occurs in some families with Alport's syndrome.

Treatment and Clinical Course

- The course is usually one of progressive deterioration.

Renal failure in affected males usually develops during the second to fifth decades of life. The rate at which renal failure develops is highly variable between different families, presumably because of different mutations in the COL4A5 gene, but progression occurs at a relatively constant rate within most families.
- Nephrotic-range proteinuria at diagnosis is considered an adverse prognostic indicator.
- There is no treatment for Alport's syndrome, except renal transplantation.
- Many patients with Alport's syndrome lack the basement membrane component against which the antibody in Goodpasture's syndrome (anti-GBM antibody disease) is directed. The normal antigen present in transplanted kidneys is therefore seen as foreign by the immune system, and an antibody to the "foreign" antigen may develop. Anti-GBM antibodies are reported to occur in up to 30% of patients after renal transplantation. However, actual glomerulonephritis occurs in only 3% to 4% of patients with Alport's syndrome overall, perhaps 5% to 7% of males. Patients with large deletions in the COL4A5 gene appear to have a higher incidence of posttransplant glomerulonephritis than do patients with the more common missense mutations.
- Posttransplant glomerulonephritis appears to be very unlikely in patients with Alport's syndrome who are not deaf and in those in whom end-stage renal disease develops after the age of 30 to 35 years. Patients in whom posttransplant anti-GBM disease develops have a high incidence of recurrence in subsequent transplants; relatives of patients who had posttransplant anti-GBM disease may have an increased chance of development of the same complication.
- Posttransplant glomerulonephritis in patients with Alport's syndrome usually results in loss of the graft. However, it appears that overall graft survival in patients with Alport's syndrome is equivalent to that in patients without Alport's syndrome.

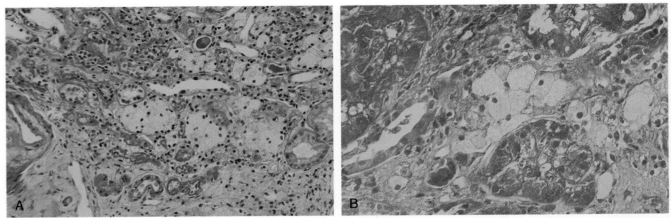

Figure 11–1. *A* and *B*, Interstitial foam cells. Foam cells in the tubulointerstitium can be seen in practically every renal disease (especially if the patient has nephrotic syndrome with hyperlipidemia/hyperlipiduria). However, if foam cells are seen in a patient without nephrotic syndrome, Alport's syndrome should be suspected (*A*, PAS reaction; *B*, Masson's trichrome stain).

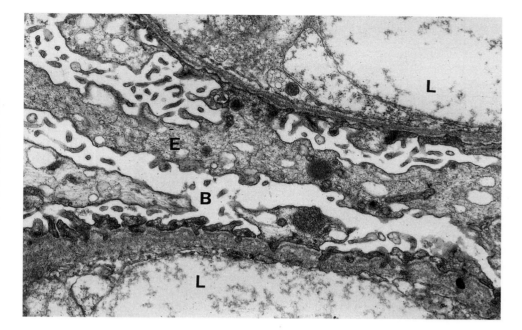

Figure 11–2. Electron micrograph of a kidney with Alport's hereditary nephropathy. The glomerular capillary basement membranes show splitting, splintering, a basket-weave appearance, lamination, and thinning. The changes must be diffuse to make the diagnosis of Alport's (hereditary nephropathy) syndrome (L, glomerular capillary lumen; E, visceral epithelial cell; B, Bowman's space).

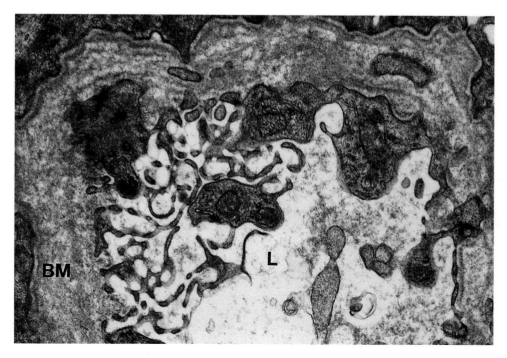

Figure 11–3. Electron micrograph of a kidney with Alport's hereditary nephropathy. Lamination and thickening of the glomerular capillary basement membrane (BM) is seen (L, glomerular capillary lumen).

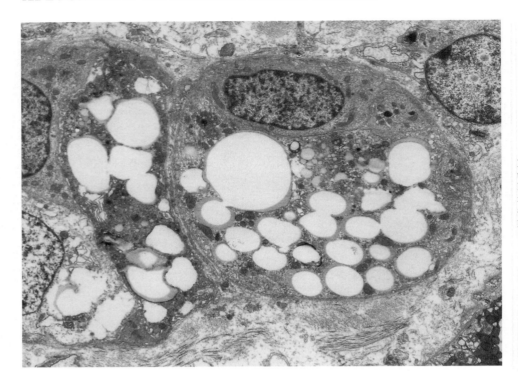

Figure 11–4. Electron micrograph of tubulointerstitial "foam" cells. These lipid-laden cells are commonly seen in patients with nephrotic syndrome and in patients with hereditary Alport's syndrome.

NAIL-PATELLA SYNDROME

Synonyms and Related Terms: Hereditary osteo-onychodysplasia; HOOD.

Biology of Disease

- The nail-patella syndrome (NPS) is an inherited disorder characterized by dysplasia of the nail beds, hypoplasia or complete absence of the patellae, deformation or subluxation of the head of the radius, abnormalities in the pelvis (iliac "horns"), and GBM abnormalities.
- Nail-patella syndrome has an autosomal dominant mode of inheritance and has been linked to the long arm of chromosome 9 (9q34), near the locus of the genes for the ABO blood group system. It may be related to abnormalities in the α1 chain of collagen type V; the *COL5A1* gene, which codes for the pro-α1(V) chain, has also been linked to 9q34.
- Nail-patella syndrome is uncommon and occurs in approximately 22 persons per million.
- Clinical evidence of renal disease is relatively uncommon in NPS; more than half of the patients have no signs or symptoms of renal disease. The characteristic ultrastructural abnormalities in the GBM are present in patients with no clinical evidence of renal disease; the degree of ultrastructural change correlates poorly with clinical manifestations of renal disease.

Clinical Features

- The most common manifestations of renal disease are proteinuria, which may reach nephrotic levels, microhematuria, edema, and hypertension.
- Nail abnormalities, the most common manifestation, occur in at least 80% to 90% of patients. A variety of changes occur; fingernails are involved more frequently than toenails.
- The iliac crests are flared, with prominent anterior and posterior iliac spines (iliac "horns") in approximately 80% of patients. Abnormalities of the patellae are present in about 60%; abnormalities in the elbow joints are less frequent.

Laboratory Values

- No laboratory results are pathognomonic in NPS.

Gross Appearance

- A variety of urinary tract abnormalities have been described in NPS, including unilateral renal hypoplasia and atrophy and calyceal dilatation associated with scarring in the upper and lower poles.

Light Microscopy

The light microscopic appearance is nonspecific; ultrastructural examination is required for diagnosis.

- Glomeruli usually appear normal in patients without clinical evidence of renal disease. There may be mild thickening of the GBM, as well as global or segmental glomerulosclerosis.
- Tubules may show protein resorption droplets and variable degrees of atrophy.
- Interstitial fibrosis and chronic inflammation may be present.

Immunofluorescence Microscopy

- Immunofluorescence is entirely negative in most cases. Staining for IgM, C3, and C1q in various combinations may be present in sclerotic areas of glomeruli.

Electron Microscopy

- Glomerular basement membranes vary in thickness from normal to increased.
- The mottled, electron-lucent areas present throughout the GBM result in a "moth-eaten" appearance. These areas are more prominent in the thickened segments of the GBM.
- Similar lucent areas may be present in the glomerular mesangium; the mesangial matrix is expanded.
- The lucent zones in the GBM contain coarse fibrils with the appearance of cross-banded collagen. These zones may not be visualized on routine heavy metal stains; phosphotungstic acid staining may be required to demonstrate the fibrils and should be performed if the standard preparation is not completely characteristic of the disease.
- Nonspecific glomerular changes such as simplification of visceral epithelial cell foot processes may be present.
- Tubular basement membranes do not show the "moth-eaten" appearance seen in GBMs.

Treatment and Clinical Course

- Renal disease is usually mild in those patients in whom it occurs. However, end-stage renal failure develops in approximately 10% of cases.
- There is no treatment for the renal disease associated with NPS. Dialysis or renal transplantation is required for the minority of patients in whom end-stage renal failure develops.

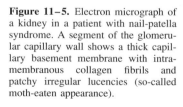
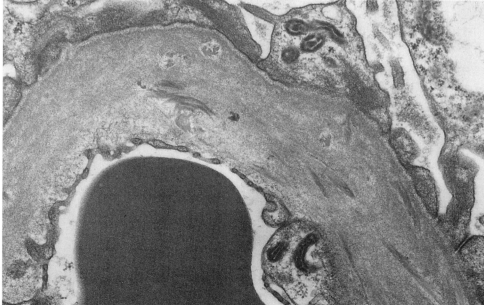

Figure 11–5. Electron micrograph of a kidney in a patient with nail-patella syndrome. A segment of the glomerular capillary wall shows a thick capillary basement membrane with intramembranous collagen fibrils and patchy irregular lucencies (so-called moth-eaten appearance).

THIN-BASEMENT-MEMBRANE NEPHROPATHY

Synonyms and Related Terms: Thin-basement-membrane disease; benign familial hematuria; benign familial nephritis.

Biology of Disease

- The terms *benign familial hematuria* and *thin-basement-membrane disease* have been applied to a group of patients with isolated microscopic hematuria who have no significant abnormalities on pathologic examination except GBM thinning and are thought to have a generally benign course.
- Both familial and sporadic forms occur; inheritance appears to follow an autosomal dominant pattern in the familial cases.
- The etiology of thin-basement-membrane nephropathy is unknown; the category may contain a heterogeneous group of conditions with different causes.
- The finding of thinning of the GBM does not guarantee a benign clinical outcome; some patients with GBM thinning follow a progressive course, with eventual development of end-stage renal failure. In some cases, thinning of the GBM may be the only finding in the workup of patients who are later found to have Alport's syndrome. In addition, thinning of the GBM may be found in other conditions such as IgA nephropathy and mesangial proliferative glomerulonephritis.
- Some families with the clinical appearance of benign familial hematuria may have normal GBM thickness.

Clinical Features

- The typical finding is microscopic hematuria, which usually begins in childhood. Hematuria is usually persistent, but it may be intermittent. Patients with episodic gross hematuria have been described, but some of them were not studied with all modern modalities and may have had another disease process such as IgA nephropathy.
- There is usually *no* or only minimal proteinuria. Proteinuria has been reported in some families but should suggest an alternative and usually more ominous diagnosis.
- The clinical features of Alport's syndrome and NPS are absent.

Laboratory Values

- Renal function (measured by serum creatinine) is normal; serum complement levels are normal, and serologic studies for autoimmune diseases are negative.

Light Microscopy

- Light microscopy is normal, with the exception of occasional erythrocytes in Bowman's space or tubular lumina.

Immunofluorescence Microscopy

- Immunofluorescence microscopy is usually negative. Small amounts of immunoglobulins or complement have been described along GBMs.

Electron Microscopy

- The characteristic finding is *widespread thinning* of the glomerular capillary basement membranes. The GBM contours are usually smooth but may be slightly irregular; some capillary loops may have GBMs with normal thickness.
- There is no single, universally accepted standard for normal GBM thickness. Glomerular capillary basement membrane thickness varies with age (usually showing a gradual increase in thickness), sex, and different methods of tissue fixation and embedding. Suggested cutoff values for adults vary from 250 to 330 nm.
- Ideally, each laboratory should establish its own means and standard deviations for different sexes and ages (as described by Dische).
- Thickness should be measured on each of several loops from at least two or more glomeruli. The usual method is to measure the right-angle distance from the outer surface of the endothelial cell to the inner surface of the overlying visceral epithelial cell on photographs of known magnification.
- The diagnosis of thin-basement-membrane nephropathy should be made very cautiously, if at all, in pediatric patients.
- Measurement of lamina densa thickness has been suggested as an alternative to measuring total GBM thickness. However, the inner and outer margins of the lamina densa may not be sufficiently well defined for accurate and reproducible measurement.

Treatment and Clinical Course

- The clinical course is generally thought to be benign, and no treatment is required. However, occasional patients initially having thin GBMs as the main morphologic change are later found to have Alport's syndrome.

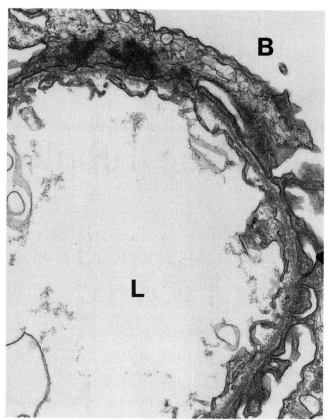

Figure 11–6. Electron micrograph of thin-basement-membrane disease in a patient with "benign" essential isolated hematuria. The picture shows a glomerular capillary loop with a very uniformly thin basement membrane; the average thickness of the membrane was 152 nm in this 8-year-old patient (normal is approximately 260 nm). Thinning of the basement membrane needs to be diffuse in order to make the diagnosis of thin-basement-membrane disease (B, Bowman's space; L, glomerular capillary lumen).

References

General

Bodziak K, Hammond WS, Molitoris BA: Inherited disorders of the glomerular basement membrane. Am J Kidney Dis 23:605, 1994.

Kashtan CE, Sibley RK, Michael AF, et al: Hereditary nephritis: Alport syndrome and thin glomerular basement membrane disease. In: Tisher CC, Brenner BM (eds): Renal Pathology: With Clinical and Functional Correlations, 2nd ed. Philadelphia, JB Lippincott, 1994, p 1239.

Alport's Syndrome

Bernstein J: The glomerular basement membrane abnormality in Alport's syndrome. Am J Kidney Dis 10:222, 1987.

Kashtan CE: Alport syndrome. Kidney Int 51(suppl 58):69, 1997.

Kashtan CE, Michael AF: Alport syndrome: From bedside to genome to bedside. Am J Kidney Dis 22:627, 1993.

Nail-Patella Syndrome

Cohen AH, Adler SG: Nail-patella syndrome (osteo-onychodysplasia), lipodystrophy, Fabry disease (angiokeratoma corporis diffusum universale), and familial lecithin-cholesterol acyltransferase deficiency. In: Tisher CC, Brenner BM (eds): Renal Pathology: With Clinical and Functional Correlations, 2nd ed. Philadelphia, JB Lippincott, 1994, p 1267.

Thin-Basement-Membrane Nephropathy

Aarons I, Smith PS, Davies RA, et al: Thin membrane nephropathy: A clinico-pathological study. Clin Nephrol 32:151, 1989.

Cosio FG, Falkenhain ME, Sedmak DD: Association of thin glomerular basement membrane with other glomerulopathies. Kidney Int 46:471, 1994.

Dische FE: Measurement of glomerular basement membrane thickness and its application to the diagnosis of thin-membrane nephropathy. Arch Pathol Lab Med 116:43, 1992.

Tina L, Jenis E, Jose P, et al: The glomerular basement membrane in benign familial hematuria. Clin Nephrol 17:1, 1982.

CHAPTER 12

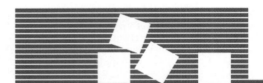

Disorders of the Tubules

ACUTE TUBULAR NECROSIS: ISCHEMIC ACUTE TUBULAR NEPHROPATHY AND TOXIC RENAL INJURY

Synonyms and Related Terms: Acute vasomotor nephropathy; shock kidney; ischemic acute tubular necrosis; acute tubular nephrosis.

Introduction

- Acute tubular necrosis is seen in two main situations: renal ischemia *(ischemic acute tubular nephropathy)* and toxic injury to the kidney. Ischemic acute tubular nephropathy is by far the more common type, and the majority of this discussion will refer to that type. Toxic acute tubular necrosis will be discussed separately.
- The term *acute tubular necrosis* is frequently a misnomer because true necrosis of the tubules is seldom marked and often not seen at all. Actual necrosis of tubules is most often seen in toxic renal injury and is uncommon in ischemic injury.

Ischemic Acute Tubular Nephropathy

Biology of Disease

- Ischemic acute tubular nephropathy, or acute vasomotor nephropathy, is seen in a variety of conditions that result in decreased renal perfusion (Table 12–1). Many but not all of these conditions are associated with hypovolemia and shock.
- Common conditions associated with ischemic acute tubular nephropathy include complications of surgery, sepsis or other infections, intravascular hemolysis, trauma, and obstetric complications.
- The histologic features of ischemic acute tubular nephropathy from any of these causes are similar.
- Ischemic acute tubular nephropathy may follow a prolonged period of prerenal azotemia. In prerenal azotemia some normal tubular function is retained; the ability to concentrate urine is maintained and the fractional excretion of sodium is low. Recovery of renal function

is rapid after correction of the condition causing the prerenal state. In contrast, in ischemic acute tubular nephropathy, the ability to concentrate urine is lost (the urine is isosthenuric or hyposthenuric when compared with serum), the urine sodium concentration is high, and recovery of renal function may take a prolonged period.
- The pathogenesis of ischemic acute tubular nephropathy is not well understood. The major postulated mechanisms are tubular dysfunction and backleak of filtered compounds through the disrupted tubular epithelium and tubular basement membrane into the interstitium, tubular obstruction by casts, and intrarenal vasoconstriction with decreased glomerular filtration pressure, possibly via tubuloglomerular feedback at the level of the macula densa. These mechanisms are not mutually exclusive, and more than one may be involved in many cases.

Clinical Features

- Ischemic acute tubular nephropathy is one of the most common causes of acute renal failure.
- Many but not all patients have a history of a precipitating event, which may precede the onset of renal failure by several days to approximately 1 week.
- The onset of ischemic acute tubular necrosis is frequently signaled by oliguria (<400 mL of urine per day), although nonoliguric renal failure occurs in as many as half of cases.

Laboratory Values

- Serum urea nitrogen and creatinine concentrations become elevated.
- Urinalysis generally shows proteinuria, usually nonselective. Significant hematuria is unusual. Casts, both hyaline and granular, may be present.
- The urine is dilute (isosthenuric or hyposthenuric relative to serum).
- The urine sodium content and fractional excretion of sodium are high.

Table 12–1
CAUSES OF ACUTE TUBULAR NECROSIS

Ischemic Acute Tubular Nephropathy	Toxic Acute Tubular Necrosis
Surgical procedures	Mercury (mercuric chloride)
Extensive trauma or burns	Carbon tetrachloride and other organic
Pancreatitis	solvents
Hemolytic transfusion reaction	Arsenic
Septicemia	Chromium
Rhabdomyolysis	Phosphorus
Obstetric accidents	Potassium dichromate
Heat stroke	Uranyl nitrate
	Ethylene glycol
	Antibiotics: aminoglycosides, amphotericin B, cephalosporins
	Nonsteroidal anti-inflammatory drugs
	Radiographic contrast material
	Anesthetics: methoxyflurane, halothane
	Cisplatin, other chemotherapy agents
	Insecticides

Gross Pathology

- The kidneys are enlarged, often tense, and may appear pale.
- On section, the parenchyma appears to bulge out of the capsule.
- The cortex is widened and appears pale, with exaggeration of the corticomedullary distinction.
- The medulla appears dark.

Light Microscopy

Glomeruli

- Glomerular changes are usually minimal. The capillary tuft may appear bloodless and contracted, and the urinary space may seem to be expanded.
- The parietal epithelial cells of Bowman's capsule may become tall and cuboidal, described as *tubularization*.

Tubules

- Necrosis of individual tubular epithelial cells, irregular spacing, and a decreased number of epithelial cell nuclei may be seen. *Extensive* necrosis of epithelial cells does *not* occur.
- Proximal convoluted tubules appear dilated, with flattening of the cells and attenuation of the periodic acid–Schiff (PAS)-positive brush border; thus they may resemble distal tubules (*distalization*). Lumina may contain eosinophilic debris, but true casts do not form in proximal convoluted tubules.
- Distal tubules are dilated, and epithelial cells become flattened.
- The cytoplasm of tubular cells may become basophilic; nuclei may become hyperchromatic or have prominent nucleoli. Mitotic figures may be present.
- Casts are often present in distal tubules. The majority of casts are usually hyaline and stain positively with PAS stain, but granular, pigmented, or nonpigmented casts may also be seen.

- Tubular lumina may contain sloughed epithelial cells, leukocytes, and cellular debris.
- Peritubular granulomas may occasionally be seen and might be a reaction to extruded casts.

Interstitium

- Interstitial edema is present with separation of tubules. The edema appears pale and loose on hematoxylin and eosin (H & E) and trichrome stains, in contrast to the dense, darker appearance of interstitial fibrosis.
- Lymphocytes and other mononuclear cells are present but are usually scant. Inflammatory cells may form rings or cluster around ruptured tubules. An extensive interstitial inflammatory infiltrate suggests acute interstitial nephritis rather than acute tubular necrosis.

Vessels

- The most prominent vascular change is the presence of numerous nucleated cells in the vasa recta of the medulla. These nucleated cells were classically described as hematopoietic precursor cells, but more recent studies suggest that nucleated erythroid precursors are not present.

Immunofluorescence Microscopy

- Staining for immunoglobulins and complement components is usually negative.
- Weak staining for fibrin/fibrinogen may be present in the interstitium or around tubules.

Electron Microscopy

- Glomeruli characteristically show minimal changes.
- Tubules show simplification of luminal cell surfaces, with loss of the brush border in proximal tubular epithelial cells. The basolateral interdigitations become simplified. Apical membrane "blebbing" may be seen early.
- Tubular cells may show cytoplasmic vacuolization, mitochondrial changes, and globular electron-dense inclusions possibly representing lipofuscin granules.
- Small gaps present in the tubular epithelial lining represent loss of individual cells, a finding described as the *nonreplacement phenomenon*.

Toxic Acute Tubular Necrosis

- Toxic acute tubular necrosis is now uncommon. Poisoning with heavy metals such as mercuric chloride or arsenicals or with organic compounds such as carbon tetrachloride were common causes in the past but are now rare.
- The majority of cases currently seen are associated with drugs such as aminoglycoside antibiotics (gentamicin and others).
- The most likely mechanism is direct toxicity against the tubular epithelium.
- Most toxins primarily affect the proximal part of the nephron (proximal tubules), in contrast to ischemic in-

128 ■ DISORDERS OF THE TUBULES

jury, which causes patchy changes or may preferentially involve the thick ascending limb of Henle.
- The clinical features and pathologic appearance of toxic acute tubular necrosis have many similarities with ischemic acute tubular necrosis (nephropathy).
- Poisoning with such compounds as mercuric chloride may be associated with obvious and extensive tubular necrosis. Cases caused by aminoglycoside toxicity, however, are often associated with much more subtle histologic changes and thus may closely resemble ischemic acute tubular nephropathy.

Treatment and Clinical Course

- No specific treatment is known for acute tubular necrosis once it is established.
- Restoration of renal perfusion during the prerenal azotemia phase of renal ischemia may prevent the development of ischemic acute tubular necrosis; however, once the stage of ischemic acute tubular necrosis is reached, treatment is supportive.
- Patients may now be supported for a prolonged time with peritoneal dialysis or hemodialysis in anticipation of recovery of normal renal function. Thus survival in acute renal failure depends on the involvement of other systems and other complications rather than the renal failure itself. Sepsis is the most common cause of death, followed by respiratory failure.

- The period of renal failure generally lasts 1 to 2 weeks. The likelihood of recovery diminishes after 4 to 6 weeks; however, recovery of renal function has been reported after periods as long as 11 months.
- Adverse indicators for recovery of renal function include severe oliguria, a prolonged period of renal failure, failure of multiple organ systems, and advanced age.

Differential Diagnosis

- The clinical differential diagnosis of acute tubular necrosis includes all causes of acute renal failure, including acute interstitial nephritis, severe acute glomerulonephritis, bilateral renal cortical necrosis, urinary tract obstruction, and others.
- By convention, the presence of glomerulonephritis excludes a diagnosis of acute tubular necrosis; in such cases the diagnosis of glomerulonephritis takes precedence.
- An important histologic differential is that between acute interstitial nephritis and acute tubular necrosis. Because there is overlap in the histologic picture of the two conditions, differentiation on pathologic grounds alone can be difficult or impossible.
- The presence of extensive or intense interstitial inflammation would favor acute interstitial nephritis over acute tubular necrosis.
- The presence of numerous neutrophils would favor acute pyelonephritis over acute tubular necrosis.

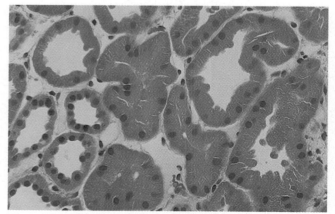

Figure 12-1. Tubules, normal. The proximal convoluted tubular epithelial cells are more eosinophilic and larger than the distal tubules.

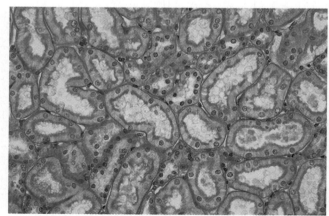

Figure 12-2. Tubules, normal. Periodic acid–Schiff reaction depicts the brush border of the proximal tubules.

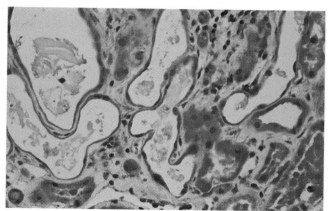

Figure 12-3. Acute tubular necrosis. Frank tubular epithelial coagulative necrosis is seen in biopsy tissue with small early renal cortical infarction. The outline of the necrotic tubular epithelial cells is still recognizable; however, no nuclear staining is seen in these tubules.

Figure 12-6. Acute tubular necrosis (ATN). Many tubules are lined by quite flattened epithelial cells, and the lumina appear to be dilated. It is difficult with severe degeneration/regeneration of the tubules to distinguish proximal from distal tubules by standard histologic examination. This is a typical pattern of ischemic ATN. (It is thought to represent a regeneration-recovery phase.)

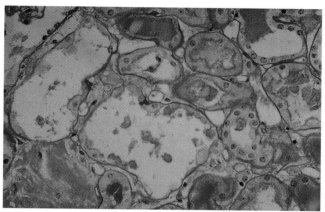

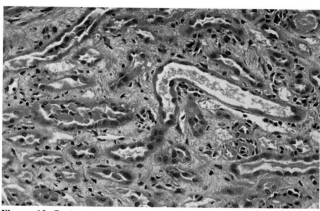

Figure 12-4. Acute tubular necrosis. Frank tubular necrosis is seen in two tubules. Many of the tubular epithelial cells are missing, whereas others appear necrotic/flattened; no nuclear staining is present in the necrotic cells. Note that the tubular basement membranes are often denuded of epithelium.

Figure 12-7. Acute tubular necrosis. The photograph displays flattening of the tubular epithelial cells, interstitial edema, interstitial inflammatory cell infiltrate, and a granular cast in one of the tubules (regeneration-recovery phase).

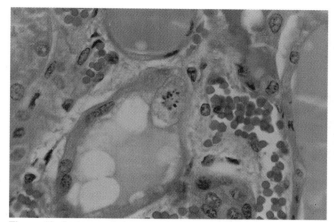

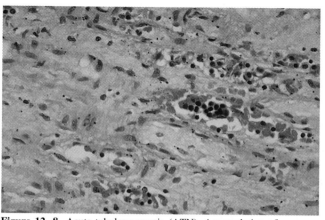

Figure 12-5. Acute tubular necrosis. The mitotic figure in the tubular epithelial cell is thought to be an indication of ongoing regeneration.

Figure 12-8. Acute tubular necrosis (ATN). Accumulation of mononuclear cells in the medullary vasa recta is frequently seen in ATN. This mononuclear cell accumulation is a good sign to distinguish ATN from postmortem autolysis in autopsy kidneys. These cells are now thought to be myeloid rather than of the erythroid series and thought to be adherent to the activated endothelial cells.

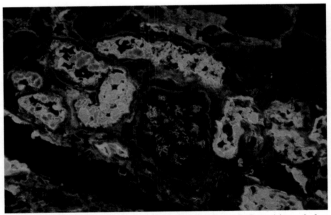

Figure 12–9. Acute tubular necrosis (ATN). These IgG-positive tubular casts in a patient with ATN might represent nonspecific nonimmunologic staining because necrotic debris has a tendency to bind antibodies nonspecifically.

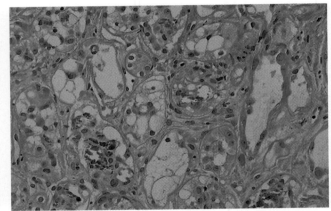

Figure 12–10. Acute tubular necrosis. Severe tubular cell vacuolization is seen in a patient who was poisoned with antifreeze (ethylene glycol).

OTHER TUBULAR ABNORMALITIES

"Hyaline" Change

- Hyaline change is caused by protein resorption droplets occurring in proximal convoluted tubular epithelial cells as a result of increased protein loss by glomeruli.
- The droplets stain eosinophilic on H & E stains and are PAS positive and silver positive on silver stains.
- On immunofluorescence microscopy, the droplets may stain for albumin, complement components (especially C3), fibrinogen, and occasionally other proteins.

Hydropic Change ("Osmotic Nephrosis")

- Hydropic change appears as a vacuolar clearing of the cytoplasm of proximal tubular epithelial cells.
- Osmotic nephrosis may be seen after the administration of hyperosmolar solutions such as hypertonic sucrose, mannitol, high-molecular-weight dextrans, or radiopaque contrast materials.

Hemosiderin in Renal Tubular Epithelium

- Hemosiderin in renal tubular epithelium can be seen in a variety of conditions leading to intravascular hemolysis such as red cell destruction by mechanical heart valves.
- This condition can be confirmed on histologic section by using a stain for iron such as Prussian blue stain.
- To detect iron in shed tubular epithelial cells, iron stain on urine is performed as a diagnostic test for intravascular hemolysis ("urine hemosiderin").
- Hemosiderin in renal tubular epithelium may appear severe but is usually associated with little or no obvious functional tubular injury.

Hypokalemic Nephrosis

- Hypokalemic nephrosis appears as large vacuoles in the cytoplasm of distal tubular epithelial cells.
- It is caused by chronic, long-standing hypokalemia, such as in patients with chronic laxative abuse.
- Hypokalemic nephrosis has been thought in the past to cause chronic interstitial fibrosis, although most experts currently believe that such complications are extremely rare if they occur at all.

Tubular Atrophy

- Tubular atrophy can result from a broad variety of conditions, including glomerulonephritis with scarring, vascular disease, chronic interstitial nephritis, and many others.
- Typically, tubular basement membranes are thickened, tubular luminal size is decreased, and the epithelium is simplified.
- Three distinct types of tubular atrophy have been described:
  - Classic or typical tubular atrophy, as just described.
  - "Thyroidization," which is often but not exclusively associated with chronic pyelonephritis.
  - "Endocrine tubules," which are usually seen in chronic ischemia. The epithelial cells are small with clear cytoplasm, and tubular lumina are inapparent.
- Dilated, hypertrophic tubules ("super tubules") may be present, presumably an attempted compensation for lost renal parenchyma.

Miscellaneous

- Numerous additional changes can be seen in the tubules, such as melanin deposition, intranuclear inclusions in lead poisoning, lipid/cholesterol accumulation, foam cell transformation, metastatic lesions, and myoglobin casts.

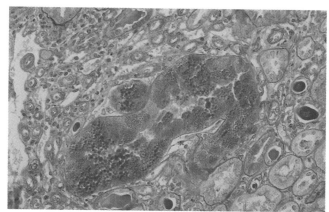

Figure 12–11. Protein resorption droplets ("hyaline" change). Tubular resorption (i.e., salvage) of protein from the abnormal glomerular ultrafiltrate is frequently seen in patients with proteinuria. The resorption droplets present in the proximal tubular epithelial cells are usually phagolysosomes (periodic acid–Schiff reaction).

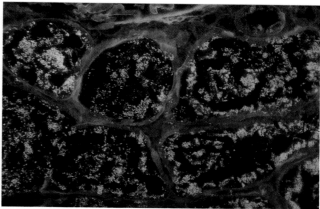

Figure 12–12. Immunofluorescence staining for albumin depicts the presence of albumin in the tubular resorption droplets from a patient with glomerular disease and proteinuria.

Figure 12–13. Electron micrograph of tubular epithelial cell protein resorption droplets. Many electron-dense protein resorption droplets are present in the tubular epithelial cells of this patient with gold therapy–associated membranous glomerulonephropathy. The dense particles (arrow) in one of the tubular epithelial cells are consistent with gold particles (BM, tubular basement membrane).

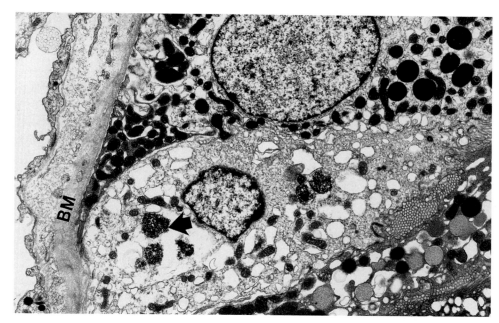

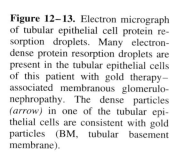

Figure 12–14. Vacuolar or hydropic degeneration ("osmotic nephrosis"). The pale swollen tubular epithelial cells show numerous fine regular vacuoles in the cytoplasm. This change is usually associated with hyperosmotic intravenous infusions but may be seen in other conditions as well (periodic acid–Schiff reaction).

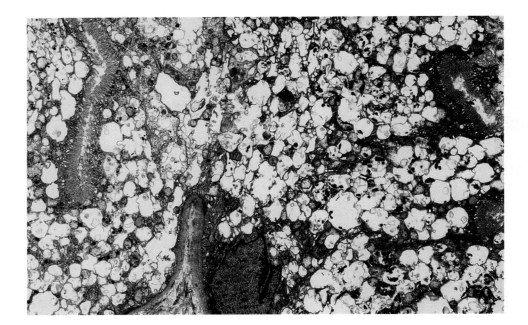

Figure 12–15. Electron micrograph of osmotic nephrosis (hydropic degeneration). The tubular epithelial cells show multiple small vacuoles. Note the well-preserved brush borders at the luminal surface of the proximal tubular epithelial cells.

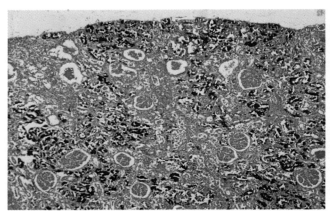

Figure 12–16. Hemosiderin deposition. Tubular deposits of hemosiderin are seen in a patient who had a metallic prosthetic aortic heart valve with severe hemolysis (Prussian blue iron stain).

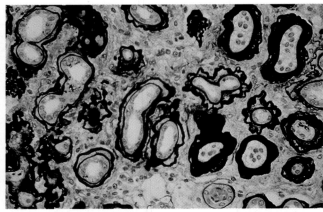

Figure 12–18. Tubular atrophy. Thickening and lamellation of the tubular basement membranes are characteristic features of "classic" tubular atrophy (methenamine silver stain).

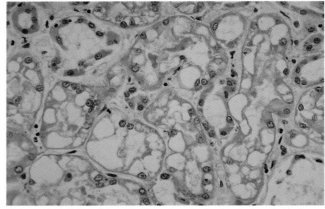

Figure 12–17. Tubular epithelial cell vacuolization in hypokalemic nephropathy. The tubular epithelial cells show large irregular cytoplasmic vacuoles, which is the characteristic morphologic change in patients with extensive prolonged K$^+$ loss (hypokalemia).

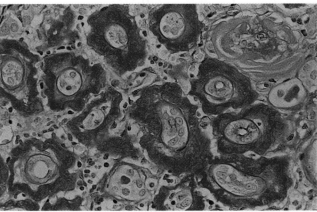

Figure 12–19. Tubular atrophy. Markedly atrophic tubules are smaller than normal, have uniform/simplified epithelium, and show thick periodic acid–Schiff (PAS)-positive basement membranes (PAS reaction).

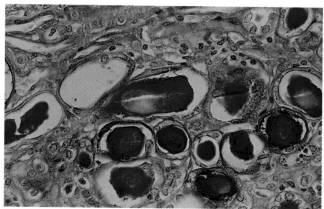

Figure 12–20. Tubular atrophy. Immunohistochemical stain for a distal tubular marker displays the "distal nature" of this "thyroidization-like" atrophy in a patient with end-stage renal disease.

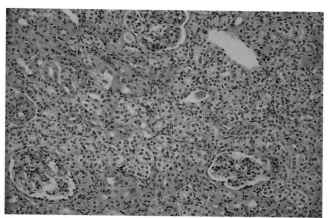

Figure 12–21. Tubular atrophy. The endocrine-type atrophic tubules depicted here are small tubules with pale-staining cytoplasm reminiscent of endocrine glands, hence the designation. The clear cells are actually full of mitochondria. This condition is usually seen in severe vascular disease (ischemia).

Figure 12–22. Electron micrograph of a tubular cast with flattened tubular epithelial lining. Most "non-specific" tubular casts have a slightly granular appearance admixed with some "debris."

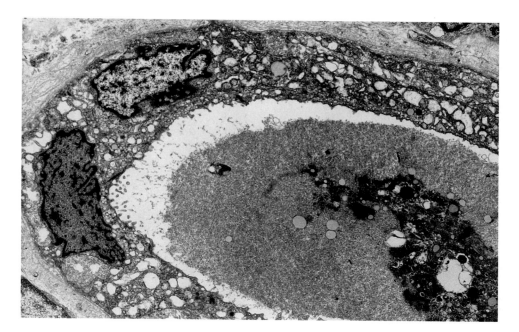

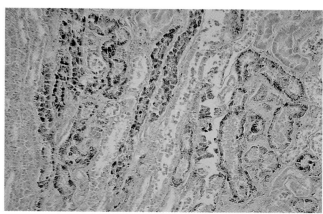

Figure 12–23. Pigment nephropathy. Melanin pigment is seen in the tubular epithelium in this patient with widespread malignant melanoma.

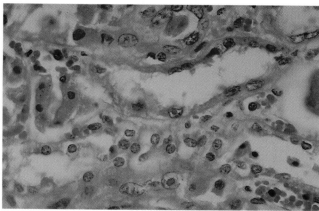

Figure 12–24. Typical intranuclear inclusions seen in a patient with lead poisoning. These red nuclear inclusions can be accentuated with acid-fast staining.

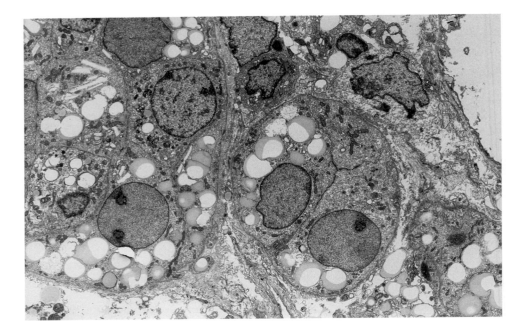

Figure 12–25. Electron micrograph of fatty change and cholesterol deposition in tubular epithelial cells. This change is seen in patients with nephrotic-range proteinuria.

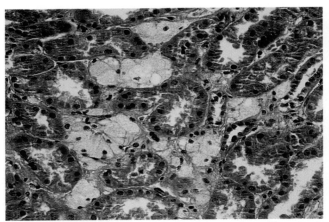

Figure 12–26. Tubulointerstitial foam cells in a patient with nephrotic syndrome. The exact nature of the foam cells is unclear; some of them may originate from tubular epithelial cells, whereas others may be interstitial (macrophagic) in origin (trichrome stain).

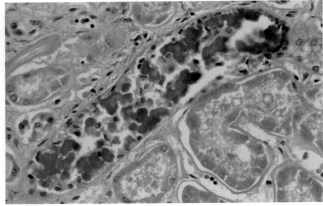

Figure 12–28. Myoglobinuria. A pigmented granular cast in the tubule is seen in a patient with myoglobinuria and acute renal failure.

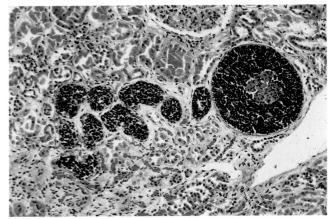

Figure 12–27. Tumor metastasis in the kidney. The metastatic tumor seen filling Bowman's space and a tubular lumen originates from an oat cell carcinoma of the lung.

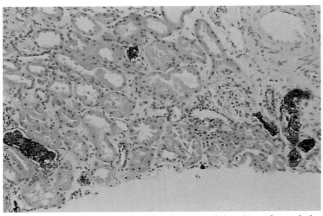

Figure 12–29. Myoglobinuria. The brown staining in a few tubules represents myoglobin positivity (immunoperoxidase, myoglobin).

REFERENCES

Cronin RE, Henrich WL: Toxic nephropathy. In: Brenner BM (ed): Brenner & Rector's The Kidney, 5th ed. Philadelphia, WB Saunders, 1996, p 1680.

Kashgarian M: Acute tubular necrosis and ischemic renal injury. In: Jennette JC, Olson JL, Schwartz MM, Silva FG (eds): Heptinstall's Pathology of the Kidney, 5th ed. Philadelphia, Lippincott-Raven, 1998, p 863.

Kelly CJ, Neilson EG: Tubulointerstitial Diseases. In: Brenner BM (ed): Brenner & Rector's The Kidney, 5th ed. Philadelphia, WB Saunders, 1996, p 1655.

Myers BD, Moran SM: Hemodynamically mediated acute renal failure. N Engl J Med 314:97, 1986.

Nadasdy T, Racusen LC: Renal injury caused by therapeutic and diagnostic agents and abuse of analgesics and narcotics. In: Jennette JC, Olson JL, Schwartz MM, Silva FG (eds): Heptinstall's Pathology of the Kidney, 5th ed. Philadelphia, Lippincott-Raven, 1998, p 811.

Nath KA: The tubulointerstitium in progressive renal disease. Kidney Int 54:992, 1998.

Olsen S, Solez K: Acute tubular necrosis and toxic renal injury. In: Tisher CC, Brenner BM (eds): Renal Pathology: With Clinical and Functional Correlations, 2nd ed. Philadelphia, JB Lippincott, 1994, p 769.

Thadhani R, Pascual M, Bonventre JV: Acute renal failure. N Engl J Med 334:1448, 1996.

CHAPTER 13

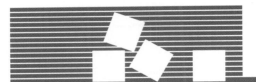

Disorders of the Interstitium
Interstitial Nephritis, Pyelonephritis, Papillary Necrosis, Analgesic Nephropathy, and Obstructive Nephropathy (Hydronephrosis)

INTERSTITIAL NEPHRITIS

Synonyms and Related Terms: Tubulointerstitial nephritis; allergic interstitial nephritis; drug-induced interstitial nephritis.

Biology of Disease

- The category of interstitial nephritis includes a variety of conditions in which the dominant pathologic feature is inflammation in the renal interstitium.
- Inflammation or injury of tubules is also often present. Therefore the term *tubulointerstitial nephritis* may be used to indicate the accompanying tubular component.
- Tubulointerstitial nephritis sometimes accompanies glomerulonephritis, most often diffuse proliferative lupus nephritis, or ANCA-related or anti–GBM-related crescentic glomerulonephritis; such cases are generally classified according to the glomerular disease and are not discussed in this chapter.
- Common causes of interstitial nephritis include medications, infections, immunologic disorders, metabolic disorders, and other systemic diseases (Table 13–1). In many cases a definite etiology cannot be determined.
- Medications are currently the most common cause of interstitial nephritis; the list of medications associated with interstitial nephritis is long and constantly growing (Table 13–2). Common medications associated with interstitial nephritis include antibiotics (various penicillins and relatives, sulfonamides, and others), nonsteroidal anti-inflammatory drugs (NSAIDs), and diuretics.
- Various mechanisms of injury may be involved in interstitial nephritis; immunologic or allergic reactions are key figures in the pathogenesis in many cases.
- Immune complexes may be deposited in the interstitium and initiate various inflammatory systems. In rare cases, strong linear staining of tubular basement membranes (TBMs) for immunoglobulins is present and indicates antibodies reacting against exogenous antigens bound to the TBM or against TBM antigens (anti-TBM antibodies).
- Many or most cases of drug-induced interstitial nephritis are believed to result from allergic or immune reactions to the medication. Methicillin (and other penicillins) can bind to TBMs, and the combination of antibiotic bound to TBM elicits an immune reaction with production of antibodies directed against the antibiotic-TBM complex.
- Inhibition of prostaglandin synthesis by NSAIDs may result in a decrease or altered distribution of renal blood flow—a nonimmunologic mechanism of interstitial nephritis.
- The clinical features of most types of interstitial nephritis are similar and rather nonspecific; a high index of clinical suspicion is needed, and renal biopsy is required for a definitive diagnosis.
- Interstitial nephritis may be either acute or chronic. The defining feature of *chronic* interstitial nephritis is the presence of *interstitial fibrosis*; the nature of the inflammatory infiltrate has no bearing on the distinction between acute and chronic interstitial nephritis because lymphocytes, plasma cells, and other "chronic" inflammatory cells are frequently present in acute interstitial nephritis. Interstitial edema is a characteristic feature of acute interstitial nephritis.
- Complete recovery of normal renal function is possible in acute interstitial nephritis, provided that the initiating cause is recognized promptly and can be removed or corrected. The presence of interstitial fibrosis (chronic interstitial nephritis) indicates some degree of irreversible renal injury.
- In general, the pathologic features of most causes of interstitial nephritis are similar. Features occurring with specific causes of interstitial nephritis are discussed in Histologic Variants.

Table 13–1
COMMON CAUSES OF INTERSTITIAL NEPHRITIS

Drugs	Infections
See Table 13–2	Bacterial
	Streptococcus
Miscellaneous	*Staphylococcus*
Anti–tubular basement mem-	*Salmonella*
brane antibody	*Escherichia coli*
Tubulointerstitial nephritis	*Legionella*
and uveitis syndrome	*Leptospira*
Kawasaki disease	*Brucella*
Systemic lupus erythematosus	Viral
Sjögren's syndrome	Measles
	Epstein-Barr virus
	Cytomegalovirus
	Hantavirus
	Polyomavirus
	Human immunodeficiency virus
	Adenovirus
	Other
	Mycoplasma
	Rickettsia
	Mycobacterium tuberculosis
	Schistosomiasis

Clinical Features

- The most common clinical finding in interstitial nephritis is renal insufficiency, detected by decreased urine output and/or rising serum urea nitrogen and creatinine levels. The onset of acute interstitial nephritis is frequently abrupt, in contrast to chronic interstitial nephritis, where the onset is often insidious.
- Nausea, vomiting, malaise, and fever may be present.
- Flank or loin pain may occur and is believed to be due to stretching of the renal capsule.
- Decreased urine output (oliguria), defined as urine output less than 400 (sometimes 500) mL/day in adults,

Table 13–2
MEDICATIONS ASSOCIATED WITH INTERSTITIAL NEPHRITIS

Antibiotics	Diuretics
Penicillins	Thiazides
Cephalosporins	Furosemide
Rifampin	Triamterene
Ciprofloxacin	Chlorthalidone
Vancomycin	
Erythromycin	**Miscellaneous**
Sulfonamides	Acetaminophen
Trimethoprim-sulfamethoxazole	Captopril
Aminoglycosides	Cimetidine
Ethambutol	Ranitidine
Tetracyclines	Phenobarbital
	Phenytoin
Nonsteroidal anti-inflammatory drugs	Phenacetin
Acetylsalicylic acid	Phenindione
Naproxen	Allopurinol
Ibuprofen	Interferon
Indomethacin	Lithium
Phenylbutazone	Interleukin-2
Sulindac	Cyclosporine
Tolmetin	Acyclovir
Mefenamic acid	
Fenoprofen	
Diflunisal	

may be present. However, approximately half of the patients are nonoliguric.

- Functional defects of renal tubules may be manifested by glycosuria and aminoaciduria, phosphaturia, renal tubular acidosis, and sodium or potassium wasting.
- Low-grade proteinuria is common; nephrotic-range proteinuria (≥ 3.5 g/1.73 m²/day) may occur in interstitial nephritis caused by NSAIDs.
- Systemic allergic symptoms may be present; however, the classic allergic triad of low-grade fever, skin rash, and arthralgias occurs in only about 15% of patients.
- Drug-induced interstitial nephritis usually develops after the patient has been taking the medication between 1 and 30 days, with a mean of approximately 1 week. Interstitial nephritis related to diuretics or NSAIDs may not manifest until the patient has been taking the medication for several months.
- Increased uptake in the kidneys bilaterally on a gallium scan (^{67}Ga) may be useful in the diagnosis of interstitial nephritis; however, increased uptake is not specific for interstitial nephritis and the sensitivity of the gallium scan for interstitial nephritis is unknown. Gallium scans may be useful in distinguishing between interstitial nephritis (which may have increased renal uptake) and acute tubular necrosis (which usually does not).

Laboratory Values

- Serum creatinine and urea nitrogen concentrations are elevated to various degrees.
- Blood eosinophilia greater than 400 cells per microliter (400×10^6/L) is present in approximately 50% of cases of allergic interstitial nephritis.
- Proteinuria and hematuria are frequently present on urinalysis. Microscopic examination of the urine may demonstrate erythrocytes, leukocytes, and granular casts; renal tubular epithelial cells may be present.
- The presence of eosinophils in the urine (*eosinophiluria*) is an important clue to the presence of interstitial nephritis; however, it is present in fewer than half of the cases. Eosinophiluria also occurs in other conditions such as upper or lower urinary tract infection, papillary necrosis, and cholesterol emboli. A Hansel stain has been reported to be more sensitive to the presence of urinary eosinophils than the standard Wright stain.

Treatment and Clinical Course

- The prognosis of acute interstitial nephritis is favorable; the majority of patients recover normal renal function provided that the precipitating cause is promptly recognized and can be removed or corrected.
- The most important treatment is recognition and discontinuation of the precipitating cause.
- Corticosteroids such as prednisone are frequently used, and many series suggest substantial benefit; however, these series have not been major randomized, controlled clinical trials.
- Full recovery of renal function may occur even in patients requiring dialysis for temporary support; the peak serum creatinine value does not appear to predict long-term outcome.

- Older patients and patients with renal failure persisting longer than 3 weeks have a lower chance of full renal recovery.
- Interstitial fibrosis on biopsy indicates irreversible scarring and probable long-term decrease in renal function. The degree of interstitial fibrosis is the best predictor of renal function.

Gross Appearance

- The kidneys are symmetrically enlarged with a tense, red-gray capsule.
- The cortex may appear pale on section; the corticomedullary junction and medullary rays may appear indistinct.
- Petechiae may be present on the capsular and cut surfaces.

Light Microscopy

Glomeruli

- Glomeruli typically appear unremarkable, with normal cellularity and patent capillary loops. Glomeruli may appear "bloodless" or swollen.

Tubules

- The degree of tubular involvement is highly variable, from minimal to marked. Tubular damage is often patchy; occasionally, extensive areas of tubular necrosis are present.
- Proximal convoluted tubules may appear dilated, with loss of the periodic acid–Schiff (PAS)-positive brush border.
- Tubular epithelial cells may appear basophilic, and there may be mitotic figures in epithelial cells; tubular cell degeneration or necrosis may occur, with subsequent sloughing of the cells into the tubular lumen. Lymphocytes or neutrophils may be seen infiltrating into the tubular epithelium ("tubulitis").
- Tubular lumina may contain degenerating tubular epithelial cells, leukocytes, and granular cast material.
- Tubular basement membranes may appear laminated or fragmented; breaks in the TBM may be present.

Interstitium

- The interstitium is expanded, with separation of tubules, by a combination of inflammation, edema, and/or fibrosis. Interstitial edema is characteristic of acute interstitial nephritis; fibrosis is characteristic of chronic interstitial nephritis.
- Edema appears pale and loose on hematoxylin and eosin (H & E) stain and pale blue or green on trichrome stain. Fibrosis is indicated by dense eosinophilic staining on H & E and darker blue or green staining on trichrome stain.
- The inflammatory infiltrate typically consists predominantly of lymphocytes and plasma cells, although macrophages, neutrophils, eosinophils, and giant cells may be present.

- Tamm-Horsfall protein may leak into the interstitium, appears eosinophilic on H & E stain and PAS-positive on PAS reaction, and is often associated with eosinophils or other inflammatory cells.

Vessels

- Blood vessels typically show little or no change.

Immunofluorescence Microscopy

- The most common finding on immunofluorescence microscopy is deposition of fibrin/fibrinogen within the interstitium, with little or no staining for immunoglobulins or complement.
- Occasional cases (perhaps 10% to 20%) show linear TBM staining for IgG, with or without staining for C3; this staining pattern was characteristic of methicillin-induced interstitial nephritis and sometimes occurs with other penicillins, cephalosporins, and other drugs.
- Granular TBM staining for IgG and C3 is occasionally present.

Electron Microscopy

- Glomeruli usually show few ultrastructural changes; there may be simplification and effacement of visceral epithelial cell foot processes.
- Tubules show a variety of nonspecific ultrastructural changes. The basal interdigitations of the proximal and distal tubular epithelial cells may be lost; arrays of actin filaments may be seen running parallel to the basement membrane. Occasional necrotic or apoptotic tubular epithelial cells may be present.
- Lymphocytes may be found within tubules in contact with epithelial cells.
- Tubular basement membranes may be laminated and thinned, with focal discontinuities.
- Granular, electron-dense deposits are occasionally seen within TBMs.

Interstitial Nephritis Variants

Drug-Induced Interstitial Nephritis

- Drug-induced interstitial nephritis in most cases resembles acute interstitial nephritis as described earlier.
- Eosinophils are frequently, although not invariably, a prominent component of the interstitial inflammation. They tend to be focal and may form clusters. Interstitial nephritis associated with NSAIDs and cimetidine (Tagamet) tends to have fewer eosinophils.
- Neutrophils are uncommon; the presence of numerous neutrophils suggests an alternative cause such as infection.
- Granuloma formation may occur in up to 30% of cases of drug-induced interstitial nephritis and can occur with virtually any drug. The granulomas are usually small and noncaseating; multinucleated giant cells may be rare. Granulomas are usually located in the interstitium but may be localized around tubules.

- Nonsteroidal anti-inflammatory drugs can cause a variety of reactions, including minimal change nephrotic syndrome and chronic interstitial nephritis characterized by interstitial fibrosis with relatively scant inflammation.

Interstitial Nephritis Associated With Bacterial Infections

- Bacteria may induce interstitial nephritis directly as a result of bacterial invasion of the kidney or indirectly, without bacteria present in the kidney. Many cases of acute interstitial nephritis with direct bacterial invasion would be classified as *acute pyelonephritis*.
- Infections with *Streptococcus* species are a common cause of acute interstitial nephritis in children. Lymphocytes and plasma cells are usually predominant; small clusters of neutrophils may be present.
- Neutrophils are a prominent component of interstitial nephritis caused by *Staphylococcus aureus* infection; microabscesses are common. Neutrophils may also be prominent in interstitial nephritis caused by *Escherichia coli* infections.
- Interstitial nephritis may be seen with numerous other bacterial infections, including typhoid fever, brucellosis, leptospirosis, and others (see Table 13–1).

Interstitial Nephritis Associated With Viral Infections

- Interstitial nephritis has been described in association with a variety of viral infections, including measles, Epstein-Barr virus (infectious mononucleosis), cytomegalovirus, human immunodeficiency virus, BK polyomavirus, Hantavirus, and others. Most of these infections are rare occurrences, with the exception of a few that commonly occur in immunocompromised hosts.
- Cytomegalovirus infection may occasionally be associated with interstitial nephritis, usually in infants or immunocompromised patients such as transplant recipients. In addition to focal mononuclear interstitial inflammation, tubular epithelial cells may show the large, eosinophilic nuclear inclusions with halos that are characteristic of cytomegalovirus. Glomeruli may show mild mesangial hypercellularity.
- The BK polyomavirus may also cause interstitial nephritis, usually in transplant recipients. Mononuclear interstitial inflammation, scattered tubular epithelial cell necrosis, and large "smudgy" epithelial cell nuclei are seen; rare nuclei may contain eosinophilic inclusions. Hemorrhagic cystitis in bone marrow transplant recipients and ureteral strictures in renal transplant recipients have also been associated with BK polyomavirus infections.

Granulomatous Interstitial Nephritis

- Granulomatous interstitial nephritis characteristically shows clusters of epithelioid histiocytes with varying numbers of lymphocytes and often multinucleated giant cells. Caseous necrosis may be present in cases caused by mycobacteria or fungi.
- Granulomatous interstitial nephritis can occur in a variety of conditions. Adverse reactions to medications are probably the most common cause; other causes include mycobacterial or fungal infections, sarcoidosis, and Wegener's granulomatosis. In occasional cases no cause can be established.
- Granulomatous interstitial nephritis can occur in association with almost any medication; allergic reactions are believed to be the most common mechanisms. Granulomas may be associated with injured or destroyed tubules. Multinucleated giant cells are relatively uncommon in drug-induced granulomatous interstitial nephritis; caseation is unusual.
- Granulomas associated with mycobacterial or fungal infections usually but not invariably show caseous necrosis. Special stains for organisms should be performed in all cases of granulomatous interstitial nephritis.
- Granulomas associated with sarcoidosis are usually small, well defined, and noncaseating. Laminated concretions (Schaumann's bodies) or asteroid bodies may be present within giant cells. Calcifications may be present within tubules, either in tubular cells or lumina, particularly in collecting ducts. Granulomas may encroach on arterial walls. Interstitial fibrosis is frequently present. Glomeruli are usually normal, but occasionally glomerulonephritis may be present. The diagnosis of sarcoidosis requires the exclusion of other causes of granulomatous interstitial nephritis; demonstration of noncaseating granulomas in other organs such as mediastinal lymph nodes or the lungs helps confirm the diagnosis.
- Wegener's granulomatosis is characterized by necrotizing glomerulonephritis and vasculitis. A granulomatous reaction may occasionally be seen around damaged glomeruli (*"granulomatous glomerulonephritis"*). Granulomas are not often found on renal biopsies, most likely because of the typical limited sample.

Interstitial Nephritis With Uveitis (Dobrin Syndrome)

- Interstitial nephritis may be associated with a rare syndrome that includes uveitis, bone marrow granulomas, hypergammaglobulinemia, and an elevated erythrocyte sedimentation rate. Originally reported in children, it is now known to occur in adults as well.
- Uveitis is frequently the initial symptom, although renal involvement may occasionally precede uveitis.
- The syndrome is more common in females than males.
- The cause of interstitial nephritis with uveitis is unknown; immunologic mechanisms may be responsible.
- The usual histologic findings are interstitial edema with variable numbers of lymphocytes, plasma cells, monocytes, neutrophils, and occasional eosinophils. Granulomas may be present. Tubules show focal necrosis, degeneration, regeneration, and dilatation. Glomeruli usually appear unremarkable.
- Immunofluorescence microscopy is usually negative or shows minimal, nonspecific findings.
- Toxoplasmosis may cause a similar clinical syndrome and must be excluded.

- The usual therapy is corticosteroids. The prognosis is generally favorable, although there may be residual renal impairment.

Differential Diagnosis of Interstitial Nephritis

- Tubulointerstitial nephritis may accompany glomerulonephritis; when the glomerular component predominates or is the primary event, the disorder should be classified according to the type and cause of the glomerulonephritis rather than the tubulointerstitial component.
- Acute tubular necrosis is frequently included in the clinical and pathologic differential diagnosis of interstitial nephritis. A predominance of interstitial inflammation over tubular changes would favor interstitial nephritis; prominent tubular changes with a relative lack of interstitial inflammation favors tubular necrosis. Because tubular injury frequently accompanies interstitial nephritis, the distinction may be difficult or impossible; the noncommittal term *tubulointerstitial nephritis* might then be preferred.
- A predominance of neutrophils in the inflammatory infiltrate, particularly aggregates of neutrophils within tubular lumina or interstitial aggregates of neutrophils, suggests acute bacterial pyelonephritis, and bacterial cultures of the urine should be recommended.

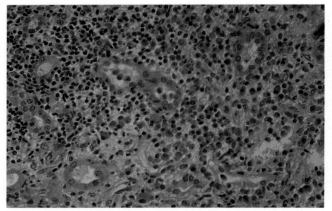

Figure 13–1. Interstitial nephritis in systemic lupus erythematosus. The markedly widened interstitium displays a heavy cellular infiltrate composed of plasma cells, lymphocytes, and a few polymorphonuclear leukocytes.

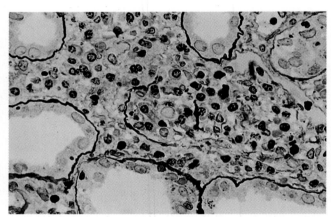

Figure 13–3. Interstitial nephritis. There is inflammatory cell invasion of the tubule in the center, along with rupture of the tubular basement membrane and destruction of the tubular epithelial cells (methenamine silver stain).

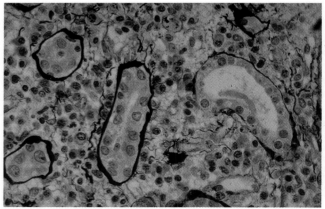

Figure 13–2. Interstitial nephritis. The tubules are widely separated from each other by a heavy interstitial cellular infiltrate composed of plasma cells and lymphocytes. There is focal loss of the tubular basement membranes (methenamine silver stain).

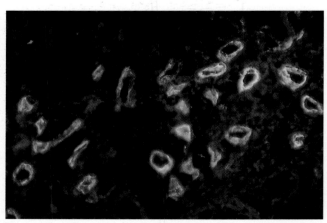

Figure 13–4. Interstitial nephritis. IgG deposition along the tubular basement membranes is seen in a patient with systemic lupus erythematosus. Immune complex deposition along the tubular basement membranes is more frequent in patients with active focal or diffuse proliferative lupus nephritis.

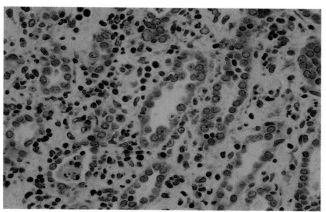

Figure 13–5. Interstitial nephritis. Marked infiltration and widening of the renal interstitium by inflammatory cells—lymphocytes and eosinophils—are seen in a case of nonsteroidal anti-inflammatory drug–induced nephritis. Eosinophils in interstitial nephritis should raise the possibility of a drug/allergy-related process.

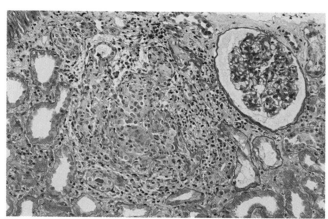

Figure 13–8. Granulomatous interstitial nephritis. Interstitial nephritis developed after treatment with sulfosalazine.

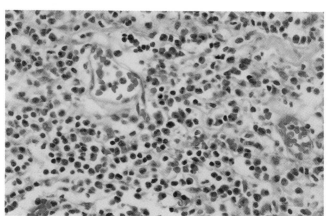

Figure 13–6. Interstitial nephritis. Eosinophilic leukocytes are seen in the interstitial cellular infiltrate.

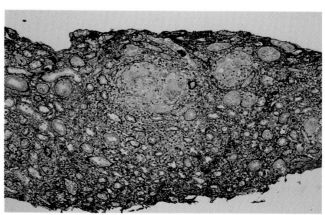

Figure 13–9. Interstitial nephritis. Interstitial giant cells and granulomas in a patient with drug-induced interstitial nephritis (methenamine silver stain).

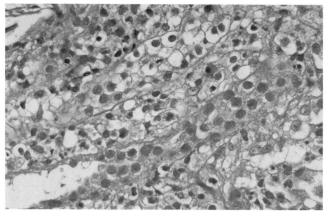

Figure 13–7. Interstitial nephritis. Cellular inflammatory infiltrate is invading the tubular epithelial cells (tubulitis). A few eosinophils are present in this case of drug-induced allergy.

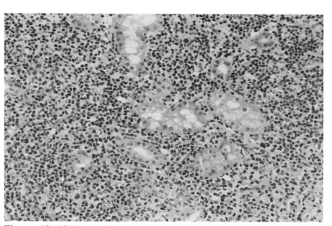

Figure 13–10. Interstitial nephritis. This 14-year-old child had severe Epstein-Barr virus infection.

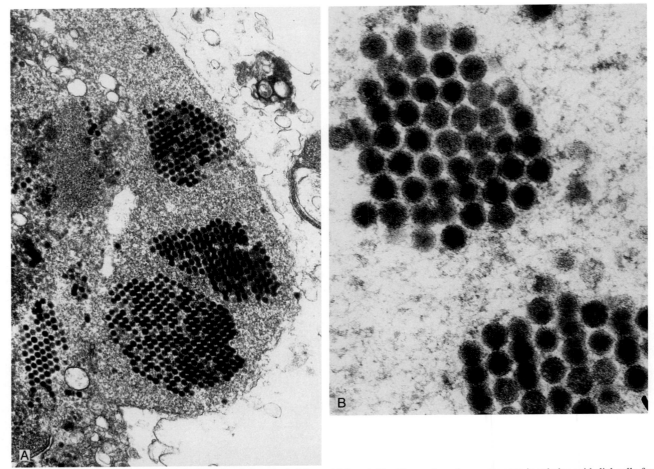

Figure 13–11. *A*, Electron micrograph of adenovirus-induced tubulointerstitial nephritis. Many adenoviruses are seen in tubular epithelial cells from an immunocompromised patient with AIDS and severe necrotizing tubulointerstitial inflammation. *B*, Electron micrograph of adenoviruses. This high-magnification picture of adenoviruses is from the case shown in *A*.

PYELONEPHRITIS

■ We define the term *pyelonephritis* as infection of the renal parenchyma with involvement of the pelvis and calyces. Thus defined, pyelonephritis is caused by bacteria that have gained access to the kidney via the ureters (*ascending infection*). Some nephrologists and renal pathologists include infections reaching the kidney by way of the bloodstream within the category of "pyelonephritis"; we would designate such infections as "multiple cortical abscesses," "diffuse suppurative nephritis," or "diffuse bacterial nephritis."

■ Two major variants are described: *acute pyelonephritis* and *chronic pyelonephritis*; obstruction of the urinary tract may be present or absent in either variant.

■ Acute pyelonephritis is common but, fortunately, resolves without serious sequelae in the majority of cases; only severe, complicated, or unusual cases come to the attention of the anatomic pathologist.

■ True chronic pyelonephritis, signifying chronic infection of the renal parenchyma, is uncommon. It is now recognized that vesicoureteral reflux plays an important role in the pathogenesis of chronic pyelonephritis, and the term *reflux nephropathy* is sometimes used synonymously with or in preference to "chronic pyelonephritis."

Acute Pyelonephritis

Biology of Disease

■ Acute pyelonephritis is an infection of the kidney and upper urinary tract, almost always bacterial.

■ In at least 95% of cases of bacterial infection of the kidney, bacteria gain access to the kidney via the ureters (ascending infection); in the remaining cases, bacteria gain access to the kidney through the blood from a source outside the urinary tract (*hematogenous infection*).

- In acute pyelonephritis caused by ascending infection, the renal pelvis and calyces are the primary sites of involvement; involvement of the cortex is secondary. In infection secondary to hematogenous dissemination (diffuse bacterial nephritis), the cortex is the predominant site of involvement; involvement of the pelvis and calyces is secondary and usually relatively minor.
- Vesicoureteral reflux and urinary tract obstruction are important factors predisposing to acute pyelonephritis; other predisposing factors include instrumentation of the urinary tract, diabetes mellitus, and pregnancy.
- The usual source of the bacteria is the gastrointestinal tract; the organisms cultured from the urine reflect that source, with Enterobacteriaceae and *Enterococcus* being the most common pathogens.
- The most common organism is *E. coli*, which causes approximately 90% of initial urinary tract infections. *Staphylococcus saprophyticus* is a common cause in young, sexually active women. Other bacteria that cause urinary tract infections include species of *Klebsiella, Proteus, Pseudomonas, Serratia,* and *Alcaligenes*. These bacteria are more common in patients with frequent urinary tract or nosocomial infections.
- Hematogenous infections are usually due to bacteremia with virulent organisms such as *Staphylococcus aureus* or species of *Pseudomonas* or *Salmonella*. The most common manifestation is multiple cortical abscesses.
- Fungi, most often *Candida* species, cause occasional cases of pyelonephritis. Predisposing factors include indwelling bladder catheters, broad-spectrum antibiotics, diabetes mellitus, and immunosuppression.

Clinical Features

- Overall, the incidence of acute pyelonephritis is higher in women than in men, but the incidence varies with age. The incidence in males is slightly higher during the neonatal period (approximately 1.5 : 1) because of a higher incidence of congenital anomalies of the urinary tract in males. After 50, the incidence in males increases as bladder outlet obstruction from prostatic hypertrophy becomes more common.
- The classic symptoms are fever, back pain, and dysuria.

Laboratory Values

- The white blood cell count is usually elevated, frequently with a shift toward band forms.
- Urinalysis shows bacteriuria, pyuria, and frequently hematuria.
- Quantitative urine culture demonstrates more than 10^5 colony-forming units per milliliter in more than 80% of patients.
- Serum urea nitrogen and creatinine values are normal unless the patient is volume depleted or has preexisting renal disease.

Gross Appearance

- The majority of patients with acute pyelonephritis recover without complications. Therefore, kidneys examined at autopsy or surgical nephrectomy represent se-

vere or complicated cases frequently associated with urinary tract obstruction.
- The kidney is usually enlarged and edematous. Yellow or white microabscesses may be present on the surface.
- On section, the microabscesses are usually confined to the cortex. Pale streaks may extend into the medulla and represent collecting ducts filled or lined with purulent material.
- The affected areas are often well circumscribed, with intervening areas of normal parenchyma.
- The mucosa of the renal pelvis is erythematous and covered by a purulent exudate.
- The pelvis is often dilated; the papillae may be blunted or flattened.
- Necrosis of one or more renal papillae is occasionally seen, most frequently in diabetics or in association with severe obstruction of the urinary tract.

Light Microscopy

- The predominant changes involve tubules and the interstitium; glomeruli and blood vessels usually demonstrate minimal alterations.
- The interstitium contains a dense inflammatory infiltrate composed of neutrophils, lymphocytes, and plasma cells in various proportions. Neutrophils may be present only transiently and are shortly replaced by lymphocytes, plasma cells, and others.
- Neutrophils predominate in microabscesses, when such lesions are present.
- Destruction of tubules is seen in the areas of microabscesses; in surrounding areas, tubules are separated by interstitial inflammation and edema.
- Aggregates of neutrophils may be present within tubular lumina; collecting ducts are filled with and distended by aggregates of neutrophils.
- Microscopically, the affected areas are usually circumscribed and separated by zones of relatively normal parenchyma.
- In later stages, interstitial fibrosis may develop; the inflammatory infiltrate consists predominantly of lymphocytes and plasma cells, and lymphoid follicles may be present.

Immunofluorescence Microscopy

- Immunofluorescence microscopy is not usually helpful in the diagnosis.

Electron Microscopy

- Electron microscopy is not usually required for diagnosis.

Differential Diagnosis

- The main clinical differential is upper urinary tract infection without involvement of the parenchyma of the kidney—the renal pelvis, calyceal system, and upper ureters (acute pyelitis)—or involvement of the lower urinary tract (acute cystitis).

■ The main histologic differential is acute interstitial nephritis of other causes. A predominance of neutrophils in the inflammatory infiltrate, aggregates of neutrophils in tubular lumina, or interstitial aggregates of neutrophils would suggest infectious pyelonephritis over noninfectious interstitial nephritis. The clinical history may also be helpful in this distinction.

Treatment and Clinical Course

■ Antibiotic therapy, guided by bacterial cultures and antibiotic sensitivities, results in complete recovery in the majority of cases.
■ Nearly all patients without underlying renal or urinary tract abnormalities recover completely with no sequelae.

Chronic Pyelonephritis and Reflux Nephropathy

Synonyms and Related Terms: Chronic atrophic pyelonephritis; chronic nonobstructive pyelonephritis.

Biology of Disease

■ "Chronic pyelonephritis" was formerly a common diagnosis; any lymphocytic infiltrate in the kidney was presumed to indicate chronic infection. However, microbial cultures of kidneys in such cases are usually negative. It is now recognized that *true* chronic pyelonephritis, implying chronic infection of the renal parenchyma or the sequela of past episodes of repeated infection, is rare.
■ Two variants of chronic pyelonephritis are described: chronic obstructive pyelonephritis, caused by obstruction of the urinary tract, and chronic nonobstructive pyelonephritis.
■ Vesicoureteral and intrarenal reflux is critical in the pathogenesis of chronic nonobstructive pyelonephritis; thus the term *reflux nephropathy* is commonly used instead of (or synonymously with) the term *chronic nonobstructive pyelonephritis*. The importance of infection in the pathogenesis of this form of chronic pyelonephritis is unclear.
■ Severe vesicoureteric reflux, which may be due to anomalies in the vesicoureteric valve, may be associated with permanent renal scarring. Such scarring usually occurs during infancy, while the kidney is growing; it is unusual for such scarring to develop after childhood. The scars in such cases probably represent failure of that segment of the kidney to grow normally rather than scarring of a segment that had attained normal size.
■ Intrarenal reflux also appears to be required for scarring to occur. Intrarenal reflux usually occurs in compound papillae, where two or three pyramids are normally fused together; such compound papillae have rounded or oval openings into the ducts of Bellini, which presumably allows reflux of urine into the renal parenchyma. Compound papillae are normally found at the upper and lower poles of the kidney, which are the most common locations of renal scars associated with chronic pyelonephritis.
■ Infection may play an important role in the pathogenesis of renal scarring and chronic pyelonephritis; antibiotic prophylaxis in children with vesicoureteric reflux may decrease the incidence of subsequent scarring and pyelonephritis.
■ The histologic features associated with chronic pyelonephritis are nonspecific and can be seen in a variety of conditions. Therefore, the diagnosis of chronic pyelonephritis cannot be made on renal biopsy alone; diagnosis requires a combination of clinical history, radiologic studies of the urinary tract or gross morphologic examination, and histologic findings.
■ Radiographic imaging studies play an important role in the diagnosis of chronic pyelonephritis. Radiographic changes include a decrease in size, dilation of the pelvis, and clubbing of one or more calyces; these changes correspond to the gross morphologic changes described later.
■ Reflux nephropathy may be associated with the lesion of focal segmental glomerulosclerosis (FSGS). Proteinuria is marked in such cases.
■ A few distinctive but relatively uncommon variants of chronic pyelonephritis are sometimes found and include xanthogranulomatous pyelonephritis, malakoplakia, and megalocytic interstitial nephritis.
■ *Mycobacterium tuberculosis* is another cause of chronic renal infection; the kidney is the most common extrapulmonary site of tuberculosis.

Clinical Features

■ Chronic nonobstructive pyelonephritis may be seen clinically in all age groups; women are more often affected than men. Some patients have a prior history of repeated urinary tract infections; however, many do not.
■ Many patients have impaired renal function with little or no history of previous renal disease.
■ Hypertension may be present at diagnosis; the presence of hypertension is associated with a higher probability of progression to chronic renal failure.

Laboratory Values

■ Serum urea nitrogen and creatinine values may be normal or increased.
■ Proteinuria may be present on urinalysis; urinalysis findings are otherwise not specific.

Gross Pathology

Chronic Nonobstructive Pyelonephritis

■ The external surface of the kidney shows single or multiple large, broad-based, U-shaped depressions. These depressions are characteristically sharply demarcated from the normal renal parenchyma. The remainder of the surface may be smooth or granular, the latter indicating the presence of arterial and arteriolar sclerosis.

- Beneath the surface scars are deformed papillae, with flattening or clubbing of the calyx or calyces; the pelvis is dilated, and the parenchyma is thinned.
- The calyces in uninvolved portions of the kidney are usually normal, and the cortex is preserved.

Chronic Obstructive Pyelonephritis

- Generalized atrophy of the parenchyma and dilatation of all portions of the pelvis are seen.
- Calculi may be present within the dilated pelvis.

Light Microscopy

Glomeruli

- Glomeruli in the affected regions may appear crowded together because of loss of the intervening tubules and interstitium.
- Capillary tufts may appear normal or collapsed.
- Generalized sclerosis of the tufts may be present and is sometimes striking.
- Bowman's capsule is often thickened; there may be concentric collagen deposition around Bowman's capsule, described as *periglomerular fibrosis.*
- Eventually the glomeruli may become completely hyalinized and merge into the surrounding fibrotic interstitium.
- Reflux nephropathy may be associated with the development of the focal segmental glomerulosclerosis (FSGS) lesion. The histologic changes of FSGS associated with reflux nephropathy are similar to those of idiopathic FSGS and will not be described here.

Tubules

- The most characteristic changes are loss or atrophy of tubules in the affected areas. Tubular basement membranes may be thickened with a decrease in lumen size and atrophy of tubular epithelial cells.
- Collections of dilated tubules lined by thinned epithelium and containing "regular" eosinophilic casts may be present. The histologic appearance resembles that of the thyroid gland and is termed *thyroidization.* Although this change is most often associated with chronic pyelonephritis, it is not pathognomonic for that condition.

Interstitium

- Fibrosis of the interstitium is seen in the affected areas. The changes are often patchy, with residual areas of intervening normal parenchyma.
- A sharp demarcation is usually found between the scarred areas and surrounding unaffected parenchyma.
- Interstitial inflammation is present and consists predominantly of lymphocytes and plasma cells.
- The presence of lymphoid follicles or accentuation of the inflammation beneath the lining of the pelvis suggests chronic infection.

Vessels

- Vascular changes are common, particularly when chronic pyelonephritis is associated with hypertension.
- Arteries show hypertrophy of the media and fibrosis of the intima.
- Arterioles are tortuous, with hypertrophy of the muscular layer. Hyaline material may be found in the intima.

Immunofluorescence Microscopy

- Findings on immunofluorescence microscopy are usually minimal and nonspecific.

Electron Microscopy

- Ultrastructural changes are nonspecific and reflect the light microscopic changes.

Differential Diagnosis

- As noted earlier, the histologic findings of chronic pyelonephritis are nonspecific, and advanced renal disease of many causes results in similar changes.
- The finding of flattened, concave or clubbed calyces and U-shaped cortical scars by imaging studies or on gross examination helps substantiate the diagnosis of reflux nephropathy/chronic pyelonephritis.
- Chronic interstitial nephritis may be indistinguishable from chronic pyelonephritis by light microscopy.
- Hypertension can cause similar histologic changes; a history of long-standing hypertension may suggest that as the cause of renal insufficiency. The differential is complicated by the fact that chronic pyelonephritis/reflux nephropathy can cause hypertension.
- Vascular disease can cause large cortical scars resembling those in reflux nephropathy, but the underlying medullary areas are usually minimally altered in vascular disease, in contrast to the striking alterations seen in reflux nephropathy/chronic pyelonephritis.
- The presence of significant glomerular deposits of immunoglobulin or complement components on immunofluorescence microscopy or immune-type deposits on electron microscopy would suggest a primary glomerulonephritis.

Treatment and Clinical Course

- No specific treatment is known for chronic pyelonephritis.
- Prevention of recurrent urinary tract infections in children may decrease the incidence of renal scarring and subsequent chronic pyelonephritis.
- The presence of hypertension or significant proteinuria with FSGS on biopsy suggests an increased likelihood of progression to chronic renal insufficiency.

Xanthogranulomatous Pyelonephritis

Biology of Disease

- Xanthogranulomatous pyelonephritis is an uncommon variant of chronic pyelonephritis characterized by granulomatous inflammaton with prominent lipid-laden macrophages.
- Obstruction of the urinary tract is almost always present, and renal calculi are usually present.
- The median age is the fifth to sixth decade, although the disease may occur at any age. The disease is twice as common in women as men.
- Involvement is almost always unilateral.
- The pathogenic mechanism(s) of xanthogranulomatous pyelonephritis is unknown; both bacterial infection and obstruction of the urinary tract appear to be important in pathogenesis.
- The most common organisms associated with xanthogranulomatous pyelonephritis are *Proteus* species, *E. coli*, and *Klebsiella* and *Pseudomonas* species; however, it has also been associated with other organisms.
- Xanthogranulomatous pyelonephritis can resemble renal cell carcinoma by gross appearance and histologically.

Clinical Features

- The most common symptoms are flank pain, fever, weight loss, and malaise; symptoms may have been present for prolonged periods, sometimes years.
- The majority of patients have a history of previous renal calculi, urinary tract obstruction, or diabetes mellitus.
- The involved kidney may be palpable in up to 60% of cases.
- Urinalysis demonstrates proteinuria and pyuria.
- Renal failure is uncommon because of the low frequency of bilateral involvement.

Gross Appearance

- The kidney is enlarged and may be adherent to the perirenal fat. The capsule is thickened.
- In most cases the entire kidney is involved; however, only a portion of the kidney may be affected.
- The pelvicalyceal system is dilated, and the papillae are usually lost. Calculi (frequently of the staghorn type) and purulent material are often present in the pelvis.
- The calyces are lined by yellow, friable material. Foci of similar material are present in the parenchyma.
- Abscesses may be present in the parenchyma.

Light Microscopy

- The yellow areas are composed of sheets of large, lipid-laden macrophages with foamy cytoplasm (*foam cells*) mixed with smaller macrophages, lymphocytes, plasma cells, and neutrophils. The smaller macrophages contain coarse, PAS-positive granules. Multinucleated giant cells may be present.
- The zones surrounding the yellow areas contain neutrophils and necrotic debris. Foci of calcification may be present.

- In the adjacent parenchyma there is diffuse tubular atrophy and loss, glomerular scarring, interstitial fibrosis, and chronic inflammation.
- The renal capsule is characteristically fibrotic and frequently adherent to the perinephric fat.

Electron Microscopy

- The foamy macrophages initially contain bacteria; subsequently they contain numerous phagolysosomes.

Differential Diagnosis

- The most important differential diagnosis is renal cell carcinoma.
- Arteriography may be helpful in the differential diagnosis; splaying of vessels around the area of inflammation and the lack of tumor "blush" suggest inflammation rather than a neoplastic process. Computed tomography and magnetic resonance imaging may also be helpful.
- The presence of renal calculi, particularly staghorn calculi, would favor xanthogranulomatous pyelonephritis over renal cell carcinoma.
- Histologically, the key is identify the foamy cells as macrophages rather than malignant epithelial cells.

Treatment and Clinical Course

- The diagnosis is made at nephrectomy in the majority of cases, although the diagnosis may sometimes be made by a combination of clinical findings and radiologic studies.
- Surgical resection usually results in cure.

Malakoplakia

Biology of Disease

- Malakoplakia is most commonly found in the urinary bladder but may occur in the renal pelvis and rarely in the parenchyma of the kidney.
- The clinical setting resembles that of xanthogranulomatous pyelonephritis. Malakoplakia occurs most often in the fifth decade, the incidence in women exceeds that in men, and it is frequently associated with infection. Unlike xanthogranulomatous pyelonephritis, calculi are seldom found in malakoplakia.
- *Escherichia coli* is the most common organism cultured from the urine.
- Malakoplakia involving the renal pelvis may result in obstruction.
- Bilateral disease is not uncommon in malakoplakia, unlike in xanthogranulomatous pyelonephritis, in which bilateral disease is rare.
- Malakoplakia may result from a defect in macrophage bactericidal capability. Approximately half of affected patients have immunodeficiency or autoimmune disorders such as hypogammaglobulinemia, immunosuppressive therapy, malignancies, rheumatoid arthritis, or the acquired immunodeficiency syndrome.

Clinical Features

- Common symptoms include fever, rigors, and flank pain.
- Urinalysis demonstrates proteinuria, pyuria, and sometimes hematuria.
- Renal failure may occasionally be present.
- Like xanthogranulomatous pyelonephritis, malakoplakia may occasionally be mistaken for a neoplasm, particularly when only part of the kidney is involved.

Gross Pathology

- The kidney may be involved diffusely or focally.
- The characteristic lesions are raised, yellow-tan plaques, usually multiple, that are present on the lining of the pelvis, sometimes on the capsular surface, and may extend into the parenchyma.

Light Microscopy

- The lesion consists of clusters of macrophages with foamy eosinophilic cytoplasm, small cytoplasmic granules, and large (4 to 10 μm) inclusions.
- The inclusions, known as *Michaelis-Gutmann bodies*, stain strongly with hematoxylin, PAS (both with and without diastase digestion), von Kossa (calcium), and iron stains. The inclusions may be laminated or homogeneous.
- The surrounding parenchyma shows loss of tubules, interstitial fibrosis, and chronic inflammation.

Electron Microscopy

- The inclusions show a crystalline structure with a central dense core, an intermediate halo, and a peripheral lamellated ring.
- Phagolysosomes or rod-shaped structures resembling bacteria may be present in the center of the inclusions.

Megalocytic Interstitial Nephritis

- Megalocytic interstitial nephritis is a rare condition that in many respects resembles malakoplakia; it may even be an early stage of malakoplakia.
- The clinical setting and features of megalocytic interstitial nephritis overlap with those of malakoplakia.
- Like malakoplakia, chronic infection and obstruction of the urinary tract appear to be important in the pathogenesis of megalocytic interstitial nephritis.
- There may be diffuse involvement of the kidney, with multiple yellow-gray foci of various sizes, or discrete nodules may be found within the cortex.
- Histologically, the disease is characterized by large numbers of polygonal cells with eosinophilic, granular cytoplasm. The granules stain strongly with PAS.
- The main distinction from malakoplakia rests on the demonstration of Michaelis-Gutmann bodies in malakoplakia in contrast with their absence in megalocytic interstitial nephritis.
- Some authors have classified cases with characteristic Michaelis-Gutmann bodies as megalocytic interstitial nephritis, thus making the distinction between the two unclear.

Tuberculosis of the Kidney

Biology of Disease

- Tuberculosis of the genitourinary tract, the most common form of extrapulmonary tuberculosis, represents approximately one fifth of extrapulmonary cases; renal tuberculosis accounts for approximately 10% of the extrapulmonary cases.
- A long latent period is often seen between the development of pulmonary and genitourinary tuberculosis.
- Spread to the kidney is believed to be occur hematogenously during the primary infection, before the development of cell-mediated immunity against the organism.
- In the majority of cases, growth of the organism is controlled and the lesions heal. In a smaller proportion of patients, infection persists in the medulla in the form of a caseating granulomatous reaction. These caseating reactions may form tumor-like masses known as *tuberculomas* or result in calyceal amputation.
- The incidence of renal tuberculosis is likely to increase because of the increased risk of tuberculosis in immunocompromised patients such as those with acquired immunodeficiency syndrome and as a result of immigration from areas of high prevalence of tuberculosis such as the Far East. The recent development of multiple drug–resistant strains of tuberculosis may also contribute to an increased incidence.

Clinical Features

- Symptoms of renal tuberculosis may be mild or absent; about one third of patients are asymptomatic. Constitutional symptoms such as fever and night sweats are rare.
- Symptoms usually relate to bladder involvement; dysuria, frequency, loin pain, and hematuria are most frequent.
- A positive tuberculin skin test (purified protein derivative) is found in approximately 90% of patients.
- Evidence of previous pulmonary tuberculosis can be seen on chest radiographs in approximately two thirds of patients.
- Renal insufficiency or hypertension is uncommon.

Laboratory Values

- Abnormalities on urinalysis are present in up to 90% of patients. The most common finding is sterile pyuria with microscopic hematuria.
- Culture of first morning urine should be performed; it may take up to 6 weeks for the organism to be cultured.
- Acid-fast stains on urine are unreliable in the diagnosis of tuberculosis because nonpathogenic, nontuberculous mycobacteria may be present in the urine and cause false-positive results.

Gross Pathology

- The initial lesion occurs in the medulla as ulceration of the transitional epithelial lining over the papillae. The papillae become clubbed and may be progressively replaced by caseous necrosis.
- Spread throughout the mucosal lining results in filling of the calyces with caseous necrotic material.
- The ureteropelvic junction may become obstructed by necrotic debris, with subsequent hydronephrosis.
- The overlying cortex becomes progressively atrophic; extensive parenchymal destruction may eventually occur.

Light Microscopy

- The initial findings are collections of neutrophils and macrophages within the medulla, followed by granuloma formation, frequently with caseation.
- Involvement of the cortex may be focal to extensive. The usual findings are glomerulosclerosis with pericapsular fibrosis, tubular atrophy, and interstitial fibrosis with an inflammatory infiltrate consisting of lymphocytes, plasma cells, and monocytes.

- Healing may result in localized interstitial fibrosis, or the parenchyma may be extensively destroyed.
- Organisms can usually be identified with acid-fast stains such as the Ziehl-Neelsen stain or with fluorochromes such as auramine-rhodamine stain.

Treatment and Clinical Course

- Therapy includes a combination of antituberculous drugs for a prolonged period; two or three medications are generally used for a minimum of 6 months. Current recommendations for antituberculous therapy should be consulted.
- Drug sensitivity testing should be performed on isolates from immunocompromised individuals and individuals at risk of having resistant strains of tuberculosis such as immigrants from Mexico, the Caribbean, or the Far East.
- Surgery may be required to relieve obstruction. Nephrectomy may be required for end-stage tuberculous kidneys if mycobacterial sepsis is present or the urine cannot be sterilized with chemotherapy.

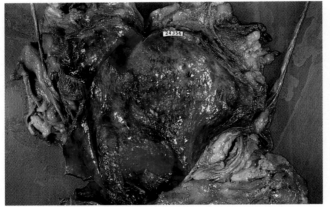

Figure 13–12. Acute hemorrhagic cystitis. Acute cystitis is often the precursor of ascending bacterial infection of the kidney.

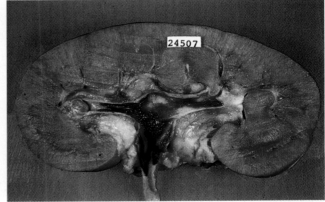

Figure 13–13. Hemorrhagic pyelitis. This patient had ascending urinary tract infection.

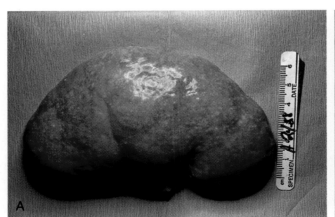

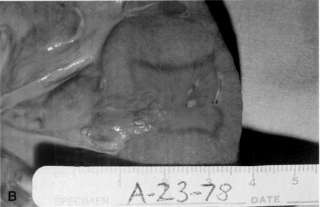

Figure 13–14. A and B, Acute pyelonephritis. A shows multiple yellow microabscesses on the surface of the kidney; the patient had ascending bacterial infection. B shows the cut surface of a kidney with a few small abscesses in the renal medulla; the cortex is pale with multiple yellow dots (microabscesses). The patient had *Candida* infection.

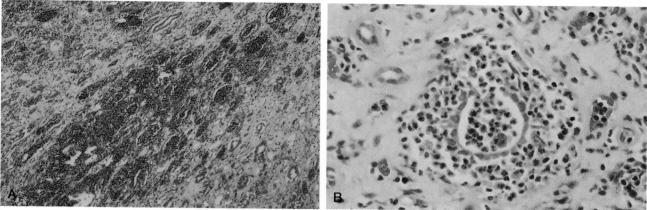

Figure 13–15. *A*, Acute pyelonephritis. Ascending infection involves many collecting ducts in the medulla. The tubular lumina are filled with acute inflammatory cells (polymorphonuclear leukocytes). *B*, Acute pyelonephritis. Polymorphonuclear leukocytes are seen in the lumen of a collecting tubule and also around the tubule in the interstitium. Note the disruption of the tubular epithelial lining at the 11-o'clock position.

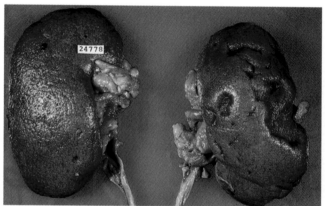

Figure 13–16. Chronic pyelonephritis. The renal cortex of the left kidney depicts deep broad-based U-shaped scars secondary to chronic pyelonephritis (although on external gross examination by itself, severe large artery disease needs to be excluded). The pelvices need to be examined.

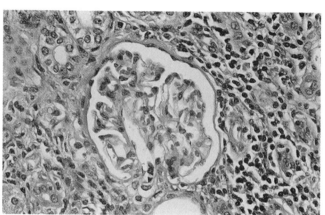

Figure 13–18. Chronic pyelonephritis. The glomerulus is histologically preserved; the interstitium shows cellular infiltrate composed mostly of lymphocytes. The glomeruli are frequently well preserved in patients with chronic pyelonephritis, even in advanced stages.

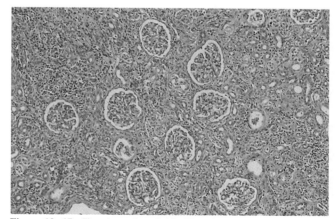

Figure 13–17. Chronic pyelonephritis. The glomeruli are closer to each other than normal because of the loss of intervening renal parenchyma/tubular atrophy. Interstitial lymphocytic infiltrate is also seen.

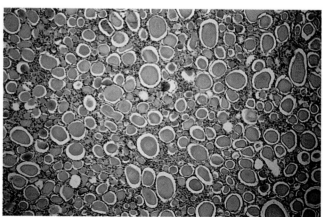

Figure 13–19. Chronic pyelonephritis, thyroidization of tubules. Atrophic tubules are filled with homogeneous eosinophil casts. This change is frequently seen in chronic pyelonephritis but is not confined to this disease.

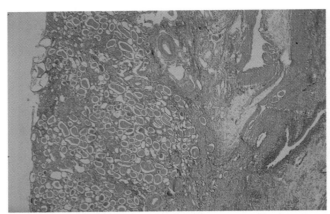

Figure 13–20. Chronic pyelonephritis. This low-magnification picture depicts a very thin renal parenchyma with markedly atrophic tubules, many of which are filled with homogeneous eosinophil casts ("thyroidization"). Interstitial inflammatory infiltrate is also present.

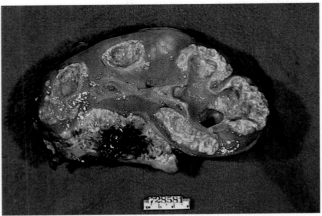

Figure 13–23. Xanthogranulomatous pyelonephritis. Large portions of the renal cortex and the renal medulla are replaced by pale tan-yellow, focally hemorrhagic inflammatory tissue. The calyces are dilated and partly destroyed. (Courtesy of Dr. Frank Vellios.)

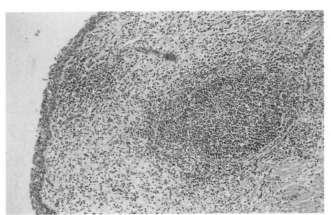

Figure 13–21. Chronic pyelonephritis. Chronic inflammation is present in and near the urothelium (transitional epithelium), along with the formation of a lymphoid follicle beneath the uroepithelium of the renal pelvis.

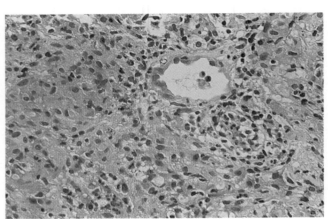

Figure 13–24. Renal malakoplakia. Heavy cellular infiltrate is seen in the tubulointerstitium with foamy histiocytes (von Hanseman's cells), lymphocytes, and scattered polymorphonuclear leukocytes. The outline of a single tubule is also seen.

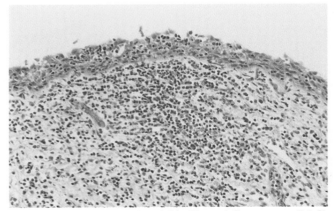

Figure 13–22. Chronic pyelonephritis. Heavy inflammatory cell infiltrate is located beneath the epithelial lining and also between the urothelial lining cells of the renal pelvis.

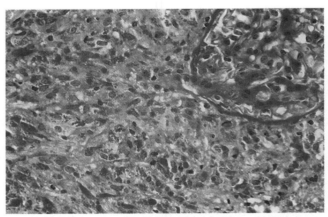

Figure 13–25. Renal malakoplakia. The tubulointerstitial histiocytes (von Hanseman's cells) reveal abundant granular periodic acid–Schiff (PAS)-positive phagolysosomes. The glomerulus is histologically unremarkable (PAS reaction).

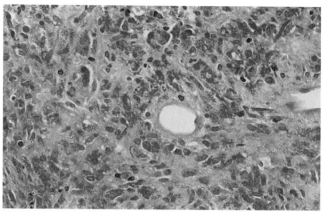

Figure 13–26. Renal malakoplakia. Granular periodic acid–Schiff (PAS) positivity is demonstrated in interstitial histiocytes (von Hanseman's cells) with high magnification (PAS reaction).

Figure 13–27. Electron micrograph of malakoplakia. The Michaelis-Gutmann body seen in an interstitial macrophage has a crystalline structure with a dense central core and outer ring (usually composed of iron and calcium). (From Laszik Z, Lajoie G, Nadasdy T, Silva FG: Medical diseases of the kidney. In: Silverberg SS, DeLellis RA, Frable WJ (eds): Principles and Practice of Surgical Pathology and Cytopathology, 3rd ed. New York, Churchill Livingstone, 1997, p 2079, with permission.)

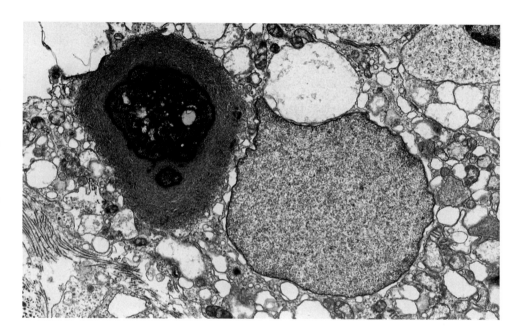

PAPILLARY NECROSIS AND ANALGESIC NEPHROPATHY

Synonyms and Related Terms: Analgesic abuse nephropathy.

Biology of Disease

- Necrosis of renal papillae occurs in three main settings: long-term consumption of combination analgesics (analgesic abuse nephropathy); acute pyelonephritis, particularly in patients with diabetes mellitus or urinary tract obstruction; and sickle cell anemia. Rare cases of papillary necrosis have been associated with use of NSAIDs, urinary tract obstruction or diabetic nephropathy in the absence of infection, and renovascular disease, renal transplant rejection, and other conditions.

- The pathophysiologic basis of papillary necrosis is complex, and different factors may be involved in different cases. Ischemia appears to be an important factor; vascular disease is also a common element in many of the conditions associated with papillary necrosis. Sickling of erythrocytes in a hypertonic and hypoxic medulla is believed to be responsible for papillary necrosis in sickle cell disease.

- Toxic effects of analgesics or their metabolites on renal tubules and interstitial blood vessels may be important in analgesic abuse nephropathy.
- Infection of the urinary tract appears to be an important factor; infections are present in most diabetics with papillary necrosis and frequently complicate analgesic nephropathy as well.
- Analgesic nephropathy occurs with prolonged, daily use of various analgesic combinations in large doses. Various combinations have been associated with analgesic nephropathy, but the majority have contained phenacetin or acetaminophen, acetylsalicylic acid, and caffeine, codeine, or barbiturates. Rarely, papillary necrosis has been reported to be associated with the use of single analgesic agents rather than combinations.
- Analgesic nephropathy was formerly common in Switzerland, Sweden, Belgium, South Africa, and Australia; it was less common in the United States. The incidence of analgesic nephropathy is now decreasing because the combination analgesics are less widely available.
- Analgesic nephropathy occurs more often in women than men; patients frequently suffer from depression or other psychiatric symptoms.
- Urothelial carcinoma of the renal pelvis is a serious potential complication of analgesic nephropathy; tobacco use appears to be a significant cofactor.
- Complications of analgesic nephropathy include chronic renal failure, hypertension, pyelonephritis, hydronephrosis, pyonephrosis, and urolithiasis.
- The lesion of focal segmental glomerulosclerosis may also occur.
- Imaging studies, usually contrast urograms, are critical in the diagnosis of papillary necrosis and analgesic nephropathy. It is rarely possible to make the diagnosis on renal biopsy, because the critical area is seldom represented in the biopsy tissue.

Clinical Features

- The clinical features of papillary necrosis are highly variable, in part because they depend on the initiating disease. In cases associated with diabetes and urinary tract obstruction, papillary necrosis usually occurs as an acute complication of pyelonephritis or another urinary tract infection. The most common manifestation of analgesic abuse nephropathy is an insidious onset of renal failure.
- Less common findings include renal colic and acute urinary tract obstruction.

Laboratory Values

- Laboratory values usually reflect chronic renal insufficiency.

Gross Appearance

- In papillary necrosis associated with diabetes mellitus or urinary tract obstruction, the kidneys are usually normal in size. Papillary necrosis may be unilateral or bilateral; several papillae may be affected, but not all. The changes usually appear to be of the same age.

- The papillae are yellow and friable and surrounded by a hyperemic border.
- In analgesic nephropathy, the kidneys are usually small and may appear ridged. Involvement is bilateral; usually all or nearly all papillae are affected, and different papillae appear to be at different stages of disease development.
- Affected papillae are firm, sclerotic, and shrunken. Necrotic papillae may slough off into the pelvis and leave a residual concave defect.
- The cortex overlying necrotic papillae may be atrophic and scarred. The columns of Bertin, which flank the papillae, are usually spared and often hypertrophied.
- Patients with chronic use of phenacetin-containing compounds may have yellow-brown pigmentation of the mucosa of the pelvis and occasionally streaks of similar color in the medullary pyramids.
- Eventually the kidneys become shrunken, heavily scarred, and distorted.

Light Microscopy

- In papillary necrosis associated with pyelonephritis, diabetes, or urinary tract obstruction, coagulative necrosis is present in affected papillae. Neutrophils are present at the interface between the necrotic area and viable tissue.
- The earliest change in analgesic nephropathy is thickening of the basement membranes of capillaries in the urinary mucosa (*capillary sclerosis*); eventually, the capillary lumina are occluded. Capillary sclerosis is most severe in the proximal third of the ureter and at the ureteropelvic junction but is also present in the mucosa overlying the calyces; in severe cases, capillary sclerosis may be found in the urinary bladder.
- Parenchymal changes are most severe in the inner medulla; the outer medulla and cortex are affected secondarily.
- The basement membranes of peritubular capillaries and the ascending limbs of the loops of Henle are thickened, and the interstitium is widened. The epithelial cells of affected tubules and endothelial cells of peritubular capillaries show degenerative changes or are necrotic; necrosis of interstitial cells may be present.
- In more advanced analgesic nephropathy, larger foci of necrosis develop in the papillae and extend upward to the border of the outer medulla. The lateral parts of the inner medulla, which receive drainage from the columns of Bertin, are usually spared, as are the vasa recta and most collecting ducts.
- In advanced analgesic nephropathy, the necrosis becomes generalized and includes the collecting ducts and vasa recta. Clefts develop within the necrotic areas, often along the interface between necrotic and viable tissue; these clefts become lined with collecting duct epithelium.
- Necrosis in analgesic nephropathy is characteristically bland; *neutrophils are conspicuously absent.*

Immunofluorescence Microscopy

- Immunofluorescence microscopy is usually not helpful in the diagnosis.

Electron Microscopy

- In analgesic nephropathy, multiple layers of basement membrane material are present around peritubular capillaries and tubules in the ascending loop of Henle and correspond to the thickened basement membranes seen on light microscopy.
- The layers of basement membrane contain polymorphous material and lipid.

Treatment and Clinical Course

- Treatment of papillary necrosis complicating diabetes or urinary tract obstruction consists primarily of relieving the acute urinary tract obstruction if present, treating the infection, and maintaining high urine volumes.
- Treatment of analgesic nephropathy includes discontinuation of analgesic use and the usual supportive measures for renal insufficiency as required.
- Analgesic nephropathy frequently runs a progressive course. The outlook for preservation of renal function has been considered good *if* the patient discontinues taking analgesics before the renal insufficiency becomes severe. However, some patients appear to have late deterioration, even after prolonged abstinence from analgesics.

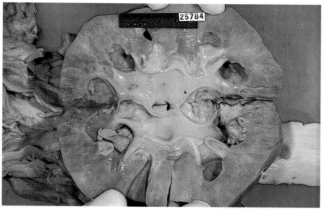

Figure 13–28. Papillary necrosis in a bisected kidney. Infarcted and detached renal papillae are seen in dilated renal calyces. A renal papilla on the *right lower* portion of the opened renal pelvis shows yellow discoloration that proved to be papillary necrosis (necrotizing papillitis or coagulation necrosis) by light microscopy from a patient with advanced diabetic nephropathy and infection.

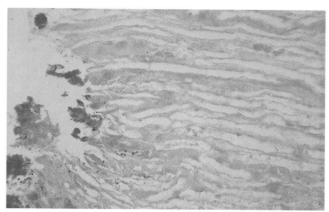

Figure 13–29. Papillary necrosis. This sloughed renal papilla in the urine shows retention of medullary tubular outlines, but no cellular epithelial structures are present.

OBSTRUCTIVE NEPHROPATHY (HYDRONEPHROSIS)

Synonyms and Related Terms: Obstructive uropathy.

Biology of Disease

- *Obstructive nephropathy* is the constellation of pathologic changes that can occur in the kidney in association with obstruction of the urinary tract. *Hydronephrosis* is generally used in a clinical sense to indicate dilatation of the renal pelvis and ureters.
- The effects of urinary tract obstruction on the kidney can be highly variable. Factors that alter the consequences of obstruction include whether the onset is sudden or gradual, whether the obstruction is complete or partial, whether the obstruction is complicated by urinary tract infection, and whether the duration of obstruction is short or prolonged.
- Often the presence or degree of hydronephrosis correlates poorly with the presence or degree of obstructive nephropathy, and vice versa. For example, approximately 70% of women will have dilatation of the renal pelvis during the third trimester of uncomplicated pregnancies, presumably because of pressure from the gravid uterus on the ureters. However, regression occurs during the first week after delivery, with no apparent sequelae.
- Much of the current knowledge about obstructive nephropathy was derived from experiments on animals, usually involving complete obstruction of the urinary tract. In clinical practice, partial obstruction is more common than complete obstruction, and relatively little is known about the morphologic changes early in the course of obstructive nephropathy in humans.

■ The causes of urinary tract obstruction are summarized in Table 13–3. Causes of urinary tract obstruction can be classified by the level of the urinary tract at which obstruction occurs, whether the lesion is congenital or acquired, whether the obstruction is intrinsic or extrinsic (external) to the urinary tract, and whether the lesion is organic (structural) or functional (resulting from neurologic diseases).

■ Ultrasonography demonstrates ureteral dilatation in up to 0.5% of fetuses; more than half of these dilatations resolve spontaneously. In childhood, urinary tract obstruction is usually congenital; although the majority of these obstructions are discovered during the first year of life, occasionally congenital urinary tract obstruction is silent until adulthood. Overall, urinary tract obstruction is more common in males than females during childhood; the most common causes include ureteropelvic or vesicoureteral obstruction or dysfunction, posterior urethral valves (usually in males), ureterocele and other congenital abnormalities, and meningomyelocele and other neurologic disorders. Congenital obstructive uropathy is frequently associated with other congenital abnormalities such as renal agenesis or ectopia, renal dysplasia, or duplicated or fused kidneys.

■ Between childhood and age 60, urinary tract obstruction is more common in women than men; the most common cause is a gynecologic tumor such as cervical or endometrial carcinoma. After approximately age 60, the incidence of urinary tract obstruction is again higher in men than women, primarily because of prostatic disease.

■ The pathophysiologic mechanisms by which urinary tract obstruction damages the kidney are not completely understood. Increased pressure inside the renal pelvis, with reflux into the collecting tubules and transmission of the increased pressure into the medulla, clearly plays a role in obstructive nephropathy. However, the pressure inside the renal pelvis in experimental models is often only slightly increased and may be normal.

■ Reflux of urine into the kidney with leakage into the interstitium (intrarenal backleak) has been demonstrated in experimental models and may be involved in inducing the interstitial fibrosis seen in obstructive nephropathy.

Table 13–3
CAUSES OF URINARY TRACT OBSTRUCTION

Intrinsic Processes	Extrinsic Processes
Nephrolithiasis	Carcinoma of the cervix or endo-
Blood clots	metrium (females)
Sloughed renal papilla (papillary	Prostatic hyperplasia or carcinoma
necrosis)	(males)
Ureteral strictures	Vascular: aneurysm of the abdom-
Congenital	inal aorta or iliac artery
Acquired: scarring from instru-	Retroperitoneal fibrosis
mentation	Idiopathic
After radiation	Drug induced (methysergide)
Urethral strictures	Inflammatory (tuberculosis, sar-
Inflammatory	coidosis)
After instrumentation	Retroperitoneal masses
Carcinoma: bladder, ureter, renal	Metastatic carcinoma
pelvis, urethra	Primary retroperitoneal neo-
	plasms
	Malignant lymphoma
	Iatrogenic: ureteral ligation

■ Ischemia is an important factor in obstructive nephropathy, particularly ischemia affecting the inner medulla. Part of the compromise in blood flow is due to direct pressure on blood vessels within the medulla; other mechanisms are clearly involved, particularly in ischemia of the cortex. Possible mediators of ischemia include the renin-angiotensin system, prostaglandins, and thromboxanes.

Clinical Features

■ The clinical picture is highly variable and depends primarily on the cause of obstruction. Sudden, complete obstruction such as that associated with obstruction of the ureter by a kidney stone elicits pain from distention of the collecting system or renal capsule (the familiar syndrome of renal colic). On the other hand, partial obstruction or obstruction that develops slowly may be clinically silent for long periods.

■ In bilateral, partial obstruction, the earliest manifestations are polyuria and nocturia, which are reflections of loss of the ability to concentrate urine. Renal tubular acidosis may be present.

■ Urinary tract infection, a common complication of urinary tract obstruction, may be the initial manifestation.

Gross Appearance

■ In the early period of sudden, complete obstruction, the only change might be slight dilatation of the renal pelvis with blunting of the calyces. The weight of the kidney is increased because of edema. After 2 to 3 days of continuing obstruction the papillae appear compressed, blunted, and flattened; small areas of necrosis may be seen in the papillary tips.

■ With continued obstruction or long-term partial obstruction, progressive dilatation of the renal pelvis, flattening of the papillae, and eventual thinning of renal tissue occur. The initial thinning occurs because of loss of the papillae and thinning of the medulla; eventually the cortex also begins to decrease in thickness.

■ The end-stage hydronephrotic kidney is pale and firm; the surface may appear slightly bosselated. Only a thin rim of renal parenchyma remains, with fibrous septa radiating outward from the hilus.

Light Microscopy

Glomeruli

■ In the acute stage, glomerular capillaries appear congested. If the obstruction persists for several weeks, focal thickening of Bowman's capsule is seen, but the capillary tuft appears unremarkable.

■ With long-standing obstruction, the size of the glomeruli tends to decrease and sclerotic glomeruli appear. Glomeruli may appear essentially unchanged despite the presence of severe tubular atrophy.

Tubules

■ The initial change is dilatation of tubules, with flattening of the tubular epithelium; loss of the brush border in proximal convoluted tubules is noted.

- The collecting ducts become dilated within the first day of obstruction. Necrosis of cells lining the ducts at the tips of the papillae may be present and is associated with the appearance of neutrophils.
- With continued obstruction, apoptotic tubular epithelial cells appear; mitotic figures may be present in tubular epithelium. Eventually the tubular epithelium becomes greatly thinned and simplified; the outline of tubules becomes irregular, with apparent outpouchings of the epithelium. The tubular basement membrane becomes thickened.
- Eventually, the tubular atrophy becomes widespread.

Interstitium

- The earliest change is interstitial edema. A leukocytic infiltrate appears in the cortex; there is less inflammation in the medulla.
- With continued obstruction, activated fibroblast-like cells appear in the interstitium and begin to lay down collagen. Tubules are separated from peritubular capillaries by interstitial fibrosis.
- Eventually, widespread interstitial fibrosis accompanies the generalized tubular atrophy.

Vessels

- In the early period, peritubular capillaries are congested; microthrombi may be present.
- Veins may be dilated; arteries generally show few changes.

Immunofluorescence Microscopy

- Immunofluorescence microscopy is not usually performed in patients with obstructive nephropathy.

Electron Microscopy

- Changes in glomeruli include effacement or loss of visceral epithelial cell foot processes. After obstruction lasting 2 to 8 weeks, the glomerular capillary basement

membranes become thickened, convoluted, and collapsed.
- Proximal convoluted tubular epithelial cells lose the apical villi that form the brush border. The cytoplasm becomes vacuolated, and increased numbers of lysosomes are present. The basal interdigitations between cells are lost. Other tubules show generally similar changes.

Treatment and Clinical Course

- Treatment depends on the primary condition causing the obstruction.
- A major clinical question is whether or how much renal function may be recovered after the obstruction is relieved. Unfortunately, that may be difficult to predict. Clearly, prompt relief of obstruction from a renal stone should result in complete recovery, and an end-stage hydronephrotic kidney with only a few remaining millimeters of renal parenchyma will have no potential for recovery. However, the situation is less clear in patients with degrees of hydronephrosis between these two extremes.
- The most important factor in determining the degree of recovery is the duration of obstruction. Animal experiments suggest that nearly complete recovery may occur if the obstruction is relieved within approximately 4 days; some recovery of renal function may occur after obstruction for up to 3 weeks, although some degree of irreversible damage will be present. Recovery may take a prolonged period (weeks to several months). The exact relevance of these experiments to the human condition is unclear, and of course, the duration of obstruction in patients is seldom known with precision.
- Additional factors that may influence the potential for recovery include whether any renal disease was present before the obstruction and whether the obstruction was complicated by infection.
- It has been suggested that the obstruction should be temporarily relieved (by a stent, percutaneous nephrostomy, etc.) and the patient monitored for a minimum of 2 weeks. Then the degree of function in that kidney should be determined with a renal isotopic scan.

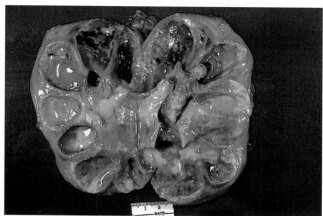

Figure 13–30. Staghorn calculi in a bisected kidney. Staghorn calculi are present in the renal calyces and in the pelvis; both the pelvis and the calyces are dilated and deformed. The cortex is thin and the pelvic mucosa is covered by gray, focally hemorrhagic inflammatory exudate.

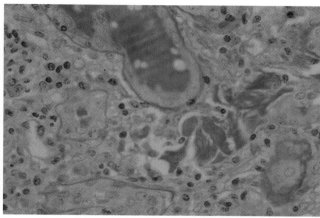

Figure 13–31. Tubular casts. A periodic acid–Schiff (PAS)-positive (probable Tamm-Horsfall protein) cast is seen in a slightly dilated distal-appearing tubule. The tubular epithelium is damaged. Some of the PAS-positive material appears to be in the interstitium.

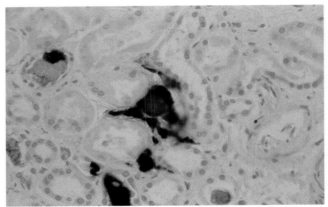

Figure 13–32. Tamm-Horsfall protein. Immunoperoxidase staining for Tamm-Horsfall protein shows a positive reaction in a few tubular lumina and also in the interstitium. Interstitial staining is related to tubular leakage of Tamm-Horsfall protein.

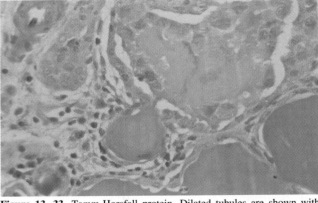

Figure 13–33. Tamm-Horsfall protein. Dilated tubules are shown with Tamm-Horsfall protein casts. Note the gap on the tubular wall with leakage of Tamm-Horsfall protein toward the interstitium. The tubular leakage induced an interstitial inflammatory reaction.

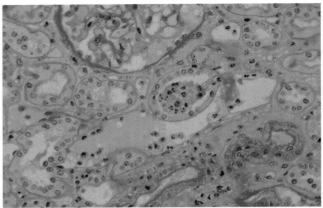

Figure 13–34. Tubulovenous reflux. Tubulovenous reflux is shown in a patient with acute renal failure and tubulointerstitial disease.

REFERENCES

General

Farrington K, Levison DA, Greenwood RN, et al: Renal biopsy in patients with unexplained renal impairment and normal kidney size. Q J Med 70:221, 1989.

Kelly CJ, Neilson EG: Tubulointerstitial diseases. In: Brenner BM (ed): Brenner & Rector's The Kidney, 5th ed. Philadelphia, WB Saunders, 1996, p 1655.

Interstitial Nephritis

Bender WL, Whelton A, Beschorner WE, et al: Interstitial nephritis, proteinuria, and renal failure caused by nonsteroidal anti-inflammatory drugs: Immunologic characterization of the inflammatory infiltrate. Am J Med 76:1006, 1984.

Cavallo T: Tubulointerstitial nephritis. In: Jennette JC, Olson JL, Schwartz MM, Silva FG (eds): Heptinstall's Pathology of the Kidney, 5th ed. Philadelphia, Lippincott-Raven, 1998, p 667.

Cohen AH, Nast CC: Renal injury caused by human immunodeficiency virus infection. In: Jennette JC, Olson JL, Schwartz MM, Silva FG (eds): Heptinstall's Pathology of the Kidney, 5th ed. Philadelphia, Lippincott-Raven, 1998, p 785.

Colvin RB, Fang LST: Interstitial nephritis. In: Tisher CC, Brenner BM (eds): Renal Pathology With Clinical and Functional Correlations, 2nd ed. Philadelphia, JB Lippincott, 1994, p 723.

Ellis D, Fried WA, Yunis J, et al: Acute interstitial nephritis in children: A report of 13 cases and review of the literature. Pediatrics 67:862, 1981.

Galpin JE, Shinaberger JH, Stanley TM, et al: Acute interstitial nephritis due to methicillin. Am J Med 65:756, 1978.

Grčevska L, Polenaković M, Ončevski A, et al: Different pathohistological presentations of acute renal involvement in Hantaan virus infection: Report of two cases. Clin Nephrol 34:197, 1990.

Heptinstall RH: Interstitial nephritis: A brief review. Am J Pathol 83:214, 1976.

Heptinstall RH: Urinary tract infection, pyelonephritis, reflux nephropathy. In: Jennette JC, Olson JL, Schwartz MM, Silva FG (eds): Heptinstall's Pathology of the Kidney, 5th ed. Philadelphia, Lippincott-Raven, 1998, p 725.

Laberke H-G, Bohle A: Acute interstitial nephritis: Correlations between clinical and morphological findings. Clin Nephrol 14:263, 1980.

Mignon F, Méry JP, Mougenot B, et al: Granulomatous interstitial nephritis. Adv Nephrol 13:219, 1984.

Nadasdy T, Racusen LC: Renal injury caused by therapeutic and diagnostic agents and abuse of analgesics and narcotics. In: Jennette JC, Olson JL, Schwartz MM, Silva FG (eds): Heptinstall's Pathology of the Kidney, 5th ed. Philadelphia, Lippincott-Raven, 1998, p 811.

Platt JL, Sibley RK, Michael AF: Interstitial nephritis associated with cytomegalovirus infection. Kidney Int 28:550, 1985.

Pusey CD, Saltissi D, Bloodworth L, et al: Drug associated acute interstitial nephritis: Clinical and pathological features and the response to high dose steroid therapy. Q J Med 52:194, 1983.

Schlondorff D: Renal complications of nonsteroidal anti-inflammatory drugs. Kidney Int 44:643, 1993.

Obstructive Nephropathy (Hydronephrosis)

Curhan GC, Zeidel ML: Urinary tract obstruction. In: Brenner BM (ed): Brenner & Rector's The Kidney, 5th ed. Philadelphia, WB Saunders, 1996, p 1936.

Hill GS: Calcium and the kidney. In: Jennette JC, Olson JL, Schwartz MM, Silva FG (eds): Heptinstall's Pathology of the Kidney, 5th ed. Philadelphia, Lippincott-Raven, 1998, p 891.

Møller JC, Djurhuus JC: Obstructive disease of the kidney (hydronephrosis) and the urinary tract. In: Tisher CC, Brenner BM (eds): Renal Pathology With Clinical and Functional Correlations, 2nd ed. Philadelphia, JB Lippincott, 1994, p 863.

Pyelonephritis

Esparza AR, McKay DB, Cronan JJ, et al: Renal parenchymal malacoplakia: Histologic spectrum and its relationship to megalocytic interstitial nephritis and xanthogranulomatous pyelonephritis. Am J Surg Pathol 13:225, 1989.

Heptinstall RH: Urinary tract infection, pyelonephritis, reflux nephropathy. In: Jennette JC, Olson JL, Schwartz MM, Silva FG (eds): Heptinstall's Pathology of the Kidney, 5th ed. Philadelphia, Lippincott-Raven, 1998, p 725.

Peterson JC, Tisher CC: Tuberculosis of the kidney. In: Tisher CC, Brenner BM (eds): Renal Pathology With Clinical and Functional Correlations, 2nd ed. Philadelphia, JB Lippincott, 1994, p 895.

Risdon RA: Pyelonephritis and reflux nephropathy. In: Tisher CC, Brenner BM (eds): Renal Pathology With Clinical and Functional Correlations, 2nd ed. Philadelphia, JB Lippincott, 1994, p 832.

Rubin RH, Cotran RS, Tolkoff-Rubin NE: Urinary tract infection, pyelonephritis and reflux nephropathy. In: Brenner BM (ed): Brenner & Rector's The Kidney, 5th ed. Philadelphia, WB Saunders, 1996, p 1597.

Papillary Necrosis and Analgesic Nephropathy

Mihatsch MJ, Brunner FP, Gloor FJG: Analgesic nephropathy and papillary necrosis. In: Tisher CC, Brenner BM (eds): Renal Pathology With Clinical and Functional Correlations, 2nd ed. Philadelphia, JB Lippincott, 1994, p 905.

CHAPTER 14

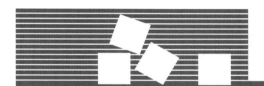

Vascular Diseases of the Kidney
Ischemic Renal Disease, Thromboembolism, Hypertension, Renal Cortical Necrosis, and Renal Vein Thrombosis

INTRODUCTION

- The kidneys receive approximately 25% of the cardiac output, the single greatest proportion of any organ. Therefore they are greatly affected by diseases of the blood vessels.
- *Ischemic renal disease* may be defined as a significant reduction in glomerular filtration rate because of hemodynamically significant renovascular occlusive disease affecting the entire functioning renal parenchyma. The result of the reduction in renal blood flow is progressive renal atrophy and decreased renal excretory function (as measured by creatinine clearance). Many causes of renal ischemia are known, and common causes of ischemic renal disease are listed in Table 14–1.
- Diseases involving the larger arteries include atherosclerosis, thrombosis, and thromboembolism; smaller arteries and arterioles are most often affected by hypertension and thromboembolism. Rarely, ischemic injury to the kidneys can result from severe hypotension or shock, without actual obstruction of vessels (*ischemic acute tubular nephropathy*). The kidneys may also be affected by vasculitides, such as Wegener's granulomatosis, polyarteritis nodosa, and others.
- Arteries of the kidneys are usually considered to be end-organ type, with no effective collateral circulation. Thus sudden occlusion of arteries usually results in infarction. However, some degree of collateral circulation can develop from retroperitoneal, adrenal, and periureteral arteries as a result of gradual narrowing of the main renal arteries.
- Renal ischemia caused by hypotension activates the renin-angiotensin-aldosterone system, which stimulates vasoconstriction, salt and water retention, and a compensatory increase in systemic blood pressure. Renal ischemia caused by stenosis of the main renal arteries or narrowing of the intrarenal arteries initiates the same process resulting in a *pathologic* increase in arterial blood pressure, or systemic hypertension.

- Systemic hypertension can be both a cause and a consequence of renal disease. Hypertension greatly accelerates the progress of arterial and arteriolar nephrosclerosis; this acceleration of arteriosclerosis may result in further activation of the renin-angiotensin-aldosterone system and a further increase in blood pressure. Thus a positive feedback loop results, with arteriosclerosis and hypertension setting the stage for progression of arteriosclerosis and a further increase in blood pressure.
- Occlusion of the renal veins also occurs, most commonly because of renal vein thrombosis occurring in the setting of nephrotic syndrome. The renal veins may also be rarely compromised by extrinsic compression by retroperitoneal masses.

RENAL ARTERY STENOSIS

Synonyms and Related Terms: Renovascular disease; renal infarction; ischemic nephropathy; fibromuscular dysplasia.

Biology of Disease

- In general, ischemic renal disease occurs when the arterial lumen is reduced by 70% or greater.
- Atherosclerosis is the most common cause of occlusion of the large renal arteries. It occurs most often in the older age groups, and men are affected about twice as often as women. Major risk factors include hypertension, hyperlipidemia, and cigarette use.
- Thromboemboli lodging in the main renal arteries and their major branches usually originate from the heart; the most common settings are cardiac arrhythmias and myocardial infarctions.
- Thrombosis of the main renal arteries may result from blunt trauma to the kidney; the left renal artery is affected approximately twice as frequently as the right. Alternatively, thrombi may form on the surface of ulcerated atheromatous plaques.

159

Table 14–1
CAUSES OF ISCHEMIC RENAL DISEASE

Renal artery atherosclerosis
Fibromuscular dysplasia of the renal arteries
Hypertensive renal vascular disease
Renal artery thromboembolism
Cholesterol embolism
Aortic or renal artery dissection
Vasculitis involving the renal artery or intrarenal arteries
Thrombotic microangiopathy
Thromboangiitis obliterans

■ *Fibromuscular dysplasia,* an interesting but relatively uncommon cause of renal artery narrowing, occurs more commonly in women than in men and at a relatively young age in comparison to atherosclerosis.
■ Several distinct forms of fibromuscular dysplasia are described and differentiated by the layer of artery involved:
  • *Intimal fibroplasia*: a rare variant that may cause severe or total stenosis; similar changes may be found in patients with chronic pyelonephritis or on long-term hemodialysis, as well as in other forms of fibromuscular dysplasia.
  • *Medial hyperplasia*: uncommon but may cause severe stenosis.
  • *Medial fibroplasia with aneurysms*: the most common variant (60% to 85%) and most often bilateral; seldom causes total arterial occlusion.
  • *Medial dissection*: probably begins in an area of intimal fibroplasia; defects in the internal elastic lamina may allow dissection of blood into the media.
  • *Perimedial fibroplasia*: 10% to 25% of the total; may be associated with severe or complete stenosis of the artery.
■ Large artery vasculitis involving the renal arteries, such as Takayasu's arteritis, is a rare cause of renal artery stenosis.
■ The consequences of occlusion of the main renal arteries or large branches depend on the size and number of vessels involved, rate of closure, presence or absence of collateral circulation, and whether involvement is unilateral or bilateral. Sudden occlusion usually results in infarction; gradual narrowing may result in diffuse atrophy, termed *ischemic nephropathy*, without infarction.
■ Renal artery stenosis is a significant cause of hypertension by activation of the renin-angiotensin-aldosterone system. Unilateral stenosis may result in the phenomenon known as the *Goldblatt kidney*; the ischemic kidney produces renin, with consequent systemic hypertension. The ischemic kidney is protected from the effects of hypertension by the renal artery stenosis; the contralateral kidney is not protected and suffers the consequences of hypertension (arterial and arteriolar nephrosclerosis).

Clinical Features

■ Ischemic nephropathy resulting from stenosis of the main renal arteries or major branches is usually asymptomatic until advanced; the first signs are usually hypertension and chronic renal insufficiency.
■ The majority of patients have widespread occlusive vascular disease, including atherosclerotic coronary artery disease, peripheral arterial occlusion, and others.

Laboratory Values

■ Ischemic nephropathy is characterized by increased serum urea nitrogen and creatinine values; urinalysis frequently demonstrates proteinuria of low to moderate degree.

Gross Appearance

■ Occlusion of the renal arteries from atherosclerosis usually involves the proximal renal arteries; the origin from the aorta is involved in approximately 50% of cases. Bilateral disease is present in up to 60% of cases.
■ Atherosclerosis causes eccentric narrowing of the artery by a yellow-white plaque (atheroma).
■ Fibromuscular dysplasia usually causes concentric narrowing of the artery; there may be thickening and fibrosis of the intima, media, or adventitia. Alternating constrictions and aneurysmal dilatations may be present.
■ Kidneys with ischemic nephropathy are usually small; large cortical scars and small cortical cysts may be present. The capsular surface is frequently finely granular because of concomitant arteriolosclerosis.
■ On section, the cortex is thin. The interlobar and arcuate arteries may appear prominent.

Light Microscopy

Renal Arteries

■ Atherosclerosis: the intima is eccentrically thickened with fibrosis, amorphous material, and lipid-laden macrophages (*foam cells*); cholesterol clefts may be present, as well as medial fibrosis.
■ Fibromuscular dysplasia:
  • Intimal fibroplasia: the intima is thickened by loose, sparsely cellular fibrous tissue; the lumen is reduced, and the internal elastic lamina is intact.
  • Medial hyperplasia: the media is thickened, with numerous smooth muscle cells; the intima, internal elastic lamina, and adventitia are unremarkable.
  • Medial fibroplasia with aneurysms: areas of thickening and fibrosis in the media alternate with aneurysmal dilatations; the internal elastic lamina is absent in the dilated areas.
  • Medial dissection: dissection of blood is present in the media.
  • Perimedial fibroplasia: mature collagen replaces the smooth muscle cells in large areas of the media; the media is irregularly thickened.

Kidneys

- The earliest change in glomeruli is modest thickening and "accordion-like" wrinkling of capillary basement membranes on periodic acid–Schiff or methenamine silver stains. The glomerular capillary tuft becomes simplified and contracts toward the vascular pole, with relative enlargement of Bowman's space.
- Collagen deposition occurs inside Bowman's capsule basement membrane in some glomeruli (*intracapsular fibrosis*); collagen deposits are often initially seen near the vascular pole and expand toward the urinary pole. Eventually, collagen completely fills Bowman's space with consequent global sclerosis. The collapsed capillary tuft may be inapparent on hematoxylin and eosin stain but will be demonstrated by periodic acid–Schiff or methenamine silver stain. "Atubular glomeruli," or residual glomeruli within fibrotic scars, may be present.
- Focal segmental glomerulosclerosis occasionally develops after long-standing hypertension and may be associated with marked proteinuria.
- Tubular atrophy and interstitial fibrosis are common; compensatory dilated tubules may be present (*super tubules*).
- One frequent histologic change is diffuse atrophy of proximal tubules, with decreased diameter, narrowed or inapparent lumen, and a lining of cuboidal epithelial cells with clear cytoplasm; this tubular appearance has been described as *endocrine change*. In experimental models, numerous mitochondria are present; other subcellular organelles are decreased.
- The juxtaglomerular apparatus may be hypertrophied.
- In unilateral renal artery stenosis, the ipsilateral ("protected") kidney shows diffuse tubular atrophy and interstitial fibrosis; glomeruli are closely approximated because of atrophy of the intervening cortex; the juxtaglomerular apparatus may be hypertrophied. Vessels are not subjected to the increased arterial pressure; therefore, artery and arteriole walls are not usually thickened (unless exposed to preexisting hypertension). The contralateral (nonstenotic or "unprotected") kidney, which is now exposed to the systemic hypertension caused by the renal artery stenosis, usually has severe arterial and arteriolar sclerosis and may show changes of "malignant" hypertension (see page 165).

Treatment and Clinical Course

- Once ischemic renal disease (with at least 70% narrowing of the renal artery lumen) has developed, it tends to progress fairly rapidly; approximately half of patients have evidence of progression (loss of renal excretory function or decrease in renal length) within 2 years. Control of blood pressure, hyperlipidemia, or serum glucose (in diabetics) appears to have little effect on slowing the progression of disease once ischemic renal disease caused by severe renal artery stenosis has developed.
- Renal artery stenosis, if detected early, may potentially be reversed by angioplasty or bypass graft. There is little hope of reversibility after chronic renal insufficiency due to ischemic nephropathy has developed.
- In long-standing unilateral renal artery stenosis, correction of the stenosis may not relieve the hypertension if advanced hypertensive changes have developed in the contralateral kidney.

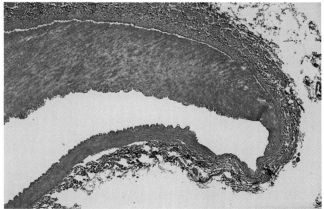

Figure 14–1. Fibromuscular dysplasia. Medial fibroplasia with aneurysms is seen in a renal artery. Medial fibroplasia is the most common variant of fibromuscular dysplasia of the renal arteries and is often bilateral.

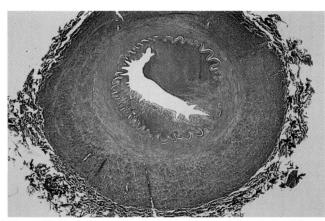

Figure 14–2. Fibromuscular dysplasia. Perimedial fibroplasia of the renal artery is shown. Some "secondary" intimal fibroplasia is seen as well.

RENAL INFARCTION

Clinical Features

- Symptoms of renal infarction are extremely variable; infarcts may be clinically silent, particularly if relatively small portions of the kidney are involved.
- Symptoms of infarcts may include chest, abdomen, flank, or back pain. Nausea and vomiting may occur; fever may be present. Gross hematuria and hypertension may also be noted.
- Acute anuria or oliguria may occur if both renal arteries are involved or the artery to a solitary kidney.
- Signs of atherosclerosis or embolic disease involving the extremities or other organs may be present.

Laboratory Values

- Leukocytosis may be noted; serum lactate dehydrogenase, transaminases, and alkaline phosphatase values may be increased.
- Urinalysis demonstrates variable amounts of hematuria and proteinuria; epithelial cells, cellular debris, and clusters of necrotic tubular cells may be present.

Gross Pathology

- Sudden occlusion of the main renal artery results in infarction of most or all of the kidney; occlusion of smaller branches results in wedge-shaped infarcts with the apex oriented toward the medulla.
- The appearance of renal infarcts varies, depending on the amount of kidney involved, the rate of occlusion, and the time since the event occurred.
- In the first 24 hours, the infarcted area appears red to gray and is surrounded by a hyperemic zone.
- Over the next 4 to 7 days the infarct begins to turn yellow and the hyperemic zone disappears; the capsular surface becomes depressed relative to uninfarcted areas.

- Eventually, the infarcted area becomes fibrotic; contraction of the affected segment leaves a deep cortical scar.
- The presence of multiple infarcts of varying age indicates recurrent thromboemboli occurring over a period of time.

Light Microscopy

- The initial change, within the first hour, is engorgement of glomerular and peritubular capillaries with erythrocytes. The glomerular and tubular cells otherwise appear preserved.
- Glomeruli around the margins of the infarct may show necrosis of the capillary tuft or crescents.
- Tubular injury and interstitial edema may be present in zones around the infarct.
- At 12 hours, a rim of neutrophils is present around the periphery of the infarct.
- Between 1 and 7 days, the nuclei of tubular and glomerular cells disappear, but the outline of the cells may still be seen. The nuclei of tubular cells are lost first; those in glomerular cells persist longer. The neutrophils disappear and are replaced by basophilic nuclear debris; granulation tissue begins to form around the periphery.
- Over several days to a few weeks the infarcted area may be replaced by granulation tissue; eventually, mature fibrous tissue may replace the infarcted area.
- Atrophic tubules, sclerotic glomeruli, and interstitial fibrosis may be present around the fibrotic infarct.

Treatment and Clinical Course

- Sudden, complete occlusion of a main renal artery may not cause immediate infarction; a short period of ischemia may ensue, during which time relief of the occlusion may prevent infarction.
- No treatment is effective once infarction has occurred; the severity depends on the size of the vessel or vessels affected and the resulting amount of renal tissue that is infarcted.

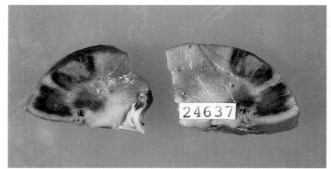

Figure 14–3. Renal infarction, acute. Sections of the kidney show cortical wedge-shaped pale tan-yellow areas (infarcts) surrounded by wide hemorrhagic borders. The term *anemic* infarction reflects the lack of hemorrhage within the infarcted area, which is the typical gross appearance of renal infarction secondary to the "end-organ" vasculature of the kidney; however, hemorrhagic infarction may also occur.

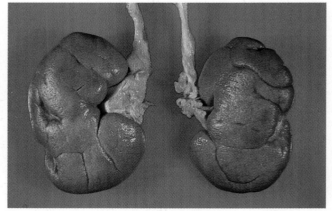

Figure 14–4. Focal infarction of the renal parenchyma, old ("healed"). Deep V-shaped scars on the renal surface on the left are consistent with the chronic sequelae of past episode(s) of renal infarction.

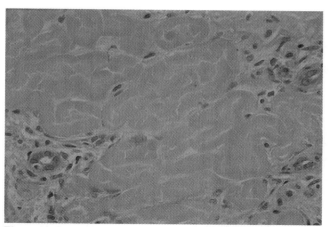

Figure 14–5. Anemic infarction of the renal parenchyma, fresh. Coagulation necrosis (loss of nuclear staining but preservation of cell outlines) is present in a large group of necrotic tubules. The nuclei of a few interstitial cells and tubular cells on the right and left are still recognizable.

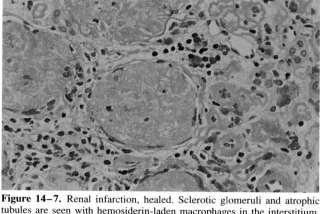

Figure 14–7. Renal infarction, healed. Sclerotic glomeruli and atrophic tubules are seen with hemosiderin-laden macrophages in the interstitium.

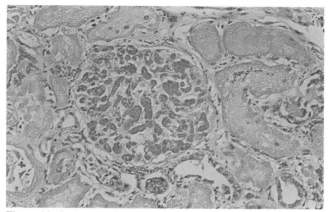

Figure 14–6. Anemic infarction of the renal parenchyma, fresh. Coagulation necrosis involves both the glomeruli (so-called glomerular paralysis) and the tubules from an autopsy kidney. The cause of the small infarction was obstruction of an interlobular renal artery by a metastatic tumor from lung cancer.

CHOLESTEROL EMBOLI

Biology of Disease

- The most common conditions affecting the smaller arteries and arterioles are hypertension (discussed later) and cholesterol emboli. These vessels may also be involved in thrombotic microangiopathies such as the hemolytic-uremic syndrome (see Chapter 7).
- Cholesterol embolism occurs in patients with atherosclerosis of the thoracic or upper abdominal aorta.
- Frequently, but not invariably, there has been a history of a previous precipitating event such as cardiac or vascular surgery, angiography, or cardiac catheterization. These procedures cause mechanical disruption of

the surface of atheromas, with release and subsequent embolization of cholesterol crystals.
- Anticoagulants such as warfarin may also predispose to cholesterol embolization. The anticoagulant is presumed to prevent the formation of a clot over the surface of an ulcerated atheromatous plaque; such a clot may prevent embolization from the exposed contents of the atheroma.
- Consequences of cholesterol emboli can include digital necrosis in the lower extremities, gastrointestinal bleeding, strokes, myocardial infarction, and renal failure.
- The kidneys are the most common organs involved by cholesterol embolization; in the past, renal involvement was considered to be progressive and irreversible, with

inevitable progression to renal failure and a high mortality rate (70% to 90%). However, in recent years patients with less severe renal failure have been described, the mortality rate has decreased, and recovery of significant renal function has occurred in some patients.

Clinical Features

- Cholesterol emboli occur in older age groups; men are more often affected than women.
- Onset frequently occurs 1 to several weeks after angiography, cardiovascular surgery, or another precipitating event.
- Common initial features include mottling of the skin of the lower extremities (*livedo reticularis*) and necrosis of the toes.
- Cholesterol emboli may occasionally be visible within retinal vessels on funduscopic examination (*Hollenhorst plaques*).
- Renal involvement is usually manifested as increased serum urea nitrogen and creatinine; urinalysis frequently shows hematuria, proteinuria, and casts but may be unremarkable.
- Hypertension may be a prominent feature.
- The diagnosis may be made by demonstrating cholesterol emboli in biopsies of skin showing livedo reticularis.

Laboratory Values

- Serum urea nitrogen and creatinine levels are elevated.
- Eosinophilia may be present.
- Urinalysis may show erythrocytes, leukocytes, and casts.
- Proteinuria may be present and occasionally reaches nephrotic levels.
- Serum complement levels may be decreased.

Gross Appearance

- If renal infarction has occurred, the gross appearance is similar to that described earlier for diseases of large vessels. Infarcts will be small, wedge shaped, and frequently multiple.

Light Microscopy

- The most characteristic finding is empty, needle-like clefts within arterioles, interlobular arteries, and occasionally arcuate arteries in association with fibrin and organizing thrombi. The clefts represent the spaces occupied by cholesterol crystals, which are dissolved out of the tissue during tissue processing and staining. The actual crystals may be visible if unstained frozen section slides are viewed under polarized light.
- Emboli may be found within glomerular capillaries, where they sometimes evoke a giant cell reaction.
- A neutrophilic infiltrate, sometimes with eosinophils, is present in the first 24 hours, followed by lymphocytes and histiocytes. Giant cells may be seen attempting to ingest the cholesterol crystals.
- Patchy acute tubular necrosis is commonly seen; small cortical infarcts may be present.
- With time, the cholesterol crystals are surrounded by a dense fibrous reaction.

Treatment and Clinical Course

- Renal involvement is variable in severity but may be progressive and result in severe renal failure requiring dialysis.
- No specific treatment is known for cholesterol embolism; anticoagulation is usually ineffective and may aggravate the condition.
- Peritoneal dialysis or hemodialysis may be required. Partial recovery of renal function has now been reported in many patients but may require a prolonged period of dialysis support.

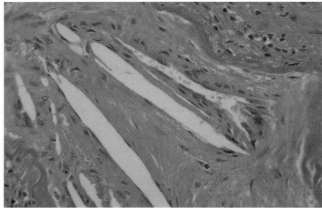

Figure 14–8. Cholesterol emboli. Jagged-edged angular cholesterol clefts of atheromatous emboli are surrounded by fibrous tissue. The cholesterol-laden material is dissolved. Giant cells are seen around the angular clefts.

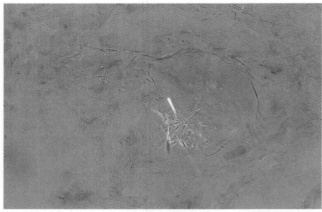

Figure 14–9. Cholesterol emboli. Birefringent cholesterol clefts are seen in an interlobular artery on a frozen unstained section. This method is excellent for detecting cholesterol emboli in renal sections.

HYPERTENSION AND THE KIDNEY

Biology of Disease

- Many causes of systemic hypertension are known, and a complete discussion is outside the scope of this text. In brief, hypertension may be divided into cases with no known cause (*primary* or *essential* hypertension) and cases caused by some other known condition (*secondary hypertension*) Primary hypertension is by far the more common; renal diseases constitute an important cause of secondary hypertension.
- As noted earlier, vascular diseases of the kidneys can be both a *cause* and a *consequence* of hypertension; hypertension of any cause significantly accelerates the progression of renal vascular disease.
- Hypertension may also be divided into mild to moderate hypertension, sometimes termed *benign* hypertension, and severe or *malignant* hypertension.
- Malignant hypertension is now uncommon. Systolic pressure is usually 190 mm Hg or greater; diastolic pressure often exceeds 120 mm Hg. However, "malignant" hypertension is best defined by the presence of associated clinical conditions rather than by a numerical value of systolic or diastolic pressure. Complications of malignant hypertension include papilledema and retinal hemorrhage, congestive heart failure, stroke, encephalopathy, proteinuria, and renal insufficiency. In the era before effective treatment for hypertension was available, the duration of the malignant phase of hypertension was usually short; survival was often a matter of months.
- "Benign" hypertension (hypertension of lesser degree and not associated with acute symptoms) is a major risk factor for cerebrovascular accidents, coronary artery disease and myocardial infarction, renal disease, and systemic arteriosclerosis in general. Unfortunately, lesser degrees of hypertension are usually asymptomatic until such a catastrophic complication occurs.
- There are also pathologic differences between benign and malignant hypertension, and therefore they will be described separately.

"Benign" Hypertension

Gross Pathology

- The kidneys may be normal or moderately reduced in size and weight.
- The capsular surface is usually granular, and there may be deep, irregular cortical scars; simple cysts may also be present.
- The cortex is frequently thinned; the interlobar and arcuate arteries may be prominent.

Light Microscopy

- Glomerular, tubular, and interstitial changes resemble those seen in ischemic nephropathy, described earlier.
- Arteries demonstrate concentric collagen deposition in the intima (*intimal fibrosis*), smooth muscle hyperplasia, and decreased lumen size. The internal elastic lamina becomes reduplicated or multilayered on elastic stains.
- The characteristic change in arterioles is *hyaline arteriolosclerosis*, seen in afferent arterioles. The medial smooth muscle is filled or replaced by homogeneous eosinophilic material, which is faintly positive on periodic acid–Schiff reaction and blue on Masson's trichrome stain. The process begins under the endothelial layer; eventually the entire media may be replaced.

Immunofluorescence Microscopy

- Staining for IgM and C3 is frequently present within the hyaline layers of arterioles; immunofluorescence staining is otherwise negative or minimal.

Electron Microscopy

- Glomerular capillary basement membranes may be thickened and wrinkled. Discrete electron-dense, immune-type deposits are absent.
- Arteriolar basement membranes show thickening and reduplication.

"Malignant" Hypertension

Gross Pathology

- The kidneys may have changes of arterial or arteriolar sclerosis, as just described, in patients with previous hypertension or renal disease; the kidneys may be normal in size in patients with no such history.
- Petechial hemorrhages may be present on the cortical surface and the mucosa of the renal pelvis.

Light Microscopy

- Interlobular arteries have intimal widening by loosely arranged connective tissue fibrils and myointimal cells within a matrix of mucoid ground substance. Erythrocytes or erythrocyte fragments may be present within the intima. The lumen is greatly reduced and may be occluded by fibrin thrombi. The internal elastic lamina may be attenuated, but it is not laminated or fragmented in the absence of preexisting hypertensive changes.
- The walls of arterioles and smaller interlobular arteries are replaced by waxy or fibrillar-appearing, intensely eosinophilic material, a condition described as *fibrinoid necrosis*. Vessel lumina may be occluded by fibrin thrombi.
- Fibrinoid necrosis may extend into the vascular poles of glomeruli in continuity with afferent arterioles. Segmental or global necrosis of the capillary tuft may be present.
- Other glomerular changes can include *mesangiolysis*, indicated by marked dilation of capillaries, usually near the vascular pole. Crescents may be present within Bowman's capsule, often but not invariably associated with glomerular necrosis.
- The juxtaglomerular apparatus may be hypertrophied.

■ Focal acute tubular necrosis and small cortical infarcts may be present.

Immunofluorescence Microscopy

■ Staining for fibrinogen, C3, and IgM may be present within small arteries, arterioles, and glomerular capillaries. This finding most likely represents leakage of plasma proteins into vessel walls (so-called "plasmatic insudation") rather than immune complex deposition.

Electron Microscopy

■ Glomerular capillary basement membranes are thickened and wrinkled.
■ Endothelial cells of arterioles, arteries, and glomerular capillaries are swollen, and the subendothelial space is widened by electron-lucent, "fluffy" material.
■ Platelet and fibrin thrombi may be present within capillary lumina and within the walls of arteries and arterioles.

Differential Diagnosis

■ The hyaline arteriolosclerosis characteristic of "benign" hypertension is not specific and can be seen in diabetic nephropathy, hyperlipidemia, and aging. In diabetic nephropathy, both the afferent and efferent glomerular arterioles may show hyaline change; in the other conditions, only the afferent arterioles are affected.
■ The vascular changes in "malignant" hypertension are also not specific; similar or identical changes are seen in conditions described as the *thrombotic microangiopathies,* such as hemolytic-uremic syndrome, thrombotic thrombocytopenic purpura, scleroderma renal crisis, and others. Clinical information is required for discrimination of these entities.
■ Vasculitis may also mimic the vascular changes of "malignant" hypertension. The presence of neutrophilic infiltrates, rupture of glomerular capillary basement membranes, and numerous glomerular crescents would favor vasculitis over malignant hypertension.

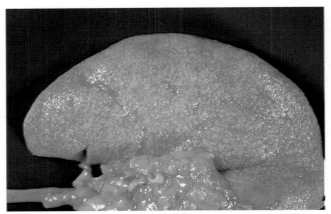

Figure 14–10. Arteriolar nephrosclerosis. The surface of the kidney is finely granular, and the weight of the kidney is slightly below normal. This gross pattern is quite typical for kidneys with arteriolosclerosis and is most commonly seen in association with "benign" essential hypertension. The depressions ("pits") represent small cortical vascular scars interposed with elevated areas of the normal (or slightly compensatorily hypertrophied) parenchyma.

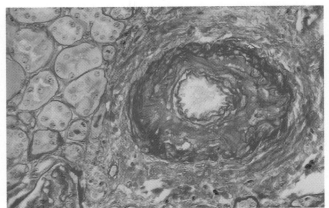

Figure 14–12. Arteriosclerosis, subarcuate/arcuate artery. Severe medial fibrosis is seen with destruction of the medial smooth muscle cells, thickening of the medial muscle cell basement membranes, and subsequent luminal narrowing. Arteriosclerosis with luminal narrowing may result in severe compromise of the blood supply downstream along with severe renal scarring (nephrosclerosis).

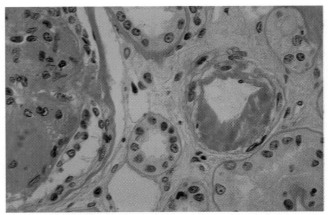

Figure 14–11. Arteriolar hyalinization. A large subendothelial hyaline deposit (homogeneous eosinophil material) is seen in an arteriole with narrowing of the lumen. Although this change is most typically caused by essential hypertension, it may be seen without hypertension as well as in diabetes and possibly aging.

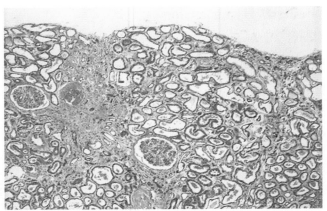

Figure 14–13. Arteriolosclerotic nephrosclerosis. This low-magnification picture of the cortical surface of the kidney depicts two small renal cortical depressions (scars), one with a globally sclerotic glomerulus and tubular atrophy *(left).* The surface of the scar is slightly indented; small cortical scars with surrounding normal tissue give a finely granular appearance to the renal cortical surface.

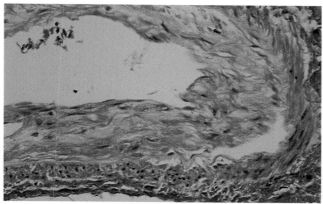

Figure 14–14. Intimal fibroplasia of an interlobar artery. The intima shows fibrous thickening and migration of fuchsinophilic medial muscle cells into the intima. The smooth muscle layer (media) appears slightly thinner than normal. The lumen is moderately narrowed (Masson's trichrome stain).

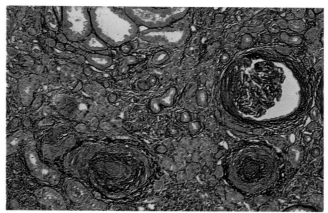

Figure 14–15. Severe arterio/arteriolonephrosclerosis from a patient with pheochromocytoma and severe hypertension. The interlobular arteries reveal marked reduplication of the internal elastic lamina with severe narrowing of the arterial lumina. Compromise of the blood supply results in interstitial fibrosis, marked tubular atrophy, and ischemic glomerular changes such as retraction and simplification of the glomerular capillary tufts, widening of Bowman's space, and fibrosis of Bowman's capsule (Masson's trichrome stain).

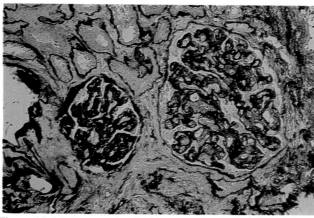

Figure 14–16. Hypertension leading to glomerular ischemic changes. Two glomeruli display advanced ischemic changes; the glomerulus on the left shows almost global collapse of the capillary lumina. The glomerulus on the right shows less advanced changes, including simplification of the tuft, thickening and wrinkling of the glomerular capillary basement membranes, and a slight increase in the mesangial matrix (sclerosis) (methenamine silver stain).

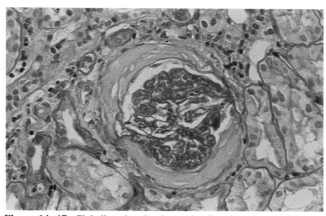

Figure 14–17. Globally sclerotic glomerulus from a patient with hypertension. The globally sclerotic glomerulus reveals collapse of the glomerular capillary lumina and periodic acid–Schiff (PAS)–positive collagen accumulation ("halo") in Bowman's space (PAS reaction).

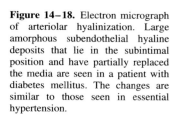

Figure 14–18. Electron micrograph of arteriolar hyalinization. Large amorphous subendothelial hyaline deposits that lie in the subintimal position and have partially replaced the media are seen in a patient with diabetes mellitus. The changes are similar to those seen in essential hypertension.

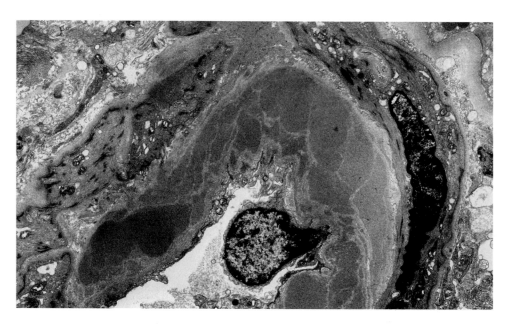

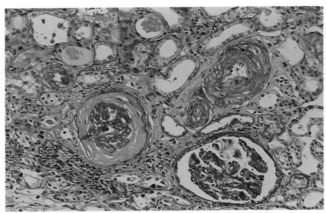

Figure 14–19. "Malignant" hypertension, late stage. Extensive reduplication (multiplication) of the elastic lamellae of the interlobular artery is seen. The glomerulus on the left is globally sclerotic and the one on the right shows features of ischemia (thickening and wrinkling of the glomerular capillary basement membranes, simplification of the tuft).

RENAL CORTICAL NECROSIS

Biology of Disease

- Renal cortical necrosis with sparing of the medulla can occur in severe circulatory failure, with or without organic renal vascular lesions such as atherosclerosis. It is frequently bilateral; however, unilateral cortical necrosis can occur.
- Arterial vasospasm may be an important component in cases occurring in the absence of renal artery narrowing.
- Renal cortical necrosis is, in general, an uncommon cause of renal failure. However, it may represent a significant fraction of cases of renal failure occurring in specific clinical situations, such as renal failure occurring in late pregnancy.
- The most common causes of renal cortical necrosis are obstetric complications such as placental abruption, eclampsia, and septic abortion; it can also occur in hemolytic-uremic syndrome and other thrombotic microangiopathies, snakebites, acute intravascular hemolysis, or severe circulatory collapse of any cause.
- Renal cortical necrosis may also be seen in the setting of renal transplant failure; the most common cause in this setting is severe allograft rejection. However, thrombosis or mechanical problems of the vascular anastomosis (i.e., constriction or torsion) may also cause similar problems.

Clinical Features

- The usual clinical finding is acute renal failure with severe oliguria or anuria after one of the predisposing conditions just described.

Gross Appearance

- The subcapsular surface is dark and mottled; on section there is a rim of pale, infarcted cortex with congestion of the medulla.

Light Microscopy

- The general histologic appearance and sequential changes resemble those of renal infarction as described earlier. The changes may be patchy, with scattered areas of nonnecrotic tissue.
- The medulla and juxtamedullary cortex are usually preserved; a rim of subcapsular cortex may also be spared.
- Arteries and arterioles may show fibrinoid necrosis and thrombosis.
- If the patient survives the acute episode, the necrotic cortex may calcify and become visible on plain radiographs.

Immunofluorescence Microscopy

- Immunofluorescence microscopy is usually not helpful; if performed, immunofluorescence is usually negative or nonspecific.

Differential Diagnosis

- At times, the distinction between renal cortical necrosis and renal infarction associated with atherosclerosis, thrombosis, or thromboemboli involving the large renal arteries may be difficult, particularly on a percutaneous biopsy specimen. The clinical situation in which renal failure occurred may suggest the most appropriate diagnosis.

Treatment and Clinical Course

- Before the availability of hemodialysis, the diagnosis of bilateral renal cortical necrosis was associated with a very high immediate mortality rate; a few patients survived with residual renal insufficiency.
- With hemodialysis, a significant number of patients survive the acute phase but are left with considerable residual renal insufficiency; many require long-term dialysis or renal transplantation.
- Less severe cases with partial renal involvement may not be recognized clinically.

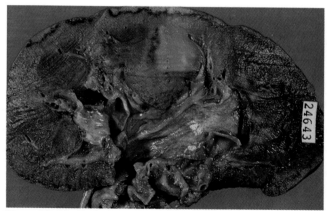

Figure 14–20. Cortical necrosis. Widespread homogeneous yellow discoloration of the subcapsular cortex with a hyperemic halo marks extensive cortical necrosis from this patient with an obstetric emergency (abruptio placentae).

RENAL VEIN THROMBOSIS

Biology of Disease

- Renal vein thrombosis occurs most commonly in patients with nephrotic syndrome, in particular membranous glomerulonephropathy. It may also occur in infants with severe dehydration.
- Although it was initially thought that renal vein thrombosis was a cause of nephrotic syndrome, it is now appreciated that the nephrotic syndrome induces a hypercoagulable state; thus renal vein thrombosis is more likely a *complication* rather than a *cause* of nephrotic syndrome.
- Patients with nephrotic syndrome have elevated levels of various clotting factors, increased α_2-antiplasmin, and decreased antithrombin III. Thus there is an increase in factors involved in coagulation and a decrease in factors involved in fibrinolysis. Collectively, these abnormalities induce a hypercoagulable state.
- The incidence of renal vein thrombosis in nephrotic syndrome is unknown. Estimates have varied from less than 2% to more than 40%; the wide variation in incidence probably depends at least in part on the indications for examination of the renal vein and the sensitivity of the method used. The actual incidence probably exceeds 10%.
- Although renal vein thrombosis is most frequently thought of in association with membranous glomerulonephropathy, it has also been found in other renal disorders, including minimal change nephrotic syndrome, membranoproliferative glomerulonephritis, IgA nephropathy, focal segmental glomerulosclerosis, lupus nephritis, diabetic nephropathy, amyloidosis, sickle cell anemia, various vasculitides, and others.
- The kidney has a rich potential collateral venous circu-

lation, including pericapsular, adrenal, ureteral, hilar, and gonadal (on the left side) veins. The kidney can therefore survive complete occlusion of the renal vein if these collaterals are able to compensate.
- The consequences and clinical manifestations of renal vein thrombosis are variable. Part of the variability probably depends on the rate and completeness of occlusion of the renal vein; sudden occlusion may lead to hemorrhagic infarction of the kidney, whereas gradual development of occlusion may allow collateral venous drainage to develop and thus be clinically silent. An additional factor may be whether the original thrombus is localized or extensive and whether it progresses.
- Thrombosis of the renal vein may extend into and induce thrombosis of the inferior vena cava.
- Pulmonary thromboembolism is a potentially lethal complication of renal vein thrombosis.

Clinical Features

- The majority of patients with renal vein thrombosis occurring in the setting of nephrotic syndrome are asymptomatic or experience mild symptoms that are not brought to the attention of a physician. Thus the majority of cases are clinically silent.
- Sudden occlusion of the renal vein produces costovertebral angle pain, which may be severe and persistent or relatively minor and transient. Some patients experience upper abdominal or epigastric pain, which may be related to thrombosis of the inferior vena cava.
- If bilateral sudden occlusion or occlusion of the vein of a solitary kidney occurs, the patient may be anuric.
- Sudden deterioration in renal function and/or a sudden increase in proteinuria in a patient with nephrotic syn-

drome should be an indication to the clinician to evaluate the status of the renal veins.

■ Pulmonary thromboembolism may be the first manifestation of renal vein thrombosis; thus the patient may have chest pain, shortness of breath, or sudden death.

Gross Appearance

■ Sudden occlusion may lead to hemorrhagic infarction of the kidney. In such instances the kidney is engorged and purple and resembles an eggplant.
■ In less catastrophic circumstances, the kidney would show relatively minor changes.

Light Microscopy

■ Biopsy in the acute phase of sudden, complete thrombosis may demonstrate increased numbers of neutrophils in glomerular capillaries (*leukocyte stasis*). Peritubular capillaries are engorged with erythrocytes, and there may be margination of neutrophils. Marked interstitial edema may be present.
■ Thrombosis of glomerular capillaries has been described as an acute change associated with renal vein thrombosis, but the frequency of this change is unclear.
■ Biopsy long after thrombosis demonstrates interstitial fibrosis and tubular atrophy.

Treatment and Clinical Course

■ The clinical outcome of renal vein thrombosis is somewhat unclear inasmuch as many cases are silent and thus never diagnosed. Undoubtedly, many patients have few or no long-term consequences. However, occasional patients may experience significant or catastrophic consequences such as pulmonary embolism.

■ Recurrent episodes occur in some patients, with deterioration in renal function, increase in proteinuria, or both.
■ Surgical thrombectomy or thrombolytic therapy may be beneficial if the patient is treated during acute onset of the symptoms.
■ The standard therapy is anticoagulation with heparin, followed by warfarin (Coumadin). This regimen appears to decrease the incidence of recurrence; however, some patients experience recurrent episodes despite therapeutic anticoagulation.

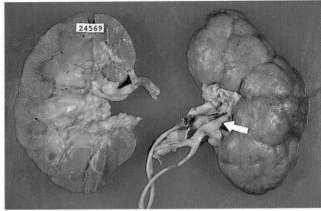

Figure 14–21. Renal vein thrombosis. The renal vein is occluded by a large thrombus (*arrow*). The patient had severe nephrotic syndrome. The multiple large scars on the cortical surface on the right are most likely related to severe vascular disease. Renal vein thrombosis in adults is usually not associated with renal parenchymal infarction as it is in infants and children; it is usually secondary to long-standing/severe nephrotic syndrome.

References

General

Greco BA, Breyer JA: Atherosclerotic ischemic renal disease. Am J Kidney Dis 29:167, 1997.
Hughson MD, Lajoie G: Vascular diseases. In: Silva FG, D'Agati VD, Nadasdy T (eds): Renal Biopsy Interpretation. New York, Churchill Livingstone, 1996, p 333.
Racusen LC, Solez K: Renal infarction, cortical necrosis, and atheroembolic disease. In: Tisher CC, Brenner BM (eds): Renal Pathology: With Clinical and Functional Correlations, 2nd ed. Philadelphia, JB Lippincott, 1994, p 810.
Kashgarian M: Acute tubular necrosis and ischemic renal injury. In: Jennette JC, Olson JL, Schwartz MM, Silva FG (eds): Heptinstall's Pathology of the Kidney, 5th ed. Philadelphia, Lippincott-Raven, 1998, p 863.

Cholesterol Emboli

Mannesse CK, Blankestijn PJ, Man in 't Veld AJ, et al: Renal failure and cholesterol crystal embolization: A report of 4 surviving cases and a review of the literature. Clin Nephrol 36:240, 1991.
McGowan JA, Greenberg A: Cholesterol atheroembolic disease: Report of 3 cases with emphasis on diagnosis by skin biopsy and extended survival. Am J Nephrol 6:135, 1986.
Smith MC, Ghose MK, Henry AR: The clinical spectrum of renal cholesterol embolization. Am J Med 71:174, 1981.

Hypertension and the Kidney

Helmchen U, Wenzel UO: Benign and malignant nephrosclerosis and renovascular disease. In: Tisher CC, Brenner BM (eds): Renal Pathology: With Clinical and Functional Correlations, 2nd ed. Philadelphia, JB Lippincott, 1994, p 1201.
Olson JL: Hypertension: Essential and secondary forms. In: Jennette JC, Olson JL, Schwartz MM, Silva FG (eds): Heptinstall's Pathology of the Kidney, 5th ed. Philadelphia, Lippincott-Raven, 1998, p 943.
Pickering TG, Blumenfeld JD, Laragh JH: Renovascular hypertension and ischemic nephropathy. In: Brenner BM (ed): Brenner & Rector's The Kidney, 5th ed. Philadelphia, WB Saunders, 1996, p 2106.

Renal Cortical Necrosis

Chugh KS, Singhl PC, Kher VK, et al: Spectrum of acute cortical necrosis in Indian patients. Am J Med Sci 286:10, 1983.

Kleinknecht D, Grünfeld J-P, Cia Gomez P, et al: Diagnostic procedures and long-term prognosis in bilateral renal cortical necrosis. Kidney Int 4:390, 1973.

Renal Vein Thrombosis

Llach F, Papper S, Massry SG: The clinical spectrum of renal vein thrombosis: Acute and chronic. Am J Med 69:819, 1980.

Pollak VE, Weiss MA: Renal vein thrombosis. In: Tisher CC, Brenner BM (eds): Renal Pathology: With Clinical and Functional Correlations, 2nd ed. Philadelphia, JB Lippincott, 1994, p 1185.

Rosenmann E, Pollack VE, Pirani CL: Renal vein thrombosis in the adult: A clinical and pathologic study based on renal biopsies. Medicine (Baltimore) 47:269, 1968.

Velasquez Forero F, Garcia Prugue N, Ruiz Morales N: Idiopathic nephrotic syndrome of the adult with asymptomatic thrombosis of the renal vein. Am J Nephrol 8:457, 1988.

Wagoner RD, Stanson AW, Holley KE, et al: Renal vein thrombosis in idiopathic membranous glomerulopathy and nephrotic syndrome: Incidence and significance. Kidney Int 23:368, 1983.

CHAPTER 15

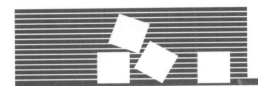

Vasculitis and the Kidney
Polyarteritis Nodosa, Wegener's Granulomatosis, Churg-Strauss Syndrome, Mixed Cryoglobulinemia, and Other Forms of Vasculitis

INTRODUCTION

- The kidney may be affected by several types of vasculitis; the most common types to involve the kidney are polyarteritis nodosa, Wegener's granulomatosis, allergic granulomatosis (Churg-Strauss syndrome), and giant cell arteritis. The majority of this section will refer to polyarteritis nodosa and Wegener's granulomatosis.
- The kidneys may be involved as one part of a multisystem disorder, or kidney involvement may be the only manifestation of the vasculitis (*renal-limited vasculitis*).
- Vasculitis in the kidney may also occur as a part of other specific conditions, including "connective tissue" or "collagen vascular" diseases (systemic lupus erythematosus, rheumatoid arthritis, and others), Henoch-Schönlein purpura, essential mixed cryoglobulinemia, intravenous drug abuse, various infections, drug reactions, and neoplasms (Table 15–1).
- Many variants of vasculitis are now known to be associated with antineutrophil cytoplasmic antibodies (ANCAs). The microscopic variant of polyarteritis nodosa is strongly associated with ANCAs that demonstrate a perinuclear staining pattern on alcohol-fixed neutrophils (P-ANCA; usually directed against myeloperoxidase), whereas Wegener's granulomatosis is associated with ANCAs that demonstrate a cytoplasmic pattern on alcohol-fixed neutrophils (C-ANCA; usually directed against proteinase 3, a serine protease). These antibodies may be of pathogenic as well as diagnostic significance; antigens recognized by the ANCAs may be expressed on the surface of neutrophils after cellular activation. The resulting reactions between ANCAs and the corresponding antigens may activate neutrophils, with release of inflammatory mediators.

POLYARTERITIS (PERIARTERITIS) NODOSA

Biology of Disease

- Renal involvement in polyarteritis nodosa is usually divided into two types: classic (macroscopic) polyarteritis nodosa, which characteristically affects larger arteries, and microscopic polyarteritis nodosa, which is usually manifested as a pauci-immune necrotizing and crescentic glomerulonephritis. The microscopic form is more common than the classic form; cases with overlapping features are not uncommon, however.
- The renal arteries involved in classic polyarteritis nodosa are interlobar and arcuate arteries; vasculitis involving arterioles and interlobular arteries may be seen in the microscopic form.
- It should be emphasized that unequivocal histologic evidence of arteritis (especially arteritis involving the larger arteries) is not common on percutaneous renal biopsy tissue because of the focal nature of the lesions by light microscopy; true vasculitis is found in fewer than half of renal biopsies, even when vasculitis is demonstrated in other sites. Therefore, *failure to demonstrate arteritis on a kidney biopsy specimen does not exclude the presence of vasculitis, either in the kidney or elsewhere.* Sites with a higher yield of vasculitis include nerve, muscle, and testis.
- *All tissue submitted should be carefully scrutinized for evidence of vasculitis.* Occasionally, unequivocal vasculitis is found in skeletal muscle or adipose tissue accidentally harvested along with the core of renal tissue, when the renal tissue shows only the effects of vasculitis, not the vasculitis itself.

Table 15–1
CONDITIONS ASSOCIATED WITH VASCULITIS IN THE KIDNEY

"Connective tissue" diseases
    Systemic lupus erythematosus
    Rheumatoid arthritis
    Dermatomyositis
    Sjögren's syndrome
    Relapsing polychondritis
Drug reactions and serum sickness
    Allopurinol
    Sulfa antibiotics
    Immune globulin
    Hyposensitization for allergy
Anti–glomerular basement membrane antibody disease
Essential mixed cryoglobulinemia
Hypocomplementemic vasculitis
Infections
    Poststreptococcal glomerulonephritis
    Endocarditis
    Hepatitis B and C viruses
Neoplasms
    Carcinomas
    Leukemias and lymphomas
    Multiple myeloma
Henoch-Schönlein purpura
Intravenous drug abuse

Clinical Features

- Classic polyarteritis nodosa is a multisystem disorder with protean manifestations. The disease commonly involves the kidneys, the gastrointestinal tract (hemorrhage, infarction), the heart (congestive heart failure, myocardial ischemia or infarction), the peripheral nervous system (neuropathy), and the musculoskeletal system (myositis, arthritis). Other systems that may be involved include the gonads, pancreas, adrenals, salivary glands, and eyes. Pulmonary involvement is less common.
- The microscopic variant is usually manifested as renal failure secondary to necrotizing and crescentic glomerulonephritis.
- Polyarteritis nodosa occurs most often in the fifth and sixth decades, although the age range is wide. Males are affected approximately twice as often as females.
- The incidence of renal involvement in polyarteritis nodosa varies from approximately 64% to 100% in different series; this wide range is due in part to selection bias inasmuch as the incidence of renal involvement will of necessity be high in series reported by nephrologists and renal pathologists.
- Renal involvement in classic polyarteritis nodosa is manifested as renal failure, hematuria, and proteinuria.

Laboratory Values

- Serum urea nitrogen and creatinine values are variably elevated.
- Urinalysis demonstrates hematuria and proteinuria; leukocytes may be present.
- Nonspecific laboratory abnormalities include elevated erythrocyte sedimentation rate, anemia, leukocytosis, and thrombocytosis; a peripheral eosinophilia may be present.

- Circulating immune complexes may be detected in 30% to 90% of patients; the rate of detection appears to be higher early in the disease course. Cryoglobulins and rheumatoid factor may be present.
- Antineutrophil cytoplasmic antibodies are detected in the serum of approximately 90% of patients with the microscopic variant of polyarteritis nodosa, mostly P-ANCA; approximately one quarter of patients with the macroscopic variant have ANCAs, again usually P-ANCA.

Gross Appearance

- The kidney in acute, severe disease characteristically has a nodular cortical surface, with the nodules corresponding to areas of better-preserved cortex surrounded by depressed areas of infarcted or atrophic tissue.
- Fresh or recent infarcts of various ages may be present.
- Thrombosis or aneurysmal dilation of the arcuate, subarcuate, and interlobar arteries may be present.

Light Microscopy

Glomeruli

- Glomeruli in classic (macroscopic) polyarteritis may show ischemic collapse of the capillary tuft, sometimes with fibrosis within Bowman's space. Other glomeruli may appear essentially unremarkable.
- Microscopic polyarteritis is characterized by segmental necrosis of capillary loops, usually associated with crescents in Bowman's space. Glomeruli without necrosis are generally histologically unremarkable.
- Necrotizing glomerulonephritis is not seen in classic polyarteritis. However, necrosis with or without crescents may be seen along with arteritis in variants that have overlapping histologic features.

Vessels

- The most striking changes in classic polyarteritis involve the arteries, predominantly medium-sized to large ones (interlobar and arcuate). Vascular changes are uncommon in microscopic polyarteritis; if present, arterioles and interlobular arteries are affected.
- The two major components of acute vasculitis are inflammation and necrosis of artery walls.
- The inflammation consists of lymphocytes, neutrophils, monocytes, and occasionally eosinophils; the infiltrate may involve the intima, the media, the adventitia of the vessel, or any combination. Inflammation may extend into the periadventitial tissue; periadventitial inflammation alone is not sufficient for the diagnosis unless accompanied by fibrinoid necrosis of the vessel wall.
- The necrosis in artery walls is usually described as "fibrinoid"; the normal components of the wall are replaced by intensely eosinophilic material, with karyorrhectic nuclear debris (leukocytoclasis). The fibrinoid material is fuchsinophilic on Masson's trichrome stain and stains with phosphotungstic acid–hematoxylin and Lendrum's stains.

- The endothelium is frequently denuded; the lumen may be occluded by fibrin thrombi.
- Elastic stains may demonstrate focal disruption or breaks in the internal elastic lamina, particularly in areas of necrosis (or in regions of a healed vasculitic process).
- Transmural necrosis may result in aneurysmal dilatation of the larger arteries (arcuate and interlobar). Rupture of such aneurysmal dilatations may result in interstitial hemorrhage.
- In the healing phase, the necrosis and inflammation disappear. The intima and media become thickened by a concentric proliferation of elongated myointimal cells embedded in a matrix of pale ground substance. The lumen of the vessel may be severely narrowed by the intimal proliferation.
- With healing, there is fibrosis of the intima and media. Intimal fibrosis may narrow the lumen of the vessel; if the vessel is patent, the endothelium is intact.
- The fibrous reaction may obliterate arteries sufficiently that trichrome or elastic stains are required for the identification of vessels.
- Elastic stains may be helpful in differentiating healed vasculitis from arteriosclerosis. Broad gaps or disruptions of the elastic lamina suggest healed vasculitis and are not seen in simple arteriosclerosis; lamination or reduplication of the elastic lamina may be seen in either condition.
- The arterial lesions in vasculitis are often focal and may be missed when only a few histologic sections are taken, even when vasculitis is present in the biopsy sample. Therefore, multiple levels of the biopsy specimen should be examined whenever vasculitis is a possibility.
- As noted earlier, true arteritis is not common on percutaneous renal biopsy tissue; *the absence of vasculitis on a biopsy specimen does not exclude the diagnosis.*

Tubules and Interstitium

- Cortical infarcts with coagulative necrosis may be present.
- Tubules in the noninfarcted areas may show degenerative and regenerative changes.
- The interstitium is edematous and contains an inflammatory infiltrate consisting of lymphocytes, monocytes, neutrophils, and plasma cells. The inflammation is usually of moderate intensity in classic polyarteritis; marked interstitial inflammation is more characteristic of the microscopic form of polyarteritis.
- In the healed phase there is interstitial fibrosis and tubular atrophy.

Immunofluorescence Microscopy

- Glomeruli are usually totally negative or demonstrate weak, segmental staining. Fibrinogen and C3 are the most common immunoreactants detected (usually in crescents or areas of necrosis); IgG and C1q are less often detected.
- Significant fluorescent staining in arteries is seen in perhaps one third of cases. Fibrinogen and C3 are also

the most common immunoreactants found in arteries; occasionally IgG and IgM, and rarely IgA, are found.
- Positive immunofluorescent staining probably represents trapping of plasma proteins in areas of endothelial or vessel wall damage rather than an indication that immunoglobulins or complement is participating in a specific immunologic reaction.

Electron Microscopy

- Glomerular capillaries show endothelial swelling and widening of the subendothelial space by "fluffy," electron-lucent material. Capillaries may be occluded by platelet-fibrin thrombi. Occasional leukocytes may be present.
- Large, discrete, electron-dense immune-type glomerular deposits are not usually present in classic polyarteritis nodosa; small, irregularly distributed mesangial deposits may be present in up to 25% of cases.
- The presence of abundant glomerular deposits suggests vasculitis occurring in the setting of some other condition such as poststreptococcal acute glomerulonephritis, lupus nephritis, cryoglobulinemic glomerulonephritis, or Henoch-Schönlein purpura.
- Arteries show degeneration or loss of the endothelium; fibrin deposits may be present between the endothelium and the underlying elastic lamina or basement membrane. Leukocytes and fibrin deposits may be present within the media. Destruction of elastic fibers may occur.
- Intraluminal platelet-fibrin thrombi and erythrocyte aggregation and hemolysis may be present in vessels.
- In the healed phase, concentric layers of collagen and elastic fibers within the thickened intima can be seen. There is focal atrophy of medial smooth muscle cells, with thickening of the basement membrane surrounding myocytes.

Differential Diagnosis

- Wegener's granulomatosis is characterized by granulomas around glomeruli with crescents; however, granulomas are not always seen on renal biopsy specimens in Wegener's granulomatosis. The clinical findings may suggest one diagnosis over the other; for example, prominent pulmonary and sinus involvement is characteristic of Wegener's granulomatosis but would be unusual in polyarteritis nodosa. Serologic information may also be helpful; polyarteritis is associated with P-ANCAs, whereas Wegener's granulomatosis is associated with C-ANCAs (although crossover exists).
- Intense immunofluorescent staining for immunoglobulins or complement or abundant electron-dense deposits on electron microscopy would be unusual in polyarteritis and would suggest vasculitis in association with one of the other conditions listed in Table 15–1.
- Healed vasculitis may be difficult to distinguish from arteriosclerosis; the presence of gaps or long breaks in the elastic lamina with elastic stains would suggest healed vasculitis.

Treatment and Clinical Course

- Before therapy was available, the majority of patients with polyarteritis nodosa followed an aggressive course, with short survival.
- Gastrointestinal involvement (bowel infarcts, gastrointestinal hemorrhage), renal failure, and cardiovascular complications are the most common causes of death.
- High-dose corticosteroids combined with cytotoxic im-

munosuppressants such as cyclophosphamide (Cytoxan) have improved the outlook of patients with polyarteritis nodosa; in some series, up to 80% of patients have sustained remission.
- Aggressive therapy may be beneficial even in patients with severe disease, including dialysis-dependent renal failure; some patients have been able to discontinue dialysis after therapy with corticosteroids and cytotoxic agents.

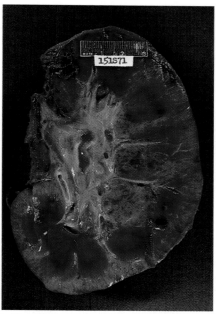

Figure 15-1. Vasculitis. A gross photograph of a bisected kidney from an autopsy shows focal hemorrhage in both the cortex and the medulla. This patient had large vessel polyarteritis and retroperitoneal hemorrhage leading to death. Note the large thrombosed intrarenal arteries.

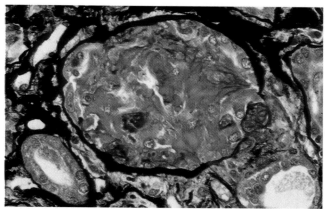

Figure 15-3. Vasculitis. The glomerulus displays global necrosis with complete disappearance of the normal glomerular capillary network (methenamine silver stain).

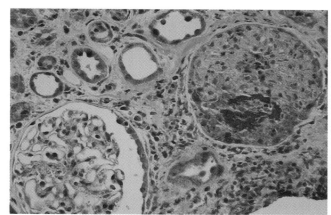

Figure 15-2. Vasculitis. A focal necrotizing glomerular lesion is shown with fibrin deposition. The other glomerulus is histologically unremarkable (Lendrum's stain). The patient had a microscopic form of polyarteritis nodosa.

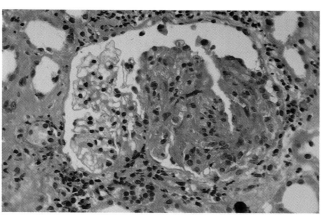

Figure 15-4. Vasculitis, focal segmental necrotizing glomerulonephritis from a patient with microscopic polyarteritis nodosa. The photograph shows an exquisite segmental glomerular necrosis with an inflammatory cell infiltrate in the necrotic segment. The segments of the glomerulus (on the left) appear histologically normal.

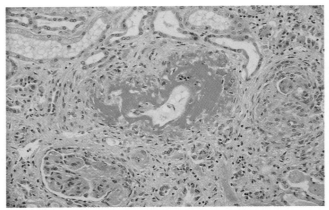

Figure 15–5. Vasculitis. The entire thickness of a large arterial wall is infiltrated by fibrin (fibrinoid necrosis); a slight, associated inflammatory reaction is seen in the necrotic wall of the vessel. A few capillary loops of a glomerulus on the right are surrounded by a large cellular crescent.

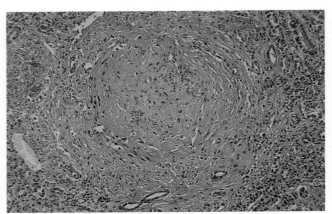

Figure 15–8. Vasculitis (healed stage). The renal interlobar/arcuate artery is seen with disruption of the wall (including the internal elastic lamellae) and fibrous closure of the lumen.

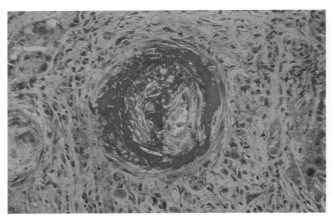

Figure 15–6. Fibrinoid necrosis, microscopic polyarteritis nodosa. The wall of an interlobular artery is infiltrated by fibrin (fibrinoid necrosis) (Fraser-Lendrum stain).

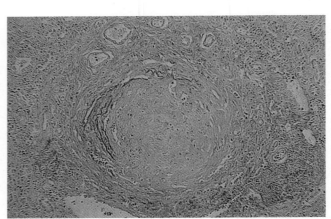

Figure 15–9. Vasculitis (healed stage). This renal interlobar/arcuate artery has focal disruption of the internal elastic lamellae—depicts old healed vasculitis. The figure depicts the same vessel as shown in Figure 15–8 at a different level (Verhoeff–Van Gieson elastic stain).

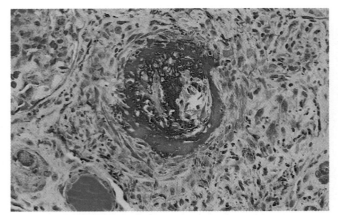

Figure 15–7. Fibrinoid necrosis, microscopic polyarteritis nodosa. Massive fibrin deposition is seen in the wall of a subarcuate artery (fibrinoid necrosis). Focal crescentic and necrotizing glomerulonephritis was seen (not shown) in the glomeruli (phosphotungstic acid–hematoxylin stain).

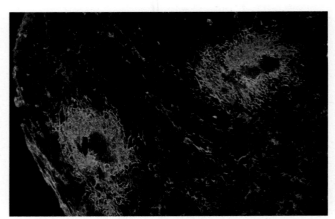

Figure 15–10. Necrotizing vasculitis. Fibrin(ogen) immunostaining reveals strong signal in two large arteries (probably interlobular) in a patient with necrotizing vasculitis and glomerulonephritis.

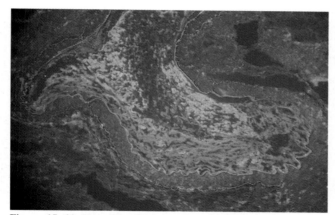

Figure 15–11. Vasculitis. Fibrin(ogen) positivity is seen in a large subarcuate artery with thrombosis.

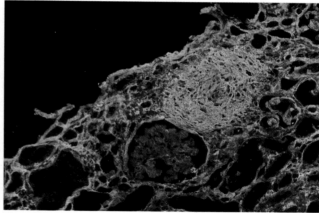

Figure 15–12. Vasculitis. Positive immunofluorescence with fibrinogen reveals strong staining in an artery. The glomerulus is negative.

WEGENER'S GRANULOMATOSIS

Biology of Disease

- Classic Wegener's granulomatosis (WG) is a triad that includes necrotizing and granulomatous inflammation of the sinuses, necrotizing granulomatous inflammation or capillaritis of the lungs, and necrotizing glomerulonephritis.
- Limited forms of WG occur, such as pulmonary or sinus involvement in the absence of renal involvement. This is thought by some nephrologists to be rare.
- Wegener's granulomatosis is strongly associated with serum ANCAs, in particular C-ANCA, as discussed earlier. A variety of disorders included in the differential diagnosis of Wegener's granulomatosis, such as pauci-immune necrotizing glomerulonephritis, are also associated with ANCAs; thus a number of conditions have been combined into a broad category of *ANCA-associated vasculitis.*
- Demonstration of *granulomatous* inflammation has always been required for a definite diagnosis of Wegener's granulomatosis. With serologic assay for ANCAs, a category of *Wegener's vasculitis* has been proposed for conditions resembling Wegener's granulomatosis but lacking true granulomatous inflammation.

Clinical Features

- Wegener's granulomatosis appears to be uncommon, although the true incidence is difficult to establish because of difficulty in diagnosis and clinical overlap with other conditions.
- Men are affected more often than women (approximately 1.5 : 1).
- Onset is most frequent between the ages of 35 and 55 years, although the age range is wide.

- The clinical features are extremely variable. The onset may be insidious, with a prolonged period of constitutional symptoms (fever, malaise) and mild respiratory tract symptoms before the diagnosis is made. Other patients may have acute, fulminant respiratory disease and renal failure.
- The upper respiratory tract is the most common area involved initially (70% to 80%). Manifestations include nasal ulceration and bleeding, sinusitis, pain in the ears, deafness, and others. The maxillary sinuses are the most commonly involved, followed by the sphenoid, ethmoid, and frontal sinuses. Sinus radiographs may demonstrate air-fluid levels.
- Lower respiratory tract involvement is present in approximately 45% to 70% of patients at diagnosis and eventually occurs in 70% to 100% of patients. Manifestations include dyspnea, cough, hemoptysis, and pleuritic chest pain; chest radiography may show evidence of involvement even when pulmonary symptoms are absent. The most characteristic radiographic finding is pulmonary nodules, usually multiple but occasionally single; nodule size ranges from 1 to 10 cm; cavitation is frequently present. Other common patterns are infiltrates and interstitial changes; small pleural effusions may be present.
- Evidence of renal disease occurs in 50% to 95% of patients over the course of their illness. Occasionally, severe renal disease precedes other manifestations by 1 to several years. Renal manifestations may vary from microscopic hematuria, erythrocyte casts, and mild proteinuria to fulminant oliguric renal failure. Renal failure probably occurs in one fifth of patients or fewer; series from referral centers suggesting a much higher incidence of renal failure probably reflect bias from selective referral of more severe cases.
- Other manifestations of Wegener's granulomatosis may

include migratory arthralgias or deforming arthritis, cutaneous purpura or rashes, myopathy, peripheral neuropathy (mononeuritis multiplex) or cranial nerve palsies, and many others. Ocular involvement may occur in up to two thirds of patients; manifestations include conjunctivitis, uveitis, episcleritis, optic neuritis, and rarely, proptosis from inflammation of retro-orbital tissues.

Laboratory Values

■ Normocytic, normochromic anemia, modest leukocytosis, and thrombocytosis are common. Eosinophilia is rare in Wegener's granulomatosis and suggests another type of vasculitis.
■ Elevated erythrocyte sedimentation rates and positive assays for rheumatoid factor are common.
■ Assay for C-ANCA is positive in approximately 80% to 90% of patients, depending on disease activity and the assay used; occasional patients have P-ANCA instead of C-ANCA.
■ Urinalysis shows microscopic hematuria, red cell casts, leukocytes, and moderate proteinuria. Nephrotic-range proteinuria is uncommon.
■ Serum urea nitrogen and creatinine values may be elevated.
■ The degree of abnormalities on urinalysis and elevation of serum creatinine may not necessarily reflect the severity of renal disease; occasionally, histologic evidence of severe renal involvement may be found with only mild laboratory abnormalities.

Gross Appearance

■ Petechial hemorrhages and small infarcts of varying age may be present on the capsular and cortical surfaces in the acute phase. The intervening parenchyma will be pale.
■ Papillary necrosis may be present in up to one fifth of cases.
■ Grossly visible aneurysmal dilatation or thrombosis of arteries is uncommon.
■ Ureteral narrowing with obstruction and hydronephrosis may be present because of vasculitis of the periureteral arteries; necrotizing urethritis may occasionally be present.
■ In the chronic phase, the kidneys are coarsely granular and decreased in size.

Light Microscopy

Glomeruli

■ The most common acute change is focal segmental necrotizing glomerulonephritis with crescents, closely resembling that seen in the microscopic variant of polyarteritis nodosa (pauci-immune necrotizing and crescentic glomerulonephritis). The proportion of glomeruli involved may vary from a small fraction to nearly 100%.
■ Endocapillary hypercellularity is usually absent or mild.
■ The appearance of the associated crescents is variable.

They may resemble typical crescents seen in other forms of crescentic glomerulonephritis, but two distinctive crescent types have been described in Wegener's granulomatosis: "sunburst" crescents and granulomatous crescents.
● "Sunburst" crescents are characterized by extensive destruction of the capillary tuft and Bowman's capsule, with exuberant cellular proliferation extending radially into the periglomerular tissue. Methenamine silver stains may be required to identify the remnants of glomeruli; on hematoxylin and eosin stain, sunburst crescents may be misidentified as interstitial granulomas.
● Granulomatous crescents contain numerous epithelioid histiocytes and giant cells. They are neither specific nor required for the diagnosis of Wegener's granulomatosis; they may occur in any form of crescentic glomerulonephritis. Granulomatous crescents are found in a minority of cases of Wegener's granulomatosis and usually in only a minority of glomeruli. They may be more frequent in cases where actual vasculitis is found in the biopsy sample.
■ Glomeruli unaffected by necrotizing glomerulonephritis usually appear histologically unremarkable.
■ Chronic glomerular lesions of Wegener's granulomatosis consist of global or segmental glomerulosclerosis, usually associated with fibrous crescents. Both acute and chronic changes may be seen within the same biopsy specimen.

Vessels

■ Vasculitic lesions are not often present on percutaneous biopsy samples in Wegener's granulomatosis. In a total of 287 cases from several series, vasculitis was described in 34 (12%). The lesions are focal, and serial sectioning through the entire biopsy specimen may increase the yield of vasculitic lesions. When vasculitis is present, usually few vessels are affected.
■ Vasculitis may affect small and medium-sized renal arteries, arterioles, capillaries, and venules.
■ The usual histologic appearance of vasculitis in Wegener's granulomatosis is similar to that of vasculitis in polyarteritis nodosa, described earlier. Granulomatous vasculitis may also be seen.

Tubules and Interstitium

■ Focal degenerative and regenerative changes may occur in the proximal convoluted tubules. Tubules may contain casts of various types, including red cell and white cell casts.
■ The interstitium is edematous and contains a dense inflammatory infiltrate consisting of lymphocytes, monocytes, plasma cells, and neutrophils; eosinophils may be present but are not common. Inflammation is often most intense around glomeruli.
■ Interstitial granulomas containing multinucleated giant cells may be present, although they are uncommon on needle biopsies. They usually represent granulomatous inflammation near glomeruli with crescents (see above).

- Interstitial hemorrhage may be present, most commonly in the medulla.
- Cortical infarcts may be present, but they are not often seen on needle biopsies.
- Necrosis of the distal portion of papillae may be present.
- In the chronic phase there is interstitial fibrosis and tubular atrophy.

Immunofluorescence Microscopy

- Immunofluorescence is usually negative in glomeruli. Weak, segmental, granular capillary wall staining for IgG, C3, or IgM is sometimes present.
- Staining for fibrinogen is present in necrotic areas, in crescents, and in Bowman's space.
- Vessels usually show no immunoreactivity but may show staining for fibrinogen, immunoglobulins, and C3. This staining pattern probably represents trapping of plasma protein within necrotic areas.

Electron Microscopy

- Some glomerular capillaries contain platelet-fibrin aggregates; fibrin deposits and electron-lucent "fluff" may be present within the subendothelial space. Endothelial cells are swollen and may become detached from the basement membrane.
- Gaps in the glomerular capillary basement membrane may be seen.
- Fibrin is present within crescents, intermixed with cells forming the crescents.
- Electron-dense, immune-type deposits are absent in the majority of cases. Deposits may be present in a variety of locations, including the mesangium and subendothelial, intramembranous, and subepithelial spaces. When present, they are usually small and sparse.
- In the chronic phase, glomerular capillary basement membranes may show wrinkling, thickening, and contraction consistent with ischemia.
- Arteries show swelling of endothelial cells, which may become detached from the underlying basement membrane. Fibrin, platelets, and amorphous electron-dense material (probably plasma proteins) may be present in the subendothelial space.
- Neutrophils are present in the media of arteries; smooth muscle cells may have dilated endoplasmic reticulum and show other degenerative changes. No electron-dense deposits are present.

Differential Diagnosis

- The main differential is that of segmental necrotizing and crescentic glomerulonephritis: immune complex diseases such as systemic lupus erythematosus, poststreptococcal acute glomerulonephritis, and severe IgA nephropathy; anti–glomerular basement membrane (GBM) antibody disease; and the microscopic form of polyarteritis nodosa (idiopathic pauci-immune necrotizing glomerulonephritis). The absence of immune complexes on immunofluorescence and electron microscopy excludes the immune complex diseases; the absence of linear GBM staining for immunoglobulins and complement excludes anti-GBM antibody disease.
- Microscopic polyarteritis may be difficult to distinguish from Wegener's granulomatosis. The presence of granulomatous inflammation would favor Wegener's granulomatosis. Clinical and serologic information may help in differentiation; the presence of pulmonary and sinonasal disease would favor Wegener's granulomatosis, as would the presence of C-ANCAs. Fortunately, because therapy for the two conditions would probably be similar, the importance of the distinction between these conditions is lessened.

Treatment and Clinical Course

- Before the availability of effective therapy, the prognosis of patients with Wegener's granulomatosis was poor, with nearly all patients having a lethal course and median survival of less than 6 months.
- An elevation in serum creatinine, indicating onset of renal insufficiency, was usually followed by rapid progression to severe renal failure.
- Corticosteroids alone usually fail to induce a complete remission, and progression of renal and pulmonary disease while receiving corticosteroid therapy has been documented.
- Combination therapy with high-dose corticosteroids and cytotoxic agents such as cyclophosphamide (Cytoxan) has dramatically altered the history of the disease. The initial trial at the National Institutes of Health resulted in marked improvement or partial remission in 90% of patients, and other series report favorable results.
- Up to half of patients relapse after complete response, so careful long-term monitoring is required.

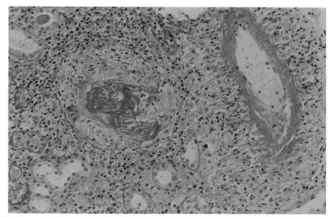

Figure 15–13. Vasculitis, Wegener's granulomatosis. Fibrinoid necrosis of a renal interlobular artery is seen. The glomerulus on the left reveals a large cellular crescent with disruption of Bowman's capsule and associated severe tubulointerstitial inflammatory cell infiltrate. The interstitial inflammatory cell infiltrate usually consists of plasma cells, lymphocytes, and polymorphonuclear leukocytes.

CHURG-STRAUSS SYNDROME (ALLERGIC GRANULOMATOSIS)

Biology of Disease

- Churg-Strauss syndrome is characterized by asthma, necrotizing granulomatous vasculitis, extravascular granulomas, peripheral eosinophilia, and eosinophilic infiltrates in numerous organs.
- The condition appears to be very rare. However, the full spectrum of the different components may be very difficult to demonstrate antemortem, and therefore the condition may be underdiagnosed. It is likely that many cases of polyarteritis nodosa diagnosed in asthmatics actually represented cases of Churg-Strauss syndrome.
- A wide variety of organs or systems may be involved, including the lungs, heart, liver, spleen, skin, peripheral nerves, gastrointestinal tract, and kidneys.
- The prevalence of significant renal disease appears to be less in Churg-Strauss syndrome than in polyarteritis nodosa or Wegener's granulomatosis. Renal disease appears to occur in approximately half of the patients. However, renal disease appears to be uncommon as a cause of death in patients with Churg-Strauss syndrome.

Clinical Features

- The peak age of onset is in the third and fourth decades, although the range is wide. The incidence in men and women is approximately equal.
- The disease typically occurs in three phases: an initial phase of asthma or allergic rhinitis, which may last for many years; a phase of peripheral blood and tissue eosinophilia, which may wax and wane over several years; and finally, the third phase, which is characterized by the appearance of systemic vasculitis.
- Occasionally, the onset of asthma, eosinophilia, and vasculitis is simultaneous rather than following the three-phase sequence.
- The lungs are involved in a high proportion of patients. Chest radiographs may show patchy infiltrates, nodules, diffuse interstitial disease, or pleural effusions.
- Other organ system involvement resembles that found in polyarteritis nodosa, described earlier.
- Renal involvement in Churg-Strauss syndrome is usually relatively minor; common manifestations include microscopic hematuria and mild proteinuria. Renal insufficiency occurs in a significant number of patients. However, renal failure is extremely rare in cases of pure Churg-Strauss syndrome.

Laboratory Values

- Eosinophilia is present by definition. The eosinophil count is usually greater than 1.5×10^3 per microliter (1.5×10^9/L); eosinophils may make up 50% or more of the leukocyte differential.
- Urinalysis demonstrates hematuria and proteinuria.
- Serum urea nitrogen and creatinine concentrations may be normal or increased.
- Several recent studies have suggested that ANCAs are present in a significant proportion of patients; both P-ANCA and C-ANCA have been reported.
- Serum IgE levels may be elevated in some patients.

Gross Appearance

- The kidneys are usually normal in size; cortical cysts may be present.
- Infarcts are occasionally present.
- The renal pelvis and ureters may have thickened, rigid walls because of inflammation and vasculitis of the periureteral and peripelvic tissues.

Light Microscopy

Glomeruli

- Glomerulonephritis in most cases is mild, with a minority of glomeruli involved, and those involved showing segmental changes.
- Focal segmental necrosis may be present, sometimes with crescents.
- Mesangial cellularity may be slightly increased.

Vessels

- Vasculitis is found in up to half of autopsy cases, but it is relatively uncommon on percutaneous biopsy samples.
- Any size artery may be involved, from arcuate arteries to afferent arterioles. Veins may also be involved, although less frequently than arteries; veins of interlobular size and venules are most often affected.
- The vasculitis differs from that seen in polyarteritis nodosa and Wegener's granulomatosis by a striking predominance of eosinophils, both intact and degenerating. Eosinophils may be present within the vessel wall and in the surrounding connective tissue. The number of eosinophils may be decreased if the patient received corticosteroid therapy before biopsy.
- Destruction of the elastic membrane, intraluminal thrombosis, and aneurysmal dilation of arteries may occur.
- Epithelioid histiocytes and giant cells may be present within the media and adventitia of vessels and in periadventitial connective tissue.
- Involvement of veins often appears granulomatous.

Tubules and Interstitium

- An interstitial infiltrate is present and consists predominantly of eosinophils, with lesser numbers of lymphocytes, plasma cells, and neutrophils.
- Interstitial granulomas may be found in a minority of cases. These granulomas have a necrotic core composed of eosinophilic or basophilic material surrounded by a rim of macrophages, giant cells, and numerous eosinophils. Degenerating eosinophils and free eosinophilic granules are prominent. These granulomas are often located adjacent to small veins.
- Tubules show nonspecific degenerative and regenerative changes.

Immunofluorescence Microscopy

- Immunofluorescence microscopy has been reported in only a few cases. In general, results are similar to those described in polyarteritis nodosa.

Electron Microscopy

- Descriptions of ultrastructural findings in Churg-Strauss syndrome are also uncommon. Electron-dense deposits are absent.

Differential Diagnosis

- Churg-Strauss syndrome, polyarteritis nodosa, and Wegener's granulomatosis may have considerable clinical and pathologic overlap. The presence of peripheral eosinophilia and the prominence of eosinophils in tissue would favor Churg-Strauss syndrome over the others.
- Churg-Strauss syndrome may enter into the clinical differential of idiopathic hypereosinophilic syndrome. The latter is associated with hepatosplenomegaly and has a striking predisposition for cardiac involvement. The presence of vasculitis in biopsy tissue would favor Churg-Strauss syndrome over a hypereosinophilic syndrome.

Treatment and Clinical Course

- With corticosteroid therapy, the clinical course of patients with Churg-Strauss syndrome has been generally favorable, with the majority of patients having long-term survival.
- Corticosteroid therapy appears to be adequate for the majority of cases; patients resistant to corticosteroids alone may benefit from cytotoxic immunosuppressive agents such as cyclophosphamide.

ESSENTIAL MIXED CRYOGLOBULINEMIA

Synonyms and Related Terms: Cryoglobulinemic glomerulonephritis; membranoproliferative glomerulonephritis; essential mixed cryoglobulinemia syndrome.

Biology of Disease

- Cryoglobulins are immunoglobulins that reversibly precipitate in cold temperatures.
- Three types of cryoglobulins are differentiated according to the component immunoglobulins contained:
  - Type I cryoglobulins consist of a single monoclonal immunoglobulin.
  - Type II cryoglobulins consist of two immunoglobulins, a polyclonal IgG and a monoclonal immunoglobulin, usually IgM, with reactivity against human IgG (in other words, an anti-IgG rheumatoid factor).
  - Type III cryoglobulins consist of polyclonal IgG and polyclonal IgM antibodies.
- Type I cryoglobulins are usually found in patients with multiple myeloma, monoclonal gammopathy of undetermined significance (sometimes called benign monoclonal gammopathy), or Waldenström's macroglobulinemia.
- Types II and III cryoglobulinemia, collectively known as the "mixed cryoglobulinemias," constitute approximately 60% to 75% of cryoglobulinemias. They are associated with rheumatologic conditions ("connective tissue" diseases), infectious diseases, lymphoproliferative disorders, and hepatobiliary diseases.
- Approximately 30% of mixed cryoglobulinemias were, until recently, of unknown etiology; these conditions were collectively described as the "essential mixed cryoglobulinemias." It is now known that a high proportion of these cases, including both type II and type III, are associated with chronic infection with hepatitis C virus (HCV).
- The "essential mixed cryoglobulinemia syndrome" is a form of systemic vasculitis usually consisting of cutaneous purpura, urticaria, weakness, arthralgias, and, in 10% to 60% of cases, renal disease.
- Renal disease usually occurs with type II mixed cryoglobulinemia and seldom occurs with type III. The monoclonal component in cases with renal disease is almost always an IgM protein with a κ light chain (IgMκ).
- Two types of renal disease occur in type II mixed cryoglobulinemia: glomerulonephritis, frequently with the morphologic appearance of membranoproliferative glomerulonephritis (MPGN), and vasculitis involving small and medium-sized arteries, which occurs in approximately one third of patients with glomerulonephritis and in some patients without glomerulonephritis.
- The glomerulonephritis associated with type II mixed cryoglobulinemia, sometimes designated "cryoglobulinemic glomerulonephritis," often has both histologic and clinical differences from typical cases of idiopathic MPGN (described later).
- Essential mixed cryoglobulinemia occurs most frequently in Italy and other Mediterranean countries. Women outnumber men in most series, including patients with renal disease.

Clinical Features

- Cutaneous purpura and urticaria are the most common clinical manifestations. Biopsy of skin lesions demonstrates leukocytoclastic vasculitis.
- Most patients have clinical manifestations of cryoglobulinemia before the onset of renal disease. However, occasionally renal disease is the first manifestation of the disease.
- The most common manifestation of renal disease, occurring in more than half of patients, is asymptomatic proteinuria with microscopic hematuria. Renal function as measured by serum creatinine is usually normal, but mild renal insufficiency may be present.
- Approximately one quarter of patients have an acute nephritic syndrome, including macroscopic hematuria, proteinuria, hypertension, and increased serum creatinine; oliguric or anuric renal failure occasionally occurs (fewer than 5% of patients). Patients with acute nephritis frequently also have signs of systemic disease.

- Approximately one fifth have nephrotic-range proteinuria or nephrotic syndrome.
- Hypertension is common and may be hard to control.

Laboratory Values

- The serum contains a cryoglobulin, almost invariably composed of IgG and IgMκ.
- The pattern of serum complement levels is highly characteristic: levels of early complement components, especially C4, are very low; C3 levels are normal or only slightly decreased.
- Serum antibodies against HCV or HCV RNA are present in the majority of patients.

Light Microscopy

Glomeruli

- In the acute phase the most common lesion is diffuse intracapillary hypercellularity with closure of glomerular capillary loops. Hypercellularity is predominantly caused by leukocytes, particularly monocytes. The predominance of leukocytes and especially monocytes in cryoglobulinemic glomerulonephritis is striking and constitutes an important feature that often assists in differentiating membranoproliferative glomerulonephritis (MPGN) secondary to cryoglobulinemia from idiopathic MPGN.
- Eosinophilic, refractile-appearing hyaline deposits may be present within and filling occasional capillary lumina ("intraluminal thrombi").
- Diffuse thickening of glomerular capillary basement membranes is apparent on periodic acid–Schiff and Jones stains; reduplication or "tram-tracking" of the GBM is often prominent and widespread.
- Extracapillary proliferation (crescents in Bowman's space) is somewhat uncommon in cryoglobulinemic glomerulonephritis; when present, crescents tend to be small and occur in a minority of glomeruli.
- Mild segmental mesangial proliferation, without monocyte infiltration or GBM alterations, occurs in approximately 10% of patients.
- Approximately 10% of patients have marked mesangial sclerosis in addition to mesangial hypercellularity; this condition is often associated with heavy proteinuria, renal insufficiency, and progression to renal failure.

Tubules and Interstitium

- Localized interstitial fibrosis and occasional atrophic tubules are common, but widespread interstitial fibrosis and tubular atrophy are rare.
- Erythrocyte casts may be present in tubular lumina during acute episodes.

Vessels

- Vasculitis, when present, involves small and medium-sized arteries; arterioles may also be involved.
- In the acute phase there is fibrinoid necrosis of the intima and media. Areas of necrosis are surrounded by a cellular reaction, which may include neutrophils and monocytes.
- Arterioles may contain intraluminal, glassy or refractile deposits similar to those seen in glomerular capillaries.
- In later stages, fibrinoid necrosis in arteries is replaced by marked intimal fibrosis.

Immunofluorescence Microscopy

- Granular staining for IgG and IgM is present in glomerular capillaries, usually in a subendothelial location; granular mesangial staining is frequently present. Staining for complement components, including C3 and C4, is often seen. The intensity of staining varies from faint to intense.
- Glomerular capillary lumina may display intense staining for IgG and IgM corresponding to the intraluminal thrombi.
- Staining for IgG and IgM may be present in arteriolar walls and intraluminal deposits in arterioles.

Electron Microscopy

- The most striking ultrastructural feature is organized, fibrillar deposits with a distinctive substructure. The deposits consist of a combination of curved cylinders with a width of 2.5 nm that are arranged in pairs and annular structures with spokes reaching 3 nm in diameter.
- These organized deposits are usually found in a subendothelial location in glomerular capillaries; they may be found within intraluminal thrombi in glomerular capillaries and can occasionally be found in an intramembranous or subepithelial location.
- Many of the cells within glomerular capillaries are monocytes; these monocytes are often found in association with the organized deposits. Monocytes often occupy a subendothelial location interposed between the glomerular capillary basement membrane and the endothelial lining; thus in cryoglobulinemic glomerulonephritis, monocytes occupy the location that mesangial cells occupy in idiopathic MPGN. They may be associated with "reduplication" of the GBM.

Differential Diagnosis

- An important differential problem is the distinction of cryoglobulinemic glomerulonephritis from idiopathic MPGN. Histologic features that would favor cryoglobulinemic glomerulonephritis include a large number of leukocytes, particularly monocytes, within the glomerular capillary tuft, the presence of intraluminal thrombi within glomerular capillaries, and the presence of vasculitis involving small and medium-sized arterioles. An assay for cryoglobulins should be performed if any of these features are noted. High magnification of the EM deposits needs to be performed (to search for the characteristic substructure of cryoglobulins).
- Cryoglobulins may be present in patients with glomerulonephritis associated with systemic lupus erythematosus, poststreptococcal acute glomerulonephritis, and

other diseases; glomerulonephritis in such patients may have histologic features resembling those of cryoglobulinemic glomerulonephritis, as described earlier.

Treatment and Clinical Course

- The course of renal disease in mixed cryoglobulinemia is variable but, at least in some series, appears to be more indolent than are the majority of cases of idiopathic MPGN.
- Progression to end-stage renal failure appears to be relatively uncommon and occurs in approximately 10% of cases, usually after several years of disease.
- Infections, cardiovascular disease, and systemic effects of vasculitis are the most common causes of death.
- Corticosteroids, cytotoxic immunosuppressive drugs

such as cyclophosphamide (Cytoxan), or a combination has been the mainstay of therapy for renal disease associated with cryoglobulinemia. Plasmapheresis may be used for relief of acute flares of renal disease.
- Recently, α-interferon has been reported to be beneficial in some patients; the activity of interferon in renal disease may relate to its antiviral effects inasmuch as decreases in the activity of renal disease appear to correlate with the elimination of HCV RNA.
- The benefit from these therapies is difficult to quantitate because of the variable course of the renal disease in individual patients and a lack of large, randomized, controlled trials. However, the survival of patients with renal disease related to cryoglobulinemia has improved and now appears equivalent to that of patients with mixed cryoglobulinemia without renal disease.

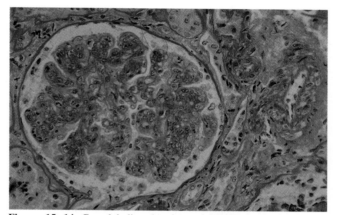

Figure 15–14. Cryoglobulinemic glomerulonephritis. The glomerulus displays intracapillary hypercellularity with intracapillary accumulation of inflammatory cells, including polymorphonuclear leukocytes and monocytes, and thickening and focal reduplication of the capillary walls (periodic acid–Schiff reaction).

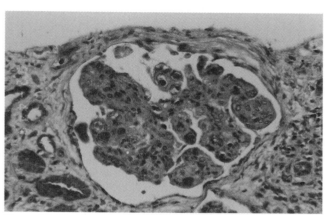

Figure 15–16. Cryoglobulinemic glomerulonephritis. Prominent intracapillary hypercellularity is seen in a glomerulus; multiple fuchsinophilic intraluminal globules representing cryoglobulins are also present. The lobular architecture is accentuated (Masson's trichrome stain).

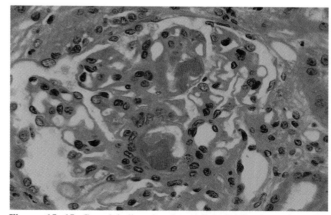

Figure 15–15. Cryoglobulinemic glomerulonephritis. A portion of a glomerulus is seen with acellular glassy refractile intraluminal protein "thrombi" representing cryoglobulins, along with a slight mesangial cellular proliferation.

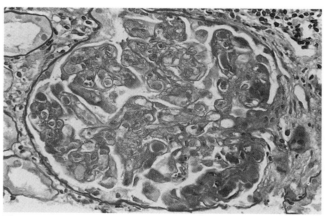

Figure 15–17. Cryoglobulinemic glomerulonephritis. The glomerular capillary basement membranes reveal extensive "reduplication"; intracapillary hypercellularity and multiple periodic acid–Schiff (PAS)–positive intraluminal acellular protein globules are also seen. This patient had malignant lymphoma and mixed cryoglobulinemia with IgG and IgM components (PAS reaction).

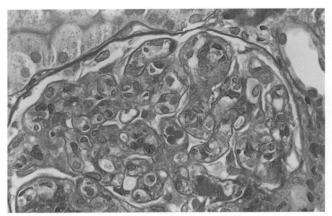

Figure 15–18. Cryoglobulinemic glomerulonephritis. The glomerular intracapillary hypercellularity consists of resident glomerular cells and blood-borne inflammatory cells, including monocytes and polymorphonuclear leukocytes. The photograph is from the same patient shown in Figure 15–17 (periodic acid–Schiff reaction).

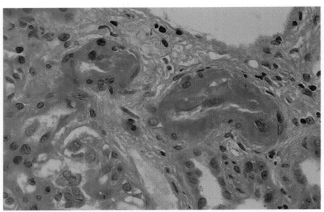

Figure 15–21. Cryoglobulinemia. Acellular hyaline refractile protein deposits are seen in small arteries. Along with the glomerular changes, the vascular deposition of "cryoglobulins" is a typical feature of cryoglobulinemia.

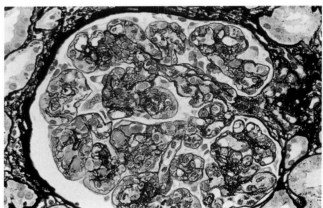

Figure 15–19. Cryoglobulinemic glomerulonephritis. The glomerulus displays mesangial sclerosis, extensive "reduplication" of the basement membranes, and multiple intracapillary silver-negative globules (methenamine silver stain).

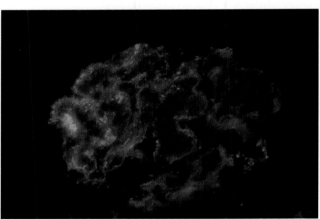

Figure 15–22. Cryoglobulinemic glomerulonephritis. IgG deposition is seen along the periphery of the glomerular capillary walls; note the few intraluminal "globules" on the left. Because the globules may be rare, recognition of these cryoglobulins can be difficult (immunofluorescence).

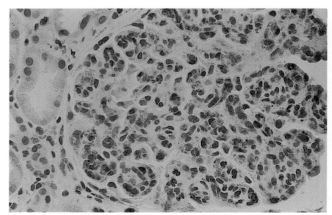

Figure 15–20. Cryoglobulinemic glomerulonephritis. Marked accumulation of KP-1 (CD68)-positive monocytes/macrophages is shown in the hypercellular glomerulus from a patient with cryoglobulinemic glomerulonephritis (streptavidin-peroxidase immunohistochemical reaction).

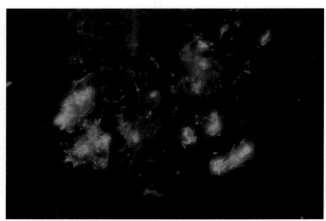

Figure 15–23. Cryoglobulinemic glomerulonephritis. Numerous glomerular intraluminal IgG-positive "globules" are seen (immunofluorescence).

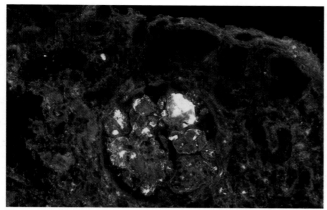

Figure 15–24. Cryoglobulinemic glomerulonephritis. Glomerular deposition of IgM is shown with segmental accentuation.

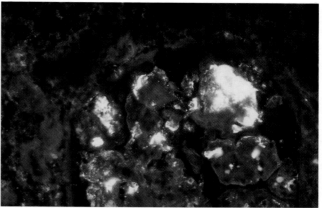

Figure 15–25. Cryoglobulinemia. The glomerular IgM deposits are seen in a subendothelial, mesangial, and probably intraluminal distribution.

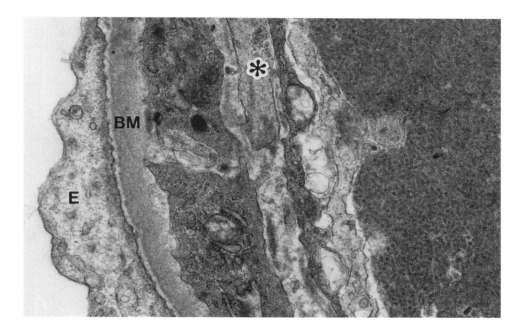

Figure 15–26. Electron micrograph of cryoglobulinemic glomerulonephritis. Note the regular substructure of the large subendothelial electron-dense immune-type deposit in the glomerular capillary loop at high magnification. There is reduplication of the glomerular capillary basement membrane and cellular mesangial interposition between the old (original) and new basement membranes (E, visceral epithelial cell; BM, glomerular capillary basement membrane; asterisk, reduplicated [new] glomerular capillary basement membrane).

THE KIDNEY IN OTHER FORMS OF VASCULITIS

Giant Cell Arteritis (Temporal Arteritis)

- Giant cell arteritis is a vasculitis of medium and large arteries that is characterized by transmural inflammation with a mixed inflammatory infiltrate including giant cells.
- Symptoms are usually related to involvement of the temporal and other cranial arteries. However, other organs may be involved, sometimes in the absence of temporal or cranial artery involvement. In some pa-

tients, the disease may be almost indistinguishable from polyarteritis nodosa.
- Renal involvement in giant cell arteritis is rare, fewer than 10% of cases, and is usually mild. Rare cases of more fulminant renal disease have been reported.
- Renal involvement is usually manifested as microscopic hematuria and proteinuria. Renal insufficiency is extremely unusual.
- Rare cases of renal involvement resembling polyarteritis nodosa have been reported.
- Renal biopsies are not usually performed in giant cell arteritis, so the renal pathology of typical cases is not well studied.

■ The rare cases of renal involvement resembling polyarteritis nodosa are associated with focal necrotizing and crescentic glomerulonephritis similar to that seen in the microscopic variant of polyarteritis nodosa.

Takayasu's Arteritis ("Pulseless Disease")

■ Takayasu's arteritis is a rare condition characterized by transmural inflammation and stenosis of medium and large arteries, with a strong tendency to involve the aortic arch and its major branches.

■ The disease characteristically affects young women. The peak age of onset is approximately 15 to 20 years, and women are affected about nine times more often than men.

■ In the United States, the most common sites of involvement are the thoracic aorta distal to the aortic arch and the abdominal aorta with its major branches. In Japan, the most common sites are the aortic arch and its major branches.

■ Acute vasculitis is characterized by transmural inflammation of elastic arteries with lymphocytes, monocytes, neutrophils, and occasionally multinucleated giant cells.

■ The chronic phase is characterized by intimal fibrosis and scarring of the media, eventually resulting in narrowing or total obliteration of the lumen.

■ Renal involvement is rare in most series. The most common manifestation is renovascular hypertension secondary to renal artery stenosis, with preservation of renal function. In this instance, the pathology is that of ischemic nephropathy.

■ Cases of Takayasu's arteritis associated with a mild mesangial proliferative glomerulonephritis have been reported. Patients have mild hematuria and proteinuria; renal function is usually normal. Immunofluorescence demonstrates mesangial staining for immunoglobulins (in various combinations of IgG, IgM, or IgA) and complement components. Electron microscopy demonstrates electron-dense mesangial deposits. Renal abnormalities usually resolve with corticosteroid therapy.

References

Vasculitis and the Kidney

Andrassy K, Erb A, Koderisch J, et al: Wegener's granulomatosis with renal involvement: Patient survival and correlations between initial renal function, renal histology, therapy and renal outcome. Clin Nephrol 35:139, 1991.

Andrassy K, Koderisch J, Rufer M, et al: Detection and clinical implication of anti-neutrophil cytoplasmic antibodies in Wegener's granulomatosis and rapidly progressive glomerulonephritis. Clin Nephrol 32:159, 1989.

Brouet J-C, Clauvel J-P, Danon F, et al: Biologic and clinical significance of cryoglobulins: A report of 86 cases. Am J Med 57:775, 1974.

Cameron JS: Renal vasculitis: Microscopic polyarteritis and Wegener's granuloma. Contrib Nephrol 94:38, 1991.

D'Agati VD, Appel GB: Polyarteritis nodosa, Wegener granulomatosis, Churg-Strauss syndrome, temporal arteritis, Takayasu arteritis, and lymphomatoid granulomatosis. In: Tisher CC, Brenner BM (eds): Renal Pathology: With Clinical and Functional Correlations, 2nd ed. Philadelphia, JB Lippincott, 1994, p 1087.

D'Amico G, Fornasieri A: Cryoglobulinemic glomerulonephritis: A membranoproliferative glomerulonephritis induced by hepatitis C virus. Am J Kidney Dis 25:361, 1995.

Gaskin G, Clutterbuck EJ, Pusey CD: Renal disease in the Churg-Strauss syndrome: Diagnosis, management and outcome. Contrib Nephrol 94:58, 1991.

Grotz W, Wanner C, Keller E, et al: Crescentic glomerulonephritis in Wegener's granulomatosis: Morphology, therapy, and outcome. Clin Nephrol 35:243, 1991.

Jennette JC: Renal involvement in systemic vasculitis. In: Jennette JC, Olson JL, Schwartz MM, Silva FG (eds): Heptinstall's Pathology of the Kidney, 5th ed. Philadelphia, Lippincott-Raven, 1998, p 1059.

Jennette JC, Falk RJ, Andrassy K, et al: Nomenclature of systemic vasculitides: Proposal of an international consensus conference. Arthritis Rheum 37:187, 1994.

Lie JT: Diagnostic histopathology of major systemic and pulmonary vasculitic syndromes. Rheum Dis Clin North Am 16:269, 1990.

Morel-Maroger Striker LJ, Preud'homme J-L, D'Amico G, et al: Monoclonal gammopathies, mixed cryoglobulinemias, and lymphomas. In: Tisher CC, Brenner BM (eds): Renal Pathology: With Clinical and Functional Correlations, 2nd ed. Philadelphia, JB Lippincott, 1994, p 1442.

Rao JK, Weinberger M, Oddone EZ, et al: The role of antineutrophil cytoplasmic antibody (c-ANCA) testing in the diagnosis of Wegener granulomatosis: A literature review and meta-analysis. Ann Intern Med 123:925, 1995.

Ritz E, Andrassy K, Küster S, et al: Wegener's granulomatosis, microscopic polyarteritis and pauciimmune crescentic necrotizing glomerulonephritis: An overview. Contrib Nephrol 94:1, 1991.

Ronco P, Verroust P, Mignon F, et al: Immunopathological studies of polyarteritis nodosa and Wegener's granulomatosis: A report of 43 patients with 51 renal biopsies. Q J Med 52:212, 1983.

CHAPTER 16

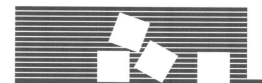

HIV-Associated Nephropathy and Intravenous Drug Abuse

INTRODUCTION

A variety of renal diseases may develop in human immunodeficiency virus (HIV)-positive patients, just as in HIV-negative individuals. However, soon after eruption of the acquired immunodeficiency syndrome (AIDS) epidemic, a unique renal disease with characteristic clinical and morphologic findings emerged in the HIV-positive population. This chapter describes this peculiar renal condition, which has been named HIV-associated nephropathy (HIVAN).

HIV-ASSOCIATED NEPHROPATHY

Synonyms: HIV nephropathy; AIDS nephropathy; HIV-associated glomerulosclerosis; HIV-associated collapsing glomerulopathy.

Biology of Disease

- The disease was first recognized in the mid-1980s. The incidence of HIVAN was continuously rising; however, it appears to have reached a plateau in recent years in the New York City area.
- Geographic differences in the incidence of HIVAN are great in the United States; the highest rates are reported along the East coast, including Florida. Along the West coast and in Europe, the incidence of HIVAN is considerably lower.
- Ninety percent of patients with HIVAN are African-Americans, 70% are male, and approximately 50% are intravenous drug abusers. In whites, HIVAN is very rare.
- The pathogenesis is obscure. No convincing evidence has been presented that direct infection of human renal parenchymal (glomerular) cells plays a role in the pathogenesis of HIVAN.

Clinical Features

- Patients generally have severe, usually nephrotic-range proteinuria and impaired renal function.
- Hypertension occurs in fewer than half of the patients.

- Ultrasonography typically shows enlarged, highly echogenic kidneys.
- Microscopic hematuria may occur.

Laboratory Values

- The serum creatinine value at diagnosis averages 5 mg/dL.
- The 24-hour urine protein excretion on average is between 6 and 7 g.
- Urine sediment is usually benign, but granular and occasional red blood cell casts may be found.
- The CD4 count does not show a good correlation with the development of HIVAN; the disease may appear at any time in an HIV-positive patient and is occasionally the first manifestation of HIV infection.

Light Microscopy

Glomeruli

- The characteristic glomerular finding is a collapsing type of glomerular sclerosis that is usually global but may be segmental. The capillary loops are collapsed, but the mesangial matrix is characteristically *not* increased.
- Prominent podocytes with many protein resorption droplets usually cover the collapsing/sclerosing glomerular capillary loops.
- Glomeruli are not necessarily small; occasionally they may be enlarged.

Tubules

- Microcystic dilatation of some tubules, characteristically with a scalloped outline, is the most typical tubular change.
- Many proximal tubules contain large numbers of protein resorption droplets.
- Tubular degenerative and regenerative features with patchy epithelial necrosis, mitotic figures, and flattened tubular epithelium are frequently seen.

- Tubular atrophy is generally prominent at the time of diagnosis.

Interstitium

- Most cases contain a prominent interstitial mononuclear cell infiltrate.
- The infiltrate consists largely of lymphocytes, mainly CD8-positive T cells, as well as plasma cells, monocytes, and some B cells.
- In most cases, a mild to moderate interstitial fibrosis is already noted at the time of diagnosis.

Vessels

- No typical vascular changes can be described; in rare cases, thrombotic microangiopathy (TMA) may be associated with HIV infection.

Immunofluorescence Microscopy

- Immunofluorescence is unrevealing; the findings are nonspecific unless concomitant immune complex glomerulonephritis or immune complex deposition is present.
- Rarely, immune complex deposits can be noted in otherwise typical HIVAN. These deposits, however, should not be considered to be part of the disease; they may be related to infections such as hepatitis C virus infection.

Electron Microscopy

- Tubuloreticular inclusions (interferon "footprints") in endothelial cells are usually abundant. These inclusions are 24-nm interanastomosing tubular structures located within dilated endoplasmic reticulum.
- Other less characteristic ultrastructural features include granular degeneration of the nuclear chromatin of interstitial or tubular cells, increased number of intranuclear electron-dense bodies, cylindrical confronting cisternae, and cytomembranous inclusions. These findings are not specific to HIVAN.
- Occasionally, electron-dense immune-type deposits can be seen in the mesangium or sometimes along the glomerular capillary basement membrane.

Differential Diagnosis

Idiopathic Focal Segmental Glomerular Sclerosis (Focal Sclerosis)

- Collapsing glomerular sclerosis with prominent podocytes, tubular microcystic dilatation, and endothelial tubuloreticular inclusions are distinctive findings in HIVAN, but they are uncommon in idiopathic focal segmental glomerular sclerosis (FSGS).
- Glomerular hyalinosis is a frequent finding in idiopathic FSGS but uncommon in HIVAN.

Heroin-Associated Nephropathy

- Findings in heroin-associated nephropathy (HAN) are similar to those of FSGS and can be distinguished from HIVAN as described earlier.
- Heroin-associated nephropathy is becoming a rare entity in comparison to HIVAN.

Idiopathic Collapsing Glomerulopathy

- Idiopathic collapsing glomerulopathy is clinically and morphologically very similar to HIVAN.
- The patients are HIV negative. Endothelial tubuloreticular inclusions are rarely seen by electron microscopy.

Lupus Nephritis

- Numerous endothelial tubuloreticular inclusions may occur in both lupus nephritis and HIVAN. The morphologic distinction may occasionally be problematic if HIVAN is associated with superimposed glomerular immune complex deposits.
- The additional typical morphologic findings in lupus, as well as the clinical and laboratory data characteristic of lupus, usually make the differential diagnosis easy.

Immune Complex Glomerulonephritis

- Immune complex glomerulonephritis may occur in HIV-infected patients. A few reports indicate an increased incidence of IgA nephropathy in white patients with HIV infection. Other forms of immune complex glomerulonephritis have also been described in HIV-positive patients. Rarely, in otherwise typical HIVAN, glomerular immune deposits may be found.

Acute Interstitial Nephritis

- Acute interstitial nephritis may occur in HIV-infected patients in the absence of HIVAN.
- A peculiar form of acute interstitial nephritis may rarely occur in HIV-infected patients as part of a systemic disease called "diffuse infiltrative lymphocytosis syndrome."

Thrombotic Microangiopathy

- The association of HIV infection and thrombotic microangiopathy (TMA) is well recognized. Rarely, TMA may occur in the setting of HIVAN.

Treatment and Clinical Course

- No treatment has been found to be definitively effective for HIVAN.
- A few data indicate that zidovudine, steroids, angiotensin-converting enzyme inhibitors, and the novel protease inhibitors may slow progression of the disease or may at least temporarily improve the proteinuria.
- Usually, HIVAN is rapidly progressive, and end-stage renal disease develops within months in most patients. Hemodialysis is the treatment of choice; renal transplantation is not usually offered to HIV-positive patients.

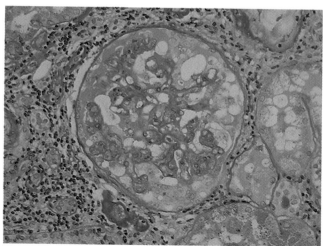

Figure 16–1. Characteristic glomerulus from a case of HIV-associated nephropathy. Note the collapsing glomerular capillary loops with only a few open lumina and the prominent glomerular epithelial cells in Bowman's space. In addition to the glomerular changes, prominent interstitial inflammatory infiltrate and tubular atrophy can be found (periodic acid–Schiff reaction).

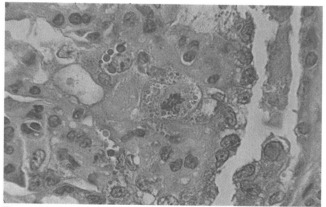

Figure 16–4. HIV-associated nephropathy (HIVAN). This glomerulus is the same as that shown in Figure 16–3, but under higher magnification. Note the eosinophilic protein droplets in the podocytes and, in particular, the mitotic podocyte in the middle of the picture. The podocyte was thought to be unable to undergo mitosis; however, in focal segmental glomerulosclerosis, particularly in HIVAN, mitotic podocytes sometimes are noted.

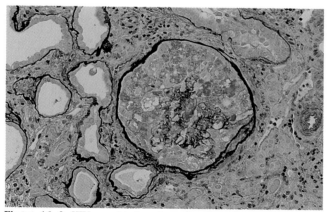

Figure 16–2. HIV-associated nephropathy. Note the extensively collapsed glomerular capillary loops surrounded by very prominent glomerular epithelial cells (mainly podocytes). These prominent epithelial cells may resemble crescents and frequently contain protein resorption droplets (methenamine silver stain).

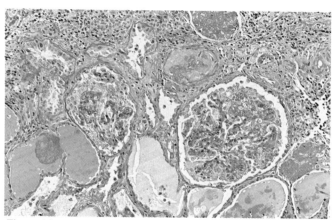

Figure 16–5. HIV-associated nephropathy. The glomerulus on the right is enlarged in spite of the capillary loop collapse. Also note the dilated tubules and interstitial mononuclear cell infiltrate. Glomeruli with collapsing capillary loops are not necessarily small; they can be large (periodic acid–Schiff reaction).

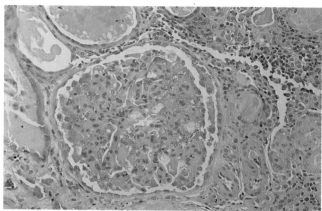

Figure 16–3. HIV-associated nephropathy. Sometimes on hematoxylin and eosin stain the glomerular capillary collapse is not obvious; however, the prominent podocytes are usually apparent.

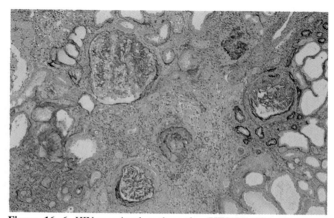

Figure 16–6. HIV-associated nephropathy (HIVAN). Note the somewhat enlarged glomerulus with collapsing features and the glomerular sclerosis with hyaninosis in the adjacent glomeruli. Glomerular hyalinosis is not a characteristic feature of HIVAN; this patient had a long history of hypertension before the development of symptoms of HIVAN (methenamine silver stain).

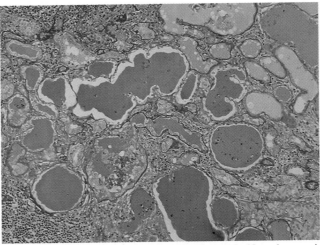

Figure 16–7. HIV-associated nephropathy (HIVAN). Note the prominent tubulointerstitial disease, including microcystic dilatation of several tubules that contain homogeneous periodic acid–Schiff (PAS)–positive casts. Microcystic dilatation of tubules, frequently with a scalloped outline, is another characteristic feature of HIVAN (PAS reaction).

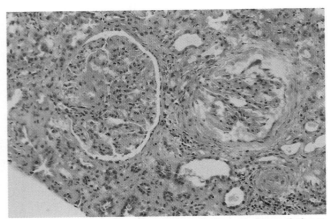

Figure 16–9. HIV-associated nephropathy with superimposed thrombotic microangiopathy. Note the mucoid arteriole in the right lower corner of the figure and the fibrin thrombus in the left (enlarged) glomerulus. Thrombotic microangiopathy is a rare, but well-known complication of HIV infection and carries a very poor prognosis.

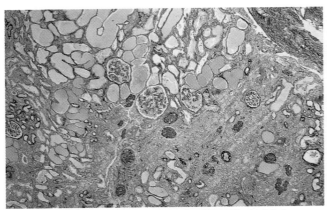

Figure 16–8. HIV-associated nephropathy (HIVAN). At this low magnification, note the prominent interstitial disease with microcystic dilatation of tubules and the glomerular sclerosis *(black globules)*. In HIVAN, involvement of the tubulointerstitium is usually at least as prominent as involvement of the glomeruli (methenamine silver stain).

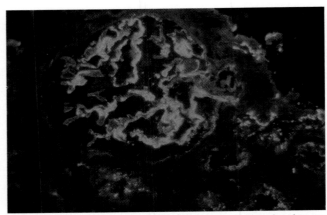

Figure 16–10. HIV-associated nephropathy. Note the granular glomerular capillary complement (C3) deposits by immunofluorescence. Occasionally, immune deposits are seen in patients with otherwise typical HIV-associated nephropathy; this patient was also positive for hepatitis C virus.

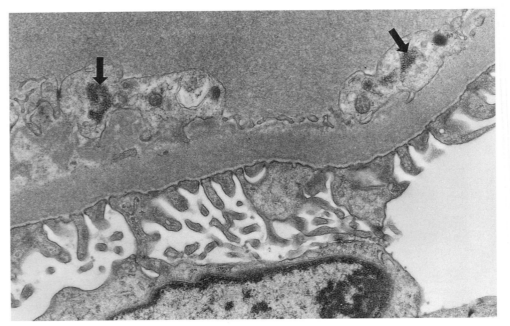

Figure 16–11. Ultrastructural findings in HIV-associated nephropathy. Note the tubuloreticular inclusions in the glomerular endothelial cells *(arrows)*. Tubuloreticular inclusions (myxovirus-like inclusions or interferon footprints) in the endothelial cells are frequently seen in HIV-infected patients. These inclusions are not specific for HIV infection and are frequently noted in patients with systemic lupus erythematosus and sometimes other conditions as well.

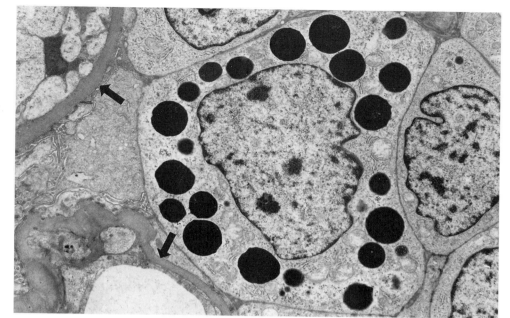

Figure 16–12. Ultrastructural findings in HIV-associated nephropathy. Note the large, swollen podocytes in Bowman's space, some of which contain large, dense, cytoplasmic granules (probably protein resorption droplets). The glomerular basement membranes of the underlying collapsing capillaries are shown by the arrows.

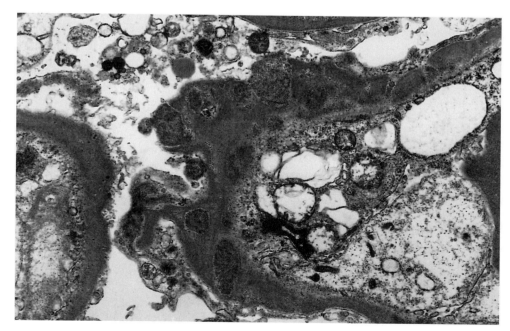

Figure 16–13. Ultrastructural findings in HIV-associated nephropathy with superimposed glomerular immune complex deposits. Note the intramembranous, subepithelial, and subendothelial discrete, electron-dense, immune-type deposits in the glomerular capillary loop. This illustration is an electron micrograph of the case shown in Figure 16–10.

HEROIN-ASSOCIATED NEPHROPATHY

Synonym: Intravenous drug abuse–associated nephropathy.

Biology of Disease

- Heroin-associated nephropathy (HAN) was described in the early 1970s and the incidence was growing during the 1980s. Starting in the early 1990s, the incidence of HAN declined and it appears that it is disappearing, at least in the New York City metropolitan area.
- The pathogenesis of HAN is obscure. Some evidence suggests that it may be associated with the purity of heroin (i.e., the vehicle with which the heroin is cut).
- In certain cases it is possible that the FSGS seen in patients with HAN may represent a healed focal glomerulonephritis secondary to infections such as endocarditis or deep-seated abscesses.
- Intravenous drug abuse–associated nephropathy can be seen in persons who are not heroin abusers, such as in intravenous pentazocine and tripelennamine (T's and Blues) abusers.
- Many intravenous drug abusers are also HIV positive, and the possibility has been raised that HAN represents HIVAN in a drug abuser. However, there is clear evidence that HAN can develop in HIV-negative patients, and the morphology and outcome are also somewhat different from that seen in HIVAN.
- Similar to HIVAN, HAN appears mostly in African-Americans.

Clinical Features

- Similar to idiopathic FSGS, patients usually have severe, usually nephrotic-range proteinuria.
- Some degree of renal impairment with elevated serum creatinine levels is usually present.
- Hypertension is a frequent long-term complication.
- The renal disease is usually advanced at diagnosis and renal insufficiency develops fairly rapidly.

Laboratory Values

- Elevated serum creatinine values and 24-hour urine protein above 3 or 3.5 g are common findings.
- Microscopic hematuria is frequently present.
- Blood cultures are negative unless infection develops because of the use of infected needles.

Light Microscopy

Glomeruli

- The glomerular changes are quite similar to those in idiopathic FSGS and are basically indistinguishable from it.
- Focal, global, and segmental glomerulosclerosis and hyalinosis are the characteristic findings.

Tubules

- A variable degree of tubular atrophy is usually present.
- Acute degenerative and regenerative changes may be seen with tubular protein resorption droplets.

Interstitium

- Focal interstitial fibrosis is commonly seen with mononuclear cell infiltrate localized to these fibrotic areas. In general, the interstitial fibrosis and the mononuclear cell infiltrate appear to be somewhat more severe in HAN than in biopsy specimens with idiopathic FSGS.

Vessels

- No specific or characteristic vascular changes are present. Arteriolar hyaline change may be seen.

Immunofluorescence Microscopy

- Immunofluorescence is usually nonspecific; segmental glomerular IgM and C3 may be present in sclerotic areas.
- Strong granular immunofluorescence with IgG, other immunoglobulins, and complement indicates immune complex deposition from endocarditis or other infections that may occur in intravenous drug abusers.

Electron Microscopy

- No specific ultrastructural lesions are described.
- Tubuloreticular inclusions may be present if the patient is HIV positive.
- Immune-type electron-dense deposits in the mesangium and along glomerular capillary loops indicate immune complex glomerulonephritis associated with endocarditis or other infections.

Differential Diagnosis

Idiopathic Focal Segmental Glomerular Sclerosis (Focal Sclerosis)

- Idiopathic FSGS is usually quite indistinguishable from HAN by morphology alone; careful clinical history and association of the disease with intravenous drug abuse are most helpful in the diagnosis.

HIV-Associated Nephropathy

- Widespread collapsing glomerulosclerosis with prominent podocytes and microcystic dilatation of tubules is not usually seen in HAN, in contrast to their characteristic occurrence in HIVAN.

Immune Complex Glomerulonephritis

- Focal glomerulonephritis may be found in intravenous drug abusers, particularly if endocarditis develops because of the use of infected needles.

- Focal glomerulonephritis may heal with focal segmental and global glomerular sclerosis and shows morphology identical to that of HAN.
- Immune deposits in FSGS in an intravenous drug abuser indicate such a healing focal glomerulonephritis or other superimposed infectious complications rather than HAN.

Treatment and Clinical Course

- No specific and effective treatment is available; therapeutic approaches used in idiopathic FSGS can be applied.
- The clinical course is usually worse than in idiopathic FSGS but considerably better than in HIVAN.

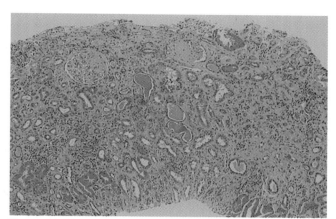

Figure 16–14. Heroin-associated nephropathy (HAN). Note the segmental sclerosis of glomeruli and the chronic tubulointerstitial disease. Histologic changes in HAN are more reminiscent of idiopathic focal segmental glomerular sclerosis than of HIV-associated nephropathy.

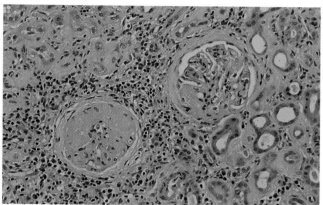

Figure 16–15. Heroin-associated nephropathy (HAN). Note the segmentally and globally sclerotic glomerulus and the prominent tubulointerstitial disease with fibrosis and tubular atrophy. In contrast to HIV-associated nephropathy, in HAN, glomerular capillary collapse, prominent podocytes, and microcystic dilatation of tubules are less common.

References

HIV-Associated Nephropathy

Cohen AH, Nast CC: HIV-associated nephropathy. A unique combined glomerular, tubular, and interstitial lesion. Mod Pathol 1:87, 1988.

D'Agati V, Appel GB: HIV infection and the kidney. J Am Soc Nephrol 8:138, 1997.

D'Agati V, Suh JI, Carbone L, et al: Pathology of HIV-associated nephropathy: A detailed morphologic and comparative study. Kidney Int 35:1358, 1989.

Kimmel PL, Phillips TM, Ferreira-Centeno A, et al: HIV-associated immune-mediated renal disease. Kidney Int 44:1327, 1993.

Seney FD, Burns DK, Silva FG: Acquired immunodeficiency syndrome and the kidney. Am J Kidney Dis 16:1, 1990.

Heroin-Associated Nephropathy

Cunningham EE, Brentjens OR, Zieleezny MA, et al: Heroin nephropathy: A clinicopathologic and epidemiologic study. Am J Med 68:47, 1980.

Friedman EA, Rao TKS: Disappearance of uremia due to heroin-associated nephropathy. Am J Kidney Dis 25:689, 1995.

Grishman E, Churg J, Porush JG: Glomerular morphology in nephrotic heroin addicts. Lab Invest 35:415, 1976.

May DC, Helderman JH, Eigenbrodt EH, et al: Chronic sclerosing glomerulopathy (heroin-associated nephropathy) in intravenous T's and Blues abusers. Am J Kidney Dis 8:404, 1986.

CHAPTER 17

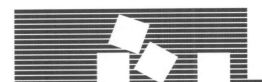

Miscellaneous Conditions Affecting the Kidney
Liver Disease, Sickle Cell Nephropathy, C1q Nephropathy, Collagen Type III Glomerulopathy, and Fibronectin Glomerulopathy

INTRODUCTION

- The conditions discussed in this chapter are a heterogeneous group that are included here primarily because they do not fit appropriately into any other section.
- The primary conditions discussed are liver disease and the kidney, and sickle cell nephropathy. Also included are three unusual, recently described variants of glomerular disease (C1q nephropathy, collagen type III glomerulopathy, and fibronectin glomerulopathy).

LIVER DISEASE AND THE KIDNEY

Introduction

- The kidney may be affected by liver disease in a variety of different ways. In some cases the effect on the kidney is primarily functional, without significant morphologic renal changes; in other cases, the kidney has morphologic or immunologic abnormalities, which may or may not be associated with abnormalities in renal excretory function.
- The hepatorenal syndrome is an example of a functional renal abnormality that is not associated with significant morphologic changes. In this condition, which has a high mortality rate, functional renal insufficiency occurs in patients with severe or end-stage liver disease. The kidneys in hepatorenal syndrome show few or no morphologic abnormalities and in fact function well if transplanted into someone with normal hepatic function.
- A less extreme example of a functional renal disorder in hepatic disease is the prerenal azotemia that occurs in patients with hypoalbuminemia caused by decreased hepatic protein synthesis. In such patients, ascites and generalized edema develop because of the decrease in plasma oncotic pressure, with a consequent decrease in circulating intravascular volume.
- Both hepatitis B virus (HBV) and hepatitis C virus may be associated with renal disease. Cryoglobulinemic glomerulonephritis caused by hepatitis C virus is discussed in Chapter 15; glomerulonephritis associated with HBV will be discussed in this chapter.
- Glomerular mesangial deposits of IgA are frequently found in patients with hepatic cirrhosis; in the majority of cases, this IgA deposition appears to be associated with few clinical consequences.

Hepatitis B Virus and the Kidney

Biology of Disease

- Hepatitis B virus (HBV) is a DNA virus that is spread by parenteral means (transfusion, blood products, shared needles among intravenous drug abusers) and by body fluids (saliva, semen, vaginal fluid). It causes both acute and chronic hepatitis, as well as a chronic carrier state. The chronic carrier state forms the reservoir for continued spread of the virus; in addition, it is estimated that 25% to 40% of chronic carriers die of complications of HBV infection, including hepatic cirrhosis and hepatocellular carcinoma.
- Hepatitis B virus is endemic in large parts of the Far East, and there is also a high prevalence in Africa and parts of eastern Europe. The prevalence of HBV in western Europe and the United States is much lower, although it is believed that there are approximately 1.5 million carriers in the United States. In endemic areas, infection with HBV is usually acquired in childhood, either vertically from the mother or horizontally from siblings. In western Europe and the United States, HBV

is usually acquired as an adult, often by a parenteral route.

- The consequences of HBV infection depend in large part on the age at which the infection is acquired. Infection during childhood is associated with a low rate of overt hepatitis, but the frequency of the chronic carrier state is high. Infection with HBV as an adult results in a high rate of overt hepatitis, but the frequency of the chronic carrier state is low.

- A variety of antigens have been associated with HBV, including the surface antigen (HBsAg), the core antigen (HBc), and the e antigen (HBe), which is a component of HBc. Antibodies to these antigens are useful in the diagnosis of HBV infection, in estimating the risk of infectivity, and also in estimating the risk of complications from HBV. Hepatitis B surface antigen and HBe are present transiently after acute infection; they disappear from the serum of most people infected but persist in the serum of chronic carriers. The presence of HBsAg and HBe in the serum indicates a chronic carrier state; the presence of HBe is considered a marker of high infectivity. The development of serum antibodies to HBsAg and HBe generally indicates the end of the chronic carrier state and loss of infectivity. Hepatitis B core antigen is not found in the serum, but antibodies to HBc (anti-HBc) are useful markers of infection during the "window period" after HBsAg is cleared from the serum and before anti-HBs is detected.

- Immune complexes composed of HBV antigens and antibodies to them are probably critical in the pathogenesis of the glomerular diseases that result from HBV infection. Hepatitis B virus antigens are frequently detected in the glomeruli of patients with HBV and glomerulonephritis.

- Several renal syndromes have been associated with HBV infection, the majority of which affect the glomeruli. A variety of morphologic patterns of glomerular disease may complicate HBV infection, including membranous glomerulonephropathy (MGN), membranoproliferative glomerulonephritis (MPGN), mesangial proliferative glomerulonephritis with mesangial IgA, and rarely, diffuse proliferative or crescentic glomerulonephritis. Systemic vasculitis resembling polyarteritis nodosa (PAN) may also occur.

- The various morphologic patterns of renal lesions that may be associated with HBV are all described in detail in other chapters. They will therefore be discussed only briefly here, with an emphasis on those features that might differ from other causes with the same morphologic pattern.

- The incidence of renal disease in people infected with HBV is low, and the relationship between HBV and some of the entities described remains controversial.

Polyarteritis Nodosa Associated With Hepatitis B Virus

- Polyarteritis nodosa associated with HBV (HBV-PAN) usually follows acquisition of HBV as an adult. It is more common in western Europe and the United States but uncommon in areas with a high prevalence of

HBV. Overall, PAN is a rare complication of HBV infection.

- Typically, HBV-PAN occurs several weeks to several months after an episode of acute hepatitis, which is usually clinically mild. Vasculitis may on occasion precede the clinical onset of hepatitis or follow it by several years.

- The initial manifestation of HBV-PAN resembles a serum sickness reaction with fever, arthralgias or arthritis, urticaria, and palpable purpura. Symptoms of systemic vasculitis develop over several weeks, and virtually any organ in the body may be involved.

- Renal involvement in HBV-PAN usually resembles the "classic" or "macroscopic" variant of PAN, with involvement of small and medium-sized muscular arteries. Necrotizing glomerulonephritis, sometimes called the "microscopic" variant of PAN, is rare.

- Renal involvement in HBV-PAN may present clinically as renin-dependent hypertension, microscopic hematuria, proteinuria that may range up to nephrotic levels, or rarely, acute renal failure.

- Laboratory tests usually demonstrate mildly elevated liver values, especially the transaminases (aspartate aminotransferase and alanine aminotransferase); both HBsAg and anti-HBc are present in the serum.

- The small and medium-sized arteries are inflamed, often at sites of branching. The inflammation involves all layers of the artery wall, with fibrinoid necrosis, leukocytic infiltration, fibrin deposition, and occasionally aneurysm formation.

- Glomeruli usually show only ischemic changes. However, diffuse proliferative glomerulonephritis, membranoproliferative glomerulonephritis, mesangial proliferative glomerulonephritis, and membranous glomerulonephropathy may occasionally be found.

Membranous Glomerulonephropathy (MGN) Associated With Hepatitis B Virus

- The morphologic pattern of MGN is the most common glomerular lesion associated with HBV. It usually occurs in chronic HBV carriers; thus it is most common in endemic areas, where the chronic carrier state occurs more frequently after HBV infection. In endemic areas, HBV has been associated with a high proportion of cases of MGN (50% to 100% of cases in different series in Africa and the Far East), although there is considerable geographic and ethnic variation. In areas of low prevalence, HBV appears to be infrequently associated with MGN. However, a study by the Southwest Pediatric Nephrology Study Group found evidence of HBV in 20% of children with MGN; it may be relevant that the majority of the cases occurred in African-Americans.

- The HBe antigen appears to be important in the pathogenesis of MGN associated with HBV (HBV-MGN). Hepatitis Be antigen has been detected in glomeruli with HBV-MGN by immunofluorescence by using antibodies against the HBe antigen.

- Usually occurring in children, HBV-MGN has an onset between the ages of 2 and 12. There is a high ratio of males to females (4 to 5 : 1), in contrast to the slight male preponderance in idiopathic MGN. In the United States, the African-American population appears to have a higher rate of HBV-MGN.

- The usual manifestation is the nephrotic syndrome, often with microscopic hematuria. Renal function as measured by serum creatinine is usually normal. Hepatitis B surface antigen and anti-HBc are almost always present in the serum; HBe is found in 60% to 80%.
- Children with HBV-MGN usually have no clinical history of preceding or ongoing hepatitis. Serum transaminase values are usually mildly elevated; liver biopsy usually shows minimal abnormalities or chronic hepatitis with little or no activity ("chronic passive hepatitis"). Adults with HBV-MGN frequently have a history of acute hepatitis, usually 6 months to several years before the onset of renal disease. Liver biopsy in adults frequently demonstrates chronic hepatitis with active changes ("chronic active hepatitis").
- The morphologic picture of glomeruli in HBV-MGN generally resembles that in idiopathic cases, with diffuse thickening of glomerular capillary walls, thickening of glomerular capillary basement membranes, and glomerular basement membrane (GBM) "spikes" on silver stains. However, the number of cells present in the glomerular mesangium is frequently increased, the mesangial area is often expanded, and mesangial sclerosis may be present. Focal membranoproliferative change in a few capillary loops may also be seen.
- On immunofluorescence, granular staining of glomerular capillary loops in a subepithelial location is seen for IgG (100%) and C3 (75%); staining for IgM (50%) and IgA (10%) may also be present. Staining may be seen in mesangial and/or subendothelial locations, in addition to subepithelial sites. Occasional cases may have prominent mesangial staining for IgA in addition to the capillary wall staining.
- On electron microscopy, electron-dense, immune complex–type deposits are present in a subepithelial location in glomerular capillary walls. The deposits may be more irregular in distribution than in typical, idiopathic MGN, with sparing of some capillary loops. Occasional subendothelial and/or mesangial deposits may be present. Visceral epithelial cells demonstrate microvillous transformation and effacement of foot processes.
- The course of HBV-MGN is relatively benign in most cases; progression to end-stage renal failure is uncommon, and children with HBV-MGN appear to have spontaneous remissions at approximately the same rate as children with idiopathic MGN. The course in adults may be less favorable, with a significant number progressing to end-stage renal disease.
- Transformation of HBV-MGN to MPGN has been noted. In one case, transformation of HBV-MGN to MPGN with crescents in Bowman's space occurred in association with acute renal failure.
- Treatment of HBV-MGN is generally conservative and supportive. There is no evidence that corticosteroids are of benefit; in fact, corticosteroids appear to prolong the chronic HBV carrier state and may be deleterious. Small numbers of patients have been treated with immunomodulating agents such as α-interferon; although there appears to be transient benefit, with clearing of

HBsAg and HBe from the serum and remission of renal disease, relapse usually follows cessation of treatment with the medication.

IgA Nephropathy Associated With Hepatitis B Virus

- The geographic area with the highest prevalence of HBV, the Far East, also has a high incidence of IgA nephropathy (IgAN). This observation raises the possibility that HBV might be a cause of IgAN. A study in Hong Kong showed a significantly higher incidence of seropositivity for HBV in patients with IgAN than in the general population (17.2% versus 9.5%); however, some other studies in the Far East and elsewhere have not supported such an association.
- The usual clinical manifestation of IgAN in HBV-positive patients is proteinuria and microhematuria; many have the nephrotic syndrome.
- The most common histologic pattern is mesangial proliferative glomerulonephritis. Some cases have had a mixed pattern, with features of both MGN and mesangial proliferation.
- Immunofluorescence microscopy shows prominent granular staining for IgA in the glomerular mesangium, frequently associated with staining for IgG and C3; staining for IgM is less common. Cases with superimposed membranous features show granular capillary wall staining for IgG in addition to mesangial staining for IgA.
- Electron microscopy demonstrates large mesangial and paramesangial electron-dense deposits; extension of the deposits into the subendothelial space of peripheral capillary loops and small subepithelial deposits may also be present. Those cases with features of both MGN and IgAN have prominent and widespread subepithelial deposits in addition to mesangial and paramesangial deposits.
- The prognostic significance of HBV seropositivity in patients with IgAN is not clear.

Other Glomerular Lesions Associated With Hepatitis B Virus

- The morphologic pattern of membranoproliferative (mesangiocapillary) glomerulonephritis has also been described in association with HBV infection, although the frequency of MPGN appears to be much lower than that of MGN.
- Membranoproliferative glomerulonephritis associated with HBV occurs in both children and adults but appears to be more common in adults. As in HBV-MGN, patients frequently have no history of preceding acute hepatitis, although serum transaminase values are often slightly elevated.
- The usual clinical manifestation of MPGN associated with HBV is the nephrotic syndrome and microhematuria. Hypertension and renal insufficiency appear to be more common at diagnosis than in HBV-MGN.
- The glomerular lesion usually resembles MPGN type I, with pronounced thickening of capillary walls, mesangial interposition, the appearance of reduplication or

"tram-tracking" of the glomerular capillary basement membrane, subendothelial deposits, and mild hypercellularity. The glomerular lesion may also resemble MPGN type III as described by Burkholder and colleagues, with subepithelial as well as subendothelial deposits. Type II MPGN, or dense deposit disease, is not associated with HBV infection.

- Immunofluorescence shows granular deposits of IgG and C3 in glomerular capillary walls. Electron microscopy shows subendothelial electron-dense deposits, with mesangial interposition and synthesis of new basement membrane–like material. Subepithelial, intramembranous, and mesangial deposits may also be present.
- Cases with features of both MGN and MPGN have been described in association with HBV. Prominent subepithelial deposits are present in addition to subendothelial deposits, mesangial interposition, and "tram-tracking" of the GBM.
- Other histologic patterns occasionally seen in patients with seropositivity for HBV include mesangial proliferative and diffuse proliferative glomerulonephritis.

Chronic Hepatitis and Renal Disease

- Renal disease is occasionally seen in association with the entity of autoimmune or "lupoid" hepatitis and other forms of chronic hepatitis with ongoing destruction of hepatocytes (formerly called *chronic active hepatitis*). Autoimmune hepatitis is a form of chronic hepatitis with active destruction of hepatocytes and clinical or serologic evidence of generalized autoimmunity (antinuclear, anti–smooth muscle, and other autoantibodies).
- Two types of renal lesions have been seen in association with autoimmune or chronic active hepatitis: glomerulonephritis and tubulointerstitial nephritis. Both are very rare.
- Patients with glomerulonephritis have the nephrotic syndrome or chronic renal insufficiency. The most common histologic patterns are MGN and MPGN.
- Patients with tubulointerstitial nephritis have polydipsia, polyuria, muscular weakness, and nausea and vomiting as a result of distal renal tubular acidosis. Histologic examination demonstrates interstitial nephritis and, in some cases, nephrocalcinosis.
- Treatment of renal disease associated with chronic hepatitis is supportive. There is no evidence that immunosuppressive therapy is beneficial.

Hepatic Cirrhosis and the Kidney

- The frequent existence of glomerular abnormalities in patients with cirrhosis was first noted during the 1940s. More recently, with the use of immunofluorescence and electron microscopy, glomerular lesions have been found in 50% to 100% of patients with cirrhosis in different series. Histologic examination may show glomerular hypercellularity, but in many cases glomeruli are morphologically unremarkable or show only minimal changes.
- Despite the high incidence of glomerular abnormalities on immunofluorescence and electron microscopy, it is uncommon to find *clinical* evidence of renal disease in patients with cirrhosis. Therefore, the association between cirrhosis and renal disease remains controversial.
- The most common abnormality, mesangial staining for IgA on immunofluorescence, is found in 30% to more than 90% of cases in different series. IgG and IgM are occasionally found but are considerably less common.
- In most cases, IgA deposits are not accompanied by significant glomerular hypercellularity. In the minority of cases with morphologic changes, the most common histologic pattern seen is that of membranoproliferative (mesangiocapillary) glomerulonephritis; mesangial proliferation, MGN, focal or lobular glomerulonephritis, or diffuse glomerulonephritis is occasionally seen.
- The incidence of *clinical* renal abnormalities in patients with cirrhosis is unknown. Urinalysis studies in patients with cirrhosis have suggested that nephritic changes (hematuria, casts, or leukocyturia) may be present in up to 10% and nephrotic-range proteinuria may be present in 1% to 2%.
- In general, the presence and degree of abnormalities on urinalysis correlate with the presence and degree of glomerular hypercellularity and other histologic abnormalities. However, significant glomerular abnormalities may be present in patients with no clinical evidence of renal disease. Renal insufficiency may be more severe in patients with the morphologic pattern of MPGN.
- The cause of glomerular disease in cirrhosis is unknown. The presence of glomerular IgA deposits in patients with cirrhosis may be related to the fact that the serum concentration of IgA is increased in patients with cirrhosis; IgA antibodies directed against albumin have been reported to develop in patients with cirrhosis. Glomerular disease occurs in cirrhosis of any cause, but it appears to be most common in patients with alcoholic cirrhosis.
- There is no established treatment for glomerulonephritis associated with cirrhosis. Renal insufficiency is generally mild, and patients' outcome probably depends more on the underlying liver disease than on the renal disease.

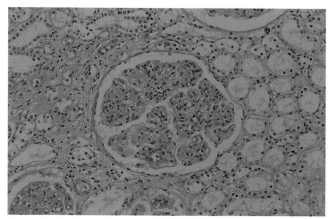

Figure 17–1. Glomerulopathy associated with liver cirrhosis. Intracapillary proliferative glomerulopathy with a membranoproliferative pattern is seen in a patient with liver cirrhosis; the patient did not have hepatitis B or hepatitis C virus infection. Immunofluorescence did not show immune deposition in the glomeruli.

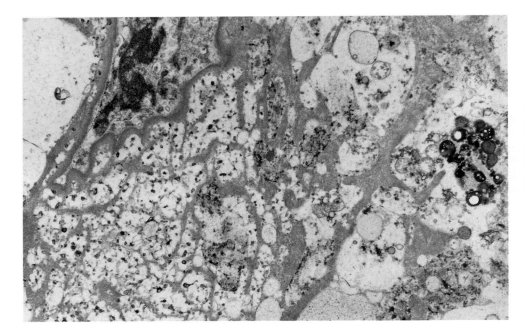

Figure 17–2. Electron micrograph of a kidney with glomerulopathy associated with liver cirrhosis. The glomerular mesangium and the basement membrane are permeated by clear lacunae with dark irregular particles. Intracapillary cells contained lipids (not shown). The ultrastructural picture is similar to that seen in lecithin-cholesterol acetyltransferase deficiency.

SICKLE CELL ANEMIA AND THE KIDNEY

Synonyms and Related Terms: Sickle cell nephropathy.

Biology of Disease

- Sickle cell anemia is due to an inherited abnormality in the gene for the β-globin chain on chromosome 11; valine is substituted for glutamic acid at position 6. Normal adult hemoglobin (hemoglobin A) is composed of two β-globin chains combined with two α-globin chains ($\alpha_2\beta_2$). Hemoglobin containing the abnormal β-globin chain, designated hemoglobin S, has a tendency to polymerize into long, rigid structures when deoxygenated. Erythrocytes containing the abnormal polymerized hemoglobin have a tendency to assume a sickle shape under conditions of low oxygen tension, high osmolality, and low pH.
- Sickled red cells are rigid and thus lack the ability of normal red cells (shaped like biconcave discs) to deform to pass through small blood vessels. Sickled red cells also have an increased tendency to adhere to endothelial cell surfaces, activate the coagulation cascade, and also activate complement; the result is a tendency to block blood flow in areas of low oxygen tension, high osmolality, and low pH. Low oxygen tension, high osmolality, and low pH are characteristic of the renal medulla, which probably explains the high incidence of renal medulla injury in patients with sickle cell disease.

- The mutation is common in parts of Africa and countries surrounding the Mediterranean, where *Plasmodium falciparum* malaria is endemic. The mutation seems to have a selective advantage in those regions because heterozygotes for the mutation appear to be resistant to falciparum malaria.
- Individuals homozygous for the mutation (*sickle cell anemia*; designated Hb SS) have anemia because of continuous hemolysis. Complications include painful vaso-occlusive crises; splenic infarction (autosplenectomy); decreased resistance to infections, particularly with encapsulated organisms such as *Streptococcus pneumoniae* and *Haemophilus influenzae*; high-output congestive heart failure and myocardial ischemia as a result of sickling in myocardial arteries; chronic restrictive lung disease; strokes; chronic leg ulcers; and a wide variety of other complications. Untreated, sickle cell anemia commonly causes death in childhood, but with advances in supportive medical care many patients with the disease are living well into their adult years.
- Individuals heterozygous for the mutation (*sickle cell trait*; Hb AS) have normal hematologic parameters, a much lower incidence of complications, and a normal or nearly normal life span. Approximately 8% of African-Americans are heterozygous for sickle cell disease.
- Patients who are double heterozygotes for sickle cell anemia and another hemoglobinopathy such as hemoglobin C disease or β-thalassemia may have a hematologic picture resembling that of homozygous sickle cell disease. They may also have the other complications seen in homozygotes, including renal disease. However,

the incidence of other complications appears to be lower in double heterozygotes than in those with homozygous sickle cell anemia.

- Patients with sickle cell anemia (Hb SS) are prone to a variety of renal complications (Table 17–1); people with sickle cell trait (Hb AS) are also predisposed to some of the renal complications, but the incidence of serious or life-threatening renal disease is lower in heterozygotes.
- An important mechanism of renal disease in sickle cell anemia is ischemia and infarction of the renal medulla. The hyperosmolar environment of the medulla strongly favors polymerization of hemoglobin S; sickling of red cells occurs even in heterozygotes. The resulting hemostasis in the vasa recta results in ischemia and eventually infarction and/or scarring of the medulla. On microangioradiographic studies, the number of vasa recta was significantly reduced in patients with Hb SS; the vessels that were present were dilated, formed spirals, or ended bluntly. In patients with Hb AS and Hb SC (sickle cell plus hemoglobin C), the vascular changes were intermediate between those of patients with Hb SS and normal kidneys.
- The vascular changes in the medulla, along with the associated ischemia and injury, result in an inability to concentrate urine, which is seen in virtually all homozygotes and the majority of heterozygotes, and distal renal tubular acidosis. Hemostasis and vascular changes in the medulla are also important factors underlying the predisposition of sickle cell patients to papillary necrosis.
- Children with sickle cell anemia have increased renal plasma flow, glomerular filtration rate (GFR), and creatinine clearance; these parameters gradually decline as the patients get older, and eventually the GFR drops

below the normal range for age. A consistent finding in children with sickle cell anemia is enlargement of glomeruli, which may be related to the increased GFR; as patients get older, however, glomeruli with segmental and global sclerosis appear. Hyperfiltration causes glomerular injury in a variety of animal models and may be involved in both diabetic nephropathy and focal segmental glomerulosclerosis; it is therefore possible that hyperfiltration is involved in initiating the glomerular injury in sickle cell patients.

- Proteinuria is common in patients with sickle cell anemia; the nephrotic syndrome may occur. The most common morphologic appearance in sickle cell patients with nephrotic syndrome is focal segmental glomerulosclerosis; a small proportion of patients have a picture resembling MPGN type I.
- Interestingly, in contrast to the defects in distal tubular function in patients with sickle cell anemia, proximal tubular function is usually increased. This situation results in increased phosphate reabsorption and increased excretion of creatinine and uric acid. Calculation of creatinine clearance may significantly overestimate GFR because of the enhanced excretion of creatinine.

Clinical Features

- The isosthenuria and renal tubular acidosis seen in sickle cell patients are not usually associated with major clinical problems inasmuch as these patients are usually able to compensate without difficulty. However, fluid restriction may result in dehydration.
- Hematuria is common in patients with both sickle cell anemia and sickle cell trait, as well as patients heterozygous for both sickle cell and hemoglobin C (Hb SC). The hematuria begins in early adulthood and appears to be more common in males than females. It is often gross, usually painless, and is spontaneous or occurs with minor trauma. On cystoscopy, bleeding is usually seen coming from only one ureter, with the left being more common than the right. Hematuria is usually self-limited but can be severe enough to require transfusion; unilateral nephrectomy has occasionally been required to stop the hemorrhage.
- Proteinuria is common and occurs in one quarter to one third of patients with sickle cell anemia. It is usually minor and detected on routine urinalysis; however, the nephrotic syndrome has been reported in up to 7% of patients.
- Renal insufficiency is a significant problem in older patients with homozygous sickle cell anemia. In an autopsy series of patients over 40 years of age with sickle cell anemia, renal insufficiency was believed to be the cause of death or a significant contributing factor in half of the cases. In a prospective study of 735 patients with Hb SS and 209 patients with Hb SC, renal failure developed in 4.2% of the Hb SS and 2.4% of the Hb SC patients.

Gross Appearance

- The kidneys are usually normal or nearly normal in size; the subcapsular surface is usually smooth.

Table 17–1
SYNDROMES OF RENAL DISEASE IN PATIENTS WITH SICKLE CELL ANEMIA

Functional or Clinical Manifestation	Anatomic Correlates
Inability to concentrate urine	Loss of the vasa recta
Distal tubular acidosis	Medullary infarction and fibrosis
Impaired potassium excretion	Papillary necrosis
Impaired acidification of urine	
Isolated hematuria	Dilatation and congestion of the vasa recta
	Congestion of the pelvic mucosa
Increased glomerular filtration rate	Glomerular hypertrophy
Increased renal plasma flow	
Proteinuria and nephrotic syndrome	Focal segmental glomerulosclerosis
	Membranoproliferative glomerulonephritis–like changes
Acute renal failure from rhabdomyolysis	Acute tubular necrosis
Chronic renal insufficiency	Interstitital fibrosis and tubular atrophy
	Glomerulosclerosis
Bacteriuria and pyelonephritis	

- Large, depressed scars on the subcapsular surface may be present. On section, these large cortical scars are associated with necrosis or loss of the underlying papillae.
- Small yellowish white infarcts may be present on the subcapsular surface; on section, these infarcts are usually shallow. Large cortical infarcts may occasionally be present.
- Glomeruli are often visible in the cortex as prominent red pinheads.
- Hemorrhage is often noted under the pelvic mucosa. The calyces may be dilated and are often associated with blunting or loss of papillae.

Light Microscopy

- The histologic appearance in sickle cell disease is highly variable and depends on the age of the patient and the genotype (Hb SS, Hb AS, or Hb SC). The appearance in the following paragraphs refers to homozygous sickle cell disease (Hb SS); changes in heterozygous sickle cell disease (Hb AS) or sickle cell–hemoglobin C (Hb SC) are variable, usually less severe, and often subtle.

Glomeruli

- Glomeruli are enlarged; glomerular capillaries are dilated and congested. Iron deposits are present in the visceral epithelial cells and parietal epithelial cells of Bowman's capsule.
- The mesangial matrix is often increased; occasionally, mesangial hypercellularity is present.
- Segmental and global sclerosis of glomeruli is often present, may be widespread, and often appears out of proportion for the age of the patient.
- In a small proportion of patients, marked thickening of glomerular capillary walls is seen. The periodic acid–Schiff (PAS) reaction and silver stains demonstrate the appearance of reduplication or "tram-tracking" of the GBM, similar to that seen in MPGN.

Tubules

- Stainable iron deposits are present in proximal tubular epithelial cells.
- Protein resorption droplets are present in proximal convoluted tubular epithelial cells in patients with proteinuria or the nephrotic syndrome.
- Focal tubular injury or necrosis may be present.
- Tubular atrophy in association with interstitial fibrosis may be present and becomes increasingly widespread in older patients.

Vessels

- Peritubular capillaries are dilated and congested and frequently contain sickled erythrocytes.
- The vasa recta in the medulla may be decreased in number. They are dilated and congested and may appear tortuous.

- Larger arteries usually appear unremarkable but may show intimal fibrosis and medial hypertrophy in patients with hypertension.

Interstitium

- The earliest change is interstitial edema, particularly in the medulla. Interstitial hemorrhage may occur and is probably caused by the abnormal vasa recta and peritubular capillaries.
- Patchy interstitial fibrosis appears in older patients, and large areas of fibrosis may be present in areas of previous infarction. Interstitial inflammation is usually scant or absent.
- Nodules of myxomatous, cellular tissue or fibrous scars may be present in the medulla.

Immunofluorescence Microscopy

- Immunofluorescence microscopy is negative or shows nonspecific changes in most cases.
- Glomeruli may show granular capillary wall staining for IgM and C3 in occasional cases; mesangial staining for IgM and C3 is sometimes present.

Electron Microscopy

- Frequently found abnormalities consist of focal effacement of glomerular visceral epithelial cell foot processes, mild thickening of glomerular capillary basement membranes, occasional mesangial interposition, and electron-dense granular material in the mesangium, probably representing iron deposits. Immune complex–type deposits are usually absent.
- The mesangial space may be expanded, with increased mesangial matrix.
- In occasional patients with the nephrotic syndrome, the mesangium extends into the peripheral glomerular capillary walls, with synthesis of new basement membrane–like material producing the appearance of reduplication or "tram-tracking" of the GBM. Subendothelial flocculent material may be present.
- Granular electron-dense material may be present within tubular epithelial cells, probably iron deposits within lysosomes.

Treatment and Clinical Course

- Children with sickle cell anemia are now frequently hypertransfused to maintain a low percentage of hemoglobin S in their blood to prevent the blood from sickling and avoid the complications related to intravascular sickling. Trials of oral hydroxyurea to increase production of hemoglobin F and thereby decrease the percentage of hemoglobin S have also been reported.
- In general, after chronic renal insufficiency begins in patients with sickle cell anemia, progression to renal failure is fairly rapid. Hypertension, proteinuria, the nephrotic syndrome, and microscopic hematuria are risk factors for the development of renal failure. In the prospective study of patients with sickle cell anemia

and sickle cell–hemoglobin C (Hb SC) cited earlier, median survival after the onset of renal failure was only 4 years despite hemodialysis.

■ The results of hemodialysis in patients with sickle cell anemia are controversial. Several studies have shown poor survival with hemodialysis, frequently with an increase in sickle cell vaso-occlusive crises and a high incidence of cardiovascular complications. Other studies have found that survival of sickle cell patients maintained by hemodialysis is similar to that of patients with renal failure from other causes.

■ Few trials of renal transplantation in sickle cell patients have been published; many nephrologists have been hesitant to consider sickle cell patients for renal transplantation because of the lack of effective treatment for their underlying disease. Initial series showed poor graft and patient survival after renal transplantation; more recent studies have had improved results, and some nephrologists and transplant surgeons believe that sickle cell patients should be considered for transplantation just as any other patient with renal failure from other causes.

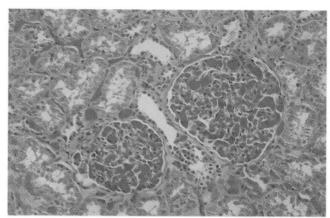

Figure 17–3. Sickle cell nephropathy. The glomerular capillary lumina are distended/congested and one glomerulus appears large.

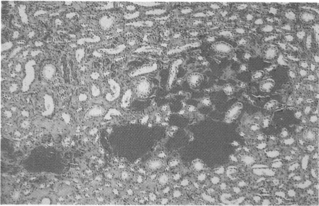

Figure 17–4. Sickle cell nephropathy. Severe congestion is seen in the interstitial capillaries. Some capillaries are severely dilated and distorted and some erythrocytes may be present in the interstitium. Other areas (not seen) showed papillary necrosis.

C1q NEPHROPATHY

Synonyms and Related Terms: Mesangiopathic glomerulonephritis with "full house" immunofluorescence.

Biology of Disease

■ C1q nephropathy is a recently described, immune complex–mediated glomerulopathy characterized clinically by heavy proteinuria or the nephrotic syndrome, resistance to corticosteroids, and an absence of systemic manifestations. Pathologically, C1q nephropathy is characterized by predominant or codominant staining for C1q on immunofluorescence, a variable glomerular appearance on light microscopy, and mesangial immune complex–type deposits on electron microscopy.

■ In two series containing both pediatric and adult patients, C1q nephropathy was found in approximately 2% of native kidney biopsy specimens. In a study limited to pediatric patients (aged 16 years or below), C1q nephropathy was found in 16% of biopsy samples harvested for nephrotic syndrome, persistent proteinuria, or persistent glomerulonephritis.

■ The cause or causes of C1q nephropathy are unknown.

Clinical Features

■ The usual clinical finding is heavy proteinuria, with half to two thirds of patients having the nephrotic syndrome. Characteristically, the proteinuria is unresponsive to oral corticosteroids, or the patients experience repeated relapses.

■ Up to 40% of patients have hematuria, with or without red cell casts.

■ The majority of patients are young; age at onset varies from 2 years to the 30s, with a median age in the teens. Some series have shown a female preponderance; however, in other series the number of males and females is approximately equal.

■ C1q nephropathy does not appear to be associated with extrarenal disease.

Laboratory Values

■ Virtually all patients have had normal renal function at diagnosis.

■ Serum complement levels are normal, and serologic assays for autoimmunity (antinuclear antibodies, anti-DNA antibodies, etc.) are negative.

Light Microscopy

Glomeruli

■ Glomeruli show a spectrum of morphologic changes; the number in each category varies in different series, possibly because of differences in patient selection criteria. Some cases (approximately half in the pediatric series and a lower proportion in series containing adult patients) show minimal histologic change and are indistinguishable from idiopathic minimal change nephrotic syndrome by light microscopy. Another pattern that is common in some series is mesangial hypercellularity with preservation of glomerular capillary lumina (mesangiopathic glomerulonephritis). Some biopsy specimens show focal segmental proliferative glomerulonephritis; others show segmental scarring in a proportion of the glomeruli (focal segmental glomerulosclerosis).

Tubules, Interstitium, and Vessels

■ In most cases, tubules show no abnormalities other than protein resorption droplets in proximal convoluted tubular epithelial cells and perhaps erythrocytes or casts within tubular lumina. In some cases, frequently those with focal segmental glomerulosclerosis, occasional atrophic tubules are seen.
■ The interstitium and vessels usually show no significant changes. Scattered areas of interstitial fibrosis may be present.

Immunofluorescence Microscopy

■ Staining for C1q is present in all glomeruli. Staining for C1q is characteristically intense (3 to 4+ out of 4); in the majority of cases it is the strongest immunoreactant. Staining is predominantly mesangial in location, although scattered capillary wall deposits may be seen in a few glomeruli in some cases.
■ Virtually all cases have immunofluorescence staining for IgG, IgM, and C3, and staining for IgA is present in a substantial number. Staining for IgG is sometimes as intense as that for C1q; staining for IgM, IgA, and C3 is usually considerably weaker.

Electron Microscopy

■ Electron microscopy shows discrete, granular, electron-dense "immune complex–type" deposits in the glomerular mesangium in all cases. These deposits are characteristically large but in some cases are confined to the zone immediately beneath the paramesangial basement membrane.
■ Some patients have small, subendothelial electron-dense deposits in the glomerular capillaries, and small subepithelial (epimembranous) deposits are occasionally present.
■ Visceral epithelial cell foot processes are characteristically widely effaced, and there may be microvillous transformation of the visceral epithelial cells.

■ Tubuloreticular structures (microtubular arrays, myxovirus-like particles) are strikingly absent in C1q nephropathy.

Differential Diagnosis

■ The most common glomerulonephritis to manifest strong staining for C1q, frequently in association with "full house" immunoglobulins and C3, is the nephritis of systemic lupus erythematosus. The histologic spectrum of C1q nephropathy also overlaps that of lupus nephritis, and the two conditions cannot be differentiated by either immunofluorescence or light microscopy. The most striking morphologic difference is the absence of tubuloreticular structures in C1q nephropathy as compared with their frequent presence in lupus nephritis. However, the two conditions should be easily differentiated on a clinical and serologic basis. Systemic lupus erythematosus has numerous extrarenal manifestations; in contrast, extrarenal manifestations have been absent in patients with C1q nephropathy. Patients with systemic lupus erythematosus also characteristically have serum autoantibodies, particularly antinuclear antibodies; these autoantibodies are absent in patients with C1q nephropathy.
■ Membranoproliferative glomerulonephritis type I can also demonstrate staining for C1q; however, the characteristic double contour or "tram-track" appearance of the glomerular capillary wall with PAS and silver stains in MPGN is not seen in C1q nephropathy, and the two conditions should be easily distinguished on that basis.
■ One patient with strong glomerular staining for C1q showed mesangial proliferation with mononuclear cell infiltration of the glomerular hilus; the same patient had mononuclear cells (primarily lymphocytes) concentrated around arterioles and invading into proximal tubules. Whether this case of "pan-nephritis" represents a different entity or a variant of C1q nephropathy is unclear at this time.

Treatment and Clinical Course

■ The number of patients in whom C1q nephropathy is diagnosed is small, and the length of follow-up of these patients has been short. Therefore, the long-term outlook for renal function in patients with C1q nephropathy is not clear. Virtually all patients with C1q nephropathy have normal renal function (serum creatinine and creatinine clearance) at diagnosis, but a slight deterioration in renal function over time has been noted in a few patients.
■ It appears that patients with focal segmental glomerulosclerosis on biopsy have a more guarded prognosis than do patients with minimal histologic alteration.
■ The proteinuria in C1q nephropathy is almost always resistant to standard oral regimens of prednisone or other corticosteroids. In pediatric series, patients with minimal histologic change on light microscopy frequently had a good response to bolus intravenous methylprednisolone (Solu-Medrol); patients with focal segmental glomerulosclerosis did not respond as well.

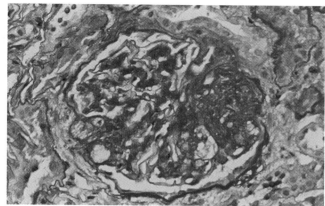

Figure 17–5. C1q nephropathy. A segmental sclerotic lesion and intracapillary foam cells are seen in a 12-year-old child with C1q nephropathy (periodic acid–Schiff reaction).

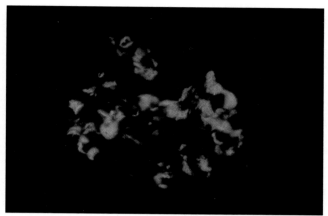

Figure 17–6. C1q nephropathy, immunofluorescence. Strong mesangial C1q staining is shown in the glomerulus. Mesangial IgG positivity is also commonly seen in patients with C1q nephropathy. One has to rule out systemic lupus erythematosus in cases like this.

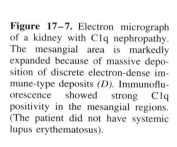

Figure 17–7. Electron micrograph of a kidney with C1q nephropathy. The mesangial area is markedly expanded because of massive deposition of discrete electron-dense immune-type deposits *(D)*. Immunofluorescence showed strong C1q positivity in the mesangial regions. (The patient did not have systemic lupus erythematosus).

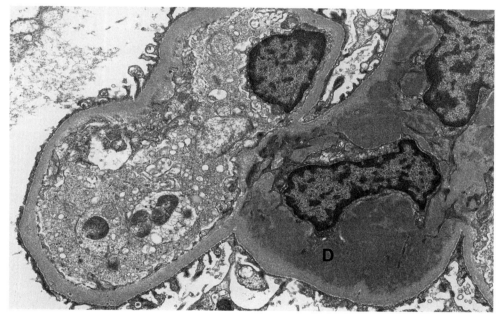

COLLAGEN TYPE III GLOMERULOPATHY

Synonyms and Related Terms: Primary glomerular fibrosis; collagenofibrotic glomerulopathy (glomerulonephropathy).

Biology of Disease

- Collagen type III glomerulopathy is a recently described, apparently rare condition characterized by the deposition of collagen type III fibers in the glomerular tuft. Clinically, it is characterized by proteinuria or the nephrotic syndrome and gradual deterioration of renal function.
- Collagen type III is normally present in hepatic sinusoids, the media of elastic arteries, and dermal papillae and may be present in the renal interstitium. However, collagen type III is not normally present in renal glomeruli; the predominant collagen types found in glomeruli are types I and IV.
- The etiology of collagen type III glomerulopathy is unknown. It has been suggested that the condition is inherited in an autosomal recessive fashion, although

the number of patients and kindreds analyzed has not allowed the inheritance pattern to be definitively established.

■ The majority of cases described thus far have been from Japan. However, cases have been described in Europe and the United States.

Clinical Features

■ The majority of patients have variable degrees of proteinuria; many have the nephrotic syndrome. Hematuria is occasionally found.

■ Renal function as measured by creatinine clearance is normal in the majority of patients when first seen. Hypertension is frequently present.

■ The cases described from Japan have been primarily in adults; many of the cases occurring in Europeans occurred during childhood. The disease appears to occur with equal frequency in both sexes.

Laboratory Values

■ Serologic studies for autoimmunity (antinuclear antibodies, etc.) are typically negative, and serum complement levels are usually within normal limits.

■ No monoclonal immunoglobulins are present in the serum or urine.

■ The serum level of procollagen III peptide, the N-terminal sequence of the precursor procollagen molecule, is characteristically markedly elevated. Elevated serum levels of the procollagen III peptide have been considered a marker of stimulated collagen synthesis in a variety of conditions; elevated serum levels have also been described in renal insufficiency from a variety of causes. However, serum levels in patients with collagen III glomerulopathy appear to be considerably higher than in patients with renal insufficiency from other causes; in addition, in patients with collagen III glomerulopathy, serum levels may be markedly elevated despite normal renal function.

Light Microscopy

Glomeruli

■ Glomerular tufts are globally expanded by eosinophilic material, with accentuation of the lobular architecture; glomerular cellularity is normal. Capillary walls are thickened, and capillary lumina are narrowed or occluded. Variable numbers of glomeruli are globally sclerotic. There are no adhesions to Bowman's capsule, and no crescents are present.

■ The eosinophilic material stains strongly with aniline blue and acid fuchsin orange G; it stains weakly with the PAS reaction and silver stains and does not stain with Congo red or fluoresce with thioflavin T.

■ The glomerulus may occasionally have a nodular appearance suggestive of a Kimmelstiel-Wilson lesion in diabetic nephropathy.

■ The glomerular capillary basement membranes appear thin and delicate with the PAS reaction and silver stains; occasional capillary loops may have a double-contour or "tram-track" appearance similar to that seen in MPGN, but this change involves only a minority of capillary loops.

Tubules, Interstitium, and Vessels

■ Patchy thickening of tubular basement membranes by amorphous eosinophilic material has been reported in a few cases; however, in the majority of cases the deposits are limited to glomeruli.

■ Proximal convoluted tubular epithelial cells may contain cytoplasmic protein resorption droplets, and occasional atrophic tubules may be present. Tubules are otherwise unremarkable.

■ Patchy interstitial fibrosis may be present, as well as arteriolar hyalinosis and thickening of the walls of arteries, probably secondary to hypertension.

■ Progressive tubular, interstitial, and vascular changes may develop over time, and these changes are generally proportional to the degree of global glomerulosclerosis.

Immunofluorescence Microscopy

■ Staining for immunoglobulins and complement components is usually negative. Scattered staining for IgM, IgG, C3, and other immunoreactants may be present in a few glomeruli and probably represents insudation of plasma proteins.

Electron Microscopy

■ Electron microscopy demonstrates expansion of the glomerular mesangium and subendothelial space by fibrillar material with the appearance and periodicity of collagen fibrils. The periodicity of the fibrils has varied from 430 to 640 nm in different series, possibly because of different fixative and staining techniques and different methods of measurement of periodicity.

■ The lamina densa of the glomerular capillary basement membranes appears normal; it is not thickened and does not contain pale areas ("lacunae") or have a "moth-eaten" appearance. New basement membrane–like material may be deposited beneath the expanded subendothelial space in a few capillary loops and corresponds to the double-contour or "tram-track" appearance seen in a few loops by light microscopy.

■ Discrete electron-dense, immune complex–type deposits are not present.

■ In one reported case (Ikeda and colleagues), the fibrils were curved or "frayed" rather than straight and formed irregularly arranged bundles that appeared "worm-like" or "comma-like" rather than circular in cross section; this appearance differs from the electron microscopic appearance described in other reports. The tissue for electron microscopy was treated with phosphotungstic acid in this case; it is possible that the phosphotungstic acid may have affected the ultrastructural appearance of the fibrils. This case may also represent a variant of collagen type III glomerulopathy.

Immunohistochemical Staining for Specific Collagen Types

- Diagnosis of collagen type III glomerulopathy can be greatly aided by immunohistochemical or immunofluorescent staining for specific collagen types, particularly types I, III, and IV. Monoclonal antibodies or polyclonal antisera for the different collagen types are available from various sources.
- In a normal glomerulus, staining for collagen types I and IV highlights the glomerular capillary basement membrane; no staining for collagen type III is seen in normal glomeruli.
- In collagen type III glomerulopathy, abundant staining for collagen type III is seen in the expanded mesangium and the thickened glomerular capillary walls; staining for types I and IV highlights the GBM, which appears to have normal thickness.

Differential Diagnosis

- Collagen type III glomerulopathy may resemble diabetic glomerulonephropathy or amyloidosis. However, the amorphous material in collagen III glomerulopathy lacks the strong PAS reaction and staining with silver stains seen in diabetic glomerulonephropathy and lacks the Congo red staining (and "apple-green" birefringence under polarized light) and fluorescence with thioflavin T seen in amyloidosis.
- The double-contour or "tram-track" appearance of the GBM seen in a few glomerular capillary loops in collagen III glomerulopathy may suggest MPGN type I. However, the "tram-track" appearance is far more extensive in MPGN; collagen type III glomerulopathy also lacks the hypercellularity of MPGN and the characteristic deposits of immunoglobulins and complement seen in MPGN with immunofluorescence microscopy.
- Collagen fibrils are also present within the glomerulus in the nail-patella syndrome. The nail-patella syndrome is inherited in an autosomal dominant fashion, unlike collagen type III glomerulopathy, and most patients will have a family history of the condition. In addition, collagen type III glomerulopathy lacks the nail and skeletal abnormalities present in nail-patella syndrome. The lamina densa of the glomerular capillary basement membrane in the nail-patella syndrome shows characteristic irregularities in width (irregular thinning and

thickening) and a characteristic "moth-eaten" appearance; the lamina densa in collagen type III glomerulopathy is normal in thickness and lacks the pale areas or "moth-eaten" appearance of the GBM in the nail-patella syndrome.

Treatment and Clinical Course

- The clinical course of collagen type III glomerulopathy appears to be one of persistent proteinuria and gradual loss of renal function; several reported patients have reached end-stage renal disease and required dialysis.
- No specific treatment is available. Supportive measures include control of hypertension and diuretics to relieve edema; dialysis may be required for patients who reach the point of end-stage renal disease.

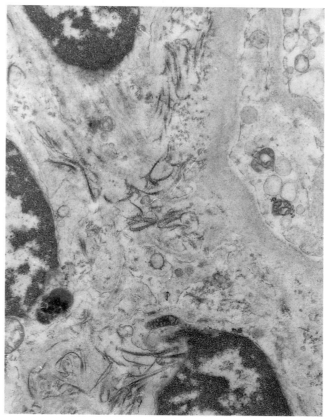

Figure 17–8. Electron micrograph of a kidney with collagen type III glomerulopathy. Type III collagen is shown in the mesangial areas admixed with mesangial matrix.

FIBRONECTIN GLOMERULOPATHY

Synonyms and Related Terms: Familial glomerulopathy with giant fibrillar (fibronectin-positive) deposits; glomerulopathy associated with predominant fibronectin deposits; familial glomerulonephritis with massive deposits of fibronectin; familial lobular glomerulopathy.

Biology of Disease

■ Fibronectin glomerulopathy is a recently described familial glomerulopathy characterized by the presence of mesangial and subendothelial deposits of fibronectin in the absence of significant deposits of immunoglobulins and complement components.

■ The condition appears to be inherited as an autosomal dominant disorder, although the inheritance pattern has not yet been definitively established. Both sexes are affected.

■ Fibronectin is a dimeric glycoprotein involved in matrix-matrix and cell-matrix interactions. It has binding sites for numerous molecules, including heparin, collagen, and cell surface proteins such as integrins.

■ Two forms of fibronectin exist: a soluble form in blood plasma and body fluids, which is secreted by the liver, and an insoluble form consisting of fibronectin multimers in basement membranes and extracellular matrices. The soluble form of fibronectin lacks a domain found in the insoluble form, and the two forms can be distinguished by using certain monoclonal antibodies that react with the domain lacking in the soluble form and others that react with both the soluble and insoluble forms. Studies using these monoclonal antibodies suggest that the majority of fibronectin in the glomerular deposits in fibronectin glomerulopathy is derived from the soluble, circulating form.

■ Fibronectin also binds to immune complexes, and it can be found in glomeruli in immune complex glomerulonephritides, together with immunoglobulins and complement. In fibronectin glomerulopathy, massive deposits of fibronectin are found in the *absence* of commensurate amounts of immunoglobulins or complement.

■ The etiology of fibronectin glomerulopathy is unknown. One family was studied for linkage to the fibronectin gene, and it was discovered that the disease did not appear to be linked to the gene, which suggests that mutations in the sequence of the fibronectin gene are not involved in pathogenesis of the disease. It is possible that an abnormality in fibronectin degradation or processing may be responsible; alternatively, an abnormality in a fibronectin-binding component may be involved.

Clinical Features

■ The majority of patients initially have proteinuria, many with the full nephrotic syndrome; hematuria is also present in a substantial number of patients. Renal function is usually normal at diagnosis; hypertension is common.

■ In the largest family studied thus far, distal renal tubular acidosis was also present (Gemperle and colleagues); it is not clear whether this condition is also present in other kindreds.

■ The usual age at diagnosis is in the 20s, although the age range is wide.

■ None of the patients appear to have evidence of extrarenal disease related to the glomerulopathy.

Laboratory Values

■ Serologic studies for autoimmunity (antinuclear antibody, anti-DNA, etc.) are negative.

■ Serum complement levels are normal; none of the patients have a monoclonal serum protein or cryoglobulinemia.

■ Serum fibronectin levels have been reported in a few patients; fibronectin levels have been variously normal or decreased.

Light Microscopy

Glomeruli

■ Glomeruli appear enlarged, with accentuation of the lobular appearance. The mesangial space is expanded, with thickening of glomerular capillary walls. Glomerular capillary lumina are often narrowed or occluded. Glomerular cellularity in most cases is normal or only slightly increased; more pronounced mesangial hypercellularity has been noted in a few cases.

■ The mesangium and subendothelial spaces contain large deposits of homogeneous material. The material is strongly positive with the PAS reaction and bright red with the acid fuchsin orange G stain; it does not stain with silver stains or Congo red and does not fluoresce with thioflavin T.

■ On silver stains the glomerular capillary basement membranes appear thin and can be distinguished from the silver-negative deposits in the subendothelial space.

■ A few globally sclerotic glomeruli may be present; in general, the more sclerotic glomeruli contain few or no deposits.

Tubules, Interstitium, and Vessels

■ The tubules, interstitium, and vessels usually show few or no changes other than cytoplasmic protein resorption droplets in proximal convoluted tubular epithelial cells.

■ There may be occasional atrophic tubules and scattered interstitial fibrosis, and vessels may show changes consistent with hypertension.

Immunofluorescence Microscopy

■ Staining for immunoglobulins and complement components is usually absent or relatively sparse.

■ Strong staining for fibronectin is present in the mesangium of all glomeruli; subendothelial staining is also usually present but may be sparse in early cases.

Electron Microscopy

■ Electron microscopy usually detects abundant osmiophilic deposits in the mesangium and subendothelial space. Scattered fibrils with a diameter of 12 nm are present in most cases; they are easy to find in some cases but may be sparse in others.

■ The lamina densa of the glomerular capillary basement membrane is usually unremarkable.

■ In one reported family (Gemperle and associates), fibrils were the predominant form of deposit present. Fibrils were found in subepithelial and intramembranous locations in glomerular capillary loops in this family.

Differential Diagnosis

■ Routine light microscopy initially suggests MPGN. However, the distinctive double-contour or "tram-track" appearance of the capillary loop on PAS and silver stains in MPGN is absent in fibronectin glomerulopathy.

■ Cases with prominent fibrillar deposits may suggest amyloidosis, fibrillary glomerulonephritis, or immunotactoid glomerulopathy by electron microscopy. However, the fibronectin deposits lack the tinctorial characteristics of amyloid on light microscopy, and the fibrils in fibronectin glomerulopathy are narrower than the fibrils in fibrillary glomerulonephritis and immunotactoid glomerulopathy (average diameter, 20 and 40 nm, respectively).

Treatment and Clinical Course

■ The majority of patients have persistent and progressive proteinuria. Some patients appear to have stable renal function; in others, renal function declines slowly, and patients may reach end-stage renal failure.

■ Treatment is supportive; at present, no specific treatment of fibronectin glomerulopathy is known.

■ Renal transplantation has been performed in several patients and appears to be successful in most. However, in the large family studied by Gemperle and colleagues, proteinuria recurred 7 months posttransplant in one man (of three patients receiving allografts); biopsy of that patient 23 months after transplantation showed subendothelial fibrillary deposits in glomerular capillaries, similar to those seen in his native kidney.

References

Hepatic Disease and the Kidney

Eigenbrodt EH, Molony DA, DuBose TD: Renal involvement in hepatic disease, rheumatoid arthritis, Sjögren syndrome, and mixed connective tissue disease. In: Tisher CC, Brenner BM (eds): Renal Pathology: With Clinical and Functional Correlations, 2nd ed. Philadelphia, JB Lippincott, 1994, p 596.

Johnson RJ, Couser WG: Hepatitis B infection and renal disease: Clinical, immunopathogenetic and therapeutic considerations. Kidney Int 37:663, 1990.

Lai KN, Lai FM: Clinical features and the natural course of hepatitis B virus–related glomerulopathy in adults. Kidney Int Suppl 40:40, 1991.

Lai KN, Lai FM, Tam JS, et al: Strong association between IgA nephropathy and hepatitis B surface antigenemia in endemic areas. Clin Nephrol 29:229, 1988.

Li PK-T, Lai FM, Ho SS, et al: Acute renal failure in hepatitis B virus–related membranous nephropathy with mesangiocapillary transition and crescentic transformation. Am J Kidney Dis 19:76, 1992.

Newell GC: Cirrhotic glomerulonephritis: Incidence, morphology, clinical features, and pathogenesis. Am J Kidney Dis 9:183, 1987.

Venkataseshan VS, Liebberman K, Kim DU, et al: Hepatitis-B–associated glomerulonephritis: Pathology, pathogenesis, and clinical course. Medicine (Baltimore) 69:200, 1990.

Sickle Cell Disease and the Kidney

Alleyne GAO, Statius van Eps LW, Addae SK, et al: The kidney in sickle cell anemia. Kidney Int 7:371, 1975.

Allon M: Renal abnormalities in sickle cell disease. Arch Intern Med 150:501, 1990.

De Jong PE, Statius van Eps LW: Sickle cell nephropathy: New insights into its pathophysiology. Kidney Int 27:711, 1985.

Elfenbein IB, Patchefsky A, Schwartz W, et al: Pathology of the glomerulus in sickle cell anemia with and without the nephrotic syndrome. Am J Pathol 77:357, 1974.

Falk RJ, Scheinman J, Phillips G, et al: Prevalence and pathologic features of sickle cell nephropathy and response to inhibition of angiotensin-converting enzyme. N Engl J Med 326:910, 1992.

Gubler M-C, Heidet L, Antignac C: Alport's syndrome, thin basement membrane nephropathy, nail-patella syndrome, and type III collagen glomerulopathy. In: Jennette JC, Olson JL, Schwartz MM, Silva FG (eds): Heptinstall's Pathology of the Kidney, 5th ed. Philadelphia, Lippincott-Raven, 1998, p 1207.

Powars DR, Elliott-Mills DD, Chan L, et al: Chronic renal failure in sickle cell disease: Risk factors, clinical course, and mortality. Ann Intern Med 115:614, 1991.

Tejani A, Phadke K, Adamson O, et al: Renal lesions in sickle cell nephropathy in children. Nephron 39:352, 1985.

Weidner N, Buckalew VM Jr: Sickle cell anemia, sickle cell trait, and the polycythemic states. In: Tisher CC, Brenner BM (eds): Renal Pathology: With Clinical and Functional Correlations, 2nd ed. Philadelphia, JB Lippincott, 1994, p 1491.

C1q Nephropathy

Imai H, Yasuda T, Satoh K, et al: Pan-nephritis (glomerulonephritis, arteriolitis, and tubulointerstitial nephritis) associated with predominant mesangial C1q deposition and hypocomplementemia: A variant type of C1q nephropathy? Am J Kidney Dis 27:583, 1996.

Iskandar SS, Browning MC, Lorentz WB: C1q nephropathy: A pediatric clinicopathologic study. Am J Kidney Dis 18:459, 1991.

Jennette JC, Hipp CG: C1q nephropathy: A distinct pathologic entity usually causing nephrotic syndrome. Am J Kidney Dis 6:103, 1985.

Shappell SB, Myrthil G, Fogo A: Renal biopsy case: An adolescent with relapsing nephrotic syndrome: Minimal-change disease versus focal-segmental glomerulosclerosis versus C1q nephropathy. Am J Kidney Dis 29:966, 1997.

Collagen Type III Glomerulopathy

Dowling JP, Forbes IK, Chou ST: Collagen type III glomerulopathy: Extension beyond the glomerulus (abstract). Kidney Int 46:937, 1994.

Ikeda K, Yokoyama H, Tomosugi N, et al: Primary glomerular fibrosis: A new nephropathy caused by diffuse intra-glomerular increase in atypical type III collagen fibers. Clin Nephrol 33:155, 1990.

Imbasciati E, Gherardi G, Morozumi K, et al: Collagen type III glomerulopathy: A new idiopathic glomerular disease. Am J Nephrol 11:422, 1991.

Tamura H, Matsuda A, Kidoguchi N, et al: A family with two sisters with collagenofibrotic glomerulonephropathy. Am J Kidney Dis 27:588, 1996.

Fibronectin Glomerulopathy

Assmann KJM, Koene RAP, Wetzels JFM: Familial glomerulonephritis characterized by massive deposits of fibronectin. Am J Kidney Dis 25:781, 1995.

Gemperle O, Neuweiler J, Reutter FW, et al: Familial glomerulopathy with giant fibrillar (fibronectin-positive) deposits: 15-year follow-up in a large kindred. Am J Kidney Dis 28:668, 1996.

Mazzuco G, Maran E, Rollino C, et al: Glomerulonephritis with organized deposits: A mesangiopathic, not immune complex–mediated disease? A pathologic study of two cases in the same family. Hum Pathol 23:63, 1992.

Strøm EH, Banfi G, Krapf R, et al: Glomerulopathy associated with predominant fibronectin deposits: A newly recognized hereditary disease. Kidney Int 48:163, 1995.

CHAPTER 18

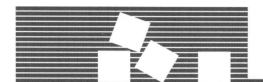

Renal Effects of Extrarenal Neoplasms

INTRODUCTION

- The kidney can be affected by extrarenal neoplasms in a variety of ways. Metastasis to the kidney is a direct, but relatively uncommon, manifestation of extrarenal neoplasms. Obstruction of the urinary tract and hydronephrosis can be seen with carcinoma of the uterine cervix, urinary bladder, prostate, and others; massive retroperitoneal lymphadenopathy from non-Hodgkin's lymphoma or other neoplasms can occasionally obstruct the ureters by external compression.
- Less direct renal effects of extrarenal neoplasms include metabolic effects, such as the tumor lysis syndrome or hypercalcemia, and complications of therapy, such as radiation nephritis or toxic effects of chemotherapy.
- A variety of glomerular effects have been described. The morphologic picture of membranous glomerulonephropathy (MGN) and the nephrotic syndrome has been described in association with carcinomas, Hodgkin's disease has been associated with the clinical and morphologic picture of minimal change nephrotic syndrome, and rare cases of other types of glomerulonephritis have been described in association with malignancies.
- Multiple myeloma and monoclonal gammopathies affect the kidney in many ways; myeloma kidney, amyloidosis, and light chain deposition disease are covered in a separate chapter.

RENAL METASTASES FROM EXTRARENAL NEOPLASMS

- Discovery of renal metastases from extrarenal neoplasms is a common finding at postmortem examination of patients dying of malignant diseases; the frequency ranges from approximately 2% to more than 10% in different series. However, *premortem* diagnosis of renal metastasis is uncommon. In exceptional cases, spread to the kidney by direct invasion from a contiguous site or metastasis from a distant site has been the initial clinical manifestation of an extrarenal neoplasm.
- Renal involvement is found in over half of patients dying of leukemia; the incidence of renal involvement

appears to be higher in lymphocytic than myelogenous (granulocytic) leukemias. Both kidneys are almost invariably affected. Involvement may range from grossly inapparent, focal or diffuse interstitial infiltrates to grossly visible, pink-white masses. The kidneys usually retain their normal shape but may be large in size. Renal excretory function is seldom significantly impaired, even in the presence of massive renal infiltration; hypokalemia resulting from renal involvement by leukemia has been described.

- The kidneys are involved in approximately one third to more than one half of patients who are dying of non-Hodgkin's lymphoma; renal involvement is less common in patients who have Hodgkin's disease. Again, premortem diagnosis of renal involvement is uncommon. Both kidneys are usually involved. There may be diffuse infiltration with generalized enlargement of the kidneys, or the neoplasm may form one or more discrete masses. Histologically, the interstitium is infiltrated by the neoplastic lymphocytes, with compression and obliteration of tubules; glomeruli are relatively spared. Neoplastic lymphoid infiltrates are characterized by cellular monomorphism and variable cytologic atypia, in contrast to the cytologically benign lymphocytes and mixture of other cells (plasma cells, eosinophils, etc.) in chronic interstitial nephritis or other benign nonneoplastic conditions. Renal excretory function is usually preserved.
- The most common solid tumors metastasizing to the kidney are lung and breast carcinomas and malignant melanoma; renal metastasis from a wide variety of sites and different types of neoplasms has been described. Metastases are usually multiple and bilateral; they form irregular, well-defined, solid nodules. There may be preferential involvement of the cortex; however, this finding is often obscured by large masses that destroy large portions of the parenchyma.

SYSTEMIC AND METABOLIC EFFECTS OF EXTRARENAL NEOPLASMS

- Ischemic acute tubular nephropathy resulting from hypotension, shock, or disseminated intravascular coagulation is probably the most common systemic effect of malignancies on the kidneys. This condition is frequently a preterminal event, discovered as an incidental finding at postmortem examination.

■ Clinical acute renal failure in patients with malignancies is most often due to acute tubular necrosis (ATN); sepsis and the use of nephrotoxic drugs (particularly aminoglycoside antibiotics) are the most common underlying factors.

■ Hypercalcemia caused by bone resorption or a paraneoplastic effect, such as the production of substances with parathyroid hormone–like activity, may result in nephrocalcinosis. Nephrocalcinosis is most frequently caused by multiple myeloma and carcinomas of the breast and lung with extensive bone metastases. Crystalline calcium precipitates are found within renal tubules. Renal function is usually normal or only moderately decreased.

■ The *acute tumor lysis syndrome* consists of a combination of metabolic abnormalities usually occurring in the setting of chemotherapy for high-grade leukemias and lymphomas. Common abnormalities include hyperphosphatemia, hyperkalemia, hypocalcemia, hyperuricemia, and azotemia. Renal insufficiency in the tumor lysis syndrome is usually due to hyperuricemia, with resulting acute uric acid nephropathy. Monosodium urate precipitates as crystals in collecting ducts, with destruction of the tubular epithelium and a surrounding foreign body reaction. The acute tumor lysis syndrome is now unusual because patients at risk for the syndrome routinely receive fluids and are treated with allopurinol before the initiation of chemotherapy.

RENAL TOXICITIES OF CANCER CHEMOTHERAPY

■ Many cancer chemotherapy drugs have potential renal toxicities, the most common toxicity being ATN. Examples of drugs that may cause ATN include streptozotocin, methotrexate, aminopterin, and cisplatin. The histologic features of ATN are described in Chapter 12.

■ Patients receiving cancer chemotherapy often receive antibiotics as well, many of which may cause ATN (aminoglycosides, amphotericin B, etc.), interstitial nephritis (penicillins, cephalosporins, etc.), or both. Thus there is a possibility of synergistic renal toxicity.

■ Cisplatin (*cis*-diamminedichloroplatinum II) is a chemotherapy agent with a broad spectrum of activity that is widely used in treating many malignancies, but has a particular propensity for nephrotoxicity. Nephrotoxicity with cisplatin is dose dependent but usually reversible. A single dose of cisplatin (2 mg/kg) produces renal insufficiency in up to 25% to 35% of patients; serum creatinine reaches a peak value approximately 8 to 12 days later. With higher or repeated doses, the renal insufficiency may become irreversible. In such cases there is patchy tubular necrosis predominantly affecting the distal tubules and collecting ducts, along with tubular dilatation and cast formation. Collecting duct epithelial cell nuclei are enlarged, and syncytia may form in collecting ducts. Interstitial fibrosis, tubular atrophy, and glomerulosclerosis have been observed in animal models of cisplatin toxicity.

■ Mitomycin C may produce renal failure by inducing thrombotic microangiopathy.

RADIATION NEPHRITIS

■ Clinical radiation nephritis may occur with doses of approximately 23 Gy (2,300 rad) to both kidneys given within 5 weeks. Acute manifestations may include proteinuria, hypertension, azotemia, and refractory anemia.

■ The primary site of injury in radiation nephritis appears to be endothelial cells.

■ In the acute stage, glomerular capillaries and afferent arterioles are narrowed by hyaline or fibrinoid material. Tubular atrophy and interstitial fibrosis may be present; interstitial inflammation is usually absent.

■ Electron microscopy studies have demonstrated widening of the subendothelial zone of glomerular capillaries by electron-lucent material; there may be focal loss of capillary endothelial cells. Deposition of material resembling fibrin may be seen in arterioles.

■ The late stage of radiation nephritis may be manifested clinically by mild proteinuria or renal insufficiency. Histologically, there is obliteration of arteries and arterioles, with resulting tubular atrophy and interstitial fibrosis.

GLOMERULAR EFFECTS OF EXTRARENAL NEOPLASMS

Biology of Disease

■ Glomerular changes are a well-described but uncommon manifestation of extrarenal neoplasms.

■ The most common glomerular morphologic pattern associated with extrarenal neoplasms is that of membranous glomerulonephropathy with the nephrotic syndrome, which has been described with a variety of carcinomas and occasionally with other neoplasms. The patterns of minimal change nephrotic syndrome, focal segmental glomerulosclerosis, membranoproliferative glomerulonephritis, and focal proliferative and focal necrotizing glomerulonephritis have also been described.

■ It is believed that the glomerular injury in many instances is due to deposition of immune complexes in the glomerular capillaries. Circulating immune complexes have been described in cancer patients; it has been suggested that these complexes may represent combinations of antigens shed from tumor cells with antibodies directed against those tumor antigens.

■ In one autopsy series, glomerular deposits were detected by immunofluorescence and electron microscopy in over 30% of patients with cancer; such findings were rare in patients without cancer. The deposits were predominantly found in the subendothelial space of glomerular capillaries. Elution of antibodies from involved kidneys in several cases demonstrated IgG antibodies that appeared to react with the patients' tumors. Notably, despite the presence of deposits at autopsy, there was little *clinical* evidence of glomerular disease in these patients before death.

- The course of illness in many cancer patients is complicated by infections. Such infections, or the immunologic reaction to them, may also be involved in the pathogenesis of glomerular injury.
- These associations between malignancy and glomerular disease remain controversial. Alternative explanations for glomerular disease have not been or cannot be excluded in many cases.

Membranous Glomerulonephropathy (MGN) and Cancer

- The association between cancer and MGN is well described, but the frequency and importance of this association remain controversial. Estimates of the frequency of malignancies in adult patients with MGN have varied from less than 2% to almost 11% in different series. On the basis of a high frequency of malignancy in their experience, some experts have suggested that all adult patients with newly diagnosed MGN should have an extensive evaluation for occult cancer; others believe that such a search for occult malignancy is not justified.
- The majority of malignancies associated with the morphologic picture of MGN have been carcinomas, with bronchogenic, gastric, and colorectal carcinomas being the most frequent. Membranous glomerulonephropathy has also been described in association with lymphomas and leukemias, malignant melanoma, Wilms tumor, and pheochromocytoma.
- The malignancy is usually found simultaneously with, shortly before, or within a short time after the diagnosis of MGN; cases in which the diagnosis of MGN is temporally distant from that of the neoplasm most likely represent chance occurrence of the two diseases in one patient.
- The significance of the association between MGN and carcinoma is strengthened by the disappearance of the nephrotic syndrome after successful treatment of the neoplasm in some cases and recurrence of nephrotic syndrome associated with recurrence of the tumor.
- The incidence of occult malignancy may be higher in patients over the age of 50 years at diagnosis of MGN.
- In most cases, survival is short after the diagnosis of malignancy in patients with MGN; some authors have suggested that MGN is an adverse prognostic factor in patients with carcinoma.
- The histologic and immunofluorescence and electron microscopic appearance of glomeruli in patients with MGN associated with malignancy resembles that seen in idiopathic MGN in most respects. Therefore, based on renal biopsy it is not possible to determine or predict which patients have malignancies or in whom they will develop.

Hodgkin's Disease and Minimal Change Nephrotic Syndrome

- Glomerular lesions have been described in many patients with Hodgkin's disease and are usually mani-

fested as nephrotic syndrome. The most common morphologic appearance is that of minimal change nephrotic syndrome (minimal change disease); MGN, focal segmental glomerulosclerosis, and membranoproliferative and focal proliferative glomerulonephritis have also been described.
- Onset of the nephrotic syndrome and the diagnosis of Hodgkin's disease usually occur within a short period.
- Successful treatment of Hodgkin's disease has frequently been associated with remission of nephrotic syndrome and relapse of Hodgkin's disease with relapse of renal disease.
- Occurrence of the nephrotic syndrome in patients with Hodgkin's disease does not appear to have the adverse prognostic implications associated with the occurrence of MGN in patients with carcinoma.

Other Associations Between Malignancy and Glomerular Disease

- Non-Hodgkin's lymphomas and lymphocytic leukemias have been associated with a variety of glomerular abnormalities, including MGN, membranoproliferative glomerulonephritis, and focal proliferative and focal necrotizing glomerulonephritis. The entity of immunotactoid glomerulopathy may also be associated with lymphoproliferative disorders (discussed in more detail in Chapter 19).
- Chronic lymphocytic leukemia has been most frequently associated with glomerular lesions of various types. The glomerular lesion is often related to production of a monoclonal protein by the neoplastic lymphocytes. In some cases, the monoclonal protein has exhibited properties of a cryoglobulin.
- Renal cell carcinoma has been associated with amyloidosis of the kidney. The amyloid is the secondary or AA type (composed of degradation products of serum amyloid–associated protein). The amyloidosis is seen both within the neoplasm and in nonneoplastic kidney tissue, outside the neoplasm itself.

References

Alpers CE, Cotran RS: Neoplasia and glomerular injury. Kidney Int 30: 465, 1986.

Brueggemeyer CD, Ramirez G: Membranous nephropathy: A concern for malignancy. Am J Kidney Dis 9:23, 1987.

Eagen JW, Lewis EJ: Glomerulopathies of neoplasia. Kidney Int 11:297, 1977.

Hande KR, Garrow GC: Acute tumor lysis syndrome in patients with high-grade non-Hodgkin's lymphoma. Am J Med 94:133, 1993.

Harris KPG, Hattersley JM, Feehally J, et al: Acute renal failure associated with haematological malignancies: A review of 10 years experience. Eur J Haematol 47:119, 1991.

Pascal RR: Renal manifestations of extra-renal neoplasms. Hum Pathol 11:7, 1980.

Peterson RO: Kidney: Neoplastic disorders. In: Peterson RO (ed): Urologic Pathology, 2nd ed. Philadelphia, JB Lippincott, 1992, p 127.

Pollock CA, Ibels LS, Levi JA, et al: Acute renal failure due to focal necrotizing glomerulonephritis in a patient with non-Hodgkin's lymphoma: Resolution with treatment of lymphoma. Nephron 48:197, 1988.

CHAPTER 19

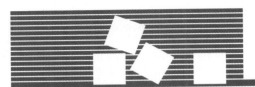

Plasma Cell Dyscrasias, Monoclonal Gammopathies, and the Fibrillary Glomerulopathies

Multiple Myeloma, Light Chain Deposition Disease, Amyloidosis, Fibrillary Glomerulonephritis, and Immunotactoid Glomerulopathy

INTRODUCTION

- Neoplasms of plasma cells *(plasma cell dyscrasias)* are a heterogeneous group of conditions associated with the proliferation of a clone of plasma cells and the production of a monoclonal immunoglobulin protein *(monoclonal gammopathy; M protein or M spike)*. The protein produced may be an intact immunoglobulin, including both heavy and light chains, a light chain only (complete or partial), or an intact immunoglobulin with excess free light chains. In rare cases of multiple myeloma, no detectable monoclonal protein is secreted (so-called nonsecretory myeloma); heavy chain disease, or the production of a heavy chain without an associated light chain, is extremely rare. The monoclonal protein may be found in the serum, the urine, or both.

- The monoclonal immunoglobulins in an individual patient all share an identical heavy chain (γ, for IgG, being the most common) and/or an identical light chain (either κ or λ but not both).

- The most common monoclonal gammopathy is *monoclonal gammopathy of undetermined significance* (previously called benign monoclonal gammopathy). This gammopathy is relatively common in the older population but is usually of no clinical consequence. Plasma cells account for fewer than 10% of the nucleated cells in the bone marrow, the amount of the monoclonal protein in serum and urine is low, patients have no lytic bone lesions, and renal function is normal. Multiple myeloma eventually develops in approximately one quarter of patients with monoclonal gammopathy of undetermined significance; however, it may not occur for many years after discovery of the monoclonal protein.

- Multiple myeloma is the second most common monoclonal gammopathy and clinically the most significant. Plasma cells make up at least 10% of the bone marrow cells or form discrete tumors (plasmacytomas) in the marrow, the amount of monoclonal protein in serum and/or urine is higher, and patients have bone lesions (either sharp, "punched out" lytic lesions or, less often, diffuse osteopenia without discrete lytic lesions). Complications of multiple myeloma include bone fractures, hypercalcemia caused by bone resorption, infections, anemia, and renal failure.

- Other monoclonal gammopathies include Waldenström's macroglobulinemia, which is associated with intact IgM in the serum. Monoclonal serum proteins may also be detected in occasional patients with non-Hodgkin's lymphomas or chronic lymphocytic leukemia; in such patients the protein is usually present in low concentrations and is seldom a significant problem in and of itself.

- The kidney is affected in a multitude of ways by monoclonal gammopathies. The most common plasma cell dyscrasia to affect the kidney is multiple myeloma, and the most common consequence of myeloma is tubular degeneration from the toxic effects of light chains on tubular epithelial cells or obstruction of tubules by casts composed of the monoclonal proteins ("myeloma kidney or myeloma cast nephropathy").

- Plasma cell dyscrasias falling short of the diagnostic criteria for myeloma (i.e., fewer than 10% plasma cells in bone marrow, low concentrations of monoclonal protein in serum and urine, and no lytic bone lesions) may cause renal disease as a consequence of amyloidosis and light chain deposition disease (LCDD).

212

- The term *amyloidosis* includes a heterogeneous group of conditions, all of which are characterized by the deposition of a protein in a β-pleated sheet configuration. One of the most common types of amyloidosis is caused by the deposition of immunoglobulin light chains or light chain fragments, designated AL amyloidosis. Such deposition can occur in the setting of multiple myeloma or in the setting of a plasma cell dyscrasia that falls short of the diagnostic criteria for myeloma ("primary amyloidosis"). Because the pathologic characteristics of all forms of amyloidosis are generally similar, they will be discussed together.
- Immunotactoid glomerulopathy (IT) and fibrillary glomerulonephritis resemble amyloidosis in some respects on ultrastructural examination and enter into the differential diagnosis of amyloidosis; some also appear to consist of a monoclonal immunoglobulin. They are therefore also included in this chapter.

MULTIPLE MYELOMA AND RENAL DISEASE (with emphasis on myeloma cast nephropathy)

Synonyms and Related Terms: Myeloma cast nephropathy; light chain cast nephropathy; myeloma kidney; Bence Jones cast nephropathy.

Biology of Disease

- Multiple myeloma occurs predominantly in the older population; men are affected more often than women. It is the most common lymphoproliferative malignancy in African-Americans and the second most common in the general population. The etiology in most cases is unknown; a small proportion of cases appear to be related to ionizing radiation or exposure to organic chemicals such as benzene.
- Renal failure is the second most common cause of death in myeloma; some degree of renal insufficiency occurs in approximately half of patients. Renal insufficiency is the most adverse prognostic indicator in patients with myeloma.
- Toxic effects of light chains on the tubular epithelium and/or obstruction of tubules by protein casts *(myeloma or Bence Jones cast nephropathy, light chain cast nephropathy, or myeloma kidney)* are the most common direct effects of myeloma on the kidney. The casts are usually composed of the intact monoclonal immunoglobulin, free immunoglobulin light chains, or both. Free immunoglobulin light chains (classically called *Bence Jones protein*) are believed to be directly toxic to renal tubular epithelial cells and may lead to obstruction downstream in the nephron.
- Dehydration, hypercalcemia, interstitial nephritis caused by nonsteroidal anti-inflammatory agents or other drugs, other nephrotoxic effects of medications, and acute tubular necrosis induced by radiographic contrast media are other potentially reversible causes of renal insufficiency in multiple myeloma. Hyperuricemia, pyelonephritis, and renal stones also may affect renal function.

- Patients with myeloma may exhibit Fanconi's syndrome, with aminoaciduria, renal glycosuria, phosphaturia, and renal tubular acidosis. These disorders are probably due to the direct toxic effects of light chains on proximal renal tubules. The onset of Fanconi's syndrome may precede other manifestations of myeloma, sometimes by several years.
- Approximately 7% to 10% of cases of multiple myeloma are associated with amyloidosis, and approximately 5% have LCDD. Patients with amyloidosis or LCDD rarely have typical myeloma cast nephropathy in our experience; the physicochemical properties of the specific monoclonal protein probably determine the form of renal disease that occurs in each case. Light chain deposition disease and amyloidosis associated with multiple myeloma are described separately.

Clinical Features

- Patients with multiple myeloma typically have some combination of anemia, back pain, or bone fracture.
- Serum creatinine levels are elevated (over 2 mg/dL) in approximately 30% of patients at diagnosis. The finding of myeloma cast nephropathy on renal biopsy performed for renal insufficiency or proteinuria may be the initial indication of myeloma.
- Acute renal failure caused by dehydration or intravenous radiographic contrast material (possibly given as part of an intravenous pyelogram) may be the initial manifestation.
- Proteinuria is present in 70% to 80% of patients with myeloma. Proteinuria in myeloma is usually predominantly due to leakage of monoclonal light chain into the urine, with little or no albumin. The presence of significant albuminuria usually indicates a glomerular disease such as amyloidosis. The amount of proteinuria is highly variable.

Laboratory Values

- A monoclonal immunoglobulin protein (M component or M spike) is found in the serum and/or urine by protein electrophoresis in virtually all patients with multiple myeloma. The specific components (heavy and light chains) should be identified by immunofixation or immunoelectrophoresis. In most cases this protein consists of an intact immunoglobulin, with or without free light chains. The concentration of monoclonal protein in the serum should be determined, and 24-hour urine protein excretion should be quantified.
- In approximately one quarter of patients the malignant clone of plasma cells secretes only light chains, with no intact immunoglobulins; this condition is sometimes called *light chain disease* but should be distinguished from LCDD, which is the deposition of monoclonal light chains or fragments in tissues. In light chain disease, routine serum protein electrophoresis does not detect a monoclonal spike because the light chain is rapidly spilled into the urine and does not accumulate to detectable levels in the serum; urine protein electrophoresis is required to demonstrate the monoclonal protein. Therefore, both serum and urine protein electro-

phoresis must be performed whenever myeloma is suspected.

■ Dipstick urinalysis may not detect proteinuria in patients excreting predominantly monoclonal immunoglobulin with little albuminuria because the routine dipstick assay for protein is primarily sensitive to albumin. Quantitative assays for urine protein will detect Bence Jones protein as well as albumin.

■ Serum immunoglobulin levels are characteristically depressed, except for the monoclonal protein when one is present. The γ-globulin fraction (i.e., total serum protein concentration minus the serum albumin concentration) is usually increased.

■ Anemia is common; the serum calcium content may be elevated. The serum β_2-microglobulin level correlates with the plasma cell load and is a useful assay for monitoring multiple myeloma except in the presence of renal insufficiency (β_2-microglobulin is normally excreted in the urine and thus accumulates in renal failure).

Gross Appearance

■ The kidneys are usually normal in size; they are enlarged in up to one third of cases. The cortical surface is smooth.

■ On section, the cortex may appear pale, but the distinction between cortex and medulla is preserved.

Light Microscopy

■ The most striking histologic finding in myeloma cast nephropathy involves the tubules, which are dilated and atrophic and contain large, distinctive casts. The casts are usually found predominantly in distal tubules and collecting tubules, but they are occasionally found in proximal convoluted tubules or even extending into Bowman's space.

■ The casts appear dense, refractile, strongly eosinophilic, and often fractured on section ("crackable"). They may appear multilamellar and sometimes contain rhomboid or needle-like crystals. The casts usually stain positively with periodic acid–Schiff (PAS), often with a darker rim of staining surrounding a pale center; they usually do not stain with silver stains.

■ The casts are surrounded by a distinctive cellular reaction consisting of mononuclear cells, multinucleated giant cells, and sometimes neutrophils, which may appear to be attempting to phagocytize the cast. The mononuclear cells and giant cells were once thought to be tubular epithelial cells but are now recognized to be derived from monocytes that enter the tubules via breaks in the tubular basement membrane (TBM).

■ The characteristic casts are not absolutely pathognomonic of multiple myeloma, and similar casts can be seen in a number of other conditions (see Differential Diagnosis later). However, in the appropriate clinical circumstances these casts are virtually pathognomonic of a plasma cell dyscrasia of some type.

■ The TBM may be disrupted, and extension of cast material into the interstitium can elicit an interstitial foreign body reaction. Eventually the cast may appear to be lying free within the interstitium.

■ Tubular epithelial cells may contain cytoplasmic protein resorption droplets. They may appear flattened or show reactive changes, even in tubules that do not contain casts. Nuclei are enlarged and hyperchromatic, and occasional mitoses may be present; the cytoplasm may appear basophilic and granular. Sloughing of epithelial cells and focal denudation of the TBM may be seen.

■ Tubulovenous communications, i.e., rupture of the tubule with extension of its contents into thin-walled veins, may be present.

■ Glomerular appearances range from normal to mild increases in mesangial cells and matrix to diffuse, uniform thickening of capillary basement membranes.

■ Interstitial changes range from diffuse edema early in the course to extensive interstitial fibrosis in advanced disease. A mixed, acute and chronic interstitial inflammatory infiltrate is often present; plasma cells are usually inconspicuous. It is rare for atypical plasma cells to be a prominent component of the interstitial infiltrate (10% of cases or fewer).

■ Arteries and arterioles show hyaline change and intimal fibrosis. Scanty deposits of amyloid material can be found in vessels in approximately one quarter of patients.

■ Other changes that can be seen include features of pyelonephritis, nephrocalcinosis, and uric acid deposits.

Immunofluorescence Microscopy

■ Casts usually stain with multiple immunoreactants, including immunoglobulins, albumin, and fibrin/fibrinogen. Staining in myeloma casts often differs from that in most casts in that myeloma casts frequently demonstrate strong peripheral staining with decreased or absent staining in the center of the casts, in contrast to the even staining seen in other casts. In the majority of cases the casts stain for *both* κ and λ light chains; less often there is staining only for the light chain found in the monoclonal protein. This may have to do with the age of the cast, or changes in the antigenic structure of the protein.

■ Tubular basement membranes are usually unreactive in our experience, although others have reported light chain staining; there may be staining in tubular epithelial cytoplasmic droplets for the immunoglobulin components in patients' monoclonal protein.

■ Glomeruli are usually negative or demonstrate weak staining; occasionally, capillary wall staining is seen for the immunoglobulins in the patient's M component.

Electron Microscopy

■ The appearance of the myeloma casts varies from dense and homogeneous to coarsely fibrillar. Casts may contain parallel arrays of large fibrils or elongated crystals of varying size.

■ Tubular epithelial cells may contain cytoplasmic crystals that have a fibrillar or lattice configuration with a periodicity of 8 to 10 nm.

■ Glomerular visceral epithelial cell foot processes may be effaced. The basement membranes may appear thickened, and mesangial spaces may be widened.

Differential Diagnosis

- The clinical differential of renal insufficiency in multiple myeloma includes amyloidosis and LCDD, dehydration, hypercalcemia, interstitial nephritis, and acute tubular necrosis.
- The characteristic casts are not completely specific for multiple myeloma, although there is some controversy regarding this. Similar casts can occasionally be seen in Waldenström's macroglobulinemia, thyroid carcinoma, and carcinoma of the pancreas. In such conditions, the number of these casts is usually less than in multiple myeloma.
- Occasional casts surrounded by macrophages are sometimes seen in patients with systemic lupus erythematosus, focal segmental glomerulosclerosis, and other conditions. The reaction is usually not as prominent or widespread as in myeloma cast nephropathy.
- Casts with the characteristic giant cell and/or neutrophilic response have been described in other conditions (pancreatic carcinoma, tuberculosis treated with rifampin) in older reports. However, a plasma cell dyscrasia was not always rigorously excluded in these cases.

Treatment and Clinical Course

- Multiple myeloma is characterized by an inexorable increase in plasma cell number, with eventual development of bone marrow failure, renal failure, or death from infection.
- The median survival in multiple myeloma is approximately 3 to 4 years, although a small proportion of patients survive 10 years or longer with few or no serious complications (*smoldering* or *indolent* myeloma).
- Multiple myeloma is considered incurable with conventional therapy, and in most patients the intent of therapy is palliation rather than cure. A variety of chemotherapy regimens are used for multiple myeloma, including phenylalanine mustard plus prednisone, VAD (vincristine, Adriamycin [doxorubicin], and dexamethasone), and others.
- Infection is the most common cause of death in patients with multiple myeloma; in particular, patients are predisposed to bacterial pneumonitis and pyelonephritis.
- Renal insufficiency develops in approximately half of patients with multiple myeloma over the course of the illness. Renal insufficiency usually develops insidiously, but dehydration or radiographic contrast material may precipitate acute renal failure.
- Renal failure in multiple myeloma was formerly considered irreversible in most cases; it now appears that some recovery of renal function may occur in up to half of patients. Recovery occurs more frequently when the renal insufficiency was relatively acute in onset, but it may occur even if the renal insufficiency had been present for several months before treatment. Recovery of renal function may take 6 months or longer; dialysis support may be required for a prolonged period.
- With dialysis support, the feature that determines survival in patients with multiple myeloma and renal disease is whether their myeloma can be controlled with chemotherapy and, if so, how long it can be controlled.
- Treatment for renal insufficiency involves control of hypercalcemia and hyperuricemia, high oral fluid intake, and alkalinization of the urine, combined with chemotherapy for myeloma.

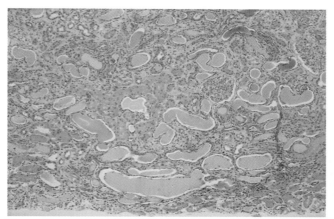

Figure 19–1. Bence Jones cast nephropathy in multiple myeloma. A low-magnification photograph depicts numerous large eosinophilic hyaline casts in the dilated tubular lumina.

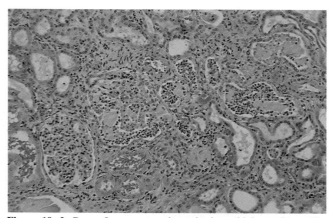

Figure 19–2. Bence Jones cast nephropathy in multiple myeloma. The picture depicts tubulointerstitial changes with large refractile "crackable" eosinophilic tubular casts admixed with polymorphonuclear leukocytes.

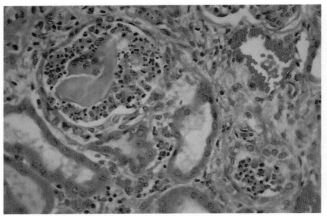

Figure 19–3. Bence Jones cast nephropathy in multiple myeloma. An irregular eosinophilic refractile hyaline tubular cast is partially surrounded by a multinucleated giant cell; many polymorphonuclear lymphocytes are in the dilated tubular lumen.

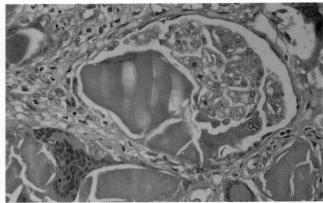

Figure 19–6. Bence Jones cast nephropathy in multiple myeloma. Material similar to that of the tubular casts is seen "regurgitated" to Bowman's space (note the giant cell apposed to the cast).

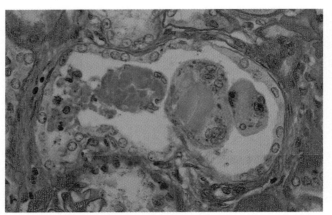

Figure 19–4. Bence Jones cast nephropathy in multiple myeloma. The picture displays tubular casts with surrounding giant cells and damaged tubular epithelial cells.

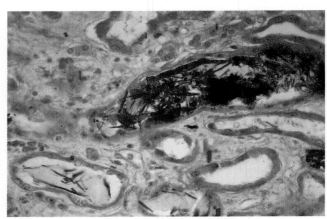

Figure 19–7. Multiple myeloma. Crystalline needle-like structures are seen in the tubular lumina and in the tubular epithelial cells in a patient with Fanconi's syndrome and myeloma.

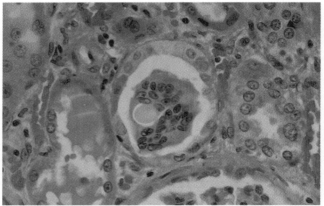

Figure 19–5. Bence Jones cast nephropathy in multiple myeloma. A small eosinophilic cast is surrounded by a large multinucleated giant cell.

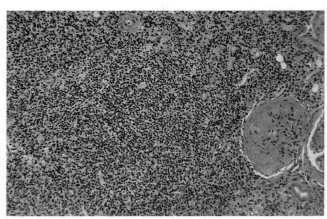

Figure 19–8. Multiple myeloma. Heavy myelomatous cellular infiltrate is in the tubulointerstitium with complete replacement of the normal structure of the kidney.

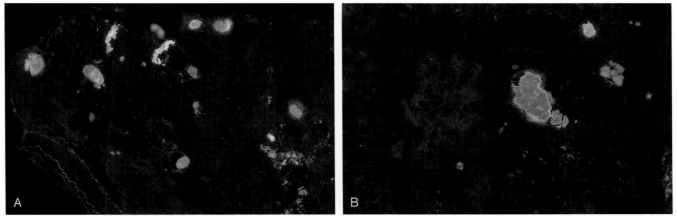

Figure 19–9. *A* and *B,* Multiple myeloma, immunofluorescence, λ light chain. Strong λ light chain staining is seen in the tubular casts. Both photographs are of the same biopsy specimen but with different magnifications. Note the strong peripheral staining in the cast in *B*.

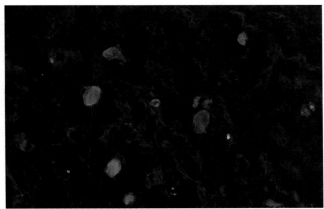

Figure 19–10. Multiple myeloma, immunofluorescence, κ light chain. The photograph shows κ light chain staining in a patient with λ light chain–positive myeloma cast nephropathy. The positivity is substantially weaker than the λ light chain staining in the same patient shown in Figure 19–9.

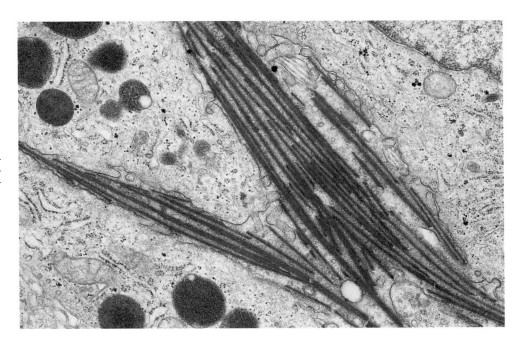

Figure 19–11. Electron micrograph, multiple myeloma. Needle-shaped crystals are located in a tubular epithelial cell.

LIGHT CHAIN DEPOSITION DISEASE (LCDD)

Synonyms and Related Terms: Systemic light chain deposition; nonamyloid light chain deposition; light chain deposition nephropathy; light chain nodular glomerulosclerosis.

Biology of Disease

- Light chain deposition disease, an uncommon complication of multiple myeloma or other plasma cell dyscrasias, occurs in approximately 5% of cases of myeloma. The majority of cases of LCDD occur in patients with multiple myeloma, but approximately one third of patients do not fulfill the diagnostic criteria for myeloma at diagnosis of LCDD.
- A monoclonal light chain of the same type found in tissue deposits is present in the serum and/or urine of approximately 90% of patients; study of the bone marrow demonstrates a clonal population of plasma cells in virtually all patients.
- Light chain deposition disease was first described in the 1970s and was initially considered to be uncommon. The diagnosis is now being made with increasing frequency as antisera specific for the individual light chains become more widely available and applied to renal tissues.
- The majority of cases involve deposition of intact κ light chains or fragments of κ light chains. The ratio of κ to λ in LCDD is at least 4:1 or higher, considerably greater than the normal ratio (approximately 2:1) and reversed when compared with the predominance of λ light chains in amyloidosis.
- Amyloidosis and LCDD have many similarities, including the sites of deposition both systemically and in the kidney. However, the deposits in LCDD do not exhibit the staining properties or ultrastructural features of amyloid.
- Glomeruli in LCDD may have prominent mesangial nodules that mimic the appearance of Kimmelstiel-Wilson nodules in diabetic glomerulosclerosis. It is likely that most and possibly all cases of "nodular diabetic glomerulosclerosis" reported in patients without diabetes actually represented LCDD.
- The kidneys are the organs most frequently involved by LCDD, and renal disease usually dominates the clinical picture. Deposits may also be found in the heart, liver, lungs, endocrine glands, skin, and other organs; cardiac and hepatic involvement follows renal disease in clinical significance.
- Protein deposits with the tinctorial characteristics of amyloid are present in a very small proportion of patients; usually the amyloid deposits are a minor component.

Clinical Features

- The mean age of onset of LCDD is approximately 57 years; the male-to-female ratio is approximately 4:1.
- Patients usually initially have renal insufficiency, which is often severe and relatively acute in onset.
- Most patients have heavy proteinuria or the nephrotic syndrome; hematuria may also be present. Proteinuria is usually nonselective, with both high- and low-molecular-weight proteins present in the urine; the monoclonal protein is the predominant component in the urine in a few patients.
- The diagnosis of myeloma is often made as a result of investigation for renal insufficiency, simultaneously with the diagnosis of LCDD.

Laboratory Values

- Laboratory values often reflect the presence of multiple myeloma or other plasma cell dyscrasia. Anemia is common, as is hypogammaglobulinemia (except for the monoclonal protein, if present); hypercalcemia may be present.
- Serum creatinine and urea nitrogen levels are elevated. Urinalysis may show microscopic hematuria.

Light Microscopy

- The most common finding is deposition of eosinophilic, refractile, ribbon-like material on the interstitial side of TBMs. The deposits are PAS-positive and Congo red–negative and appear brown on silver stains. The TBM appears thickened and laminated.
- Deposits are most prominent in the medulla, around distal tubules and the loop of Henle, and sometimes around collecting tubules. Deposits may be seen around the vasa recta and lying free in the interstitium.
- Occasionally the TBM deposits are surrounded by multinucleated giant cells, apparently attempting to phagocytize the deposits.
- The tubular epithelium often appears flattened and atrophic. Occasionally the epithelium is proliferative, with multiple infoldings and apparent subdivisions of the original lumen.
- Occasional tubules contain casts, which sometimes resemble those of myeloma kidney. There appears to be an inverse relationship between the presence of myeloma-like tubular casts and glomerular deposits in LCDD.
- Glomerular lesions in LCDD are heterogeneous. In some cases, glomeruli appear unremarkable. The prototypic glomerular finding, present in approximately 60% of cases, is multiple mesangial nodules resembling diabetic nodular glomerulosclerosis (Kimmelstiel-Wilson lesions). Characteristically the nodules are rather evenly distributed, with several nodules present in each glomerulus; the nodules often appear relatively homogeneous in size. The nodules are strongly PAS-positive but do not stain with silver stains, unlike the Kimmelstiel-Wilson nodules in diabetes.
- Less advanced cases may show an increase in glomerular mesangial cells and matrix, without distinct nodules; occasional small, PAS-positive mesangial deposits may be present.
- Peripheral loops of glomerular capillaries appear thickened; the lumina may be compressed by mesangial deposits.

- Occasionally, glomeruli show an endocapillary proliferative response. This response may range from focal glomerulonephritis with closure of capillary loops to an MPGN-mesangiocapillary glomerulonephritis; extracapillary (crescentic) glomerulonephritis has been described.
- The interstitium often appears fibrotic; PAS-positive deposits may be present in the interstitium.
- Similar deposits may be present within the walls of arteries and arterioles, along with atrophy and progressive dissolution of smooth muscle cells.

Immunofluorescence Microscopy

- The majority of cases exhibit strong, linear, ribbon-like staining for κ light chains around tubules; there may be fainter, diffuse staining in the interstitium. Occasionally, staining for an immunoglobulin heavy chain is present; a minority of cases show staining for λ rather than κ.
- Glomeruli usually show linear staining of capillary walls for κ light chain, with or without staining of the mesangium. Staining of Bowman's capsule may be present. Not infrequently, glomeruli are negative on immunofluorescence or demonstrate only weak staining for complement.

Electron Microscopy

- The tubular deposits are finely granular and quite electron dense. Deposits are present around the interstitial aspect of the TBMs and also within them.
- The most common finding in glomeruli is finely granular, electron-dense deposits distributed throughout the mesangium and along the subendothelial aspects of glomerular capillary basement membranes. On occasion, the entire thickness of the glomerular basement membrane (GBM) is permeated by very finely granular material; the GBM appears more electron dense than usual, but otherwise normal ("dense transformation"). In many cases, no distinct glomerular deposits are recognizable; this may be more common in λ deposition.
- Deposits are uniformly distributed within the media of arteries and arterioles, closely applied to the smooth muscle cells.

Differential Diagnosis

- In some cases the diagnosis is straightforward and based on the histologic appearance. However, in many cases the diagnosis cannot be established without immunofluorescence and the use of antisera specific for the individual light chains.
- Diabetic glomerulosclerosis with Kimmelstiel-Wilson nodules can be a problematic differential. Both LCDD and diabetic glomerulosclerosis can exhibit mesangial nodules, thickening of glomerular capillary walls, and arterial and arteriolar hyaline deposits. Some of the histologic and staining characteristics can help in the differential (Table 19–1). Immunofluorescence staining with antisera specific for κ and λ light chains will make the correct diagnosis in most cases; TBMs and

Table 19–1

CHARACTERISTICS OF NODULES IN DIABETES VERSUS LIGHT CHAIN DEPOSITION DISEASE

Characteristic	Diabetes	Light Chain Deposition Disease
PAS reaction	Positive	Positive
Silver stains	Positive	Negative
Size	Variable within glomeruli	Uniform within glomeruli

PAS, periodic acid–Schiff.

GBMs stain for *both* κ and λ in diabetes but only one (usually κ) in LCDD. Clinical history is also of considerable assistance.
- The TBM deposits may be mistaken for the TBM thickening seen in simple tubular atrophy. The deposits in LCDD differ in being brightly refractile; the tubular outline usually appears less wrinkled and shrunken, for any given degree of TBM thickening, in LCDD than in simple atrophy.
- The glomerular appearance may resemble lobular or membranoproliferative glomerulonephritis (MPGN). However, in LCDD the mesangial nodules do not stain with silver stains, whereas they are silver positive in lobular glomerulonephritis or MPGN.

Treatment and Clinical Course

- No specific therapy for LCDD is known. When present, myeloma is treated with the usual chemotherapy regimens.
- The clinical course in LCDD is usually dominated by the renal disease. The general tendency is a progressive decline in renal function, which may be rapid. However, some patients exhibit a slower decline in glomerular filtration over the course of years.

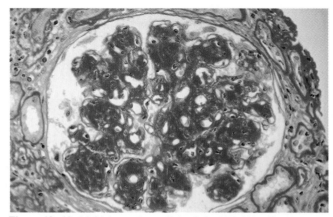

Figure 19–12. Multiple myeloma, light chain deposition disease (nodular glomerulopathy). The glomerulus displays many strongly periodic acid–Schiff–positive hypocellular mesangial nodules. The light microscopic appearance of the glomerular changes is quite reminiscent of nodular diabetic glomerulosclerosis. Additional differential diagnosis includes amyloidosis, advanced membranoproliferative (lobular) glomerulonephritis, and idiopathic lobular glomerulonephritis.

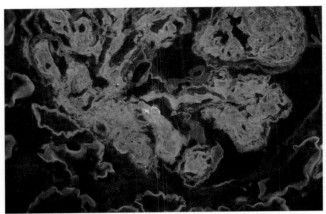

Figure 19–13. Multiple myeloma, light chain deposition disease (nodular glomerulopathy), immunofluorescence. Strong κ light chain staining is seen along the glomerular capillary basement membranes, in the mesangial areas, and along the tubular basement membranes.

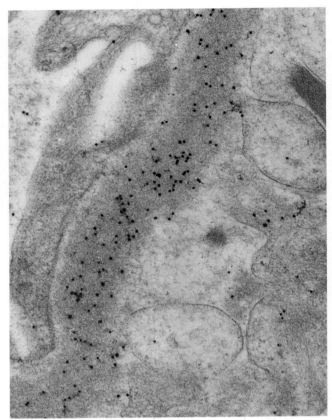

Figure 19–15. Immuno-electron microscopy, κ light chain deposition disease, κ light chain. Immunogold staining for κ light chain reveals positivity in the glomerular capillary basement membrane.

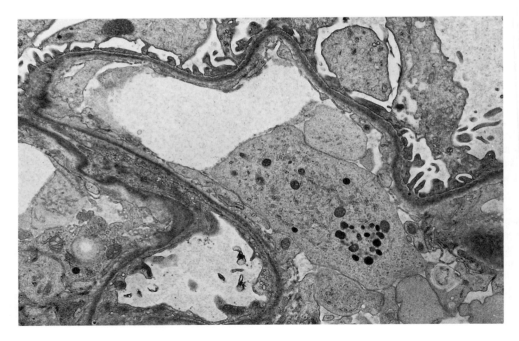

Figure 19–14. Electron micrograph, κ light chain deposition disease. Finely granular electron-dense deposits (looks dark linear) are shown along the glomerular capillary basement membrane. This ultrastructural pattern is virtually diagnostic of light chain disease, although one has to rule out dense deposit disease.

WALDENSTRÖM'S MACROGLOBULINEMIA

■ Waldenström's macroglobulinemia is an uncommon, indolent lymphoproliferative disorder associated with a monoclonal serum IgM protein. Common sites of involvement include lymph nodes, spleen, and bone marrow. The cytologic appearance varies from small lymphocytic to plasmacytoid cells.

■ The most common renal lesion of Waldenström's macroglobulinemia is glomerular intracapillary "hyaline thrombi"; these thrombi are usually positive with antibodies against IgM on immunofluorescence or immunohistochemical stains. Unlike cryoglobulinemic glomerulonephritis which also has glomerular intracapillary "hyaline thrombi," the glomeruli in Waldenström's macroglubulinemia are usually not hypercellular.

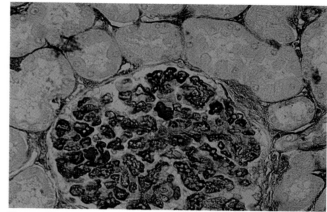

Figure 19–16. Waldenström's macroglobulinemia. Immunoperoxidase staining demonstrates glomerular (luminal and endocapillary) deposition of IgM (immunoperoxidase, IgM).

AMYLOIDOSIS

Biology of Disease

■ The category of amyloidosis includes a heterogeneous group of conditions, all of which feature the deposition of one of a variety of proteins in a β-pleated sheet configuration. The β-pleated sheet configuration gives the deposits the typical histologic appearance, the affinity for Congo red and thioflavine T fluorescence, and the characteristic ultrastructural appearance of amyloid.

■ The term *amyloid* ("starch-like") refers to the fact that tissues with amyloid turn blue after treatment with iodide followed by sulfuric acid, as starch does.

■ In the past, cases were classified primarily according to the clinical setting and the pattern of organ involvement. Cases were classified as "primary" if there was no obvious underlying cause, "secondary" if there was a predisposing condition such as chronic infection or inflammation, "myeloma associated" if the patient had multiple myeloma, and "hereditary" if there was a family history of amyloidosis. However, the distinction between the different types was not always clear, and there was overlap in the patterns of organ involvement between the different categories.

■ At present, the most logical classification appears to be based on the protein that makes up the deposits (Table 19–2). However, no single classification system has yet been universally accepted, and terms are used inconsistently by different experts. In particular, the term *primary amyloidosis* is used by some to indicate all cases composed of immunoglobulin light chains (AL amyloid), whereas others exclude from the category those cases associated with myeloma. In addition, it may be difficult to determine the exact nature of the protein component in some cases.

■ Overall, approximately 90% of cases of systemic amyloidosis are the AL type; most of the remainder are the AA type.

■ The protein in AL amyloid is a monoclonal immunoglobulin light chain or a fragment of a light chain. This category includes most cases formerly classified as "primary" amyloidosis, as well as amyloidosis associated with multiple myeloma. There is a preponderance of λ light chain over κ (approximately 4:1), contrary to the normal ratio and the reverse of the ratio of κ to λ in LCDD. Certain segments of the λ gene are overrepresented in amyloidosis, probably because light chains containing those specific segments are predisposed to precipitate in the β-pleated sheet configuration. Approximately one third of cases of AL amyloidosis are associated with overt multiple myeloma; the remaining cases also represent a plasma cell dyscrasia; however, the number of plasma cells in the bone marrow is lower (fewer than 10%) and the patients do not have the other stigmata of myeloma. Study of bone marrow plasma cells in these patients demonstrates an imbalance of light chain expression, and a monoclonal protein containing the same light chain type present in the deposits can also be found in the serum and/or urine of most patients.

■ The protein in AA amyloid is derived from a serum protein known as "serum amyloid–associated" (SAA) protein. This protein acts as an acute phase reactant and is present in elevated levels in the serum of patients with chronic inflammatory conditions such as chronic infections (tuberculosis, syphilis, osteomyelitis, parasitic infections, and others), chronic rheumatologic diseases (rheumatoid arthritis, adult Still's disease [juvenile rheumatoid arthritis], ankylosing spondylitis, Behçet's syndrome, and others), and other conditions (chronic inflammatory bowel disease, familial Mediterranean fe-

Table 19–2
CLASSIFICATION OF AMYLOIDOSIS BASED ON THE PROTEIN COMPONENT

Designation	Component Protein	Examples
AL (primary amyloidosis)	Monoclonal immunoglobulin light chain (usually λ)	Primary amyloidosis without myeloma Myeloma associated
AA (secondary amyloidosis)	Serum amyloid–associated protein degradation products	Chronic infections Rheumatoid arthritis, other rheumatologic disorders Neoplasms: Hodgkin's, renal cell carcinoma Familial Mediterranean fever
AF (familial)	Transthyretin (prealbumin)	Familial amyloidotic polyneuropathy Familial amyloid cardiomyopathy Senile systemic amyloidosis
AE (endocrine)	Hormones or prohormones	Medullary carcinoma of the thyroid: calcitonin Islet cell tumors (insulinoma, gastrinoma)
$A\beta_2M$	β_2-Microglobulin	Hemodialysis-associated myeloma

ver). Rheumatoid arthritis and similar diseases have replaced tuberculosis and syphilis as the most common conditions predisposing to AA amyloidosis in the United States, but chronic infections remain the most common conditions predisposing to AA amyloidosis worldwide. Cutaneous injections ("skin popping") of heroin or other narcotics may cause amyloidosis in drug abusers. AA amyloidosis can also be seen in patients with malignancies, including carcinomas (most often renal cell carcinoma) and Hodgkin's disease. In only a minority of patients with such chronic inflammatory conditions does amyloidosis develop; it is believed that either a defect in macrophage processing of SAA or a mutation in the sequence of the protein causes the protein to accumulate and precipitate as amyloid.

■ Other forms of amyloidosis are uncommon. Examples include the familial variants, most of which are due to abnormalities in the serum protein *transthyretin* (also known as *prealbumin*), and the endocrine variants caused by production of hormones or hormone precursors by neoplasms of endocrine cells (such as the production of calcitonin by medullary carcinomas of the thyroid).

■ A new form of amyloidosis that is of particular interest to nephrologists is hemodialysis-associated amyloidosis, which is due to the accumulation of β_2-microglobulin. β_2-Microglobulin is normally excreted by the kidneys but is not cleared by hemodialysis. Therefore it accumulates in the serum of patients maintained on long-term hemodialysis. β_2-Microglobulin is closely related to the immunoglobulin light chains and has the capacity to precipitate as β-pleated sheets. Carpal tunnel syndrome is a common manifestation of dialysis-associated amyloidosis.

■ A wide variety of organs and tissues can be involved by amyloid deposits, including the kidneys, heart, liver, spleen, gastrointestinal tract, tongue, adrenal glands, nerves, skin, and many others—in essence, every organ and tissue in the body. The organs of most clinical importance are the kidneys, the heart, and the liver.

■ Tissue biopsy is required to establish the diagnosis of amyloidosis. The rectum, skin, and gingiva may be fruitful sites to biopsy; aspiration of the abdominal fat pad and staining for amyloid have been advocated as a

noninvasive way to make the diagnosis, but this technique has been disappointing in our experience. Renal biopsy has a high probability of being diagnostic if proteinuria or renal insufficiency is present.

■ The histologic and ultrastructural appearance of the deposits in all types of amyloid is the same. Identification of the specific type of amyloid in an individual case can be difficult. The clinical setting (pattern of involvement, existence of underlying conditions, family history of amyloidosis) may be helpful. Serum and urine protein electrophoresis and bone marrow examination should be done to identify or exclude a plasma cell dyscrasia. Antibodies are available for immunohistochemical identification of specific amyloid components such as immunoglobulin light chains and the AA protein; however, the results may be difficult to interpret in some cases.

■ Amyloid of the AA type loses its affinity for Congo red after treatment with potassium permanganate in the majority of cases (approximately 85%), whereas AL amyloid is generally resistant. However, rather massive accumulation of amyloid is required to demonstrate this phenomenon, and both false-positive and false-negative results for AA amyloid can occur.

Clinical Features

■ The common forms of amyloid (AL and AA) typically exhibit widespread involvement, and renal disease is frequent. The inherited forms of amyloid are often associated with neuropathy or other limited involvement, and amyloid associated with endocrine tumors is often manifested as localized disease; renal involvement is less common in these forms, and they will not be discussed further.

■ Renal involvement in amyloidosis usually takes the form of proteinuria, which is present in up to 80% of patients and may be massive; the nephrotic syndrome may be present in up to one third of patients. Serum creatinine levels are increased in up to half of patients when initially evaluated.

■ Cardiac involvement causes congestive heart failure and cardiac dysrhythmias.

Laboratory Values

- Laboratory values are usually nonspecific.
- Routine serum protein electrophoresis demonstrates a monoclonal protein in fewer than half of patients with AL amyloidosis; immunoelectrophoresis or immunofixation may detect a monoclonal protein in up to two thirds.
- A monoclonal protein is present in the urine in approximately two thirds of patients with AL amyloidosis; again, immunoelectrophoresis or immunofixation on concentrated urine may be more sensitive than routine electrophoresis.

Gross Appearance

- The kidneys are typically enlarged and pale, with a smooth cortical surface.
- In up to 10% of patients the kidneys are normal sized or small, and the surface may be scarred or finely granular because of preexisting vascular disease.
- On section, the parenchyma appears pale, and the distinction between cortex and medulla may be poorly defined.

Light Microscopy

- Amyloid appears amorphous, pink, and acellular on hematoxylin and eosin (H & E) stain. It characteristically does not stain with the PAS reaction or with silver stains.
- Amyloid has high affinity for Congo red; under polarized light, sections stained with Congo red demonstrate a characteristic "apple-green" or yellow-green birefringence. (It should be noted here that sections to be stained with Congo red should be 6 to 8 μm in thickness, much thicker than the usual histologic sections required for diagnosis of renal disease.)
- Amyloid is metachromatic; methyl violet stains amyloid purple against a blue background. Unfortunately, relatively large amounts of amyloid must be present to demonstrate this property.
- Amyloid stained with thioflavine T fluoresces under ultraviolet light; fluorescence with thioflavine T is not totally specific for amyloid, but it is sensitive.

Glomeruli

- Glomeruli are involved in virtually all cases of AA amyloidosis but are said to be involved in only one third of cases of AL amyloidosis. The appearance of involved glomeruli is identical in the two conditions.
- In most cases the initial amyloid deposits occur in the mesangium (described as the *mesangial form* of amyloidosis); involvement of glomerular capillary loops occurs relatively late. In a minority of cases, mesangial and capillary involvement is simultaneous (*diffuse form*).
- Initially, mesangial deposits may be segmental and irregularly distributed within and between glomeruli and may appear most prominent near the vascular pole. With progressive accumulation the deposits may form nodules, and the distribution becomes more uniform both within and between glomeruli. Mesangial cells may appear pushed to the periphery of the deposits, but mesangial cellularity is usually normal.
- The initial capillary loop deposits are primarily located in the subendothelial space; in more advanced cases there may be large, irregular subepithelial deposits in addition to subendothelial deposits. On silver stains, the GBM usually appears continuous between subepithelial and subendothelial deposits, but in some cases deposits apparently span the width of the capillary wall.
- Subepithelial deposits tend to form parallel spicules oriented perpendicularly to the basement membrane. In this location they demonstrate increased affinity for silver stains (probably related to the time course of amyloid deposition) and produce a spike-like appearance that may mimic membranous glomerulonephropathy (MGN).
- Eventually the glomerulus is overwhelmed and replaced by amyloid deposits, with the appearance of global glomerular sclerosis. In contrast to typical sclerotic glomeruli, which are small, in amyloidosis the obliterated glomeruli are often large. Residual deposits of amyloid may be visible; however, these tend to lose their usual amyloid staining characteristics over time.
- Occasionally, proliferation of visceral and parietal epithelium may give the appearance of a crescent in Bowman's space. In other cases, multinucleated giant cells may surround amyloid deposits, apparently attempting to phagocytize the amyloid.
- The glomeruli in amyloidosis may appear essentially normal by routine light microscopy; electron microscopy is required for diagnosis in such cases.

Tubules

- Initially, tubules may show no recognizable changes or show only cytoplasmic protein resorption droplets. However, examination of sections stained with thioflavine T under ultraviolet light may reveal minute deposits along the TBMs.
- Progressive accumulation of amyloid may result in thickened, wrinkled TBMs associated with tubular atrophy. Distal tubules and the loops of Henle are characteristically most prominently involved.
- Tubular casts are often present, but they usually do not resemble the casts seen in myeloma kidney. Occasionally (most often in patients with myeloma), the casts may appear laminated; the outer layers of casts may demonstrate the staining characteristics of amyloid. The appearance of atrophic tubules with hyaline casts may suggest "thyroidization" as seen in chronic pyelonephritis.
- In occasional cases tubular deposits predominate, with inconspicuous deposits in glomeruli and vessels.
- Tubular casts may occasionally demonstrate affinity for Congo red and even "apple-green" birefringence under polarized light. In the absence of *tissue* deposits of amyloid-like material with the appropriate tinctorial characteristics, this appearance in casts should not be interpreted as representing amyloid.

Vessels

- Vessels of all sizes, both arteries and veins, may be involved; involvement of arcuate and interlobular arteries is often striking. Amyloid deposits occur in all layers of vessel walls; the lumen may be occluded.
- Thrombosis of branches of the renal vein may occur and extend into the main renal veins. This situation may precipitate acute renal failure.
- Vascular involvement may predominate, with minimal or no glomerular deposits, particularly in AL amyloidosis. When both are present, there is usually a general correlation between the degree of glomerular and vascular involvement, but massive vascular deposits may be present in the presence of mild glomerular disease and vice versa.

Interstitium

- Deposits of amyloid in TBMs and vasa recta may extend into the interstitium. In addition, masses of amyloid may accumulate in the interstitium, particularly in the inner medulla.

Immunofluorescence Microscopy

- In the experience of many pathologists, immunofluorescence in amyloidosis is often difficult to interpret because of the nonspecific absorption of multiple immunoreactants by the deposits.
- Others have reported a high degree of concordance between immunofluorescence staining for κ or λ immunoglobulin light chains or for AA protein and the type of amyloidosis as determined by other methods.
- Antibodies are available for the AA protein and for the amyloid P protein, which is found in all varieties of amyloid.
- Immunohistochemical staining for κ and λ on fixed, paraffin-embedded tissue may be more variable and more difficult to interpret than immunofluorescence on frozen tissue.

Electron Microscopy

- The characteristic ultrastructural feature of amyloidosis is linear, rigid-appearing, nonbranching fibrils. The fibrils have a diameter of 8 to 10 nm and may be up to 1 μm in length. The fibrils may appear beaded, with a periodicity of 5.5 nm. The fibrils are randomly arranged, reminiscent of children's jackstraws or "pick up sticks." They tend to form compact arrays when adjacent to cell membranes and more loose arrays when away from cell surfaces.
- In the glomerulus, fibrils are first found in the mesangium. They appear to spread from the mesangium into the peripheral capillary wall, eventually encompassing the entire circumference. Fibrils are initially seen in the subendothelial space, but in more advanced cases they are found within the substance of the GBM and the subepithelial space.
- In the subepithelial space, fibrils are often arranged in bundles oriented perpendicularly to the GBM. These bundles may be quite long; in some cases the appearance has been likened to that of "church spires."

- In active cases the glomerular capillary basement membrane is frequently fragmented and attenuated or may be completely absent in areas. In cases in which progress of the disease has been arrested, the GBM may have a double-contour, lattice-like arrangement with new basement membrane material on the epithelial side of the deposits. The fibrils appear to sit in lacunae; the fibrils themselves may appear to be partially reabsorbed.
- Glomerular visceral epithelial cell foot processes may be effaced, and often, multiple zones of foot process detachment from the GBM can be seen.

Differential Diagnosis

- The presence of nodules in the glomerular mesangium may suggest diabetic glomerulosclerosis. However, capillary loops are characteristically involved early in the course of diabetic glomerulosclerosis, whereas capillary loop involvement tends to be relatively late in amyloidosis. In diabetes, the mesangial regions tend to be hypercellular early in the course of the disease, whereas in amyloidosis, the mesangial regions tend to be hypocellular. The mesangial nodules in diabetes stain with PAS and silver stains, whereas those in amyloidosis do not. The affinity of amyloid for Congo red and the characteristic birefringence under polarized light should also assist in differentiating the two.
- Light chain deposition disease may also resemble amyloidosis on H & E stain. However, LCDD does not demonstrate affinity for Congo red; immunofluorescence and ultrastructural examination should distinguish amyloidosis from LCDD.
- Fibrillary glomerulonephritis and immunotactoid glomerulopathy (IT) may resemble amyloidosis both on H & E stain and under the electron microscope. The reaction with Congo red is an important differentiating feature; both fibrillary glomerulonephritis and IT lack the characteristic affinity demonstrated by amyloid. Measuring the diameter of the fibrils on electron microscopy is also important in differentiating these conditions.
- The presence of subepithelial spikes on silver stains in amyloidosis may mimic membranous glomerulonephropathy (MGN). The appearance of the spikes in amyloidosis tends to be more variable than in MGN; the presence of similar spikes in Bowman's capsule and along the inner side of TBMs would indicate amyloidosis rather than MGN.

Treatment and Clinical Course

- No specific treatment is known for amyloidosis. Efforts to control the disease depend on control of the primary disease process causing the amyloid. Cases of AL amyloidosis associated with multiple myeloma are usually treated with chemotherapy regimens for myeloma; the same regimens are sometimes used in patients with AL amyloidosis not associated with myeloma ("primary" amyloidosis). Renal transplantation has been performed in some cases of amyloidosis, with reasonable results.
- The prognosis of AL amyloid is generally poor. Median survival in cases associated with multiple myeloma is usually 1 year or less; patients without mye-

loma do slightly better, with median survivals of approximately 2 to 2.5 years.

■ The prognosis of AA amyloid depends on the primary disease process and whether it can be controlled. The prognosis also depends on the sites of organ involve-

ment in a specific case; cardiac and renal involvement in particular have very adverse prognostic implications.

■ Cardiac disease is the most common mechanism of death in patients with amyloidosis, followed by renal disease.

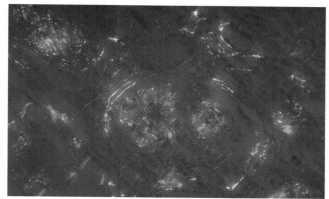

Figure 19–17. Amyloidosis. A Congo red–stained section reveals apple-green birefringence under polarized light. This stain is the most specific for amyloid.

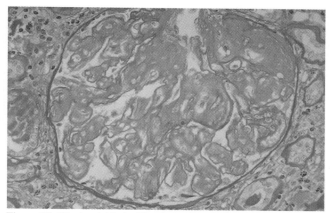

Figure 19–20. Amyloidosis. The glomerulus displays replacement of the glomerular tuft with mesangial widening and thickening of the capillary walls because of deposition of the homogeneous eosinophilic acellular amyloid material. The capillary lumina are totally narrowed/occluded.

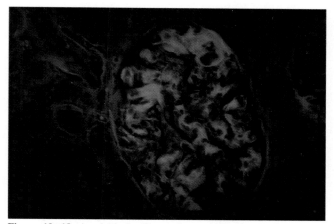

Figure 19–18. Amyloidosis. Glomerular positivity is seen in a Congo red–stained section under fluorescent light.

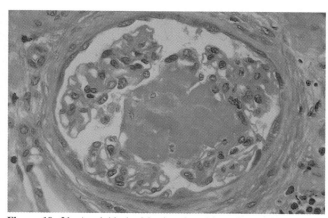

Figure 19–21. Amyloidosis. Massive deposition of amyloid (homogeneous eosinophil material on hematoxylin and eosin–stained sections) in the glomerulus produced a large nodule in the center of the glomerulus.

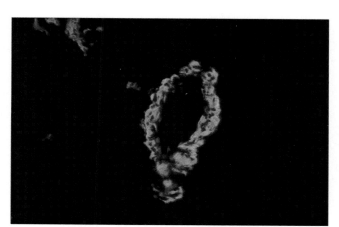

Figure 19–19. Amyloidosis. A thioflavine T–stained section under fluorescein light depicts amyloid deposition in an artery. This stain is the most sensitive for amyloid.

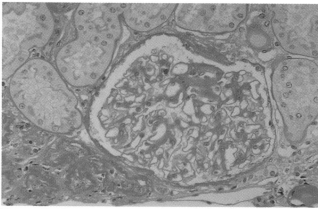

Figure 19–22. Amyloidosis. The glomerulus depicts the mild/early change in glomerular amyloidosis: slight mesangial widening without cellular proliferation. A few capillary walls are also thickened. The disease may be so mild that the diagnosis can be missed without special stains (Congo red) and/or EM.

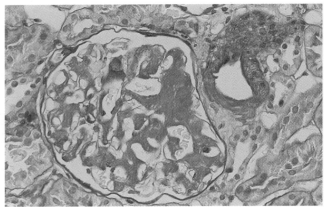

Figure 19–23. Amyloidosis. The widened mesangial areas reveal periodic acid–Schiff (PAS)-positive deposition of homogeneous acellular material (amyloid). A few capillary walls are also widened (PAS reaction).

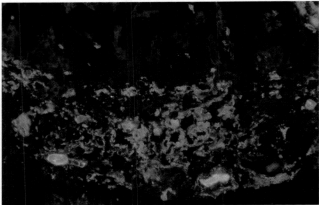

Figure 19–26. Amyloidosis (AL-type), immunofluorescence. Massive κ light chain–positive interstitial amyloid deposits are seen in a patient with κ light chain–positive multiple myeloma. Light chain amyloid in the kidney is, however, more commonly λ light chain positive.

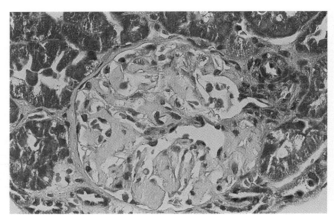

Figure 19–24. Amyloidosis. On trichrome-stained sections amyloid shows pale blue reactivity (Masson's trichrome stain).

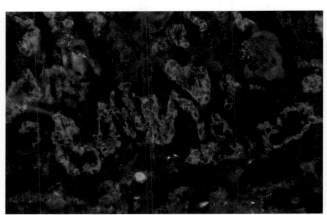

Figure 19–27. Amyloidosis, immunofluorescence. λ light chain staining is completely negative in the same case shown in Figure 19–26.

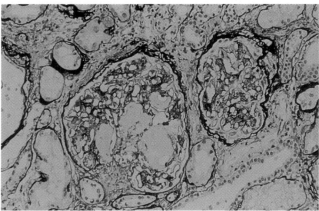

Figure 19–25. Amyloidosis. A methenamine silver–stained section depicts two glomeruli with large mesangial acellular silver-negative amyloid deposits.

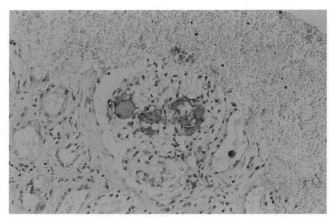

Figure 19–28. Amyloidosis, streptavidin peroxidase method. AA amyloid is seen in the glomerular mesangial amyloid deposits in a transplanted kidney. This is suggestive of "secondary" amyloidosis (i.e., associated with inflammation).

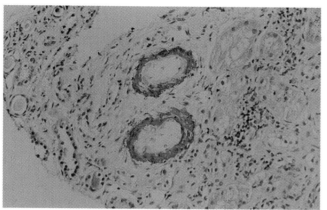

Figure 19–29. Amyloidosis, streptavidin peroxidase method. Interlobular arteries reveal strong reactivity with antibodies against AA amyloid in a transplanted kidney from the same case as shown in Figure 19–28.

Figure 19–30. Electron micrograph, renal amyloidosis. The bulk of the amyloid is present in the mesangium *(M)*; amyloid fibrils are also seen outside the basement membrane with the typical spikes *(S)*. The outline of the original basement membrane is still visible as a pale linear structure *(arrows)*. Note the narrowed glomerular capillary lumen with largely intact basement membrane *(C)*.

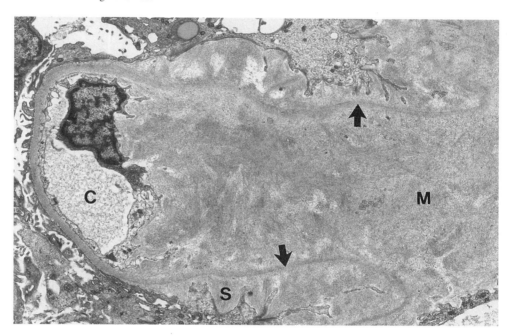

Figure 19–31. Electron micrograph, renal amyloidosis. Massive mesangial deposition of amyloid *(A)* is seen with significant mesangial widening and severe narrowing of the glomerular capillary lumina. In advanced stages of the disease the rigid-appearing, nonbranching long amyloid fibrils appear on both sides of the glomerular capillary basement membranes as well as within the basement membranes *(C, glomerular capillary lumina)*.

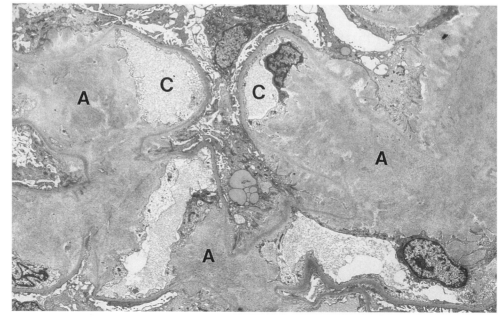

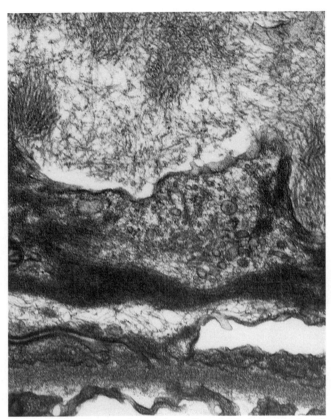

Figure 19–32. Electron micrograph, renal amyloidosis. Randomly oriented, extracellular, rigid-appearing, long nonbranching amyloid fibrils (8 to 12 nm in width) are seen beneath the visceral epithelium in a patient with advanced disease. Ultrastructural differentiation of amyloid fibrils from other fibrillary structures in the kidney is primarily based on the size of the fibrils.

THE FIBRILLARY GLOMERULOPATHIES: FIBRILLARY GLOMERULONEPHRITIS AND IMMUNOTACTOID GLOMERULOPATHY (IT)

■ Fibrillary glomerulonephritis and IT are recently described, relatively uncommon entities characterized by the presence of fibrillar or microtubular deposits on ultrastructural examination.

■ It is controversial whether fibrillary glomerulonephritis and IT represent two distinct diseases, different variants of a single disease, or merely ultrastructural appearances that may be caused by a variety of conditions. No classification or definition of the entities is universally accepted as yet; clinicopathologic studies are difficult to interpret because of heterogeneous patient populations. The clinical features of the two are very similar, but it is not clear whether the outlook for renal survival differs; no therapy has yet been shown to be beneficial for either condition. Therefore it is not yet clear whether the different ultrastructural appearances are clinically sufficient to mandate retention of the distinction. We believe that the morphologic differences between the two conditions are sufficient to justify maintaining them as separate entities, at least for the present, and therefore they will be discussed individually. As additional clinicopathologic studies accumulate, a preponderance of evidence may come to favor one opinion over the other, and either the "lumpers" or the "splitters" will triumph.

■ Differences between amyloidosis, fibrillary glomerulonephritis, and IT are summarized in Table 19–3.

Fibrillary Glomerulonephritis

Synonyms and Related Terms: Congo red–negative amyloid-like glomerulonephropathy.

Table 19-3

SUMMARY OF THE FEATURES OF AMYLOIDOSIS, FIBRILLARY GLOMERULONEPHRITIS, AND IMMUNOTACTOID GLOMERULOPATHY

Characteristic	Amyloid	Fibrillary Glomerulonephritis	Immunotactoid Glomerulopathy
Deposit structure	Fibrillar	Fibrillar	Microtubules
Arrangement	Random	Random	Parallel arrays
Diameter (nm)	Average, 8–10	Average, 20	Average, 40
		Range, 15–30	Range, >30
Component	Various	IgG, C3	IgG, C3
Monoclonal	AL amyloid	Minority (10%)	Majority (90%)
Light chain	$\lambda > \kappa$	κ (monoclonal cases)	κ
Extrarenal deposits	Majority of cases	Rare	Occasional

Biology of Disease

- The cause or causes of fibrillary glomerulonephritis are unknown. The fibrils appear to represent immune complexes, but the reasons why they are deposited in glomeruli and the mechanisms that lead to their characteristic fibrillar structure are unknown.
- The immunoglobulins in the deposits in fibrillary glomerulonephritis are usually polyclonal; light chains of both the κ and λ type are present in the majority of cases. A minority of cases contain a single light chain type, which suggests a clonal plasma cell disorder.
- Studies by Iskandar, Falk, and Jennette found that even in patients with deposits composed of polyclonal IgG, the IgG4 subclass was the exclusive or predominant subclass present. Because IgG4 is the least common subclass of IgG in serum, the predominance of that subclass in deposits suggests that some characteristic of IgG4 molecules predisposes to the ultrastructural appearance of the fibrils.
- In most cases, fibrillary glomerulonephritis is not associated with plasma cell dyscrasias, other lymphoproliferative disorders, or other systemic illnesses. This finding is in contrast with amyloidosis, which is frequently associated with lymphoproliferative disorders or other systemic diseases.
- The fibrillar deposits usually appear to be confined to the kidneys; in rare cases, deposits have been described in other organs such as the lungs.

Clinical Features

- The average age at onset is approximately 50 years, but the age range is wide.
- The majority of patients have heavy proteinuria; many have the nephrotic syndrome. Microhematuria is common.
- Many have renal insufficiency at diagnosis; hypertension is frequent.

Laboratory Values

- The usual serologic screening tests (antinuclear antibodies, antinuclear cytoplasmic antibodies, etc.) are absent. Serum complement levels are usually normal.
- No monoclonal proteins are present in the serum or urine.

Gross Appearance

- The gross appearance of kidneys with fibrillary glomerulonephritis has not been well described.

Light Microscopy

Glomeruli

- The glomerular changes are quite heterogeneous. The glomerular appearance on sections stained with H & E may vary from mesangioproliferative glomerulonephritis to MGN, MPGN, or crescentic glomerulonephritis.
- The most common changes are mesangial matrix expansion, thickening of peripheral capillary walls, and variable mesangial hypercellularity, which are found in the majority of cases.
- Deposits that are PAS positive may be visible in the mesangium and sometimes in peripheral capillary loops.
- A pattern resembling MPGN with circumferential mesangial interposition in peripheral capillary loops occurs in up to half of cases in some series.
- Crescents in Bowman's space may be found in up to one quarter of cases; the proportion of glomeruli involved varies from 10% to 80%. In some series, most crescents are primarily fibrous and associated with glomerular scarring.
- A variable proportion of globally obsolescent glomeruli are usually present.
- The glomerular deposits do not stain with Congo red, crystal violet, or thioflavine T.

Tubules and Interstitium

- Protein resorption droplets are present in proximal convoluted tubular epithelial cells.
- A variable amount of tubular atrophy, interstitial fibrosis, and interstitial lymphocytic infiltration is present, generally in proportion to the degree of glomerular obsolescence.

Vessels

- Arteries and arterioles may show hyalinization and thickening, usually commensurate with the proportion of obsolescent glomeruli.

Immunofluorescence Microscopy

■ Intense staining for IgG is seen in glomeruli in virtually all cases. Staining for IgM and IgA is less common and usually much less intense. In most cases there is strong staining for *both* κ and λ light chains; rarely, staining for a single light chain, usually κ, is seen. Staining for C3 is almost always present, usually slightly less intense than the staining for IgG; weak staining for early complement components (C1q or C4) is seen in a minority of cases.

■ In most cases there is staining in the glomerular mesangium, with diffuse or segmental staining of peripheral capillary loops. Mesangial staining is confluent, with irregular margins; capillary staining usually appears linear or ribbon-like rather than granular.

■ Tubules and vessels usually do not show significant immunofluorescent staining.

Electron Microscopy

■ The key ultrastructural feature is nonbranching, linear, randomly arranged fibrils resembling those of amyloid but approximately twice as thick. The diameter of the fibrils, measured on electron microscopic pictures, averages approximately 20 nm, with a range of approximately 10 to 30 nm (the diameter measured in different laboratories may vary depending on the method of measurement used). The fibrils do not have an inner core or an organized substructure. Ill-defined areas of greater density or granular electron-dense deposits may be present and admixed with the linear fibrils.

■ Abundant fibrils are present in the glomerular mesangium in all cases and extend into peripheral capillary loops in most cases. Deposits may also be found in Bowman's capsule. In glomerular capillaries, fibrils may be found in the subendothelial space, in the subepithelial space, and within the capillary basement membrane itself. The capillary wall deposits distort the GBM; sometimes synthesis of new basement membrane material is seen at the periphery of subepithelial or subendothelial deposits.

■ Glomerular visceral epithelial cell foot processes are diffusely effaced and there is microvillous transformation of visceral epithelial cells, both of which are consequences of the proteinuria.

■ Fibrillar deposits are not seen in tubules or vessels.

Differential Diagnosis

■ The most important differential diagnosis is amyloidosis. The deposits in fibrillary glomerulonephritis do not demonstrate the usual staining with Congo red, methyl violet, and thioflavine T seen with amyloid, and sections stained with Congo red do not demonstrate "apple-green" birefringence under polarized light. The fibrils in fibrillary glomerulonephritis average approximately 20 nm in diameter as opposed to the average 8- to 10-nm diameter of amyloid fibrils.

■ Immunotactoid glomerulopathy may resemble fibrillary glomerulonephritis histologically. However, on ultrastructural examination, the deposits in IT are cylindrical or tubular and average approximately 40 nm in diameter.

■ Small, scattered accumulations of fibrils may be seen in the glomerular mesangium in a variety of sclerosing processes and could be confused with the fibrils of fibrillary glomerulonephritis. These reactive nonspecific fibrils average approximately 10 nm in diameter (range, 5 to 20 nm) and tend to be more irregular than the fibrils of fibrillary glomerulonephritis.

Treatment and Clinical Course

■ Approximately half of patients with fibrillary glomerulonephritis progress to end-stage renal disease within a short time from diagnosis (median time, approximately 2 years); the remainder of patients tend to have relatively stable renal function. Patients who are older or have established renal insufficiency at diagnosis have a high probability of progressing to renal failure.

■ No effective treatment of fibrillary glomerulonephritis is known. Corticosteroids have been tried in small groups of patients, with little or no apparent benefit.

■ Recurrence of fibrillary glomerulonephritis in a transplanted kidney has been noted in at least one patient. Recurrent proteinuria developed in that patient approximately 5.5 years posttransplant; biopsy of the transplant showed histologic and ultrastructural features similar to those of the native kidney pretransplant.

Immunotactoid Glomerulopathy (IT)
Biology of Disease

■ Immunotactoid glomerulopathy is a poorly understood disorder characterized by glomerular deposits consisting of organized microtubules, which most likely represent immune complexes.

■ The deposits in IT differ from those in fibrillary glomerulonephritis in several respects. The average size of the deposits in IT is larger than that of the fibrils in fibrillary glomerulonephritis, although there is overlap between the two conditions. The deposits in IT often have a definite structure consisting of organized microtubules with a hollow core, frequently arranged in parallel arrays, in contrast to the linear, randomly arranged fibrils of fibrillary glomerulonephritis.

■ On immunofluorescence only a single immunoglobulin light chain (usually κ) is present in the majority of cases of IT, thus suggesting the presence of an underlying monoclonal gammopathy.

■ In some series, cases in which the diagnosis of IT was based on the presence of characteristic microtubules have been associated with lymphoproliferative disorders (chronic lymphocytic leukemia) or other systemic diseases (Sjögren's syndrome, leukocytoclastic vasculitis). In the opinion of some experts (Dr. Melvin Schwartz and colleagues), such an association *precludes* the diagnosis of IT; those experts would include such cases in the category of the primary illness (for example, glomerular disease associated with chronic lymphocytic leukemia) rather than IT.

- The appearance of the organized deposits resembles that of the deposits often seen in cryoglobulinemia, and similar deposits are sometimes seen in patients with systemic lupus erythematosus. Therefore, cryoglobulinemia and systemic lupus should be excluded before a diagnosis of IT is made.

Clinical Features

- The average age at diagnosis is approximately 60 years, about 10 years older than the average age of patients with fibrillary glomerulonephritis at diagnosis. However, there is a wide age range in both conditions, with considerable overlap.
- The majority of patients have heavy proteinuria; in some series, more than half have nephrotic syndrome.
- Some series have suggested that patients with IT have better preservation of renal function at diagnosis than do most patients with fibrillary glomerulonephritis; however, this suggestion requires confirmation.

Laboratory Values

- Routine serologic screening tests for autoimmune disease are negative, as is assay for serum cryoglobulins.

Gross Appearance

- The gross appearance of the kidneys in IT has not been well characterized.

Light Microscopy

- The glomerular appearance in IT is heterogeneous, and there is considerable overlap with fibrillary glomerulonephritis.
- The various glomerular appearances can include mesangial expansion alone, mesangial expansion with variable mesangial hypercellularity, MGN, mesangial expansion with thickening of capillary walls similar to MPGN, and diffuse proliferative glomerulonephritis.
- The glomerular capillary basement membranes may appear thickened, irregular, or reduplicated ("tram-track") on PAS or silver stains.
- Staining with Congo red is usually absent, and "apple-green" birefringence is not present under polarized light. Staining for thioflavine T is usually absent.
- Nonspecific tubular atrophy, interstitial fibrosis and chronic inflammation, and arterial and arteriolar sclerosis may occur, generally in proportion to the degree of glomerular injury and scarring.

Immunofluorescence Microscopy

- Typically, strong mesangial and capillary wall staining for IgG is noted; staining for C3 is present in the same distribution, but usually of slightly less intensity. Staining for other immunoglobulins is occasionally present. In some series, capillary wall staining with little or no mesangial staining is described.
- Approximately 90% of cases demonstrate strong staining for κ immunoglobulin light chain and no staining

for λ light chain. Staining for *both* κ and λ is seen in the remaining cases.
- Tubules and vessels usually exhibit no immunofluorescence staining or nonspecific staining only.

Electron Microscopy

- The defining feature of IT is the presence of electron-dense microtubules within glomeruli. The microtubules usually have a hollow core and are often arranged in parallel arrays.
- The microtubules average approximately 40 nm in diameter; they are almost always 30 nm or greater in diameter. Thus there is little overlap with the usual range in diameter of the fibrils in fibrillary glomerulonephritis. However, microtubules as small as 20 nm in diameter have been described. The microtubules in a single case appear to be relatively uniform; however, the diameter of the microtubules varies between cases.
- Microtubules are usually present in the mesangium. They are often present in a subendothelial location in peripheral glomerular capillary loops and may also be present in a subepithelial (epimembranous) location.
- Synthesis of new basement membrane–like material may be seen beneath subendothelial deposits or covering subepithelial deposits.
- Deposits of microtubules may occasionally be seen in the interstitium.

Differential Diagnosis

- The differential diagnosis with amyloidosis and fibrillary glomerulonephritis was discussed earlier.
- The ultrastructural appearance of the microtubules may strongly resemble that of the immune complex deposits seen in cryoglobulinemia; the histologic appearance of glomeruli in IT can also resemble that in cryoglobulinemia. The most common glomerular appearance in cryoglobulinemic glomerulonephritis is that of MPGN, often with an exuberant glomerular infiltration of leukocytes (mostly monocytes); this appearance can also occur in IT and is the most common appearance in some series. Hyaline intraluminal thrombi may be seen in glomerular capillaries in cryoglobulinemia. Ultimately, a serum assay for cryoglobulins may be required to distinguish IT from cryoglobulinemia.

Treatment and Clinical Course

- No treatment has been shown to be effective in IT. Corticosteroids have been tried, but results have generally been disappointing.
- The outlook for renal survival in patients with IT is not clear. In some series, patients with IT have appeared to have better preservation of renal function than did patients with fibrillary glomerulonephritis. However, other series have found little difference in long-term renal function between the two conditions, with a significant proportion of cases of IT progressing to chronic renal insufficiency.

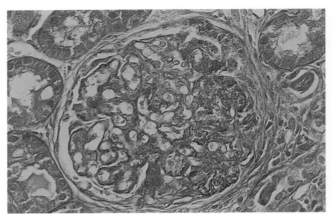

Figure 19–33. Fibrillary glomerulonephritis. Segmentally accentuated sclerosis is present in the glomerulus; the nonsclerotic glomerular segments have thickened capillary walls (Masson's trichrome stain).

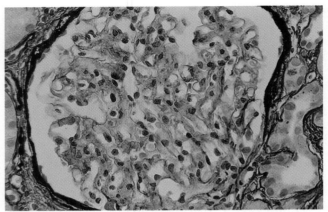

Figure 19–34. Fibrillary glomerulonephritis. The widened mesangium and the thickened glomerular capillary walls are silver negative (methenamine silver stain).

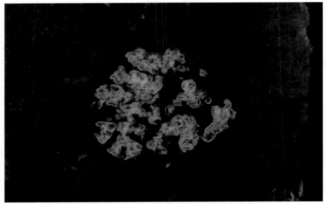

Figure 19–35. Fibrillary glomerulonephritis, immunofluorescence. IgG staining is seen in the glomerular mesangium and also along the glomerular capillary walls. The most commonly seen IgG subset in fibrillary glomerulonephritis is IgG4.

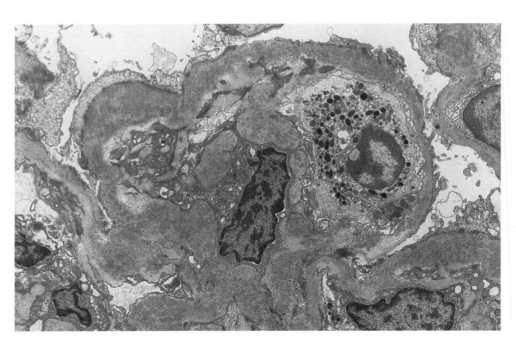

Figure 19–36. Electron micrograph, fibrillary glomerulonephritis. This low-magnification photograph shows randomly arranged fibrils in the mesangial areas and within the glomerular capillary basement membranes.

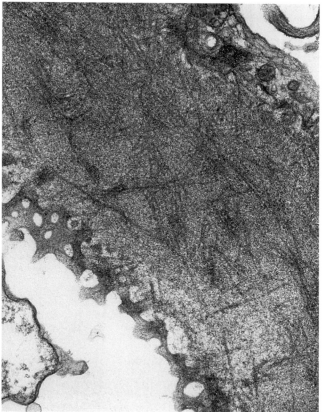

Figure 19–37. Electron micrograph, fibrillary glomerulonephritis. Randomly oriented fibrils about 20 nm in diameter are seen in the glomerular capillary basement membrane. No microtubular substructure can usually be recognized in the fibrils. The size of the fibrils is usually helpful to differentiate fibrillary glomerulonephritis and amyloidosis, as well as other renal diseases with fibrillary structures.

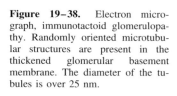

Figure 19–38. Electron micrograph, immunotactoid glomerulopathy. Randomly oriented microtubular structures are present in the thickened glomerular basement membrane. The diameter of the tubules is over 25 nm.

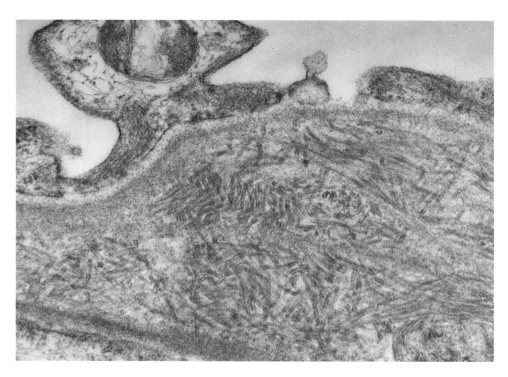

References

General

Feiner HD: Pathology of dysproteinemia: Light chain amyloidosis, non-amyloid immunoglobulin deposition disease, cryoglobulinemia syndromes, and macroglobulinemia of Waldenström. Hum Pathol 19: 1255, 1988.

Korbet SM, Schwartz MM, Lewis EJ: The fibrillary glomerulopathies. Am J Kidney Dis 23:751, 1994.

Morel-Maroger Striker LJ, Preud'homme J-L, D'Amico G, et al: Monoclonal gammopathies, mixed cryoglobulinemias, and lymphomas. In: Tisher CC, Brenner BM (eds): Renal Pathology: With Clinical and Functional Correlations, 2nd ed. Philadelphia, JB Lippincott, 1994, p 1442.

Shwartz MM: The dysproteinemias and amyloidosis. In: Jennette JC, Olson JL, Shwartz MM, Silva FG (eds): Heptinstall's Pathology of the Kidney, 5th ed. Philadelphia, Lippincott-Raven, 1998, p 1321.

Myeloma Cast Nephropathy

Kyle RA, Greipp PR: "Idiopathic" Bence Jones proteinuria: Long-term follow-up in seven patients. N Engl J Med 306:564, 1982.

Rota S, Mougenot B, Baudouin B, et al: Multiple myeloma and severe renal failure: A clinicopathologic study of outcome and prognosis in 34 patients. Medicine (Baltimore) 66:126, 1987.

Solomon A, Weiss DT, Kattine AA: Nephrotoxic potential of Bence Jones proteins. N Engl J Med 324:1845, 1991.

Light Chain Deposition Disease

Buxbaum JN, Chuba JV, Hellman GC, et al: Monoclonal immunoglobulin deposition disease: Light chain and light and heavy chain deposition diseases and their relation to light chain amyloidosis. Clinical features, immunopathology, and molecular analysis. Ann Intern Med 112:455, 1990.

Ganeval D, Noël L-H, Preud'homme J-L, et al: Light chain deposition disease: Its relation with AL-type amyloidosis. Kidney Int 26:1, 1984.

Iványi B: Frequency of light chain deposition nephropathy relative to renal amyloidosis and Bence Jones cast nephropathy in a necropsy study of patients with myeloma. Arch Pathol Lab Med 114:986, 1990.

Venkataseshan VS, Faraggiana T, Hughson MD, et al: Morphologic variants of light-chain deposition disease in the kidney. Am J Nephrol 8:272, 1988.

Amyloidosis

Cohen AS, Connors LH: The pathogenesis and biochemistry of amyloidosis. J Pathol 151:1, 1987.

Gertz MA, Kyle RA: Primary systemic amyloidosis—a diagnostic primer. Mayo Clin Proc 64:1505, 1989.

Jadoul M, Garbar C, Noël H, et al: Histological prevalence of β2-microglobulin amyloidosis in hemodialysis: A prospective post-mortem study. Kidney Int 51:1928, 1997.

Kyle RA, Greipp PR: Amyloidosis (AL): Clinical and laboratory features in 229 cases. Mayo Clin Proc 58:665, 1983.

Tan SY, Pepys MB: Amyloidosis. Histopathology 25:403, 1994.

The Fibrillary Glomerulopathies: Fibrillary Glomerulonephritis and Immunotactoid Glomerulopathy

Alpers CE: Immunotactoid (microtubular) glomerulopathy: An entity distinct from fibrillary glomerulonephritis? Am J Kidney Dis 19:185, 1992.

Devaney K, Sabnis SG, Antonovych TT: Nonamyloidotic fibrillary glomerulopathy, immunotactoid glomerulopathy, and the differential diagnosis of fibrillary glomerulopathies. Mod Pathol 4:36, 1991.

Fogo A, Qureshi N, Horn RG: Morphologic and clinical features of fibrillary glomerulonephritis versus immunotactoid glomerulopathy. Am J Kidney Dis 22:367, 1992.

Iskandar SS, Falk RJ, Jennette JC: Clinical and pathologic features of fibrillary glomerulonephritis. Kidney Int 42:1401, 1992.

Jennette JC, Iskandar SS, Falk RJ: Fibrillary glomerulonephritis. In: Tisher CC, Brenner BM (eds): Renal Pathology: With Clinical and Functional Correlations, 2nd ed. Philadelphia, JB Lippincott, 1994, p 553.

Korbet SM, Schwartz MM, Lewis EJ: Immunotactoid glomerulopathy. Am J Kidney Dis 17:247, 1991.

CHAPTER 20

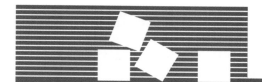

Cystic Renal Diseases and Renal Dysplasia

INTRODUCTION

- The cystic renal diseases include both hereditary and acquired conditions, with great variety in terms of clinical onset, manifestations, and effect on renal function. A summary of cystic renal diseases is given in Table 20–1.
- *Renal dysplasia* is a congenital, but not inherited, abnormality in renal development that is frequently associated with other congenital anomalies of the genitourinary tract. Renal dysplasia is included in this section because of the frequent presence of cysts in the condition.
- The hereditary forms of cystic kidney diseases vary in terms of pattern of inheritance, age at clinical onset of symptoms, and types of extrarenal manifestations that may occur. The most common inherited renal cystic disease is autosomal dominant polycystic kidney disease (ADPKD), formerly called adult polycystic kidney disease. Autosomal recessive polycystic kidney disease (ARPKD), formerly known as infantile polycystic kidney disease, is far less common.
- The common acquired forms of renal cysts are simple renal cysts, which are usually innocuous, and acquired cystic kidney disease, which occurs primarily in patients undergoing long-term dialysis but may occasionally be seen in patients with chronic renal failure who are not undergoing dialysis.
- The pathogenesis of renal cysts was long considered simply a matter of obstruction of tubules, which then become distended and cystic because of the continued flow of urine. It is now clear that although obstruction may be a component of the process, obstruction by itself is not responsible for renal cyst formation.
- Three fundamental processes are thought to be required for renal cyst formation:
  - Abnormal proliferation and/or lack of differentiation of renal epithelial cells
  - Continued fluid formation
  - Abnormalities in the tubular basement membrane and/ or extracellular matrix
- Recent, remarkable advances in our knowledge of the mechanisms and genetics of inherited renal cystic diseases have culminated in identification and cloning of the genes responsible for the majority of cases of ADPKD.

Table 20–1
CATEGORIES OF RENAL CYSTIC DISEASE

Inherited Renal Cystic Diseases	Acquired Renal Cystic Diseases
Autosomal dominant polycystic kidney disease	Simple renal cysts
Autosomal recessive polycystic kidney disease	Acquired renal cystic kidney disease (associated with dialysis or chronic renal failure)
Nephronophthisis–medullary cystic disease complex	Medullary sponge kidney
von Hippel–Lindau disease	

AUTOSOMAL DOMINANT POLYCYSTIC KIDNEY DISEASE:

Synonym: Adult polycystic kidney disease.

Biology of Disease

- Autosomal dominant polycystic kidney disease is apparently the most common *potentially lethal* single-gene disease. It is found worldwide, with an estimated prevalence of approximately 1 in 200 to 1 in 1,000 persons. It is estimated that approximately 500,000 people in the United States are affected by ADPKD and that ADPKD accounts for 8% to 10% of the patients receiving renal replacement therapy (dialysis or renal transplantation).
- At least three different genes have been implicated in ADPKD. The first gene associated with ADPKD (designated *PKD1*) was linked to the short arm of chromosome 16 and appears to cause 85% to 90% of cases of ADPKD in white families of European origin. A second gene, designated *PKD2*, is located on chromosome

4 and appears to cause the majority of cases not linked to chromosome 16. There is evidence for a third gene for ADPKD, which at present has not been linked to a specific chromosome.

■ The severity of disease associated with mutations in *PKD1* and *PKD2* appears to differ, with disease linked to *PKD2* tending to have a more indolent course than disease linked to *PKD1*. The incidence of hypertension and renal failure is lower in families linked to *PKD2*, and the age of onset of renal failure tends to be later.

■ The *PKD1* gene was cloned in 1995, and the protein was named *polycystin*. Polycystin is a large transmembrane protein with multiple functional domains; it is probably involved in cell adhesion and cell-matrix interaction and appears to be important in maturation of tubular epithelial cells. The *PKD2* gene was cloned in 1996; interestingly, the PKD2 protein has considerable homology to polycystin (approximately 25% of the PKD2 protein is identical to polycystin). The PKD2 protein appears to be involved in ion exchange.

■ Cysts can develop from any part of the nephron in ADPKD kidneys, including both proximal and distal tubules, as well as Bowman's space (glomerular cysts). Cysts involve only a small proportion of nephrons in ADPKD kidneys; one estimate suggests that cysts involve fewer than 1% of the nephrons.

■ Small cysts become detectable on imaging studies during childhood, and the number and size of cysts progressively increase with age.

■ Extrarenal manifestations are prominent in ADPKD and at times may dominate the clinical picture. The most common extrarenal manifestations are hepatic cysts, intracranial aneurysms, colonic diverticula, and cardiac valvular abnormalities (Table 20–2).

Clinical Features

■ The clinical manifestations of ADPKD tend to be worse in men than in women for unknown reasons. The severity of disease can vary within families, which suggests that some factors other than possession of the mutated gene are involved in determining the severity of disease.

■ Hypertension is common in patients with ADPKD and is usually present before any evidence of renal insufficiency. The renin-angiotensin-aldosterone system appears to be involved in the pathogenesis of hyperten-

Table 20–2
EXTRARENAL MANIFESTATIONS OF AUTOSOMAL DOMINANT POLYCYSTIC KIDNEY DISEASE

Manifestation	Approximate Incidence (%)
Hepatic cysts	40–70
Intracranial aneurysms	4–40
Colonic diverticula	40–80
Cardiac valvular abnormalities (mitral valve prolapse)	0–30
Pancreatic cysts	5–10
Arachnoid cysts	5–8

sion, possibly by compression of intrarenal vessels by cysts.

■ The mainstay in diagnosis of ADPKD is ultrasound; computed tomography (CT) may be more sensitive and is useful in atypical or equivocal cases. In families linked to *PKD1,* cysts are present in 64% of affected children by the age of 10 and in up to 90% between the ages of 10 and 19 years.

■ The most common renal manifestations of ADPKD are hematuria, flank or abdominal pain, infection, nephrolithiasis, enlarged and palpable kidneys, and end-stage renal disease (ESRD). Another possible association is the development of renal cell carcinoma (discussed in Treatment and Clinical Course, later).

■ Hematuria may be due to hemorrhage into a cyst, nephrolithiasis (which occurs in approximately 20% of patients with ADPKD), or renal neoplasia. Hemorrhage into cysts may or may not be associated with hematuria.

■ Acute exacerbations of pain can be caused by hemorrhage into or infection of cysts. Chronic flank pain appears to be related to cyst or kidney size; pain control can be a significant management problem in patients with ADPKD.

■ Infection of the renal parenchyma (pyelonephritis) or infection of the cysts themselves may occur in patients with ADPKD. The distinction of parenchymal versus cyst infection is clinically significant inasmuch as many antibiotics used for pyelonephritis are lipophobic, do not penetrate into cysts, and are not effective in treating infections in cysts.

■ End-stage renal disease occurs in approximately half of patients with ADPKD by age 60. Age at development of ESRD is substantially variable and ranges from 3 to 80 years; however, renal failure is typically manifested around the fifth decade of life.

■ The most significant, although not the most common, extrarenal manifestation of ADPKD is the development of intracranial arterial ("berry") aneurysms. These aneurysms probably occur in approximately 10% of patients overall, although a wide range in the frequency of aneurysms is seen in different series. There appears to be familial clustering of intracranial aneurysms, which suggests that there may be variation in the risk associated with different gene mutations. Rupture of an intracranial aneurysm is associated with a 50% mortality rate in patients with ADPKD, and half of the survivors are left with significant disability. The mortality rate associated with rupture of an intracranial aneurysm in patients with ADPKD is greater than the mortality rate in patients without ADPKD, and rupture tends to occur at an earlier age in patients with ADPKD than in patients without ADPKD. Patients with ADPKD are also at increased risk for hypertensive cerebral hemorrhage and ischemic cerebral infarcts; in fact, the risk of hypertensive cerebral hemorrhage or ischemic infarcts probably exceeds that of rupture of a "berry" aneurysm.

■ The most common extrarenal manifestation is the development of hepatic cysts. The prevalence of hepatic cysts increases with age and reaches 70% in patients older than 60 years. In general, hepatic cyst disease is more severe in patients with the most severe renal cystic disease and the worst renal function. However, severe hepatic cyst disease primarily affects women, particularly those who have had multiple pregnancies or exposure to exogenous female sex steroids. Hepatic cysts are usually asymptomatic, liver synthetic function is generally well preserved, and serum transaminases and bilirubin levels are usually normal. However, occasional patients do have significant complications from hepatic cyst disease, including cyst infection, obstructive jaundice, portal hypertension with esophageal varices, and hepatic neoplasms.

■ The other extrarenal manifestations of ADPKD are not usually associated with significant morbidity or mortality.

Gross Appearance

■ The kidneys are bilaterally enlarged, but the size of the two kidneys may differ up to 30% in a single patient. The kidneys usually retain a semblance of the normal reniform or "bean-shaped" outline. Kidney size and weight vary greatly, depending on the age, sex, and severity of disease in the individual patient. The weight of single kidneys ranges from slightly greater than the normal 150 g to 3 kg or more; football-sized kidneys weighing a kilogram or more are probably the exception rather than the rule. Multiple cysts are visible on the surface and vary in size from a few millimeters to several centimeters in diameter.

■ On section, multiple to innumerable cysts of various size are diffusely scattered throughout the kidney, in both the cortex and the medulla; the largest cysts are usually in a subcapsular location. The renal parenchyma may appear to be entirely replaced by cysts, with only lacy fibrous septa left, or considerable normal renal parenchyma may remain. The cysts are usually spherical and unilocular; the inner lining is usually smooth but may contain small irregularities or papillations.

■ The majority of cysts contain clear fluid resembling urine; some contain blood or clot, and a few may contain purulent material.

■ The papillae and pyramids may be difficult or impossible to identify, and the calyces and pelvis may be greatly distorted.

Light Microscopy

■ The cells lining the majority of the cysts are flattened and simplified, and it is not usually possible to identify the type of tubule from which the cyst arose. Focal areas of epithelial hyperplasia or small polyps with fibrovascular stalks are present in some cysts in almost all patients. Occasionally, the presence of a residual glomerular capillary tuft within a cyst indicates origin from Bowman's capsule.

■ Areas of identifiable residual renal parenchyma are *always* present and are in fact required for the diagnosis of ADPKD. The residual renal parenchyma may demonstrate interstitial fibrosis, tubular atrophy, and glomerulosclerosis, probably from compression by the cysts.

Differential Diagnosis

■ In a typical patient with a family history of the disease, the diagnosis is not difficult. The presence of multiple, bilateral renal cysts on ultrasound or CT establishes the diagnosis; the presence of cysts in other organs such as the liver provides additional diagnostic confidence.

■ Up to 25% of patients do not have a family history of renal cysts. Such cases were previously thought to be new mutations; however, in the majority of cases, appropriate imaging studies demonstrate previously unknown disease in one of the parents. Such cases illustrate the variability in clinical severity of the disease.

■ Mild cases may be difficult to distinguish from multiple simple cysts; the presence of cysts in other organs or a family history of the disease favors ADPKD.

■ It may be difficult to distinguish mild (late onset) cases of ARPKD from ADPKD; investigation of the parents for evidence of renal cysts may be helpful in this distinction. The presence of hepatic cysts, or cysts in other organs, favors the autosomal dominant over the autosomal recessive form.

■ The presence of cartilage or other heterotopic tissue suggests renal dysplasia rather than ADPKD.

■ A cystic renal cell carcinoma may occasionally mimic ADPKD; distinction is based on the presence of carcinoma in the residual tissue, unilateral rather than bilateral cystic disease, or the presence of large amounts of normal renal parenchyma.

Treatment and Clinical Course

■ No specific treatment is known for ADPKD. Control of hypertension is important and may delay or slow the progression of renal disease; it may also lower the risk of rupture of intracranial berry aneurysms and decrease the incidence of cardiovascular disease and other complications.

■ Dialysis or other renal replacement therapy is required in the half of the patients who reach end-stage renal failure. In general, patients with ADPKD survive longer on dialysis than do patients with end-stage renal failure secondary to other causes. Renal transplantation is also successful in patients with ADPKD.

■ Chronic pain or acute exacerbations of pain caused by hemorrhage into a cyst may be a major problem. Cyst puncture with aspiration of cyst contents may be very effective in relieving pain.

■ Patients with ADPKD have previously been considered to be at increased risk for the development of renal cell carcinoma; more recently, this increased risk has been disputed. However, it does appear that the incidence of *bilateral* renal cell carcinoma is higher in patients with ADPKD than in patients with renal cell carcinoma but no ADPKD; approximately 20% of patients with ADPKD and renal cell carcinoma have bilateral disease as compared with 1.4% to 5% of patients with renal cell carcinoma but no ADPKD. The average age at diagnosis of renal cell carcinoma in patients with ADPKD is also less than that in patients without ADPKD (approximately 46 years versus approximately 65 years).

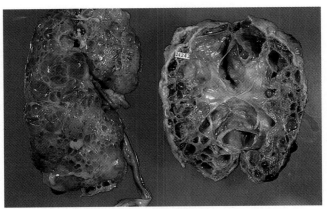

Figure 20–1. *Autosomal dominant (adult) polycystic kidney disease, advanced. The cut surface of the kidney on the right shows numerous large cysts with a smooth inner surface in both the renal cortex and medulla. The renal parenchyma appears completely replaced by the cysts. The kidney on the left has cysts throughout the surface.*

AUTOSOMAL RECESSIVE POLYCYSTIC KIDNEY DISEASE

Synonym: Infantile polycystic kidney disease.

Biology of Disease

■ Autosomal recessive polycystic kidney disease is far less common than the autosomal dominant form, with the former having a reported incidence ranging from 1 in 6,000 to 1 in 55,000. A gene for ARPKD has recently been linked to chromosome 6. It was once thought that there were four distinct genetic variants that differed in the age of onset of renal disease; it is now believed that these variants represent merely variability in clinical manifestation of the disease rather than genetic variability.

■ Because inheritance is recessive, neither parent is affected and there is often no family history of the disease. Each full sibling of an affected patient has a 1 in 4 chance of development of the disease.

■ The main extrarenal manifestation of ARPKD is congenital hepatic fibrosis; cysts do not occur in the liver or other organs in ARPKD.

■ The etiology of ARPKD is unknown.

Clinical Features

■ The disease can occur at any age from newborn to early adult years. In fact, the age range of "infantile" (autosomal recessive) polycystic kidney disease overlaps that of the "adult" (autosomal dominant) form.

■ All affected children have both kidney disease and hepatic disease, but renal disease tends to dominate the clinical picture in children affected at a younger age whereas liver disease is usually the dominant feature in patients affected later in childhood or as adolescents.

■ Autosomal recessive polycystic kidney disease is usually manifested at birth as abdominal distention caused by grossly enlarged kidneys. In some cases the diagnosis is made prenatally by ultrasonography. Pulmonary hypoplasia is common in such infants and is presumed to be due to compression of the lungs by the massively enlarged kidneys. The combination of oligohydramnios, pulmonary hypoplasia, and other anomalies (Potter's syndrome) may be present.

■ Children who survive the neonatal period may have a remarkably variable course. In some, ESRD may develop; in others, renal function is relatively preserved and hepatic disease is the main clinical problem.

■ Hepatic synthetic function is usually well maintained. In patients with clinical evidence of liver disease, the primary manifestation is portal hypertension with splenomegaly and bleeding from esophageal varices.

Gross Appearance

■ In children in whom ARPKD is diagnosed at birth, the kidneys are symmetrically enlarged and fill the abdominal cavity; the combined weights of the kidneys may range from 200 to 600 g. The kidneys retain the normal renal outline and lobulation. The capsular surface is studded with innumerable tiny cysts (1 to 2 mm in diameter).

■ On section, the kidneys are diffusely and uniformly involved. Numerous narrow, elongated, radially oriented cystic spaces extend the full thickness of the cortex. Similar dilated spaces are present in the medulla; however, dilated spaces in the medulla are more often sagittally or transversely oriented.

- In patients surviving the neonatal period, the appearance of the kidneys is variable. The kidneys may be enlarged, normal, or even decreased in size. They contain fewer but larger cysts (up to 1 or 2 cm) that are irregularly distributed. In some cases the appearance strongly resembles that of autosomal dominant polycystic disease; in other cases, the kidneys may be indistinguishable from medullary sponge kidney.

Light Microscopy

- In a young kidney, the parenchyma is made up almost entirely of dilated tubules. These tubules appear elongated in the cortex and round or oval in the medulla. They are predominantly lined by a single layer of cuboidal cells but may contain small foci of hyperplastic epithelium and small polyps.
- The cysts are composed of dilated collecting ducts. Glomeruli and proximal tubules are crowded between the dilated collecting ducts or grouped into subcapsular wedges. Glomerular cysts are not found.
- The appearance differs in patients affected by renal disease after the childhood period. The cysts take up less of the parenchymal area (only 15% to 20%) and may be larger, more spherical, and more irregularly distributed. Glomerulosclerosis, tubular atrophy, and interstitial fibrosis may be present.
- In patients affected during the adult years, the primary histologic feature may be dilated ducts in the medulla; there may be few or no larger cysts.

Differential Diagnosis

- A typical case with onset at birth and massively enlarged kidneys is not a diagnostic problem. Cases occurring later in childhood or early adulthood may be less straightforward.
- Cases with fewer, but larger cysts may be difficult to distinguish from ADPKD. The presence of glomerular cysts indicates the autosomal dominant form. Evidence of hepatic cysts would also favor the autosomal dominant form, whereas hepatic fibrosis without cysts favors the autosomal recessive variety. Ultrasonography of the parents may be helpful in the distinction; discovery of renal cysts in one of the parents would favor the autosomal dominant type.
- Cases with a predominance of medullary ductal ectasia may be difficult to distinguish from medullary sponge kidney; the presence of hepatic disease would favor ARPKD.

Treatment and Clinical Course

- Patients with severe disease usually die within the first few days after birth; death is usually due to respiratory failure or other complications of pulmonary hypoplasia rather than being directly due to renal failure.
- Children surviving into late childhood or early adulthood may have a remarkably varied clinical course. Some have a progressive drop in creatinine clearance that culminates in end-stage renal failure and require dialysis or renal transplantation. In other cases, renal function remains relatively stable; complications of the hepatic disease, particularly portal hypertension, may then become the major problem.
- Overall actuarial survival is reported to be approximately 46% at 15 years for all children and 79% at 15 years for those children surviving the first year of life.

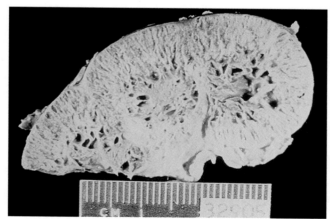

Figure 20–2. Autosomal recessive (infantile) polycystic kidney disease. The gross photograph shows a portion of a kidney from a newborn; small cylindrical tubules (cysts) are seen throughout the renal cortex. Note that the normal kidney shape is intact and that many of the cysts run in parallel from the surface of the kidney.

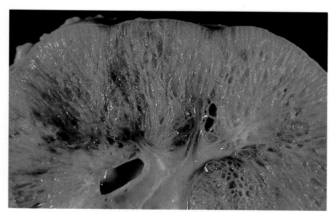

Figure 20–3. Autosomal recessive (infantile) polycystic kidney disease. The gross photograph shows a portion of a kidney from a newborn; small cylindrical tubules (cysts) are visible in the renal cortex.

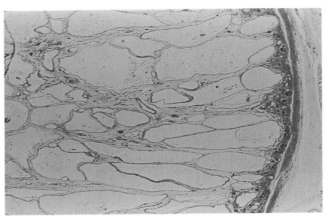

Figure 20–4. Autosomal recessive (infantile) polycystic kidney disease. Dilated collecting tubules extending to the capsular surface (right) have replaced the normal renal parenchyma.

NEPHRONOPHTHISIS–MEDULLARY CYSTIC DISEASE COMPLEX

Synonyms and Related Terms: Familial juvenile nephronophthisis; nephronophthisis–uremic medullary cystic disease; medullary cystic disease.

Biology of Disease

- The nephronophthisis–medullary cystic disease complex includes two conditions that were originally considered to be distinct: juvenile nephronophthisis and medullary cystic disease. They are now considered to be related, with variable modes of inheritance.
- The apparent modes of inheritance are:
  - Sporadic occurrence, with no family history of the disease, which accounts for approximately one sixth of the total.
  - A recessively inherited form, which makes up approximately half of the cases; in some families, ocular abnormalities ("renal-retinal dysplasia"), skeletal anomalies, or central nervous system defects are inherited with the renal disease.
  - A form with a dominant inheritance, probably autosomal, which makes up the remainder.
- The characteristic features are interstitial fibrosis and tubular atrophy, renal failure, and renal medullary cysts.
- The nephronophthisis–medullary cystic disease complex may be responsible for 1% to 5% of cases of renal failure requiring dialysis or transplantation; it may cause 10% to 20% of cases of renal failure in childhood.
- The etiology is unknown.

Clinical Features

- The stigmata of chronic renal failure usually occur during the first or second decades of life but may be delayed until well into adulthood.
- Hematuria, nephrolithiasis, pain, and infection are uncommon, unlike the other cystic renal diseases.

Gross Appearance

- At autopsy or at nephrectomy before renal transplantation, the kidneys are small, symmetrically shrunken, and firm.
- On section, the cortex and medulla are thin; a variable number of cysts are present at the corticomedullary junction. The cysts are typically thin walled, filled with clear fluid resembling urine, and range in size from a few millimeters up to perhaps 2 cm.
- Cysts are absent in up to 25% of cases.

Light Microscopy

- Glomeruli show variable degrees of sclerosis, often with periglomerular fibrosis.
- Marked tubular atrophy is mixed with compensatory hypertrophy of other tubules. The interstitium shows fibrosis and a mild chronic inflammatory infiltrate.
- Tubular atrophy is most striking in the distal segments and is accompanied by marked thickening of tubular basement membranes by periodic acid–Schiff (PAS)-positive material.
- Cystically dilated tubules and larger cysts are present primarily at the corticomedullary junction.

Electron Microscopy

- On electron microscopy, the thickened tubular basement membranes variously show homogeneous thickening, splitting into fine lamellae, "net-like transformation," thinning, disintegration, or complete disappearance. Some tubules may show an abrupt transition from thick to thin basement membranes.

Differential Diagnosis

- The morphologic changes seen are nonspecific. The family history and other clinical characteristics are critical in the differential diagnosis.
- Medullary cysts are seldom found on renal biopsy; even when present, they are not specific.
- The most striking feature is the tubular basement membrane thickening, which exceeds that seen in most conditions except diabetes mellitus.

Treatment and Clinical Course

- No specific treatment is known for the nephronophthisis–medullary cystic disease complex. Dialysis or renal transplantation may be required; the condition does not recur after transplantation.

MEDULLARY SPONGE KIDNEY

Synonyms and Related Terms: Renal tubule ectasia; cystic disease of the renal pyramids; precaliceal canalicular ectasia.

Biology of Disease

- Medullary sponge kidney is characterized by dilatation of collecting ducts in the renal pyramids, usually without significant compromise of renal function.
- The majority of cases appear to be sporadic; autosomal dominant inheritance has been suggested in a few cases.
- The condition has been considered to be caused by a developmental abnormality, although there is little strong evidence supporting such an origin. Tubular ectasia is not a common finding in stillborn infants, and medullary sponge kidney is rarely found in children.
- Medullary sponge kidney has been associated with the unusual condition of congenital hemihypertrophy of the body.

Clinical Features

- The majority of cases are asymptomatic. The condition is usually an incidental finding on excretory urography (intravenous pyelography), which demonstrates linear striations or spherical cystic lesions in the renal papillae.
- Occasional cases are detected as a result of complications, which can include hematuria, infections, and nephrolithiasis.

Gross Appearance

- The majority of affected kidneys appear normal on external examination; approximately one third are diffusely or irregularly enlarged, and a few are shrunken (because of chronic pyelonephritis).
- On section, small cysts and ectatic papillary ducts are present in the pyramids. These structures are usually most prominent near the papillary tips; the corresponding calyx may appear flattened and splayed out.
- The condition may involve a few, many, or all papillae; it is bilateral in approximately three fourths of patients.
- The cysts usually measure 1 to 3 mm in diameter; occasionally, cysts up to 5 mm or greater are present.

Light Microscopy

- The ectatic collecting ducts and cysts are lined by multilayered transitional, columnar, or occasionally stratified squamous epithelium. Some cysts may contain PAS-positive material.
- The medullary interstitium usually shows fibrosis and chronic inflammation; occasionally, acute inflammatory cells are present.
- The renal cortex appears unremarkable or shows nonspecific secondary changes.

Differential Diagnosis

- Because medullary sponge kidney is usually asymptomatic and not associated with renal failure, it should seldom enter into the *clinical* differential of the other renal cystic diseases.
- The most likely *pathologic* differential diagnosis is between medullary sponge kidney and the nephronophthisis–medullary cystic disease complex. The distribution of the cysts on gross examination of the kidney is a key feature in this distinction. In the nephronophthisis–medullary cystic disease complex, the cysts are located predominantly at the corticomedullary junction; in medullary sponge kidney, the cysts are located in the tips of the papillae.

Treatment and Clinical Course

- Medullary sponge kidney is usually an incidental finding or discovered during evaluation of hematuria, nephrolithiasis, or infection. Provided that nephrolithiasis and infection are adequately managed, renal function will remain normal and no specific treatment is necessary.

ACQUIRED CYSTIC KIDNEY DISEASE

Synonyms and Related Terms: Dialysis kidney; acquired renal cystic disease in azotemia and maintenance dialysis.

Biology of Disease

- The term *acquired cystic kidney disease* is usually restricted to the development of renal cysts in patients with end-stage renal failure *not* caused by primary renal cystic diseases such as ADPKD.

■ Acquired cystic kidney disease is most common in patients undergoing long-term dialysis, although it also occurs in patients with chronic renal failure who have not undergone dialysis. The development of renal cysts is not limited to patients maintained on hemodialysis; it also occurs in patients maintained on peritoneal dialysis. Cysts have less of a tendency to develop in the native kidneys of patients who have successfully undergone renal transplantation; there have been reports of regression of preexisting cysts after kidney transplantation in some patients.

■ The incidence increases with increasing duration of support by dialysis; acquired renal cysts have been found in approximately 44% of patients maintained on dialysis for less than 3 years, 80% of patients maintained on dialysis for more than 4 years, and 90% of patients maintained on dialysis for 5 to 10 years.

■ One definition of acquired cystic kidney disease requires at least five cysts per kidney. The number of cysts present is usually considerably greater than five; hundreds of cysts may be present.

■ Acquired cystic kidney disease occurs in both males and females, although some reports describe a higher incidence in males; several series have reported a disproportionately high incidence in African-Americans. Acquired cystic kidney disease occurs in both adult and pediatric dialysis patients.

■ The etiology of acquired cystic kidney disease is unknown. It occurs in patients with ESRD of all types (with the exception, by definition, of patients with primary renal cystic diseases).

■ The most serious complication of acquired cystic kidney disease is renal cell carcinoma (discussed in Treatment and Clinical Course, later).

Clinical Features

■ The majority of cases of acquired cystic kidney disease are asymptomatic and discovered on screening ultrasonography or CT.

■ Painful cyst hemorrhage, retroperitoneal hemorrhage, or infection can occur.

■ Occasionally, the cystic kidneys can become so large that they cause abdominal discomfort similar to that experienced with the enlarged kidneys of ADPKD.

Gross Appearance

■ Kidney size is variable. The majority of kidneys are decreased in size; however, some may be enlarged.

Kidneys may occasionally approach the size of kidneys in ADPKD.

■ Multiple cysts are present and range in size from a few millimeters to several centimeters in diameter. The cysts are usually filled with clear fluid resembling urine.

■ On section, the cysts may have a smooth inner lining, or the lining may be irregular or have small papillations.

Light Microscopy

■ The cyst walls usually consist of a single layer of flattened to cuboidal epithelial cells resting on a basement membrane. Two or more cell layers may be present, and there may be papillary ingrowths into the center of the cyst.

■ In some cases *(atypical cysts)*, the cyst lining consists of multiple layers of columnar cells. The cells may have finely granular cytoplasm or coarsely granular cytoplasm containing hyaline cytoplasmic droplets. Significant nuclear atypia may be present. Such atypical cysts are generally microscopic or small in size; the larger, macroscopic cysts are usually lined by a single layer of simple cells.

■ The remaining kidney shows glomerulosclerosis, tubular atrophy, interstitial fibrosis, and arteriosclerosis and arteriolosclerosis.

Treatment and Clinical Course

■ No specific treatment is known for acquired cystic renal disease.

■ The annual incidence of renal cell carcinoma appears to be increased approximately three to six times in dialysis patients when compared with the general population. The risk of renal cell carcinoma appears to increase with increased duration of chronic renal failure and with increased severity of acquired cystic kidney disease; the risk also appears to be several times higher in men than in women. Survival after diagnosis of renal cell carcinoma is usually poor; the median survival after diagnosis in one series was only 14 months.

■ It is controversial whether dialysis patients should be screened for the development of acquired cystic disease or renal cell carcinoma. Renal cell carcinoma is an uncommon cause of death in dialysis patients; in addition, many dialysis patients are not good candidates for aggressive surgical resection because of chronic illness, and management of such patients might therefore not be altered by the discovery.

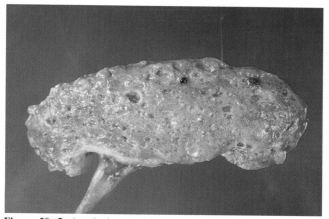

Figure 20–5. Acquired cystic kidney disease. Multiple cysts are seen on the surface of the kidney. This patient had undergone hemodialysis for several years. (Courtesy of Dr. Michael Hughson.)

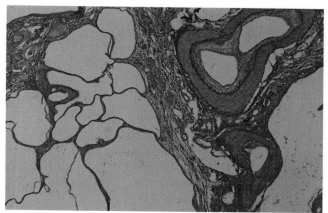

Figure 20–6. Acquired cystic kidney disease. The micrograph depicts multiple thin-walled cysts lined by flattened epithelial cells. (Courtesy of Dr. Michael Hughson.)

SIMPLE RENAL CYSTS

- Simple renal cysts, those that occur outside the settings of chronic renal insufficiency or inherited renal cystic disease, are common incidental findings at autopsy or on CT scans of the abdomen. They are seldom associated with symptoms or significant complications; the major significance of the discovery of simple renal cysts is the need to exclude a renal neoplasm.
- Renal cysts are uncommon in children, but the incidence rises progressively with increasing age; they may be present in up to half of individuals older than 40 years of age. The prevalence of cysts is probably equal in men and women.
- The etiology of simple renal cysts is unclear; it is believed that they originate from preexisting nephron segments, possibly diverticula off distal nephrons. The mechanism or mechanisms for such diverticula to become cystically dilated are not known. Some authors have suggested that there is a direct relationship between the presence of hypertension or vascular disease and the likelihood and number of cysts.
- Simple renal cysts may be solitary or multiple, unilateral or bilateral. Patients with multiple and bilateral simple cysts can be difficult to distinguish from milder cases of ADPKD; a family history of cysts or the presence of cysts in other organs would favor ADPKD over simple cysts.
- Simple cysts may be found anywhere in the kidney, including the cortex and medulla. They do not connect with the pelvis or calyceal system, although occasionally a cyst may project into the pelvis rather than toward the external surface of the kidney.
- On gross examination, simple cysts are usually spherical or ovoid. Many cysts project from the outer surface of the kidney (cortical cysts); the free wall of such a cyst is usually smooth, thin, and translucent. Most cysts contain clear, slightly yellowish fluid with a low specific gravity and low protein content; occasional cysts may contain old hemorrhage.
- Approximately half of simple cysts are less than 1 cm in diameter; cysts greater than 5 cm in diameter are rare, but cysts up to 28 cm in diameter have been described. In kidneys with multiple cysts, the size of individual cysts may vary greatly.
- Simple cysts are usually unilocular, with a smooth inner lining, but occasionally they may have internal septations or prominent lobulations.
- On light microscopy, the lining usually consists of a single layer of flattened epithelial cells; the lining may be discontinuous. The wall usually consists of nondescript fibrous tissue with occasional smooth muscle cells.
- The majority of cysts are asymptomatic and not associated with significant complications; renal excretory function is usually normal. Cysts may occasionally become infected, or there may be hemorrhage into a cyst. Peripelvic cysts may occasionally cause obstruction, with subsequent hydronephrosis and nephrolithiasis.
- The major concern regarding a cyst is the exclusion of a renal neoplasm. Fortunately, a simple cyst can usually be recognized as innocuous by CT scan or ultrasonography by its thin wall and lack of calcification; cyst aspiration for cytologic examination may be helpful in those rare cases that remain diagnostic problems.
- An association between simple renal cysts and renal neoplasms has been reported in several series, with neoplasms being reported in 2% to 4% of kidneys with cysts. There is little evidence for a *causal* association between simple cysts and neoplasms. Tumors may also on very rare occasion arise within a simple cyst.

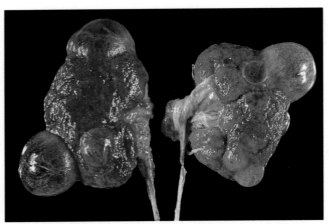

Figure 20–7. Simple cysts. The cysts were incidental autopsy findings.

RENAL DYSPLASIA

Synonyms and Related Terms: Renal adysplasia; multicystic dysplasia; aplastic dysplasia; hypoplastic dysplasia; segmental dysplasia; diffuse cystic dysplasia.

Biology of Disease

■ The term *renal dysplasia* indicates a group of conditions characterized by abnormal development and differentiation of the kidney (metanephric differentiation). As used here, "dysplasia" has no connotation of cellular atypia or preneoplastic potential, in contrast to use of the term in connection with the uterine cervix.

■ The majority (approximately 90%) of cases of renal dysplasia are associated with other abnormalities of the genitourinary tract, usually with obstruction. It is believed that normal development of the kidney requires the production and passage of urine; urinary tract obstruction during embryogenesis therefore interferes with normal development and maturation of the kidney. The obstruction can be complete or partial and can occur at any level of the urinary tract.

■ The appearance of the kidney in renal dysplasia may be highly variable. A variety of subtypes of dysplasia have been described, including multicystic dysplasia, hypoplastic dysplasia, diffuse cystic dysplasia, and others. Certain features are common to all types of dysplasia; these common features will be emphasized here, in preference to the features specific to the different subtypes of dysplasia.

■ The gross appearance of renal dysplasia overlaps with the appearance of kidneys with acquired scarring or atrophy caused by postnatal events such as vesicoureteral reflux and chronic pyelonephritis, and distinction can at times be difficult.

■ Histologic features that are considered clearly dys-

plastic are metaplastic cartilage and primitive ducts. Primitive ducts are small ducts or cysts lined by undifferentiated columnar epithelium and surrounded by fibromuscular collars. An additional feature that is characteristic but not diagnostic of renal dysplasia is *lobar disorganization*. In lobar disorganization, the lobar units of the kidney lack the normal medullary structure; the calyces and fornices are not open, the pyramids are not clearly defined, and the usual arrangement of vasa recta and recurrent loops of Henle in relation to the collecting ducts is lacking.

■ Renal dysplasia occurs more often in males than in females.

■ The majority of cases of renal dysplasia are sporadic and not associated with chromosomal abnormalities or inherited gene mutations. However, renal dysplasia may be a feature of hereditary conditions such as the chondrodysplasia syndromes, and dysplasia may be associated with chromosomal abnormalities such as trisomy of chromosomes 9 or 13. Renal dysplasia may also be associated with abnormalities in other organs, including the central nervous system (the cerebrohepatorenal syndrome of Zellweger), the liver, and the pancreas (renal-hepatic-pancreatic dysplasia). Renal dysplasia can be a feature of *Potter's syndrome*, which includes oligohydramnios, abnormal facies, pulmonary hypoplasia, and sometimes other abnormalities.

Clinical Features

■ Renal dysplasia is often found during postmortem examination of spontaneous abortions, stillborn infants, or infants dying in the early postnatal period. In most cases, renal dysplasia is found as one of multiple congenital anomalies, and death was due to other abnormalities rather than renal dysplasia directly.

- Enlarged, multicystic dysplastic kidneys may be detected as a palpable abdominal mass in childhood.
- In older patients, renal dysplasia can be discovered as a result of complications such as nephrolithiasis or urinary tract infection.

Gross Appearance

- Renal dysplasia can be unilateral or bilateral; if unilateral, the left kidney is involved more often than the right.
- The dysplastic kidney can be small, normal, or increased in size. Cysts are frequently present, are usually multiple, and may vary in size from a few millimeters to several centimeters.
- The normal medullary architecture, with pyramids and papillae, is partially or completely absent.
- Small islands of cartilage may be visible on section.

Light Microscopy

- Islands of cartilage are present. Primitive ducts are present; these ducts are surrounded by a dense collar of fibrous tissue and lined by a single layer of columnar epithelium, which is often ciliated.
- Cysts of various sizes are usually present and lined by flattened to cuboidal to columnar epithelial cells.
- The interstitium is fibrotic. A few glomeruli may be recognizable; if present, they are small and have a poorly developed capillary tuft.

Differential Diagnosis

- Renal dysplasia can be confused with hypoplasia of the kidney. A hypoplastic kidney is small for age; the number of lobes may be reduced. However, hypoplastic kidneys show relatively normal maturation and organization of the renal parenchyma, and islands of metaplastic cartilage and primitive ducts are absent.
- Enlarged, multicystic dysplastic kidneys can be misdiagnosed as ARPKD. The presence of ureteral atresia or other anomalies of the genitourinary tract would favor renal dysplasia, as would the finding of islands of cartilage or primitive ducts on histologic examination.
- In an older child or adult it may be difficult to differentiate renal dysplasia from acquired scarring caused by chronic pyelonephritis, reflux, or other scarring conditions. A dysplastic kidney that has a patent connection to the urinary bladder may have many of the secondary changes seen in nondysplastic kidneys subjected to reflux. Again, the presence of metaplastic cartilage or primitive ducts would favor renal dysplasia.

Treatment and Clinical Course

- Dysplastic kidneys are usually nonfunctional. Bilateral, severe renal dysplasia is incompatible with life; in many cases, associated anomalies are present and may be incompatible with postnatal survival.
- Dysplastic kidneys that have patent ureters may be subjected to reflux, which causes secondary scarring; such kidneys are also prone to infections or nephrolithiasis.

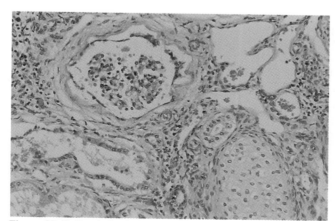

Figure 20–8. Renal dysplasia. Metaplastic cartilage (lower right) and normal glomeruli and tubules are seen.

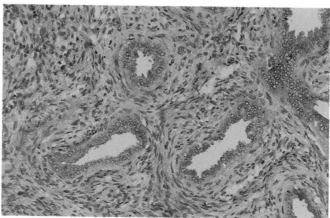

Figure 20–9. Renal dysplasia. Immature or "primitive" ducts are surrounded by mantles of concentrically arranged mesenchymal cells admixed with inflammatory cells.

References

General

Fick GM, Gabow PA: Hereditary and acquired cystic disease of the kidney. Kidney Int 46:951, 1994.

Risdon RA, Woolf AS: Developmental defects and cystic diseases of the kidney. In: Jennette JC, Olson JL, Schwartz MM, Silva FG (eds): Heptinstall's Pathology of the Kidney, 5th ed. Philadelphia, Lippincott-Raven, 1998, p 1149.

Welling LW, Grantham JJ: Cystic diseases of the kidney. In: Tisher CC, Brenner BM (eds): Renal Pathology: With Clinical and Functional Correlations, 2nd ed. Philadelphia, JB Lippincott, 1994, p 1312.

Autosomal Dominant Polycystic Kidney Disease

Gabow PA: Autosomal dominant polycystic kidney disease—more than a renal disease. Am J Kidney Dis 16:403, 1990.

Grantham JJ: The etiology, pathogenesis and treatment of autosomal dominant polycystic kidney disease: Recent advances. Am J Kidney Dis 28:788, 1996.

Perrone RD: Extrarenal manifestations of ADPKD. Kidney Int 51:2022, 1997.

Watson ML: Complications of polycystic kidney disease. Kidney Int 51:353, 1997.

Acquired Cystic Kidney Disease

Hughson MD, Hennigar GR, McManus JFA: Atypical cysts, acquired renal cystic disease, and renal tumors in end stage dialysis kidneys. Lab Invest 42:475, 1980.

Matson MA, Cohen EP: Acquired cystic kidney disease: Occurrence, prevalence, and renal cancers. Medicine (Baltimore) 69:217, 1990.

Renal Dysplasia

Bernstein J: Developmental abnormalities of the renal parenchyma—renal hypoplasia and dysplasia. Pathol Annu 3:213, 1968.

Bernstein J, Gilbert-Barness E: Congenital malformations of the kidney. In: Tisher CC, Brenner BM (eds): Renal Pathology: With Clinical and Functional Correlations, 2nd ed. Philadelphia, JB Lippincott, 1994, p 1355.

CHAPTER 21

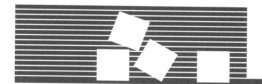

Pathology of Renal Transplantation

INTRODUCTION

The ratio of renal transplant biopsies to nontransplant (i.e., native renal) biopsies in most renal pathology laboratories is close to 1 : 1 because renal biopsy is the accepted standard for diagnosing transplant rejection. The pathologic changes in renal allografts may be quite complex, and in addition to rejection, a variety of recurrent, de novo, and donor-transmitted diseases may occur. This chapter concentrates on changes related to rejection of transplanted kidneys and on renal pathologic complications of antirejection (immunosuppressive) therapy.

HYPERACUTE REJECTION

Biology of Disease

- Hyperacute rejection is considered to be the prototype of humoral immune response–mediated rejection.
- The presence of preformed circulating antibodies against donor endothelial antigens plays the most important role.
- Presensitization is probably important; such presensitization may occur in multiparous women, in patients with prior blood transfusions, or in recipients who have already rejected previous grafts.
- The preformed antibodies react with antigens on the graft endothelium, and an Arthus-type reaction develops with subsequent necrosis of the graft.

Clinical Features

- Hyperacute rejection is now quite rare because of cross-matching (testing the recipients for antidonor antibodies).
- The affected transplanted kidney never functions. Characteristic changes are already apparent on the operating table. The kidney turns dusky and cyanotic. There is no good blood flow.
- Rarely, hyperacute rejection occurs after a delay of 1 or 2 days (delayed hyperacute rejection).

Laboratory Values

- Primary anuria is present (the transplanted kidney never functions); no specific laboratory findings can be noted. Preformed antidonor antibodies may be detected.

Light Microscopy

Glomeruli

- Prominent leukocyte margination in the glomerular capillaries is characteristic.
- Glomerular intracapillary thrombi are frequently seen.
- If the kidney is not removed, necrosis of the glomerular tuft develops.

Tubules

- If the kidney is not removed immediately, the tubular epithelium becomes necrotic.

Interstitium

- Leukocyte margination in peritubular capillaries is usually prominent with or without thrombus formation.
- Interstitial hemorrhage and interstitial edema may be seen.

Vessels

- Leukocyte margination and thrombi may be noted in small arterioles and venules. The arteries usually do not show prominent changes.

Immunofluorescence Microscopy

- Immunoglobulin and complement deposits may be present along the endothelium of the entire renal vasculature, including the glomerular and peritubular capillaries.

Electron Microscopy

- Polymorphonuclear leukocytes, platelets, fibrin, and necrosis of the endothelium may be noted.

Differential Diagnosis

■ Leukocyte margination in glomerular and peritubular capillaries may occur as a nonspecific finding in immediate posttransplant biopsy specimens.

■ Glomerular intracapillary thrombi may develop in cadaveric donor kidneys if the donor had disseminated intravascular coagulation at the time of death. These thrombi usually resolve without consequence.

Treatment and Clinical Course

■ The only treatment is immediate removal of the graft.

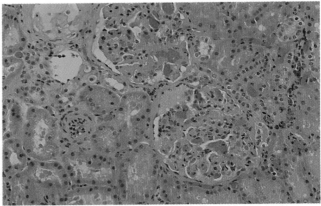

Figure 21–1. Hyperacute rejection. Note the neutrophil margination, which in this figure is particularly prominent in the arteriole, and the occlusion of glomerular capillaries by eosinophilic material (fibrin and platelets) and red blood cells. Hyperacute rejection invariably leads to graft loss.

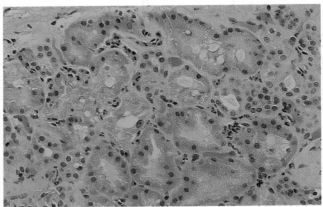

Figure 21–2. Hyperacute rejection. Note the large numbers of neutrophils filling the lumina of peritubular capillaries. The lesion usually develops within minutes after release of the vascular clamps after renal allograft transplantation.

ACUTE INTERSTITIAL (CELLULAR) REJECTION

Biology of Disease

■ Acute interstitial rejection is the most frequent type of rejection.

■ Cellular immune responses play the most important role, but humoral immune responses also participate in this type of rejection.

■ T-cell receptors recognize specific foreign antigens bound within the groove of a major histocompatibility complex molecule on the surface of an antigen-presenting cell (monocyte/macrophage, dendritic reticulum cell, etc.). This T-cell receptor signal defines the specificity of the immune reaction. It appears that other costimulatory signals initiated through the binding of ligands on the T-cell surface with costimulatory molecules on antigen-presenting cells also play an important role and may involve the humoral immune response.

■ Both CD4-positive helper and CD8-positive cytotoxic T cells play an important role. T_H1 helper cells appear to be more prevalent than T_H2 helper cells. T_H1 helper cells produce interleukin-2, interferon-γ, and other lymphokines that promote cytotoxic T-cell responses, de-

layed-type hypersensitivity, and also humoral immune responses.

Clinical Features

■ Acute interstitial rejection usually develops after the first week of transplantation and is uncommon after the first 3 months. However, it may appear at any time.

■ Graft swelling and tenderness may occur with deterioration of graft function (increased serum creatinine with or without decreased urine output).

Laboratory Values

■ No laboratory values are specific for rejection. An elevation in serum creatinine level is seen.

Light Microscopy

Glomeruli

■ The glomeruli are typically normal; a mild increase in glomerular intracapillary mononuclear cells (transplant glomerulitis) may occasionally be noted.

Tubules

- The most characteristic and one of the most important findings is infiltration of the tubular epithelium by inflammatory cells coming from the interstitium *(tubulitis)*. Most of these inflammatory cells infiltrating the tubules are T lymphocytes and macrophages. Tubulitis is the hallmark of acute interstitial rejection. Tubular epithelial degenerative changes and patchy tubular necrosis secondary to the rejection are frequently seen.

Interstitium

- An interstitial mononuclear cell infiltrate consisting mainly of lymphocytes and macrophages is invariably present. Tubulitis is always associated with this infiltrate. A mild, patchy, perivascular or periglomerular infiltrate does not necessarily mean rejection.
- In mild acute interstitial rejection, up to one third of the renal parenchyma contains infiltrating mononuclear cells. In moderate rejection, up to two thirds of the parenchyma is involved. In severe acute interstitial rejection, at least two thirds of the renal parenchyma shows peritubular mononuclear cell infiltrate with tubulitis.
- A variable degree of interstitial edema is frequently associated with the inflammatory cell infiltrate of rejection.
- Scattered polymorphonuclear leukocytes, plasma cells, and eosinophils may occur. Sometimes, large numbers of plasma cells are seen in late acute rejection episodes (occurring several months or years posttransplant). Occasionally a larger number of eosinophils are present. This feature is considered by some to be an indicator of a relatively unfavorable outcome.

Vessels

- Typically, the vasculature is not involved in acute interstitial rejection.
- Margination of mononuclear cells in capillaries, arteries, and veins may occur. The presence of only a few scattered subendothelial inflammatory cells does not warrant a definite diagnosis of acute vascular rejection.

Immunofluorescence Microscopy

- No immunofluorescence findings are specific for acute interstitial rejection. C3 deposition along tubular basement membranes and arterioles is commonly seen, but it is most likely without practical significance. Some interstitial fibrinogen may be present, particularly if interstitial edema is prevalent.

Electron Microscopy

- Electron microscopy is not contributory to the diagnosis of acute interstitial rejection.

Differential Diagnosis

- A mild, patchy, perivascular or periglomerular infiltrate in the absence of tubulitis does not warrant the diagnosis of acute interstitial rejection.
- Posttransplant lymphoproliferative disorder (PTLD) may resemble acute interstitial rejection, and the differential diagnosis can be difficult, particularly in a small biopsy specimen. Detection of Epstein-Barr virus (EBV) by in situ hybridization and a prevalence of B cells in the infiltrate are highly suggestive of PTLD. (For more detail, see the section on PTLD.)
- In acute pyelonephritis, polymorphonuclear leukocytes are seen within tubular lumina, usually filling the tubules, and neutrophils are also present in the interstitium. Interstitial microabscesses may be noted. Sometimes there may be concomitant acute rejection. The presence of a few intratubular and interstitial neutrophils does not warrant the diagnosis of acute pyelonephritis; they may occur in acute interstitial or vascular rejection and in acute tubular necrosis.
- Acute interstitial nephritis not related to rejection is extremely difficult to differentiate from acute interstitial rejection. In such cases, eosinophils may be prevalent; however, eosinophils may be present in rejection as well. As a rule of thumb, in a transplant kidney a mononuclear cell infiltrate with eosinophils should be considered rejection until proved otherwise. In occasional cases, acute interstitial nephritis may be caused by viruses (adenovirus, herpes virus, BK virus, etc.); in such cases, in situ hybridization or immunohistochemistry with specific probes against these viruses is helpful. The role of cytomegalovirus infection of renal parenchymal cells in the induction of rejection is debated. The nuclei of tubular epithelial cells in a variety of viral disorders are enlarged or smudgy or have intranuclear inclusions.

Treatment and Clinical Course

- In its pure form (in the absence of vascular rejection), acute interstitial rejection is the most benign or treatable form of rejection, and it generally responds well to therapy.
- Corticosteroids, cyclosporine, and azathioprine (Imuran) are the most frequently used immunosuppressants to avoid rejection; these drugs are mostly used in combination (triple therapy).
- A new potent immunosuppressive drug, FK-506, is now available and can be used instead of cyclosporine (but not in combination with cyclosporine).
- Monoclonal antibodies against T cells and various T-cell subsets are useful in the management of acute interstitial rejection; the most frequently used of these antibodies now is OKT3, a monoclonal antibody against T cells. Antilymphocyte globulins are also used.
- Other new immunosuppressive agents such as mycophenolate mofetil (CellCept) are now available and can be used as adjunctive or alternative therapies.

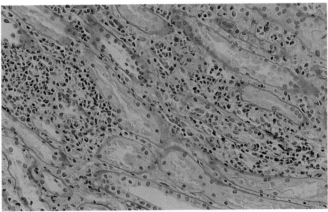

Figure 21–3. Acute interstitial rejection. Note the disruption of tubular basement membranes and infiltration of tubular epithelium by mononuclear cells (tubulitis). Tubulitis is the hallmark of acute tubulointerstitial rejection (periodic acid–Schiff reaction).

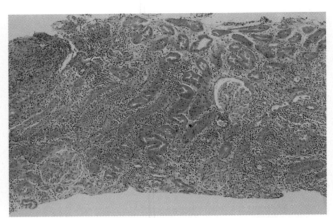

Figure 21–6. Severe acute interstitial rejection. Note that in this case, most of the renal parenchyma is involved by mononuclear cell infiltrate with prominent tubulitis.

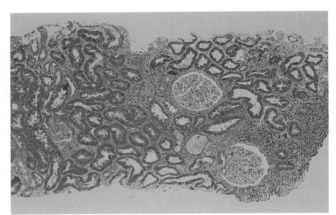

Figure 21–4. Mild acute interstitial rejection. Note the focal infiltrate present in the peritubular space and, occasionally, infiltrating tubules as well (tubulitis). In mild acute interstitial rejection, usually not more than one third of the renal parenchyma is involved by inflammatory infiltrate.

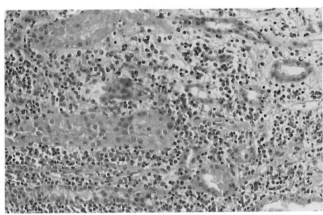

Figure 21–7. Late acute interstitial rejection. Note the dense infiltrate containing many plasma cells, a frequent finding in late acute rejection. Late acute rejection usually develops months or years after transplantation and is frequently associated with noncompliance.

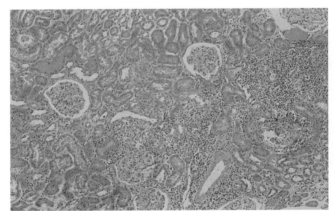

Figure 21–5. Moderate acute interstitial rejection. When compared with Figure 21–4, the cellular infiltrate is more prominent and interstitial edema is also noted, but the artery is not involved. In moderate acute interstitial rejection, the infiltrate usually does not involve more than two thirds of the renal parenchyma.

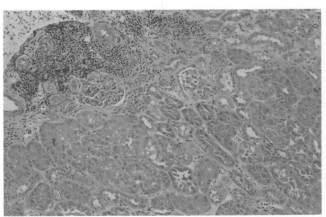

Figure 21–8. Renal allograft with normal function. Note the patchy perivascular infiltrate. No prominent peritubular infiltrate with tubulitis is present. This type of focal perivascular or periglomerular infiltrate should not be overinterpreted as rejection.

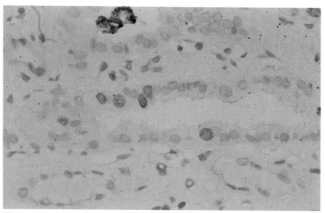

Figure 21-9. Polyoma (BK) virus infection in a transplant kidney, in situ hybridization. The enlarged nuclei of the tubular epithelial cells are positive with a probe against polyomavirus. (Courtesy of Dr. E. O. Major, National Institutes of Health.)

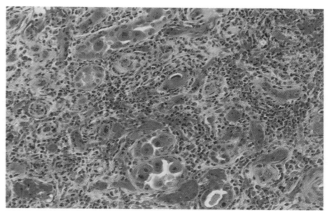

Figure 21-10. Cytomegalovirus (CMV) infection of a renal allograft. Note the characteristic intranuclear CMV inclusions in several tubular epithelial cells. Cytomegalovirus infection is a feared complication of immunosuppressive therapy. Interestingly, even in prominent systemic CMV disease, characteristic CMV inclusions are rarely found in renal transplant biopsy specimens.

ACUTE VASCULAR (HUMORAL) REJECTION

Biology of Disease

- Acute vascular rejection was once thought to be the consequence of primarily humoral immune responses. Today it is obvious that acute vascular rejection is the result of a mixture of cellular and humoral immune responses; thus "acute humoral rejection" is a misnomer and the term *acute vascular rejection* should be used.
- Antiendothelial immune responses are probably of major importance.
- Acute vascular rejection, particularly the more severe form, responds poorly to therapy, and if prominent arterial fibrinoid necrosis is present graft failure usually occurs within a few months.

Clinical Features

- Acute vascular rejection usually appears after the second week of transplantation, most frequently within the first 2 or 3 months; however, it may appear any time.
- Renal biopsy is the only way to differentiate acute vascular rejection from acute interstitial rejection and other forms of graft disease.

Laboratory Values

- No laboratory values can be used to reliably diagnose acute vascular rejection specifically. The serum creatinine level increases.

Light Microscopy

Glomeruli

- Margination of mononuclear cells and leukocytes (transplant glomerulitis) can be noted. In severe cases, fibrinoid necrosis of the glomerular tuft may occur in some glomeruli.

Tubules

- Some degree of interstitial rejection with tubulitis is almost always present in acute vascular rejection. Patchy subcortical infarcts are commonly seen in severe cases. In these areas, the tubular epithelium is necrotic. Ischemic changes with tubular epithelial degenerative and regenerative changes are commonly seen.

Interstitium

- A variable degree of interstitial mononuclear cell infiltrate is present. The number of macrophages is usually larger than in acute interstitial rejection.
- Patchy interstitial hemorrhage reflecting microvascular injury is commonly seen.
- Areas of anemic infarcts with focal vascular occlusion are frequently present in severe cases.

Vessels

- The hallmark changes are the presence of inflammatory cells in the subendothelial space (*intimal arteritis*) and fibrinoid necrosis of the arterial wall.

- In mild cases, one to two layers of mononuclear cell infiltrate are noted in the subendothelial space without fibrinoid necrosis.
- In moderate cases, two or more layers of inflammatory cells are present in the intima with possible patchy fibrinoid change in the arterial wall.
- In severe cases, transmural arteritis is noted along with fibrinoid necrosis of the arterial wall. Secondary thrombus formation with luminal occlusion may occur.

Immunofluorescence Microscopy

- Fibrin/fibrinogen deposition can be noted within arterial walls and glomerular and peritubular capillary lumina. Sometimes complement and, rarely, immunoglobulin deposition may be present along the endothelium.
- No other characteristic immunofluorescence findings are seen, and immunofluorescence is not usually helpful in the routine diagnosis of vascular rejection.

Electron Microscopy

- Fibrin deposition within the arterial and capillary walls with patchy necrosis of the endothelium may be seen.

No other characteristic electron microscopic findings are noted.

Differential Diagnosis

- Thrombotic microangiopathies developing in the graft, including cyclosporine- or FK-506–induced thrombotic microangiopathy and recurrent hemolytic-uremic syndrome, may sometimes pose a differential diagnostic problem. In thrombotic microangiopathy, subendothelial mucoid intimal thickening, the distinctive glomerular changes ("bloodless glomeruli"), and luminal thrombi in small arterioles and glomerular capillaries are the characteristic findings; however, fibrinoid necrosis of arteries or arterioles may occur in thrombotic microangiopathies as well.

Treatment and Clinical Course

- Acute vascular rejection responds poorly to treatment with steroids, cyclosporine, or other immunosuppressants. We have seen a few patients who appeared to benefit from plasmapheresis, and other preliminary data also indicate that in certain cases plasmapheresis may be helpful.

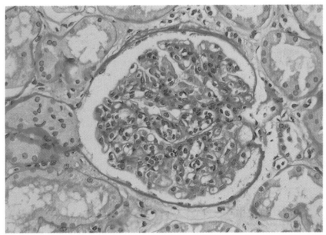

Figure 21–11. Transplant glomerulitis. Note the large numbers of mononuclear cells within glomerular capillary lumina. Transplant glomerulitis can be considered an indirect sign of at least some degree of vascular rejection because the mononuclear cell margination is most likely a consequence of prominent endothelial activation (periodic acid–Schiff reaction).

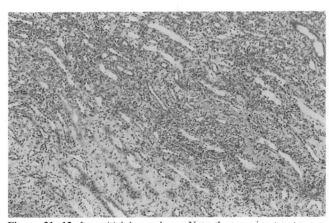

Figure 21–12. Interstitial hemorrhage. Note the prominent extravasation of red blood cells into the interstitial space. Interstitial hemorrhage in renal transplants most likely represents microvascular injury and can be considered an indirect sign of vascular (humoral) rejection. It is generally thought to be a harbinger of a poor prognosis.

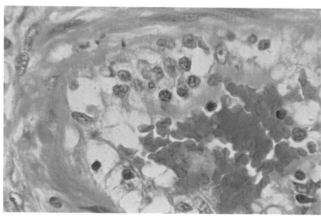

Figure 21–13. Mild acute vascular rejection. Note the swollen endothelium and infiltration of the subendothelial space by mononuclear cells (intimal arteritis). Intimal arteritis is the hallmark of mild to moderate acute vascular rejection.

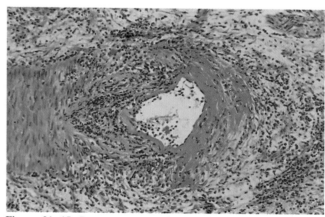

Figure 21–15. Severe acute vascular rejection. Note the transmural fibrinoid necrosis of the arterial wall and the prominent mononuclear cell infiltrate within the vascular wall. Acute vascular rejection with fibrinoid necrosis is associated with poor graft survival.

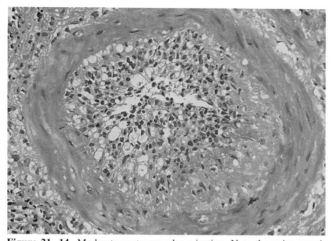

Figure 21–14. Moderate acute vascular rejection. Note the quite prominent infiltration of the intima by mononuclear cells. In this artery, a segmental area of old (probably donor transmitted) fibrous intimal thickening is also present.

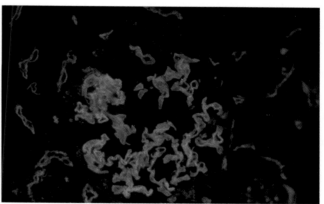

Figure 21–16. Acute vascular (humoral) rejection. Immunofluorescence picture shows prominent complement deposition along the endothelium of glomerular and peritubular capillaries. Such endothelial complement and rarely immunoglobulin deposition can occasionally (but not always) be detected by immunofluorescence in acute vascular rejection.

CHRONIC REJECTION

Synonyms and Related Terms: Obliterative transplant arteriopathy; chronic transplant nephropathy.

Biology of Disease

- Chronic rejection is the most frequent cause of graft loss today.
- The pathogenesis is not entirely clear; smoldering, ongoing, low-grade rejection or repeated acute rejection episodes are probably important factors.
- Nonimmunologic causes such as hemodynamic factors (including hypertension), ischemia, drug toxicity, the recipient's race and sex, the recipient's body weight, etc., may be contributing factors to the chronic changes.

Clinical Features

- A gradual increase in serum creatinine is a characteristic finding. Renal blood flow usually decreases in more advanced cases. Otherwise, no specific clinical symptomatology is apparent in chronic rejection.
- In some cases of chronic rejection with transplant glomerulopathy, significant, sometimes even nephrotic-range proteinuria may develop.

Laboratory Values

■ Except for gradually increasing serum creatinine levels, no laboratory findings are characteristic of chronic rejection.

Light Microscopy

Glomeruli

■ Changes of glomerular ischemia with glomerular capillary wrinkling are frequently seen.
■ In some kidneys with chronic rejection (in about 25% of kidneys transplanted 10 or more years previously), a peculiar glomerular lesion called transplant glomerulopathy develops. Light microscopic changes in transplant glomerulopathy resemble membranoproliferative glomerulonephritis or thrombotic microangiopathy. Frequently, a mixture of these two patterns is noted. A mild glomerular hypercellularity that is primarily mesangial may be present.
■ In advanced chronic rejection, glomeruli may undergo sclerosis or obsolescence.

Tubules

■ Tubular atrophy with thickened, wrinkled tubular basement membranes and simplified tubular epithelium is the most characteristic finding. Occasionally, mononuclear cells may infiltrate these atrophic tubules, the significance of which is uncertain.
■ Some tubules may undergo compensatory hypertrophy.

Interstitium

■ A variable degree of interstitial fibrosis is invariably present, usually with an uneven distribution. A patchy mononuclear cell infiltrate consisting mainly of T lymphocytes, macrophages, and plasma cells is frequently noted.

Vessels (Arteries)

■ Obliterative transplant arteriopathy is perhaps the most important change in chronic rejection. Fibrous intimal thickening with abundant extracellular matrix is seen. Some degree of intimal inflammatory cell infiltrate is frequently noted, and occasionally intimal foam cells are present.
■ The lamina elastica interna is usually lamellated and disrupted. The media is frequently thinned and has decreased layers of smooth muscle cells.
■ Sometimes in advanced, old cases, a new media-like smooth muscle layer forms around the prominently narrowed arterial lumen (vessel-in-vessel phenomenon).

Immunofluorescence Microscopy

■ Immunofluorescence is applied primarily to exclude recurrent or de novo glomerular disease.
■ Weak or segmental glomerular deposition of C3 and IgM, as well as mild linear staining for IgG along the glomerular capillary loop, is a common, but nonspecific, finding. Arteriolar IgM and C3 deposits are frequently seen.

Electron Microscopy

■ Electron microscopy is not helpful in the diagnosis of chronic rejection.
■ In transplant glomerulopathy, electron microscopy is helpful to exclude a true immune complex glomerulonephritis; in transplant glomerulopathy, subendothelial electron-lucent widening and mesangial cell interposition can be noted in the absence of discrete electron-dense immune-type deposits.

Differential Diagnosis

■ The most common differential diagnostic problem is chronic cyclosporine (or FK-506) toxicity. Arteriolar changes (hyaline change) are more prevalent than obliterative arterial changes in cyclosporine toxicity. In contrast, in chronic rejection, obliterative transplant arteriopathy is the most characteristic change, with relatively little involvement of the arterioles.
■ Donor-transmitted chronic changes are impossible to differentiate from chronic rejection after a few months unless an immediate peritransplant biopsy is available for comparison.
■ Any disease causing chronic renal changes, such as reflux nephropathy in the transplanted kidney, recurrent disease, hypertension, etc., could be mentioned in the differential diagnosis.
■ If it is difficult to decide whether the chronic changes are due to chronic rejection or some other cause, the terminology of chronic transplant nephropathy can be used.

Treatment and Clinical Course

■ The changes in chronic rejection are thought to be irreversible; no effective specific therapy is known.
■ The prognosis depends on the severity of the chronic changes. Some degree of chronic rejection (or chronic change) will eventually develop in every renal allograft.

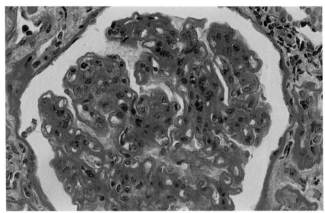

Figure 21–17. Transplant glomerulopathy. Note the lobulation of the glomerulus with some mesangial expansion and occasional double contours of the capillary loops. The morphologic pattern in transplant glomerulopathy frequently resembles membranoproliferative glomerulonephritis (periodic acid–Schiff reaction).

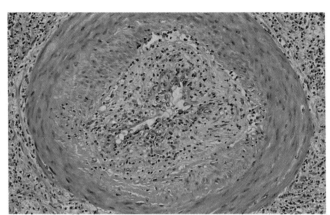

Figure 21–19. "Active" obliterative transplant arteriopathy in chronic rejection. Note the prominent thickening of the intima because of the presence of myointimal cells, abundant extracellular matrix, and inflammatory cells. Obliterative transplant arteriopathy is probably the most characteristic feature of chronic rejection.

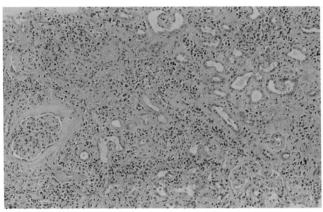

Figure 21–18. Advanced chronic rejection. Note the tubular atrophy, the interstitial fibrosis with patchy areas of inflammatory cell infiltrate containing many plasma cells, and the glomeruli showing signs of ischemia. Many of the tubulointerstitial and glomerular changes in chronic rejection are probably related to ischemia secondary to obliterative arterial changes.

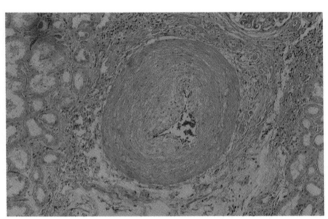

Figure 21–20. Advanced obliterative transplant arteriopathy in chronic rejection. Note the prominent fibrous intimal thickening in this artery. In advanced "burned-out" cases of chronic rejection, very few or no inflammatory cells are present in the thickened intima.

Figure 21–21. Ultrastructure of transplant glomerulopathy. Note the circumferential mesangial cell interposition in the glomerular capillary on the right side and the subendothelial, slightly electron-lucent, fluffy material in the glomerular capillary on the left side of the picture. Immunofluorescence and electron microscopy are important for distinguishing transplant glomerulopathy from immune complex glomerulonephritis, particularly from membranoproliferative glomerulonephritis; in transplant glomerulopathy, no or only a few discrete electron-dense immune-type deposits are present.

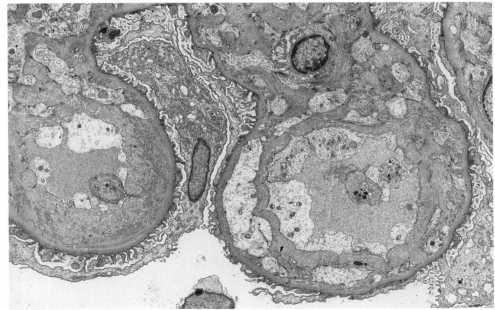

BANFF CLASSIFICATION OF RENAL TRANSPLANT REJECTION

- A recently introduced, new classification, the Banff classification is becoming more and more popular. This classification tries to overcome the overlap between the various types of rejection and is an attempt to standardize criteria to classify renal transplant rejection.
- The Banff classification consists of six diagnostic criteria:
  NORMAL
  HYPERACUTE REJECTION
  BORDERLINE CHANGES
  - Mild to moderate focal mononuclear interstitial infiltrate with occasional mild tubulitis.
  ACUTE REJECTION
    Grade I
    - At least moderate interstitial infiltrate with moderate tubulitis; no arterial changes.
    Grade II
    - At least moderate interstitial infiltrate with severe tubulitis, mild to moderate intimal arteritis, or both.
    Grade III
    - Severe intimal arteritis or transmural arteritis (or both) with fibrinoid necrosis, focal infarction, and interstitial hemorrhage (the severity of tubulointerstitial changes is not considered here).
  CHRONIC REJECTION
    Grade I
    - Mild interstitial fibrosis and tubular atrophy.
    Grade II
    - Moderate interstitial fibrosis and tubular atrophy.
    Grade III
    - Severe interstitial fibrosis and tubular atrophy with tubular loss.
  OTHER CHANGES
  - Changes not related to rejection (such as cyclosporine toxicity, acute tubular necrosis, etc.).

CYCLOSPORINE AND FK-506 NEPHROTOXICITY

Biology of Disease

- Cyclosporine and FK-506 are structurally unrelated but have very similar nephrotoxic effects. Cyclosporine is a cyclic undecapeptide of the fungus *Tolypocladium inflatum*; FK-506 is a macrolid antibiotic.
- The intracellular binding proteins for FK-506 and cyclosporine are different. However, their immunosuppressive effect is very similar, primarily suppression of T-cell responses.
- Both cyclosporine and FK-506 decrease the glomerular filtration rate and urinary excretion of nitric oxide (a potent vasodilator). It is well known that cyclosporine induces endothelin synthesis (a potent vasoconstrictor). Thus vasoconstriction is probably an important pathogenic factor in nephrotoxicity.
- Both drugs appear to have a direct tubulotoxic effect, and they are most likely inhibitory to tubular epithelial cell regeneration.

Clinical Features

- In acute nephrotoxicity in the posttransplant period, acute renal failure may occur or the normal posttransplant decrease in serum creatinine has an abnormally slow pace.
- In chronic nephrotoxicity, a gradual increase in serum creatinine concentration is noted. Chronic nephrotoxicity usually occurs several months after transplantation.

Laboratory Values

- Serum levels of cyclosporine and FK-506 should be measured and the therapeutic doses adjusted to reach appropriate serum levels.
- It is important to note that nephrotoxicity may occur even with normal cyclosporine and FK-506 levels.

Light Microscopy

Glomeruli

- The glomerular changes are not usually striking; ischemic glomeruli with capillary loop wrinkling may occur.
- In chronic nephrotoxicity, sclerotic glomeruli and occasionally even segmentally sclerotic glomeruli may be noted.
- In rare cases, the characteristic picture of thrombotic microangiopathy can be seen in the glomeruli.

Tubules

- Isometric vacuolization (small cytoplasmic vacuoles of approximately the same size) of proximal tubular epithelium is commonly seen in both cyclosporine and FK-506 toxicity.
- Although changes of acute tubular necrosis are not characteristic of cyclosporine or FK-506 toxicity, because of the tubulotoxic effects of these drugs, the doses of cyclosporine or FK-506 should be reduced if acute tubular necrosis is present.
- Tubular epithelial microcalcification is commonly noted.
- Sometimes, giant mitochondria can be seen in the tubular epithelium. However, these mitochondria are not truly useful in the diagnosis because electron microscopy is needed for definite detection.
- Tubular atrophy occurs in chronic nephrotoxicity in areas of interstitial fibrosis.

Interstitium

- Peritubular capillary congestion is commonly seen in acute nephrotoxicity, but this sign is unreliable.
- Patchy interstitial fibrosis with atrophic tubules in the fibrotic areas is commonly seen in both chronic cyclosporine and FK-506 toxicity. Because of the focal zonal distribution of this fibrosis, it is frequently designated as "striped-form" interstitial fibrosis.

Vessels

- Vacuolization of smooth muscles cells in arteries and arterioles is commonly seen; however, in our opinion this finding is fairly nonspecific.
- In chronic nephrotoxicity due to cyclosporine/FK-506, arteriolar hyaline change is very characteristic. This hyalin is frequently nodular and replaces single necrotic smooth muscle cells, and characteristically the hyaline nodules have a pearl necklace–like pattern and often protrude toward the adventitia or outer portion of the vessel wall.
- Subendothelial mucoid widening in small arteries and arterioles may also occur.
- In typical cases, unlike the situation in chronic rejection, arcuate and larger arteries are not involved.
- In rare cases of cyclosporine and FK-506 toxicity, small arterial and arteriolar changes of thrombotic microangiopathy are noted (thrombi, etc.).

Immunofluorescence Microscopy

- Immunoflourescence is not helpful in the diagnosis; the findings are mostly nonspecific. Arteriolar C3, C1q, and IgM deposition is commonly seen. Occasionally, glomerular IgM and C3 staining is also seen, particularly if glomerular sclerosis is present.

Electron Microscopy

- Electron microscopy is not helpful in the diagnosis. In occasional cases, giant mitochondria can be seen in the tubular epithelium.

Differential Diagnosis

- The aforementioned changes are generally nonspecific, and careful clinicopathologic correlation is very impor-

tant to arrive at the diagnosis of probable cyclosporine or FK-506 toxicity (e.g., where patients are on the drug with high levels in the absence of rejection or response to lowering cyclosporine/FK-506 levels).
- Isometric vacuolization of tubular epithelium can be seen in a variety of conditions, including osmotic nephrosis, contrast media–induced tubular changes, etc.
- Chronic rejection can be very difficult, if not impossible, to differentiate from chronic cyclosporine or FK-506 toxicity in a small biopsy specimen, particularly if the specimen does not contain arteries. In addition, chronic rejection and nephrotoxicity can coexist.
- Donor-transmitted nephrosclerosis can be very similar to chronic nephrotoxicity; a pretransplant or immediate posttransplant baseline biopsy may be very helpful in excluding donor-transmitted changes.
- Cyclosporine- or FK-506–induced thrombotic microangiopathy cannot be differentiated from other forms of thrombotic microangiopathy by morphology alone. From a practical point of view, these cases should be considered to be FK-506 or cyclosporine induced if the patient is taking these medications.

Treatment and Clinical Course

- Dose reduction or discontinuation of cyclosporine or FK-506 therapy with the administration of alternative immunosuppressive agents is the appropriate management.
- If the renal failure was truly due to nephrotoxicity, renal function will improve or at least deterioration in graft function will stop after dose reduction or discontinuation of cyclosporine or FK-506 therapy.
- Cyclosporine- or FK-506–induced thrombotic microangiopathy frequently has a poor outcome, with approximately a 50% short-term graft loss rate.

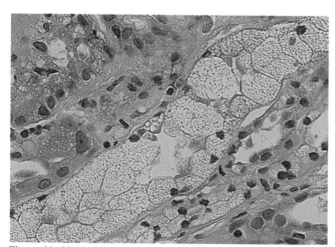

Figure 21–22. Acute cyclosporine toxicity. Note the isometric vacuolization of the tubular epithelium. Isometric vacuolization (tubular epithelial cytoplasmic vacuoles of similar small size) is a nonspecific change but characteristic of cyclosporine toxicity in renal transplants.

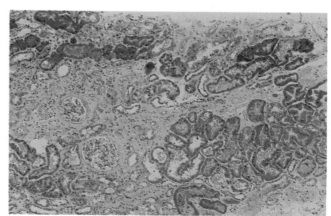

Figure 21–23. Chronic cyclosporine nephrotoxicity. Note the focal zonal ("striped-form") interstitial fibrosis with relatively well-preserved adjacent renal parenchyma. This type of fibrosis is characteristic, but not specific for chronic cyclosporine nephrotoxicity (trichrome stain).

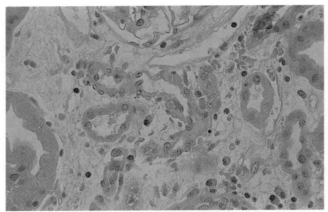

Figure 21–24. Chronic cyclosporine nephrotoxicity. Note the nodular hyaline deposits in the arterioles. Nodular pearl-like hyaline deposits, particularly along the adventitial sides of arterioles, are thought to be characteristic of cyclosporine nephrotoxicity.

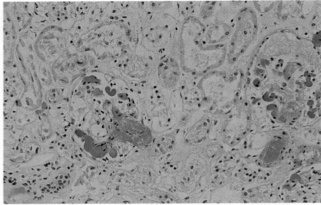

Figure 21–26. Cyclosporine-associated thrombotic microangiopathy. Note the necrosis of the afferent arteriole and the thrombi in the arterioles and glomerular capillaries. Thrombotic microangiopathy is a rare complication of cyclosporine or FK-506 treatment; it usually has a poor outcome but can be reversible after discontinuation of treatment with the responsible drug.

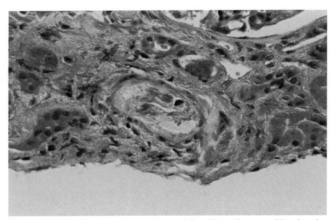

Figure 21–25. Cyclosporine nephrotoxicity. Note the mucoid subendothelial widening in this arteriole. This widening is the other type of arteriolar change (somewhat resembling the arteriolar changes in thrombotic microangiopathy) that can be seen in chronic cyclosporine nephrotoxicity (trichrome stain).

POSTTRANSPLANT LYMPHOPROLIFERATIVE DISORDERS (PTLD)

Biology of Disease

- The incidence of PTLD in the renal transplant population is about 1% to 2%, but with more potent immunosuppressive agents (particularly with the extensive use of monoclonal antibodies such as OKT3), PTLD becomes more frequent.
- The disease is caused by Epstein-Barr virus (EBV).

EBV infection may be either primary or the reactivation of a latent infection because of the immunosuppressed state.
- PTLD may be monoclonal or polyclonal.

Clinical Features

- If the transplanted kidney is involved, deterioration of graft function may occur.
- Lymphadenopathy and bone marrow involvement may be seen.

Laboratory Values

- Serologic tests for EBV infection may be useful but do not necessarily exclude the possibility of EBV infection resulting from the immunosuppressive state.

Light Microscopy

Glomeruli

- Glomeruli are not usually involved.

Tubules

- Tubules in the involved area are usually pushed apart by the dense lymphomatous infiltrate, with no or little tubulitis.

Interstitium

- The interstitium is typically densely infiltrated with polymorphous or monomorphous lymphoid or lymphoplasmacytic infiltrate.
- Most of the lymphocytes are B cells.
- Apoptosis is common in the lymphoid infiltrate, and occasionally necrosis is seen as well.
- Epstein-Barr virus is almost always detectable in many infiltrating cells by in situ hybridization.

Vessels

- No characteristic vascular changes are noted.

Immunofluorescence Microscopy

- The routine panel of antibodies used for renal immunofluorescence is not useful in the diagnosis. The cytoplasm of the plasma cells may be positive for immunoglobulins and light chains.

Electron Microscopy

- Electron microscopy is not helpful.

Differential Diagnosis

- Posttransplant lymphoproliferative disorder should be differentiated primarily from acute interstitial rejection.
- Lymphomatous infiltrate with relatively little tubulitis, predominance of B cells, and detection of EBV in the infiltrating cells are helpful in distinguishing PTLD from acute cellular/interstitial rejection.

Treatment and Clinical Course

- In many patients, PTLD will regress after reduction or cessation of immunosuppressive therapy.
- In some patients, PTLD may behave as a true lymphoma and chemotherapy or irradiation may be necessary.
- Antiviral therapy is somewhat controversial. Preventive acyclovir may be beneficial.

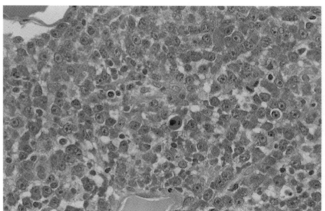

Figure 21–27. Posttransplant lymphoproliferative disorder. Note the bulky lymphoma-like infiltrate with many plasmacytoid cells pushing the tubules apart. Posttransplant lymphoproliferative disorder is frequently reversible after cessation of the immunosuppressive therapy; however, some cases behave as true progressive lymphomas.

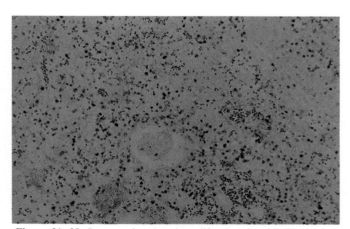

Figure 21–28. Posttransplant lymphoproliferative disorder. In situ hybridization for EBV with EBER probe (detecting EBV small nuclear RNA) shows many positive (blue) nuclei in the intersittial infiltrate. This is the best ancillary methodology for differentiating between acute rejection and PTLD involving the kidney.

References

Transplant Rejection

Colvin RB: Clinical applications of monoclonal antibodies in renal allograft biopsies. Am J Kidney Dis 11:126, 1988.

Colvin RB: The renal allograft biopsy. Kidney Int 50:1069, 1996.

Massy ZA, Guijarro C, Wiederkeihr MR, et al: Chronic renal allograft rejection: Immunologic and nonimmunologic risk factors. Kidney Int 49:518, 1996.

Nadasdy T: Transplantation. In: Silva FG, D'Agati VD, Nadasdy T (eds): Renal Biopsy Interpretation. New York, Churchill Livingstone, 1996.

Pavlakis M, Lipman M, Strom TB: Intragraft expression of T-cell activation genes in human renal allograft rejection. Kidney Int 49(suppl): 7, 1996.

Porter KA: Renal transplantation. In: Heptinstall RH (ed): Pathology of the Kidney, 4th ed. Boston, Little, Brown, 1992.

Solez K, Axelsen RA, Benekiktsson H, et al: International standardization of criteria for the histologic diagnosis of renal allograft rejection: The Banff working classification of kidney transplant pathology. Kidney Int 44:411, 1993.

Cyclosporine/FK-506 Toxicity

Bergstrand A, Bohman SO, Farnsworth A, et al: Renal histopathology in kidney transplant recipients immunosuppressed with cyclosporin A: Results of an international workshop. Clin Nephrol 24:107, 1985.

Mihatsch MJ, Ryffel B, Gudat F: The differential diagnosis between rejection and cyclosporine toxicity. Kidney Int 48(suppl):63, 1995.

Nizze H, Mihatsch MJ, Zollinger HU, et al: Cyclosporine-associated nephropathy in patients with heart and bone marrow transplants. Clin Nephrol 30:248, 1988.

Randhawa PS, Shapiro R, Jordan ML, et al: The histopathological changes associated with allograft rejection and drug toxicity in renal transplant recipients maintained on FK506. Am J Surg Pathol 17:60, 1993.

Randhawa PS, Tsamandas AC, Magnone M, et al: Microvascular changes in renal allografts associated with FK506 (tacrolimus) therapy. Am J Surg Pathol 20:306, 1996.

Young BA, Marsh CL, Alpers CE, et al: Cyclosporine-associated thrombotic microangiopathy/hemolytic uremic syndrome following kidney and kidney-pancreas transplantation. Am J Kidney Dis 28:561, 1996.

Posttransplant Lymphoproliferative Disorders

Nalesnik MA, Jaffe R, Starzl TE, et al: The pathology of posttransplant lymphoproliferative disorders occurring in the setting of cyclosporin A–prednisone immunosuppression. Am J Pathol 133:173, 1988.

Purtilo DT, Strobach RS, Okano M, et al: Epstein-Barr virus–associated lymphoproliferative disorders. Lab Invest 67:5, 1992.

Randhawa P, Demetris AJ, Pietrzak B, et al: Histopathology of renal posttransplant lymphoproliferation: Comparison with rejection using the Banff schema. Am J Kidney Dis 28:578, 1996.

CHAPTER 22

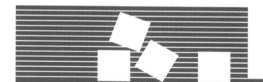

Pediatric Tumors and Tumor-Like Conditions of the Kidney

INTRODUCTION

- Accurate diagnosis and staging of pediatric neoplasms require thoughtful attention to the proper handling and sampling of biopsy and resection specimens. Perirenal fat should not be dissected from the kidney and tumor in nephrectomy specimens. In cases of penetrating tumor, suspicious areas and areas in which the tumor appears closest to the margin should be inked before opening the specimen. Reviewing the orientation of the specimen, sites of adhesions to other organs, and questionable sites of capsular rupture or penetration by the tumor with the operating surgeon may be helpful.
- The initial incision should ideally bisect the specimen so as to optimally reveal the tumor and its relation to the kidney, renal capsule, and renal sinus. This incision should avoid areas in which capsular or margin involvement is suspected. Several additional cuts made parallel to the initial cut can then be made to divide the specimen into "slabs" for fixation. Representative portions of fresh viable tissue should be snap-frozen, placed in special fixatives, or procured for any special diagnostic or research studies prior to placing the specimen in fixative.
- Sections for histologic study should generally be cut from well-fixed, rather than fresh, tissue. Allowing the tissue slabs to fix in cold formalin prior to dissection will firm the outer layers of the specimen, help prevent capsule retraction, and reduce artifactual tumor displacement.
- The weight of the nephrectomy specimen, tumor size and location, and all information important in the pathologic staging of the patient should be included in the gross and final pathology report.
- The site from which each tumor section is obtained should be carefully documented; a diagram, photograph, or other illustrative representation of the block sampling is recommended.
- It is important to sample pediatric renal neoplasms adequately. The National Wilms Tumor Study (NWTS) recommends a minimum of one block of tumor for each centimeter of the tumor's largest dimension. An alternative method for ensuring adequate systematic sampling is to submit one block for every 20 g of tumor.
- The NWTS has established and recently revised the staging system for nephroblastoma and other pediatric renal neoplasms (Table 22–1).

NEPHROBLASTOMA (WILMS TUMOR)

Synonyms: Embryoma; carcinosarcoma; adenosarcoma; adenomyosarcoma.

Note: When the eponym is used as an alternative to nephroblastoma, it is recommended that it be used in the nonpossessive form as "Wilms tumor."

General Features

- Nephroblastoma is derived from embryonic renal blastema and often recapitulates various stages of kidney development.
- Nephroblastoma is the most common malignant urinary tract tumor in children and the fifth most common malignant neoplasm of childhood (exceeded only by leukemia, lymphoma, brain tumors, and neuroblastoma as a cause of cancer-related death in this age group).
- A "premalignant" or precursor lesion, nephroblastomatosis (multicentric or diffuse foci of immature glomeruli and tubules) is identified in many cases.
- Stage and tumor histology (favorable versus unfavorable) are the most important prognostic determinants (Tables 22–1 and 22–2).

Clinical Features

- Nephroblastoma occurs primarily in children (50% of cases before 3 years of age and 90% before age 6).
- This tumor is rare in neonates and infants in the first 6 months of life; it occurs sporadically in adolescents and adults.

Table 22–1
NATIONAL WILMS TUMOR STUDY (NWTS) SYSTEM FOR STAGING PEDIATRIC RENAL TUMORS (NWTS-5)

Stage	Extent of Tumor
Stage I	Tumor confined to kidney and completely resected Requirements: No penetration of renal capsule No invasion of vessels (venous or lymphatic) of renal sinus Minor invasion of sinus soft tissues is acceptable if the medial sinus margin is free of tumor No prior open or core needle tumor biopsy (fine-needle aspiration is acceptable)
Stage II	Tumor extends locally beyond kidney but is completely resected Requirements: Tumor penetrates renal capsule or involves sinus vessels Specimen margins negative Extensive soft tissue invasion of sinus approaches (but does not definitely involve) the medial sinus margin Prior open or core needle biopsy Local rupture with spillage that does not contaminate the peritoneum
Stage III	Residual tumor confined to abdomen without hematogenous spread Includes cases with any of the following after resection: Residual tumor in abdomen Tumor in abdominal lymph nodes Diffuse peritoneal contamination by direct tumor growth, implants, or spillage Specimen margins positive
Stage IV	Hematogenous metastasis present (includes intra-abdominal organs) or involvement of lymph nodes beyond renal drainage region (e.g., mediastinal nodes)
Stage V	Bilateral renal tumors *Comment:* Tumors in each kidney should be individually substaged as I–IV. The case stage includes both stage and the substage of the most advanced tumor (e.g., stage V, substage III).

Modified from Beckwith JB: National Wilms Tumor Study: An update for pathologists. Pediatr Dev Pathol 1:79, 1998.

- A palpable abdominal mass is the classic and most common initial symptom (90%); hematuria, abdominal pain, gastrointestinal obstruction, hypertension (secondary to renin production), and symptoms related to traumatic rupture may also be present.

Table 22–2
DEFINITION OF FOCAL VERSUS DIFFUSE ANAPLASIA (NATIONAL WILMS TUMOR STUDY-5)

Focal Anaplasia
All of the following criteria must be met:
Anaplasia is confined to the primary intrarenal tumor and is not present in any invasive or extrarenal sites.
Significant cytologic atypia not quite attaining the criteria for anaplasia is not present outside the anaplastic focus/foci.
Anaplasia is sharply demarcated from adjacent non-anaplastic tumor. Size of the anaplastic foci is not important as long as they are localized. Multiple anaplastic foci are acceptable, if each focus meets the above criteria.

Diffuse Anaplasia
One or more of the following features are present:
Non-localized anaplasia
Anaplastic tumor in intrarenal or extrarenal vessels
Anaplasia outside the kidney
Anaplasia in a random biopsy
Anaplasia extending to the edge of one or more sections (e.g., the edges of the anaplastic region cannot be evaluated or the site from which the section was taken is unclear).
Anaplasia associated with severe nuclear atypia elsewhere in the tumor.

Modified from Beckwith JB: National Wilms Tumor Study: An update for pathologists. Pediatr Dev Pathol 1:84, 1998.

- There is no appreciable sex predilection.
- Stable incidence throughout the world suggests that environmental factors are not of major significance.
- Racial variation indicates a genetic predisposition (African-Americans > whites > Asians).
- The tumor is usually sporadic but is associated with several syndromes or congenital abnormalities. Hereditary anomalies that increase the risk of nephroblastoma include
  - *WAGR syndrome*—nephroblastoma (33%), aniridia, genital anomaly, mental retardation.
  - *Beckwith-Wiedemann syndrome*—omphalocele, macroglossia, hemihypertrophy, renal medullary cysts, adrenal cytomegaly.
  - *Hemihypertrophy.*
  - *Denys-Drash syndrome*—nephroblastoma, pseudohermaphroditism, glomerulonephritis.
- Hereditary (familial) nephroblastoma is uncommon (about 1% of patients registered in the NWTS have a family history positive for nephroblastoma).
- The genetic basis of Wilms tumor is complicated. Tumor development in some cases has been linked with two distinct chromosomal loci (putative tumor suppressor genes), Wilms tumor–associated genes *WT1* and *WT2* located on the short arm of chromosome 11 (*WT1* at 11p13 and *WT2* at 11p15.5).
- Regional lymph nodes, lungs, and liver are the most common sites of metastasis. Metastases to other sites, including brain and bone metastases are unusual.
- Radiologic studies, including computed axial tomography, magnetic resonance imaging, and ultrasound, are useful in staging.

Gross Pathology

- The kidney is the most common site of origin; unusual sites include inguinal, retroperitoneal, and gonadal regions.
- The tumor is usually unicentric and unilateral; multicentric masses may occur in a single kidney, and tumors are bilateral in about 5% of cases.
- Tumors are usually large (>5 cm and >500 g), solid, circumscribed (pseudoencapsulated), soft, fleshy, and friable, gray-white to tan, with or without necrosis, hemorrhage, or cystic change. A lobulated appearance is often created by prominent septa.
- Polypoid protrusions of tumor into the pelvicaliceal system may occur and produce a gross resemblance to botryoid rhabdomyosarcoma.

Microscopic Pathology

- Tremendous histologic variability is seen in nephroblastoma. Three major components are usually identified:
  - *Blastema*—consists of undifferentiated small cells with hyperchromatic nuclei, coarse and evenly distributed chromatin, inconspicuous nucleoli, and scant cytoplasm; mitotic figures are frequent. The pattern of growth may be serpentine (cord-like), diffuse, nodular, or basaloid (with peripheral palisading).
  - *Epithelial*—primitive tubules, glomerular structures, and rare rosettes or well-developed tubular and papillary structures are common; foci of mucinous, squamous, neural, or endocrine differentiation may be seen, and ciliated cells can occur.
  - *Mesenchymal*—fibroblastic, myxoid, and fibromyxoid spindle cell patterns are most common; stroma may differentiate toward skeletal muscle (striated muscle is the most common differentiated mesenchymal component), smooth muscle, fat, bone, cartilage, or neuroglial tissue. These differentiated types of mesenchymal components are often referred to collectively as heterologous elements.
- Most nephroblastomas show varying proportions of all three components (triphasic); biphasic or monophasic tumors also occur. If one component comprises more than two thirds of the tumor sample, the tumor is designated accordingly (blastemal, epithelial, or stromal predominant).
  - Uncommonly, tumors may show diffuse and predominant differentiation toward mature skeletal muscle (so-called fetal rhabdomyomatous nephroblastoma) or combinations of mature differentiated epithelium and stroma (so-called teratoid nephroblastoma).
- Histologic assessment for nuclear anaplasia is critical in terms of favorable versus unfavorable prognosis and appropriate treatment.
- Unfavorable histology (anaplasia) is defined by the presence of
  - Enlarged hyperchromatic nuclei that are at least three times the size of nuclei of the same cell type. Histologic features should suggest triaxial nuclear enlargement and not simply nuclear elongation within a single plane. *Note:* Multinucleated and enlarged nuclei

in rhabdomyoblasts are not indicative of anaplasia unless atypical mitotic figures are present.
- Multipolar mitotic figures that are structurally abnormal and enlarged and appear hyperdiploid. Enlargement of the mitotic figure is required to indicate increased DNA content.
- Both enlarged hyperchromatic nuclei and multipolar mitotic figures must be present to fulfill the criteria for anaplasia.
- Anaplasia may be focal or diffuse (Table 22–2).

Challenges and New Pathologic Concepts in Renal Pediatric Neoplasms

- The NWTS staging system has recently incorporated some new definitions and concepts of critical importance in determining therapy and prognosis. Assignment to the proper therapeutic regimen depends primarily on tumor stage and histologic category (presence or absence of anaplasia).
- Stage:
  - The distinction between stage I and II in the renal sinus is no longer defined by the hilar plane, but by the presence or absence of venous or lymphatic invasion. Tumors with lymphatic or venous invasion within the renal sinus are stage II (regardless of whether the involved vessels lay within the hilar plane).
  - Evaluation of the renal capsule is often difficult owing to formation of fibrous pseudocapsules (intrarenal and perirenal), which may fuse with the true capsule. Stage II tumors can sometimes be detected by sampling the tumor capsule near its intersection with the renal capsule to find tumor cells within perirenal fat.
- Anaplasia (Favorable Versus Unfavorable Histology):
  - Anaplasia is associated with increased resistance to chemotherapy and is not a marker of increased tumor aggressiveness.
  - The NWTS has made recent changes in the criteria for focal versus diffuse anaplasia. The original definition was based on a quantitative criterion (nephroblastoma with <10% of microscopic fields containing anaplastic features was classified as focal anaplasia). Table 22–2 outlines the revised criteria for focal versus diffuse anaplasia.

Special Studies

- Immunohistochemical studies are not generally of diagnostic value. The blastema component expresses vimentin but is generally negative for other differentiation markers; the mesenchymal components stain according to type of differentiation (e.g., muscle markers in skeletal muscle).
- Ultrastructural findings are dependent on the component present and degree of differentiation.
  - Ultrastructural studies may be helpful in biopsy specimens in which the blastemal component predominates and the differential diagnosis includes nephroblastoma and other "small blue cell tumors" (e.g., neuroblastoma and lymphoma).

- Features most helpful in confirming blastema cells include well-formed desmosomes and characteristic flocculent, electron-dense material coating the cell surface.

Differential Diagnosis

- Nephroblastoma can morphologically resemble other renal and nonrenal pediatric tumors. The differential diagnosis between nephroblastoma and other primary renal neoplasms of infancy and childhood is considered in detail in the sections describing those lesions (Table 22–3).
- The differential diagnosis may be especially challenging in large retroperitoneal tumors in which the site of origin cannot be determined or in metastatic foci.
- Clinical features are statistically important clues to the most likely diagnosis.
  - The presence of lung metastasis in a child with a retroperitoneal tumor strongly favors nephroblastoma over neuroblastoma. Neuroblastoma typically has elevated levels of catecholamine metabolites and stippled calcification on imaging studies and may show widespread metastases to bones and organs other than the lungs, liver, and lymph nodes.
  - The presence of bone metastasis in a child with an intrarenal tumor favors clear cell sarcoma over nephroblastoma.
- *Neuroblastoma and renal primitive neuroectodermal tumor (PNET):* Neuroblastoma and renal PNET may resemble blastemal predominant Wilms tumor. Histologically, the rosettes seen in some neuroblastomas and PNETs may resemble the epithelial tubules in some nephroblastomas. Tubules formed in nephroblastoma have a single parallel layer of nuclei, while classic Homer-Wright rosettes in neuroblastoma show nuclei arranged around a central fibrillary core without a distinct parallel layer of nuclei. Immunohistochemically, neuroblastoma usually shows reactivity for neuron-specific enolase and ultrastructurally has neuritic processes with neurofilaments, neurotubules, and dense-core neurosecretory granules, which are generally sparse. Renal PNET is described in Chapter 23.

Table 22–3
DIFFERENTIAL DIAGNOSIS AND
RELATIVE FREQUENCY OF PEDIATRIC
RENAL TUMORS

Tumor	Estimated Relative Frequency (%)
Nephroblastoma (favorable histology)	80
Nephroblastoma (anaplastic)	5
Mesoblastic nephroma	5
Clear cell sarcoma	4
Rhabdoid tumor	2
Miscellaneous	4
Neurogenic tumors	
Renal cell carcinoma	
Oncocytoma	
Angiomyolipoma	
Lymphoma	
Other rare neoplasms	

- *Intra-abdominal desmoplastic small round cell tumor:* This tumor typically affects adolescents and young adults. The small cell component associated with desmoplastic stroma may resemble the serpentine blastemal pattern of nephroblastoma. Nephroblastomas do not usually contain abundant collagen. Immunohistochemistry will show expression of keratin, epithelial membrane antigen, desmin, and neuron-specific enolase in the small cell component of intra-abdominal desmoplastic small round cell tumor.
- *Lymphoma:* Lymphoma cells may resemble the diffuse blastemal pattern of nephroblastoma. Immunohistochemistry with leukocyte common antigen and pan–T- and pan–B-cell markers may be helpful.
- *Other uncommon tumors:* Nephroblastoma with heterologous mesenchymal components may resemble synovial sarcoma, hepatoblastoma, pancreatoblastoma, or mesothelioma. Immunohistochemistry may be required to resolve difficult cases.
- *Renal cell carcinoma (RCC):* Nephroblastoma with a predominant monophasic epithelial component may be confused with RCC. Evaluation of nuclear features can be helpful; epithelial nuclei in nephroblastoma are often elongated, molded, and wedge shaped, in contrast to the spheroidal nuclei more characteristically seen in RCC. The diagnosis of RCC in a young patient should be made only after an unusual epithelial variant of nephroblastoma has been excluded.

Treatment and Clinical Course

- The NWTS currently includes a trial of nephrectomy alone for certain stage I favorable histology Wilms tumors (patient < 2 years of age; nephrectomy specimen < 550 g).
- Therapy for stage I tumors with favorable histology (patient ≥ 2 years of age; nephrectomy specimen ≥ 550 g), stage I tumors with anaplasia, and stage II tumors with favorable histology includes nephrectomy and double-agent chemotherapy (dactinomycin and vincristine) without radiotherapy.
- Therapy for stage III, IV, and V tumors with or without anaplasia and stage II with anaplasia includes surgery, radiotherapy, and more toxic chemotherapy.
- The majority of nephroblastomas are low stage (stage I and II), have favorable histology, and have an excellent prognosis. The most significant unfavorable prognostic factors are age of more than 2 years, high stage, and diffuse anaplasia.
- The presence of anaplasia indicates a significantly increased risk of treatment failure and poor prognosis. Anaplasia is most consistently correlated with poor prognosis when it is diffusely distributed.
  - Focal anaplasia (involving one or multiple sharply demarcated areas restricted to the intrarenal tumor) is associated with a prognosis similar to that for tumors of favorable histology.
  - Anaplasia (focal or diffuse) has no effect on prognosis for tumors confined to the kidney (stage I tumors).
  - Anaplasia is found in about 5% of nephroblastomas.

- Anaplasia is rare in children younger than 1 year of age; >80% of patients with anaplasia are older than 2 years.
■ For stage I tumors (confined to kidney and completely resected), other features associated with an increased rate of relapse include the following:
  - Presence of an inflammatory pseudocapsule

- Invasion of the renal sinus
- Extensive infiltration of the renal capsule without extracapsular penetration
- Tumor infiltration of intrarenal vessels
■ Rare cases of RCC arising within nephroblastoma have been reported; the presence of high-grade RCC indicates a worse prognosis.

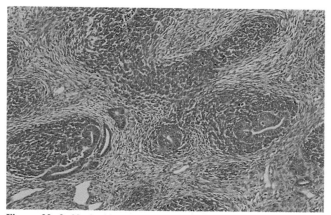

Figure 22–1. Nephroblastoma. The characteristic gross appearance of a well-circumscribed, bulging, tan-brown tumor with a lobulated appearance and areas of hemorrhage is shown.

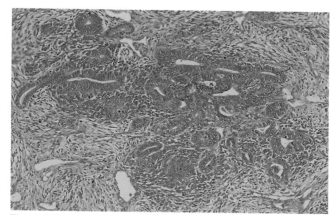

Figure 22–4. Nephroblastoma. The epithelial component shows variable stages of tubular differentiation.

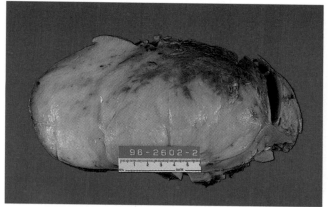

Figure 22–2. Nephroblastoma. The triphasic pattern consists of undifferentiated blastema and epithelial and mesenchymal components.

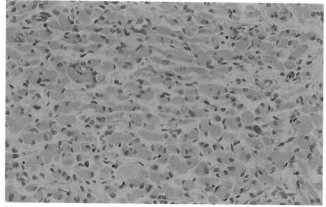

Figure 22–5. Nephroblastoma with rhabdomyoblastic differentiation. The mesenchymal component is differentiated toward skeletal muscle.

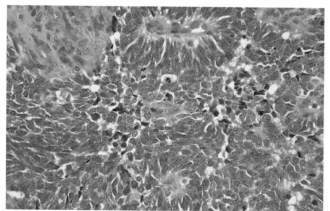

Figure 22–3. Nephroblastoma. A diffuse blastemal pattern has cohesive sheets of small cells containing hyperchromatic nuclei that are slightly elongated, molded, and wedge shaped.

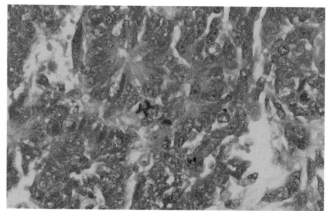

Figure 22–6. Anaplastic nephroblastoma. Unfavorable histology (anaplasia) is characterized by marked nuclear enlargement, hyperchromatism, and an enlarged multipolar mitotic figure.

NEPHROGENIC RESTS AND NEPHROBLASTOMATOSIS

General Features

- Nephrogenic rests are abnormally persistent foci of embryonal tissue; when these foci are multifocal or diffuse, the term *nephroblastomatosis* is used.
- Beckwith and colleagues have proposed the following classification:
  - Perilobar nephrogenic rests—located at the periphery of the renal lobes; composed predominantly of blastema and tubules with scanty stroma; often single with sharply demarcated margins.
  - Intralobar nephrogenic rests—located randomly in the cortex or medulla; stroma often predominates over blastemal and tubular structures; admixed irregularly with renal tissue and often multifocal.
  - Combined nephroblastomatosis—the presence of both perilobar and intralobar nephrogenic rests.
  - Universal nephroblastomatosis—rare variant in which renal tissue consists entirely of embryonal structures.
  - Nephrogenic rests are subclassified with respect to their development and morphologic appearance as dormant, incipient, involuting (sclerosing), obsolescent, hyperplastic, and neoplastic.

Significance

- Persistent foci of embryonal tissue are found in up to 40% of kidneys harboring nephroblastoma and are found in about 1% of infant autopsies.

- Careful examination of grossly uninvolved kidney in cases of nephroblastoma is important because the presence of nephrogenic rests indicates an increased risk for the development of nephroblastoma in the opposite kidney (either synchronous or metachronous).

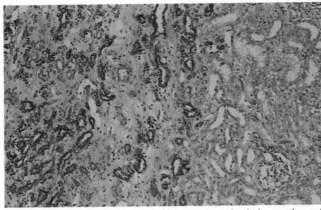

Figure 22–7. Nephroblastomatosis. Immature renal tubules are located in the subcapsular cortex in this example of perilobar nephroblastomatosis.

CYSTIC NEPHROMA (MULTILOCULAR CYST) AND CYSTIC PARTIALLY DIFFERENTIATED NEPHROBLASTOMA

Synonyms: Benign multilocular cystic nephroma; benign cystic differentiated nephroblastoma.

General and Clinical Features

- Cystic nephroma (CN) and cystic partially differentiated nephroblastoma (CPDN) are controversial lesions that are seen in both children and adults. Diagnostic criteria have been variably defined by different authors, and their pathogenesis remains debated. Some authors speculate that cases occurring in children may represent an entity distinct from those occurring in adults, while others consider CN, CPDN, and nephroblastoma to be histogenetically related. Both CPDN and CN could evolve from nephroblastoma (Joshi and

Beckwith, 1989) or from nephrogenic rests (Madewell and colleagues, 1983). Kajani and associates (1993) concluded that the presence of blastema within septa was of no clinical significance and suggested that all cases are morphologic variants of the same entity.
- CN and CPDN have two peak age distributions occurring in both children and adults.
  - These lesions are most common in children younger than 2 years with a male preponderance of 2:1.
  - Adults are most often middle-aged or elderly females (the adult form will be discussed in Chapter 23).
- Most tumors in children are asymptomatic or present as palpable masses; hematuria may be an initial symptom.
- Radiologic studies (computed tomography or ultrasound) readily identify these cystic lesions and may show progressive enlargement over time.

Gross Pathology

- CN and CPDN are both usually unilateral, solitary, well-circumscribed, multicystic masses, often with a bulging and bosselated external surface; they are usually 5 to 10 cm in size and characteristically without hemorrhage, necrosis, or calcification.

- Individual cysts range from several millimeters to several centimeters in size and are usually filled with clear serous fluid. The cysts have a smooth lining, are separated by septa composed of fibrovascular stroma, and do not communicate with one another or with the renal pelvis.
- Septa do not contain nodular expansile tumor masses (the latter would suggest cystic nephroblastoma).
- These lesions may extend beyond the renal capsule.
- The gross appearance of lesions with and without blastema is identical.

Microscopic Pathology

- Joshi and Beckwith classify these tumors according to the presence (CPDN) or absence (CN) of blastema and other immature elements in the septa between the cysts; they allow the presence of mature tubules in septa in CN. Almost 40% of tumors from patients younger than 2 years contain blastema.
- Cysts are partially lined by a single layer of epithelial cells with eosinophilic cytoplasm; the epithelium may appear cuboidal or "hobnail" and may be flattened and attenuated in larger cysts.
- Septa consist predominantly of fibrous tissue and do not contain solid masses of blastema.
- The presence of clear cells is acceptable for the diagnosis if they are restricted to the single layer of lining epithelium and do not form nests within the septa.
- According to Joshi and Beckwith, heterologous nephroblastomatous elements (e.g., skeletal muscle,

smooth muscle, and fat) are found only in lesions containing blastema.

Special Studies

- Immunohistochemical and lectin-binding studies show variable expression of proximal and distal nephron and collecting duct markers in cyst epithelium.

Differential Diagnosis

- *Cystic nephroblastoma:* The presence of expansile solid masses of primitive nephroblastomatous tissue in the cyst wall causing compression of the cysts indicates a diagnosis of Wilms tumor.
- *Clear cell sarcoma, mesoblastic nephroma,* and *renal cell carcinoma* may also be predominantly cystic and must be excluded.
- *Localized cystic disease* and *polycystic kidney disease:* The paucity of mature renal parenchymal elements in the fibrous septa of CN is the most important distinguishing feature.

Treatment and Clinical Course

- In line with the aforementioned gross and histologic definitions, CN and CPDN are benign neoplasms effectively treated by complete surgical resection. The presence or absence of blastema appears to have no impact on outcome.
- CPDN may recur if incompletely excised.
- No cases of metastasis involving CN or CPDN have been documented.

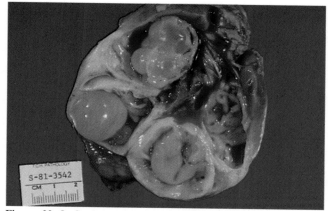

Figure 22–8. Cystic partially differentiated nephroblastoma. Grossly, the cut surface has variably sized cysts and the septa lack solid expansile tumor nodules. (Courtesy of Dr. Edith Hawkins, Houston.)

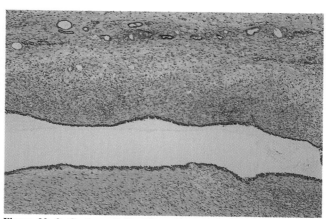

Figure 22–9. Cystic partially differentiated nephroblastoma. Embryonal elements are present within and conform to the fibrous septa between cysts. (Courtesy of Dr. Edith Hawkins, Houston.)

MESOBLASTIC NEPHROMA

Synonym: Leiomyomatous hamartoma.

General and Clinical Features

- The histogenesis of mesoblastic nephroma remains controversial; most experts favor a neoplasm of early nephrogenic mesenchyme rather than a hamartoma.
  - One theory proposes tumor origin from metanephric blastema capable of forming epithelial structures that are part of the tumor and not just entrapped. This theory regards mesoblastic nephroma as a cytodifferentiated or maturing form of nephroblastoma in which the stromal component predominates.
  - The current favored theory contends that mesoblastic nephroma is derived from secondary mesenchyme that is incapable of forming epithelial structures; according to this theory, epithelial structures are entrapped and are not part of the tumor.
- This neoplasm is usually congenital and diagnosed at birth or within the first 3 months of infancy; it is uncommon after 12 months of age. Because of the widespread use of ultrasound studies, many cases are recognized before birth.
- Rare tumors have been reported in children and adults; some experts believe that the adult form may represent a clinicopathologic entity distinct from the infantile lesion (see Chapter 23).
- Males and females are equally affected.
- Infants have an abdominal mass. Polyhydramnios and prematurity have been associated with these tumors; hypercalcemia (because of excess prostaglandin E production) and hyperreninism are also reported.
- This tumor is occasionally associated with Beckwith-Wiedemann syndrome but has not been reported in other congenital anomalies associated with nephroblastoma.

Gross Pathology

- Tumors are solitary, unilateral, gray-tan, and often large (reported size, <1 to 14 cm).
- The cut surface is often bulging, soft, or firm, with a whorled or bosselated appearance reminiscent of leiomyoma.
- Necrosis, cystic change, and hemorrhage are common findings; cysts may occasionally dominate the gross appearance.
- Most tumors are centered near the hilus of the kidney, involve the renal sinus, and may extend beyond the renal capsule. The tumor often has poorly defined infiltrative borders and tends to spread medially along the major renal vessels.

Microscopic Pathology

- Mesoblastic nephroma consists of well-defined interlacing bundles of spindled to plump polygonal cells that resemble fibroblasts or myofibroblasts.

- Several distinctive histologic subtypes are recognized on the basis of cellularity and mitotic activity. Cellularity and mitotic activity are variable but often parallel one another.
- In the classic pattern (one third or less of cases), the tumor has a relatively low cell density and low mitotic rate and resembles infantile myofibromatosis.
- Cellular variants (50% or more of cases) with substantially increased cellular density and mitotic figures more closely resemble fibrosarcoma. Two major histologic subgroups of cellular mesoblastic nephroma (not associated with clinical or biologic differences) have been described.
  - "Plump cell" mesoblastic nephroma is composed predominantly of rather large cells with vesicular nuclei that often have prominent nucleoli. Most will also contain clearly spindled areas.
  - "Blue cell" mesoblastic nephroma is composed of thinner, more closely packed spindled cells that have less vesicular nuclei and inconspicuous nucleoli.
- Classic and cellular patterns may coexist (approximately 20% of cases).
- The tumor edges are ill defined with finger-like projections that often infiltrate well beyond the grossly apparent tumor.
- Tumor commonly entraps normal renal tubules and glomeruli at the periphery; tubules may occasionally appear hyperplastic or immature and dysplastic.
- Foci of hyaline cartilage and extramedullary hematopoiesis may be seen.

Special Studies

- Immunohistochemically, the fibroblastic or myofibroblastic component is immunoreactive for vimentin, desmin, and actin; keratin and other epithelial markers are positive only within entrapped epithelium.
- Ultrastructural studies show mesenchymal differentiation.
- Cytogenetic studies have reported frequent polysomies, especially for chromosome 11 (also encountered in extrarenal infantile fibrosarcoma).

Differential Diagnosis

- *Nephroblastoma:* Unlike Wilms tumor, mesoblastic nephroma occurs most commonly in the first 6 months of life; it does not contain blastema, and the mesenchymal component does not show heterologous differentiation.
- *Clear cell sarcoma:* Differentiating mesoblastic nephroma from clear cell sarcoma can be challenging because both tumors are mesenchymal. Helpful features supporting mesoblastic nephroma include irregular tumor margins radiating into renal and perirenal tissue, an interlacing fascicular growth pattern, dilated "staghorn" vessels, coarse nuclear chromatin, high cell density with overlapping nuclei, high mitotic rate, desmin or muscle-specific actin positivity, and absence of a classic clear cell sarcoma cord pattern.

- *Renal rhabdoid tumor:* Cellular variants of mesoblastic nephroma composed of plump polygonal cells can mimic rhabdoid tumor. The presence of foci resembling rhabdoid tumor in a neoplasm that otherwise fulfills the clinicopathologic criteria of mesoblastic nephroma should not cause misdiagnosis.

Treatment and Clinical Course

- Mesoblastic nephroma usually behaves in a benign fashion; local recurrences and distant metastases are uncommon.
- The completeness of resection (rather than cellularity)

is the most important prognostic factor. Wide surgical resection with negative margins is the treatment of choice.
- Local recurrence to the abdomen (usually occurring within 1 year after nephrectomy) is the most common complication.
- Metastases usually to the lungs and brain have been reported.
- Recurrence and metastases are higher in children diagnosed beyond 12 months of age.
- Frequent radiologic evaluation to identify relapse is recommended for 1 year following nephrectomy in most cases. Relapsed disease is treated optimally, when possible, by complete surgical resection.

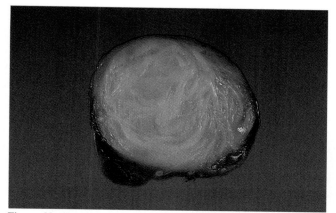

Figure 22–10. Mesoblastic nephroma. The cut surface typically has a whorled appearance resembling leiomyoma.

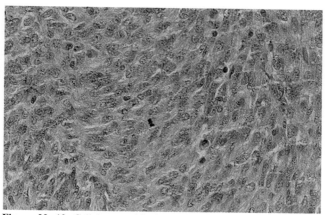

Figure 22–12. Cellular mesoblastic nephroma. The mitotic rate is increased and parallels the increased tumor cellularity.

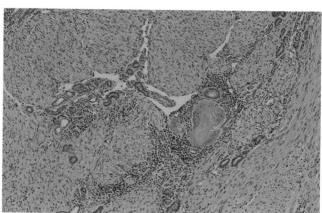

Figure 22–11. Mesoblastic nephroma. Interlacing bands of spindle cells with infiltrative borders entrap normal renal elements at the periphery of the tumor.

CLEAR CELL SARCOMA OF THE KIDNEY

Synonym: Bone-metastasizing renal tumor of childhood.

General and Clinical Features

- Also known as "bone-metastasizing renal tumor of childhood," clear cell sarcoma of the kidney (CCSK) is a rare renal neoplasm that was originally recognized and named for its marked propensity to metastasize to bone.
- The histogenesis of CCSK remains uncertain; assumed differentiation is toward primitive nephrogenic mesenchyme.
- It accounts for approximately 5% of pediatric renal neoplasms.
- The incidence of CCSK is highest between 1 and 3 years of age; it is rare in infants less than 6 months of age, and no cases in adults are well documented.
- There is a male preponderance (3 : 2).
- No racial or geographic predisposition has been observed.
- There is no known familial incidence or association with congenital anomalies.
- Patients usually have an abdominal mass.
- Widespread metastases are often present at the time of diagnosis; metastatic sites in addition to bone include regional lymph nodes, brain, lung, liver, and soft tissue, including periorbital fat.

Gross Pathology

- Tumors are usually well circumscribed, single, and unilateral, often larger than 500 g.
- The cut surface usually appears firm, variably homogeneous, gray, and lobular or variegated gray and pink with prominent cystic change; production of mucosubstances may impart a glistening appearance.
- Tumors are usually confined within the renal capsule.

Microscopic Pathology

- The classic pattern has monomorphous cords or nests of cells separated by vascular septa containing prominent small branching blood vessels.
  - Cells have nuclei with finely dispersed chromatin, small nucleoli, and pale or vacuolated cytoplasm with indistinct borders.
  - Depending on the fixative used, the vacuoles may appear empty or filled with pale or granular mucopolysaccharides; these abundant mucosubstances account for the "clear cell" appearance.
  - Despite the name, cytoplasmic clarity should not be required for the diagnosis; most tumors contain areas in which the cytoplasm appears more condensed and eosinophilic.
- Variant patterns include spindle cell proliferations, prominent collagenous sclerosis, and myxoid, epithelioid, cystic, palisading, sinusoidal (hemangiopericytoma-like), and pleomorphic areas that are often admixed with the classic pattern.

- Mitotic activity is variable; it may appear deceptively lower than that in other malignant pediatric renal tumors.
- Infiltrative borders between tumor and adjacent kidney with entrapment of benign renal tubules are characteristic (the entrapped tubules may appear embryonal or hyperplastic).

Special Studies

- Immunohistochemistry and electron microscopy are chiefly helpful in excluding other pediatric renal neoplasms.
  - Immunohistochemistry is positive for vimentin in some cases of CCSK.
  - Electron microscopy shows scant intermediate filaments and incompletely formed cell junctions.

Differential Diagnosis

- The variant CCSK patterns may cause diagnostic confusion with other pediatric renal neoplasms, but most CCSKs have the classic pattern at least focally. Helpful diagnostic features include the pale, homogeneous appearance on hematoxylin and eosin stain, the tendency for the tumor to entrap and isolate nephrons at its periphery, and the prominent collagen background.
- *Nephroblastoma:* Foci of blastema and heterologous mesenchymal components such as muscle and cartilage are not identified in CCSK.
- *Rhabdoid tumor:* CCSKs may occasionally contain focal areas reminiscent of rhabdoid tumor. CCSK is characterized by inconspicuous nucleoli, more lucent cytoplasm, and a less infiltrative tumor interface.

Treatment and Clinical Course

- Treatment includes surgery and chemotherapy.
- The tumor is resistant to conventional therapy for nephroblastoma but is often responsive to doxorubicin chemotherapy regimens.
- A propensity for late recurrence is characteristic; relapses after intervals of 5 years have been reported.

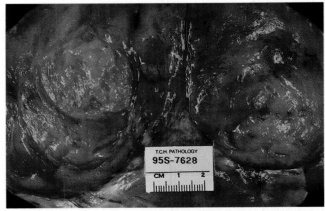

Figure 22–13. Clear cell sarcoma of the kidney. This large tumor has an irregular homogeneous light cut surface and extensively replaces normal kidney. (Courtesy of Dr. Edith Hawkins, Houston.)

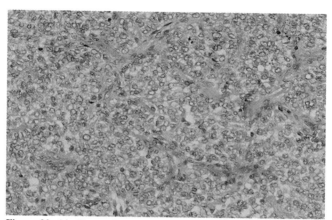

Figure 22–14. Clear cell sarcoma. The classic pattern has nests of cells with pale vacuolated cytoplasm associated with prominent small branching vessels.

RHABDOID TUMOR

General and Clinical Features

- Rhabdoid tumor is a rare tumor of uncertain histogenesis (although the name refers to the resemblance of tumor cells to immature skeletal muscle, there is no evidence of myogenic differentiation).
- Rhabdoid tumor accounts for approximately 2% of renal tumors in childhood.
- Most cases (approximately 90%) occur in children younger than 2 years of age; it is rare after 4 years of age.
- Tumors are more common in males, with a preponderance of 1.5 : 1.
- Patients usually have an abdominal mass and often metastasis at the initial diagnosis.
- Association with primitive neuroectodermal tumors of the central nervous system (15%) and paraneoplastic hypercalcemia has been reported.
- Extrarenal rhabdoid tumors with morphologic features substantially similar to their renal counterparts have been reported over a wider age range. A more heterogenous group of extrarenal and renal tumors with "rhabdoid features" which mimic renal rhabdoid tumor are also encountered.

Gross Pathology

- Tumors are soft, fleshy, yellow-gray to pale tan, and often large, and lack encapsulation; smaller satellite nodules may be present; hemorrhage and necrosis are common.
- The main tumor mass is usually located medially in the kidneys and generally involves the renal sinus and pelvis.

Microscopic Pathology

- The classic pattern consists of diffuse monotonous sheets of poorly cohesive cells with a large, eccentric nucleus, thick nuclear membrane, large central nucleolus, and abundant eosinophilic cytoplasm containing a typical large hyaline inclusion that displaces the nucleus. The cytoplasmic inclusions may be sparse.
- A wide range of other patterns (sclerosing, epithelioid, spindled, lymphomatoid, vascular, pseudopapillary, and cystic) may occur, typically mixed with the classic pattern.

Special Studies

- Ultrastructural and immunohistochemical studies indicate primitive epithelial differentiation.
- Immunohistochemical studies have provided conflicting results. According to Wick et al (1995), tumor cells are consistently reactive for vimentin and usually reactive for cytokeratins and epithelial membrane antigen; muscle and neural (including CD99) markers are usually negative.
- Ultrastructurally, the cytoplasmic inclusions consist of whorled aggregates of intermediate filaments 6 to 10 nm in thickness.
- No consistent cytogenetic abnormalities have been reported; cytogenetic abnormalities involving chromosome 11 (characteristic of Wilms tumors) have not been identified in renal rhabdoid tumors.

Differential Diagnosis

- A wide range of renal tumors with filamentous cytoplasmic inclusions, prominent nucleoli, and rhabdoid differentiation, including *nephroblastoma, renal cell carcinoma, mesoblastic nephroma, transitional cell carcinoma of the renal pelvis, renal medullary carcinoma, and rhabdomyosarcoma* may mimic rhabdoid tumor and need to be excluded.

■ *Nephroblastoma with extensive skeletal muscle differentiation (fetal rhabdomyomatous nephroblastoma)* may be confused with rhabdoid tumor or rhabdomyosarcoma.

■ The differential diagnosis can usually be resolved with thorough tissue sampling and conventional light microscopy; immunohistochemistry and electron microscopy are sometimes also necessary.

Clinical Course

■ Rhabdoid tumor is the most malignant of all pediatric renal neoplasms.

■ It usually metastasizes widely (lungs, abdomen, lymph nodes, liver, brain, and bone) and causes death within 12 months of diagnosis.

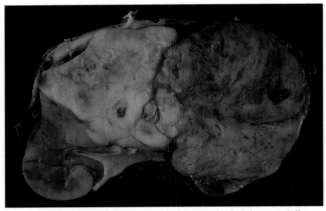

Figure 22–15. Rhabdoid tumor. This large, pale, bulging, partially necrotic tumor appears irregularly demarcated from the adjacent kidney.

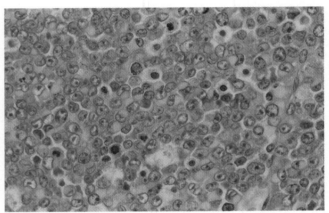

Figure 22–16. Rhabdoid tumor. Sheets of tumor cells have large vesicular nuclei, prominent nucleoli, and cytoplasmic inclusions that displace the nucleus.

METANEPHRIC ADENOFIBROMA

Synonym: Nephrogenic adenofibroma. Metanephric adenofibroma is the preferred nomenclature for avoiding confusion with nephrogenic adenoma, a lesion that is usually found in the urinary bladder or urethra.

General and Clinical Features

■ Metanephric adenofibroma is a recently described and very uncommon renal tumor of children and young adults (range, 3.5 to 23 years; mean age, 13 years).

■ Patients may have systemic manifestations, including polycythemia, hypertension, or hematuria, that resolve following nephrectomy.

■ These tumors are believed by some experts to derive from multiple nephrogenic rests that persist after birth, undergo slow maturation, and differentiate into mesenchymal elements. This composite epithelial and stromal tumor may be related histogenetically to metanephric adenoma (see Chapter 23) and may be part of a spectrum of tumors with varying proportions of stromal and epithelial components.

Gross Pathology

■ Metanephric adenofibroma forms firm, pale tan, spheroidal or irregular nonencapsulated masses with or without cystic change; margins are ill defined.

Microscopic Pathology

■ Fascicles of fibroblast-like spindle cells that lack nuclear atypia or mitotic figures surround discrete nodules of an embryonal-appearing epithelial component.

■ The epithelial component consists of small cuboidal to columnar epithelial cells with darkly staining nuclei, scant cytoplasm, inconspicuous nucleoli, and no significant mitotic activity; these cells are arranged in sheets or in papillary, tubular, or glomeruloid patterns that contain frequent psammoma bodies.

■ The margins of the spindle cell proliferation are irregularly infiltrative and entrap adjacent normal renal tubules and glomeruli.

■ Two reported cases were associated with small well-circumscribed papillary tumors located near the renal pelvis that resembled so-called low-grade collecting duct carcinomas.

Differential Diagnosis

- *Nephroblastoma:* Metanephric adenofibroma lacks the active proliferative growth features and mitotic activity characteristic of Wilms tumor; unlike nephroblastoma, the tumor is unencapsulated and interdigitates with uninvolved renal parenchyma.
- *Mesoblastic nephroma:* The mesenchymal cells of metanephric adenofibroma histologically mimic the spindle cell proliferation and infiltrative growth pattern seen in the classic type of mesoblastic nephroma. The mesenchymal cells in metanephric adenofibroma lack immunoreactivity for actin or desmin and also lack the myofibroblastic features of mesoblastic nephroma.
- Clinical features are also helpful in that metanephric adenofibroma tends to occur at a later age than mesoblastic nephroma and nephroblastoma.

Treatment and Clinical Course

- Treatment has included complete surgical resection; two patients were also treated with adjuvant chemotherapy appropriate for nephroblastoma.
- Preliminary data suggest a nonaggressive clinical course; no recurrence or metastasis has been reported to date, but the number of reported cases is few and the period of follow-up is short. Close clinical follow-up is indicated.

OSSIFYING RENAL TUMOR OF INFANCY

General and Clinical Features

- Ossifying renal tumor of infancy is a very rare tumor of uncertain histogenesis that has been reported in four male infants less than 6 months of age evaluated for hematuria.
- Radiologic studies often reveal a calcified mass in the pelvicalyceal system that may mimic renal calculus clinically and radiologically.

Gross and Microscopic Pathology

- The tumor forms a hard, calcified mass that projects into the renal pelvis and has ill-defined borders with adjacent medullary tissue.
- The tumor consists of poorly cellular nests of plump cells with small round to oval nuclei and variable amounts of pale cytoplasm that are embedded within a matrix of dense bone; mitotic figures are infrequent.
- Osteoclasts and cartilaginous tissue are not present.

Treatment and Clinical Course

- Treatment consists of surgical resection.
- The clinical course is benign, with no reported recurrences or metastases to date.

LYMPHANGIOMA

- Lymphangioma is a rare cause of renal enlargement, either unilateral or bilateral, that can be confused with infantile polycystic disease, nephroblastomatosis, or renal vein thrombosis.
- Lymphangioma shows predominantly cortical involvement but usually also involves medullary tissue.
- Renal lymphangioma may actually represent diffuse or pericalyceal lymphangiectasia rather than a true neoplasm.

INTRARENAL TERATOMA

- Intrarenal teratoma is a very rare primary pediatric renal neoplasm. Many of the reported cases may actually represent nephroblastoma with teratoid differentiation.
- Nonrenal tissues (such as brain, gastrointestinal, skin, etc.) should be identified in true renal teratomas, and their presence represents the major differentiating feature from teratoid nephroblastoma.

OTHER UNCOMMON PEDIATRIC NEOPLASMS

- Renal cell carcinoma is uncommon in the pediatric age group but is histologically identical to tumors in adults.
- Lymphoreticular and hematopoietic tumors (see Chapter 18) may be manifested as unilateral or bilateral renal masses in children and must be differentiated from nephroblastoma, neuroblastoma, and other "small blue cell tumors."

REFERENCES

Nephroblastoma

Beckwith JB: Wilms' tumor and other renal tumors of childhood: A selective review from the National Wilms' Tumor Study Pathology Center. Hum Pathol 14:481, 1983.

Beckwith JB: National Wilms' Tumor Study: An update for pathologists. Pediatr Dev Pathol 1:79, 1998.

Breslow NE, Sharples K, Beckwith JB, et al: Prognostic factors in nonmetastatic, favorable histology Wilms' tumor. Cancer 68:2345, 1991.

Charles AK, Vujanic GM, Berry PJ: Renal tumors of childhood. Histopathology 32:293, 1998.

Faria P, Beckwith JB, Mishra K, et al: Focal versus diffuse anaplasia in Wilms' tumor—new definitions with prognostic significance: A report from the National Wilms Tumor Study Group. Am J Surg Pathol 20:909, 1996.

Green DM, Beckwith JB, Weeks DA, et al: The relationship between microsubstaging variables, age at diagnosis and tumor weight of children with stage I/favorable histology Wilms' tumor. Cancer 74:1817, 1994.

Murphy WM, Beckwith JB, Farrow GM: Tumors of the Kidney, Bladder, and Related Structures, 3rd ed. Washington, DC, Armed Forces Institute of Pathology, 1994.

Re GG, Hazen-Martin DJ, Sens DA, et al: Nephroblastoma (Wilms' tumor): A model system of aberrant renal development. Semin Diagn Pathol 11:126, 1994.

Weeks DA, Beckwith JB, Luckey DW: Relapse-associated variables in stage I favorable histology Wilms' tumor, a report of the National Wilms' Tumor Study. Cancer 60:1204, 1987.

Zuppan CW: Handling and evaluation of pediatric renal tumors. Am J Clin Pathol 109(Suppl 1):S31, 1998.

Nephroblastomatosis

Beckwith JB: Precursor lesions of Wilms' tumor: Clinical and biological implications. Med Pediatr Oncol 21:158, 1993.

Beckwith JB, Kiviat NB, Banadio FJ: Nephrogenic rests, nephroblastomatosis, and the pathogenesis of Wilms' tumor. Pediatr Pathol 10:1, 1990.

Bove KE, McAdams AJ: The nephroblastomatosis complex and its relationship to Wilms' tumor: A clinicopathologic treatise. Perspect Pediatr Pathol 3:185, 1976.

Machin GA: Persistent renal blastema (nephroblastomatosis) as a frequent precursor of Wilms' tumor: A pathological and clinical review. Part 1. Nephroblastomatosis in the context of embryology and genetics. Am J Pediatr Hematol Oncol 2:165, 1980.

Cystic Nephroma (Multilocular Cyst) and Cystic Partially Differentiated Nephroblastoma

Castillo OA, Boyle ET Jr: Multilocular cysts of kidney, a study of 29 patients and review of the literature. Urology 37:156, 1991.

Eble JN: Cystic nephroma and cystic partially differentiated nephroblastoma: Two entities or one? Adv Anat Pathol 1:99, 1994.

Joshi VV, Beckwith JB: Multilocular cyst of the kidney (cystic nephroma) and cystic, partially differentiated nephroblastoma. Cancer 64:466, 1989.

Kajani N, Rosenberg BF, Bernstein JL: Multilocular cystic nephroma. J Urol Pathol 1:33, 1993.

Madewell JE, Goldman SM, Davis CJ, et al: Multilocular cystic nephroma: A radiographic-pathologic correlation of 58 patients. Radiology 146:309, 1983.

Mesoblastic Nephroma

Beckwith JB, Weeks DA: Congenital mesoblastic nephroma. When should we worry? (editorial). Arch Pathol Lab Med 110:98, 1986.

Bolande RP: Congenital mesoblastic nephroma of infancy. Perspect Pediatr Pathol 1:227, 1973.

Bolande RP, Brough AJ, Iaant RJ Jr: Congenital mesoblastic nephroma of infancy: Report of eight cases and the relationship to Wilms' tumor. Pediatrics 40:272, 1967.

Gonzalez-Crussi F, Sotelo-Avila C, Kidd JM: Malignant mesenchymal nephroma of infancy: Report of a case with pulmonary metastases. Am J Surg Pathol 4:185, 1980.

Gormley TS, Skoog SJ, Jones RV, et al: Cellular congenital mesoblastic nephroma: What are the options? J Urol 142:479, 1989.

Howell CG, Othersen HB, Kiviat NE, et al: Therapy and outcome in 51 children with mesoblastic nephroma: A report of the National Wilms' Tumor Study. J Pediatr Surg 17:826, 1982.

Joshi VV, Kasznica J, Walters TR: Atypical mesoblastic nephroma. Arch Pathol Lab Med 100:106, 1986.

Pettinato G, Manivel JC, Wick MR, et al: Classical and cellular (atypical) congenital mesoblastic nephroma: A clinicopathologic, ultrastructural, immunohistochemical and flow cytometric study. Hum Pathol 20:682, 1989.

Schofield DE, Yunis EJ, Fletcher JA: Chromosome aberrations in mesoblastic nephroma. Am J Pathol 143:714, 1993.

Clear Cell Sarcoma

Marsden HB, Lawler W: Bone metastasizing renal tumor of childhood: Histopathological and clinical review of 38 cases. Virchows Arch 387:341, 1980.

Marsden HB, Lawler W, Kumar PM: Bone metastasizing renal tumor of childhood: Morphological and clinical features, and differences from Wilms' tumor. Cancer 42:1922, 1978.

Mierau GW, Weeks DA, Beckwith JB: Anaplastic Wilms' tumor and other clinically aggressive childhood renal neoplasms: Ultrastructural and immunocytochemical features. Ultrastruct Pathol 13:225, 1989.

Rhabdoid Tumor

Bonnin JM, Rubinstein LJ, Palmer NF, et al: The association of embryonal tumors originating in the kidney and in the brain, a report of seven cases. Cancer 54:2137, 1984.

Haas JE, Palmer NJ, Weinberg AG, et al: Ultrastructure of malignant rhabdoid tumor of the kidney, a distinctive renal tumor of children. Hum Pathol 12:646, 1981.

Palmer NF, Sutow W: Clinical aspects of the rhabdoid tumor of the kidney: A report of the National Wilms Tumor Study Group. Med Pediatr Oncol 11:242, 1983.

Sotelo-Avila C, Gonzalez-Cruzzi F, deMello D, et al: Renal and extrarenal rhabdoid tumors in children: A clinicopathologic study of 14 patients. Semin Diagn Pathol 3:151, 1986.

Weeks DA, Beckwith JB, Mierau GW, et al: Renal neoplasms mimicking rhabdoid tumor of kidney, a report from the National Wilms' Tumor Study Pathology Center. Am J Surg Pathol 15:1042, 1991.

Weeks DA, Beckwith JB, Mierau GW, et al: Rhabdoid tumor of kidney, a report of 111 cases from the National Wilms' Tumor Study Pathology Center. Am J Surg Pathol 13:439, 1989.

Wick MR, Ritter JH, Dehner LP: Malignant rhabdoid tumors: A clinicopathologic review and conceptual discussion. Semin Diagn Pathol 12:233, 1995.

Metanephric Adenofibroma

Hennigar RA, Beckwith JB: Nephrogenic adenofibroma, a novel kidney tumor of young people. Am J Surg Pathol 16:325, 1992.

Ossifying Renal Tumor of Infancy

Chatten J, Cromie WJ, Duckett JW: Ossifying tumor of infantile kidney, report of two cases. Cancer 45:609, 1980.

Jerkins GR, Callihan TR: Ossifying renal tumor of infancy. J Urol 135:120, 1986.

Renal Lymphangioma

Pickering SP, Fletcher BD, Bryan PJ, et al: Renal lymphangioma: A cause of neonatal nephromegaly. Pediatr Radiol 14:445, 1984.

Intrarenal Teratoma

Dehner LP: Intrarenal teratoma occurring in infancy: Report of a case with discussion of extragonadal germ cell tumors in infancy. J Pediatr Surg 8:367, 1973.

CHAPTER 23

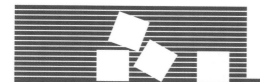

Adult Renal Tumors and Tumor-Like Conditions

INTRODUCTION

- Protocols for handling adult tumor-bearing nephrectomy specimens usually recommend that the perirenal fat and capsule overlying the tumor be left intact to optimize evaluation of the tumor-fat interface.
- Gross examination should determine the inking of margins near areas of suspected extracapsular tumor penetration. The renal vein and regional lymph nodes should be examined grossly for evidence of tumor involvement.
- Histologic sections should be representative of any areas having unusual gross features and should be submitted to provide all the information required for accurate pathologic staging.
- The gross and final surgical pathology report should contain information regarding tumor size, location, histologic type, and nuclear grade; status of the capsule and surgical margins; presence or absence of renal vein invasion; and lymph node involvement.

CLASSIFICATION OF RENAL EPITHELIAL NEOPLASMS

- The classification of renal epithelial tumors has been the subject of considerable controversy and change during the past two decades (Table 23–1).
- The World Health Organization classification system (1981) categorized tumors on the basis of cell type (clear, granular, oncocytic, spindle, and mixed), architecture (tubular, papillary, solid, cystic, sarcomatoid, etc.), and presumed site of origin (proximal versus distal tubular origin).
- Thoenes and colleagues (1986—Mainz, Germany) proposed a classification of renal epithelial tumors based on morphologic, histochemical, and electron microscopic features. The basic tumor cell types included clear, chromophilic (basophilic, eosinophilic), chromophobe, oncocytic, and spindle shaped/pleomorphic and subsequently included categories of collecting duct carcinoma and mixed tumors.
- Recent cytogenetic and molecular information (Kovacs and others) has demonstrated consistent patterns of

cytogenetic abnormalities which differentiate various adult renal epithelial tumors (Table 23–2). The proposed cytogenetic classification of renal tumors shows considerable correlation with the cytologic subtypes outlined by Thoenes et al.

- A contemporary classification of renal epithelial neoplasms based on morphology and current knowledge of genetic and molecular information was proposed following two international workshops on renal cell carcinoma held independently in Heidelberg, Germany, and Rochester, Minnesota, during 1997. These workshops resulted in substantially similar classifications (referred to as the Heidelberg and Rochester Classifications in Table 23–1). Granular renal cell carcinoma (RCC) is no longer a diagnostic category in these classifications. Oncocytoma and subsets of chromophobe RCC, papillary RCC, collecting duct carcinoma, and clear cell RCCs with cytoplasmic eosinophilia have been removed from this heterogeneous group of tumors formerly known as granular RCCs.
- Cytogenetic and molecular techniques are sure to provide further refinement of these classification systems.

RENAL CELL CARCINOMA

Synonyms: Renal adenocarcinoma; hypernephroma; Grawitz's tumor.

General Features

- Renal cell carcinoma (RCC) accounts for about 2% of all human cancers; the most common malignant renal tumor, RCC accounts for about 90% of all primary malignant renal tumors in adults.
- Grawitz (1883) favored origin of these tumors from ectopic adrenal rests (hence the term *hypernephroma*).
- Modern morphologic, immunohistochemical, and ultrastructural studies have shown the vast majority of RCCs to demonstrate differentiation toward mature renal tubular epithelium.
- The incidence of RCC varies among countries, with the highest rates being in North America and Scandinavia;

Table 23–1
COMPARISON OF VARIOUS CLASSIFICATION SYSTEMS
FOR RENAL EPITHELIAL TUMORS

WHO (1981)	Mainz (Thoenes et al)	Cytogenetic	Heidelberg/ Rochester (1997)
Adenoma	Adenoma	Papillary tumors	Benign
Renal cell carcinoma	Renal cell carcinoma	Adenoma	Papillary adenoma
Clear cell type	Clear cell	Carcinoma	Oncocytoma
Granular cell type	Chromophilic	Nonpapillary (clear cell)	Metanephric adenoma and
Spindle cell type	Basophilic	Chromophobe	adenofibroma
Others	Eosinophilic	Oncocytoma	Malignant
Bellini duct carcinoma	Duophilic		Clear cell carcinoma
	Chromophobe		Papillary carcinoma
	Typical		Chromophobe carcinoma
	Eosinophilic		Collecting duct
	Collecting duct		carcinoma
	Oncocytoma		Renal cell carcinoma,
			unclassified

WHO, classification system proposed by Mostofi et al in the World Health Organization Histologic Typing of Kidney Tumours in 1981; Heidelberg/Rochester Classifications, see Kovacs G et al. J Pathol 183:131, 1997 and Störkel S et al. Cancer 80:987, 1997.

the incidence has been steadily rising over the past three decades, predominantly because of improved radiologic diagnostic techniques.

■ Renal cancer can be induced in animals with a variety of agents, including viruses, hormones, x-rays, and various chemicals such as aromatic hydrocarbons.
  • None of these agents has been proved to be an important etiologic factor for RCC in humans (with the exception of the factors listed next).
  • The most important etiologic factor for RCC in humans is tobacco smoking.
  • Obesity (particularly in females) and occupational exposure to petroleum products, heavy metals, or asbestos are additional risk factors in humans.

Clinical Features

■ Renal cell carcinoma occurs in all ages but increases in incidence with advancing age; the incidence peaks in the sixth decade of life; it is reported rarely in children and infants as young as 6 months.
■ Renal cell carcinoma is more common in men, with most studies showing a 2:1 male preponderance.
■ Most cases are sporadic (without a recognizable hereditary pattern).

• Several rare familial (hereditary) forms occur and are characterized by autosomal dominant inheritance, younger age at diagnosis (the third to fifth decades), and bilateral and multifocal tumors.
• There is also a familial incidence associated with von Hippel–Lindau disease, a multiple-cancer syndrome with a predisposition to a variety of neoplasms, including RCCs (clear cell type), renal cysts, angiomyolipomas, retinal hemangiomas, hemangioblastomas of the central nervous system, pheochromocytomas, pancreatic cysts and carcinomas, and cystadenoma of the epididymis; RCC develops in about 40% of patients with von Hippel–Lindau disease and is a major cause of death.
• Renal cell carcinoma is also associated with acquired renal cystic disease arising in patients with chronic renal failure and with autosomal dominant polycystic kidney disease.
■ The most common initial symptoms in all RCCs are hematuria (60%), flank pain (50%), or an abdominal mass (33%), symptoms often indicative of an advanced stage of disease at diagnosis.
  • A combination of all three of the aforementioned symptoms (the classic triad) is present in about 10% of all cases.

Table 23–2
CYTOGENETIC CHARACTERISTICS AND RELATIVE FREQUENCY OF ADULT RENAL EPITHELIAL TUMORS

Neoplasm	Cytogenetic Abnormality Major	Minor	Frequency* (%)
Clear cell RCC	$-3p$	$+5q, +7, +12, -6q, -8p, -9, -14q, -Y$	75
Papillary RCC	$+7, +17, -Y$	$+12, +16, +20, -14$	10–15
Chromophobe RCC	$-1, -2, -6, -10, -13, -17, -21$		5
Collecting duct carcinoma	No consistent abnormality		<1
Oncocytoma	-1 and $-Y$; translocations involving 11q13		5
RCC, unclassified	Heterogeneous		<1

*Relative frequency of adult renal epithelial tumors in surgical series.
RCC, renal cell carcinoma.

- Other common systemic manifestations include fever, night sweats, malaise, weight loss, anemia, and gastrointestinal symptoms.
- A metastasis of RCC may be the initial manifestation of a clinically unsuspected renal primary in about 10% to 25% of all patients.
- Systemic metastases are identified in 25% to 30% of patients at initial evaluation.
  - The most common sites of distant metastases include lung, bone, liver, adrenal gland, and brain.
  - Unusual sites of metastases are common for renal cancer; virtually any organ or tissue can be involved, including the thyroid, pancreas, skeletal muscle, skin, soft tissue, heart, ovaries, salivary glands, and oral mucosa.
- Renal cell carcinoma is known as one of the great masqueraders in medicine because of its ability to produce a diversity of systemic symptoms and paraneoplastic effects that are attributable to inappropriate or ectopic hormone production or immunologic or unknown mechanisms. These paraneoplastic manifestations include
  - Polycythemia (from production of an erythropoietin-like substance).
  - Hypertension (from increased renin production).
  - Hypercalcemia (associated with parathormone-like secretion).
  - Masculinization or feminization (associated with secretion of gonadotropins and placental lactogen).
  - Ectopic production of glucagon, prolactin, prostaglandin A, and insulin-like substances.
  - Hepatic dysfunction, neuromyopathy, leukemoid reactions, and amyloid production.
- Radiologic studies, including intravenous pyelography, ultrasound, and computed tomography (CT), aid in the diagnosis, evaluation, and staging of renal masses.
  - With the widespread use of newer imaging techniques, 25% to 40% of diagnoses are made after the detection of an incidental renal mass.
  - Angiography shows characteristic tumor vascularity in more than 95% of cases; now it is rarely used in diagnosis and is performed mainly in selected cases for preoperative angiographic mapping when nephron-sparing surgery is planned.

Pathology

- The gross, microscopic, and specific cytogenetic, immunohistochemical, and ultrastructural features of the various subtypes of RCC and its variants will be discussed in further detail in later sections.

Pathologic Staging of Renal Cell Carcinoma

- The most commonly used staging systems include the modified Robson system and the tumor node metastasis (TNM) system recommended by the American Joint Committee on Cancer (Table 23–3). Both systems have their advantages and disadvantages, and both pro-

Table 23–3
STAGING OF RENAL CELL CARCINOMA

Modified Robson System	TNM System (1997)	
Stage I Tumor confined within the renal capsule	T1	Tumor 7 cm or less, limited to kidney
	T2	Tumor >7 cm, limited to kidney
Stage II Tumor confined by Gerota's fascia	T3a	Tumor invades adrenal gland or perinephric adipose tissue, but not beyond Gerota's fascia
Stage III A Gross renal vein or inferior vena cava involvement	T3b	Tumor grossly involves renal vein or vena cava below diaphragm
	T3c	Tumor involves vena cava above diaphragm
B Lymphatic invasion	N1	Metastasis in a single regional lymph node
	N2	Metastasis in >1 regional lymph node
C Both vascular and lymphatic involvement		
Stage IV A Invasion of adjacent organs (other than ipsilateral adrenal gland)	T4	Tumor invades beyond Gerota's fascia
B Distant metastasis	M1	Distant metastasis (includes ipsilateral adrenal gland)

vide useful prognostic information regarding survival based on patterns of tumor growth and dissemination. The new 1997 TNM classification is the result of efforts aimed at developing a common international staging system. Because staging classifications are subject to ongoing re-evaluation, additional systems will certainly be proposed as our knowledge of renal cancer advances.

- Challenges may arise in the staging of RCC because of problems involved in interpretation of the capsule or pseudocapsule and renal vein invasion.
  - Tumors that bulge into perinephric adipose tissue but remain limited by the renal capsule or pseudocapsule should be regarded as pathologic (p)T1 or pT2. Bulging above the renal contour does not qualify as invasion beyond the confines of the kidney. Obvious gross extracapsular tumor extension or histologic evidence of infiltrative growth into perirenal and/or renal sinus adipose tissue should be required for classification of tumor as pT3a.
  - Renal vein invasion is defined by grossly evident tumor within the renal vein or its segmental (muscle-containing) branches or within the vena cava; vascular invasion of smaller intrarenal veins identified at the microscopic level may be indicative of a worse prognosis in the pT2 cases but should not upstage the tumor.
  - The distinction between direct invasion of the adrenal (pT3a) and metastasis to the adrenal gland (M1) is prognostically important. The surgical pathology report should document whether the presence of carcinoma in the adrenal gland is direct extension or metastasis.

Grading of Renal Cell Carcinoma

■ Several grading systems are currently in use throughout the world, with no consensus regarding the optimal system. Although grading systems are subject to interobserver variation and lack of reproducibilty, most experts agree that grading provides useful prognostic information. The most widely accepted grading scheme in North America is that of Fuhrman and colleagues, in which nuclear features are the main criteria for tumor grading (Table 23–4).
  • In the Fuhrman system, the tumor is classified by the highest-grade nuclear component, regardless of its prevalence.

Treatment and Clinical Course

■ The clinical course of RCC is notoriously unpredictable, with documented recurrences 10 or more years

Table 23–4
NUCLEAR GRADING OF RENAL CELL CARCINOMA*

Grade 1	Round uniform nuclei (approximately 10 μm); nucleoli not visible or inconspicuous (at 400×)
Grade 2	Larger nuclei (approximately 15 μm) with irregular contours; small nucleoli present (at 400×)
Grade 3	Larger nuclei (approximately 20 μm) with more irregular contours; prominent nucleoli (at 100×)
Grade 4	Grade 3 features plus pleomorphic or multilobated nuclei, with or without spindle cells

*Criteria of Fuhrman et al. Grading is based on the most malignant features, even if only focal.

after nephrectomy seen in more than 10% of patients who survive that long. Spontaneous regression of metastasis has been documented rarely (< 1%) after surgical excision of the renal primary and also in the absence of nephrectomy.
■ Radical nephrectomy (removal of the kidney, perinephric fat, Gerota's fascia, and ipsilateral adrenal gland) is the standard therapy for localized RCC.
■ Partial nephrectomy may be performed for bilateral RCC, in the surgical treatment of patients with anatomically or functionally solitary kidneys, and in selected patients with compromised renal function.
■ Preoperative angioinfarction (using an embolus of absorbable gelatin sponge, steel coils, or autologous muscle) performed a few days preoperatively may reduce tumor vascularity and facilitate the resection of large renal tumors.
■ Surgical resection may also be of value in the treatment of solitary metastases to the lung, liver, brain, or elsewhere.
■ Present systemic chemotherapeutic agents and hormones, used singly and in combination, have little or no effect against RCC.
■ Immunotherapy with interferon and interleukin-2 has shown promising clinical results.
■ The therapeutic benefit of regional lymphadenectomy remains controversial.
■ Preoperative or postoperative radiation therapy has not been conclusively documented to be of value in the treatment of disseminated disease.
■ Tumor stage and grade (see earlier) are the most important determinants of clinical outcome.

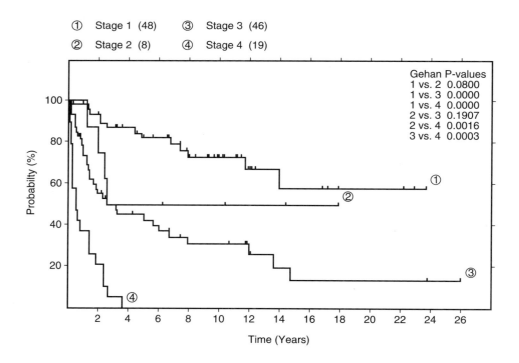

Figure 23–1. Actuarial disease-free survival of patients with renal cell carcinoma according to stage. (From Medeiros LJ, Gelb AB, Weiss LM, et al: Renal cell carcinoma. Prognostic significance of morphologic parameters in 121 cases. Cancer 61:1639, 1988, with permission.)

CLEAR CELL RENAL CELL CARCINOMA

General and Clinical Features

- Clear cell carcinoma, the most common type of RCC, accounts for about 75% of all surgically resected adult renal epithelial tumors (benign and malignant).
- This group includes the conventional clear and granular (clear cell-eosinophilic variant of Thoenes et al) RCCs not included in other groups.

Gross Pathology

- Most tumors appear to be centered on the cortex and are usually solitary and unilateral.
  - In early stages, most tumors appear to be circumscribed by a pseudocapsule composed of compressed fibrotic non-neoplastic renal tissue.
  - In more advanced stages, tumors may largely replace renal parenchyma and show a marked tendency for invasion of the renal vein; tumors may invade the inferior vena cava and rarely extend into the right atrium of the heart.
- Gross features are highly variable with respect to size, color variegation, consistency, and extent of secondary alterations such as hemorrhage, necrosis, and cystic change.
  - Bright yellow areas correspond histologically to tumor cells rich in lipid, pale tan-white areas may indicate tumors cells containing more glycogen and less lipid, and brown areas may reflect tumor cells rich in subcellular organelles.
  - Areas of recent hemorrhage are red-violet, and rusty discoloration corresponds to old hemorrhage.
  - Cystic spaces may contain gelatinous semitranslucent amber material.
  - Firm white to pale gray semitranslucent areas often indicate hyaline fibrosis.
  - Fleshy, pale tan-white areas may indicate a sarcomatoid component.
  - Tumors may be multifocal.
- Bilateral tumors occur in 1% of cases and are more common in patients with von Hippel–Lindau disease and tuberous sclerosis.

Microscopic Pathology

- Clear cell tumors characteristically have transparent cytoplasm in formalin-fixed sections and distinct cell membranes. The cell cytoplasm appears lucent because of variable amounts of glycogen and lipid.
  - Some cells may have a perinuclear or diffuse cytoplasmic distribution of eosinophilic material that may appear finely to more coarsely granular (clear cell eosinophilia), a feature often associated with high nuclear grade; this type of cell may predominate in some areas of the tumor. Clear cell eosinophilia accounts for the prior classification of some tumors as granular and mixed clear and granular cell types.

- Tumors occasionally may have extensive cytoplasmic deposits of hemosiderin or numerous cytoplasmic hyaline globules that are brightly eosinophilic in hematoxylin and eosin stain.
- Some tumors may have large cells with eccentric nuclei and abundant eosinophilic cytoplasm with "rhabdoid" features (i.e., features vaguely resembling rhabdomyoblastic differentiation).
- Multinucleated giant cells are an uncommon histologic feature.
- Architecturally, the most common tumor patterns are alveolar, trabecular, tubular and microcystic. Although a single histologic pattern may predominate in some tumors, a diverse combination of growth patterns is often identified when multiple sections from any given tumor are examined.
  - The fibrous stroma typically contains numerous thin-walled or ectatic blood vessels that may partition the tumor into compact alveolar or trabecular patterns. This rich vascular network is a diagnostically valuable feature. The fibrous and vascular stroma may be less conspicuous in areas of tumor with a more solid appearance.
  - Whereas the compact alveolar and trabecular patterns lack luminal differentiation, the tubular and microcystic patterns have central spaces that may be empty or filled with eosinophilic serous material or red blood cells.
  - Papillae lined by clear cells may be present focally. A predominant papillary architecture composed of clear cells is very rare (further cytogenetic and molecular studies will be useful in determining whether such tumors are best classified as clear cell or papillary carcinomas).
- Hemorrhage into stroma and areas of necrosis and fibrosis are common.
- The nuclei in clear cell RCCs range from round, small, and hyperchromatic with invisible or inconspicuous nucleoli to large and pleomorphic with prominent nucleoli. Considerable nuclear heterogeneity can exist in a single tumor.
  - Most clear cell RCCs are nuclear grades 2 and 3.
  - Grade 4 tumors account for 5% to 10% of cases, and grade 1 tumors are uncommon (<5%).
- Mitotic rate is highly variable. Mitotic figures are rare in grade 1 and 2 tumors, but are usually more easily identified in grade 3 and 4 tumors.

Special Studies

- Histochemical, immunohistochemical, and lectin-binding studies provide evidence that clear cell RCCs usually differentiate toward proximal tubular epithelium.
- The neutral lipids that are typically dissolved during routine tissue processing can be identified in frozen sections (or in formalin-fixed tissue that has not been processed through alcohol and xylene) using oil red 0 or other fat stains. Glycogen can be identified by the periodic acid–Schiff reaction. Clear cell RCCs generally do not stain for mucin and do not show strong or diffuse staining with Hale's colloidal

iron (hemosiderin, which is often present, will stain with Hale's colloidal iron).

■ Immunohistochemically, clear cell RCCs are characteristically immunoreactive for broad-spectrum cytokeratin, epithelial membrane antigen, or both and also coexpress vimentin; they express low-molecular-weight cytokeratins (8/18, 19, and 7) and are negative for high-molecular-weight cytokeratin and carcinoembryonic antigen. Dedifferentiation leads to increasing expression of vimentin and decreased expression of keratin. Use of a broad-spectrum cocktail of several monoclonal anticytokeratins (e.g., AE1/AE3, CAM 5.2, MAK-6) will maximize the identification of epithelial differentiation.

■ Immunohistochemistry may provide information useful in differentiating clear cell RCCs from other clear cell neoplasms with similar histologic appearance (e.g., adrenocortical carcinomas, melanomas with "balloon cell" features, clear cell hepatocellular carcinomas, clear cell adenocarcinomas of the müllerian tract, clear cell germ cell tumors, clear cell chondrosarcoma, and clear cell osteosarcoma) and may be useful in the study of metastatic disease. However, RCC is an immunohistochemical "have-not" in that it expresses few, if any, antigenic determinants that allow specific localization of an occult tumor primary with metastasis.

■ Ultrastructurally, tumor cells show numerous cell junctions and often show a glandular arrangement around microlumina, demarcation of groups of cells by basal lamina, and varying numbers of microvilli located on the luminal aspect of cell membranes (the presence of brush border is considered indicative of differentiation toward proximal tubular epithelium); abundant lipid vacuoles and glycogen are characteristic features, and hyaline globules 5 to 7 μm in diameter may be present. Organelles such as Golgi and rough endoplasmic reticulum are sparse.

■ Cytogenetic and restriction fragment length polymorphism analysis reveals a consistent deletion involving the short arm of chromosome 3, del(3)(p25), in 97% of clear cell RCCs. Other frequent aberrations include numerical or structural alteration in the long arm of chromosome 5 ($+$5q) and the long arm of chromosome 14 ($-$14q).

■ About 50% of clear cell RCCs show somatic mutations in the von Hippel–Lindau (*VHL*) gene, and an additional 10% to 20% show inactivation of the *VHL* gene by epigenetic changes (hypermethylation). Identification of the gene for VHL disease on chromosome 3p25 and its mutation in the majority of clear cell RCCs provide strong evidence that the *VHL* gene is the tumor suppressor gene whose inactivation contributes to tumor development in both RCC associated with VHL disease and sporadic cases of clear cell RCC.

Differential Diagnosis

■ *Papillary renal cell carcinoma:* Clear cell RCCs may show prominent cytoplasmic eosinophilia and may have a focal papillary architecture; such tumors should not be included in the papillary (chromophil) group of RCCs.

■ *Chromophobe cell carcinoma:* Renal cell carcinomas of the clear cell type that contain numerous cells showing clear cell eosinophilia may be confused with the eosinophilic variant of chromophobe cell carcinoma. Adequate tumor sampling will usually identify areas of more classic clear cell appearance.

■ *Xanthogranulomatous pyelonephritis and malakoplakia:* These unusual inflammatory disorders can be confused both clinically and pathologically with RCC. The initial symptoms of flank mass, pain, weight loss, and hematuria overlap with those of RCC. The characteristic gross appearance of large, yellow, tumor-like masses that may infiltrate perinephric fat may also be confused with RCC. Histologically, the inflammatory infiltrate of foamy macrophages in xanthogranulomatous pyelonephritis may be confused with the clear cells of RCC. The large eosinophilic macrophages (Von Hansemann cells) observed in malakoplakia may be confused with the clear cells with cytoplasmic eosinophilia of RCC. Attention to the foamy character of the macrophage cytoplasm, the presence of an associated inflammatory infiltrate (composed mostly of lymphocytes and plasma cells), and lack of the vascular network and architectural patterns characteristic of RCC should enable a correct diagnosis of xanthogranulomatous pyelonephritis. Identification of characteristic intracytoplasmic inclusions known as Michaelis-Gutmann bodies (containing calcium and sometimes iron salts) within the macrophages establishes the diagnosis of malakoplakia.

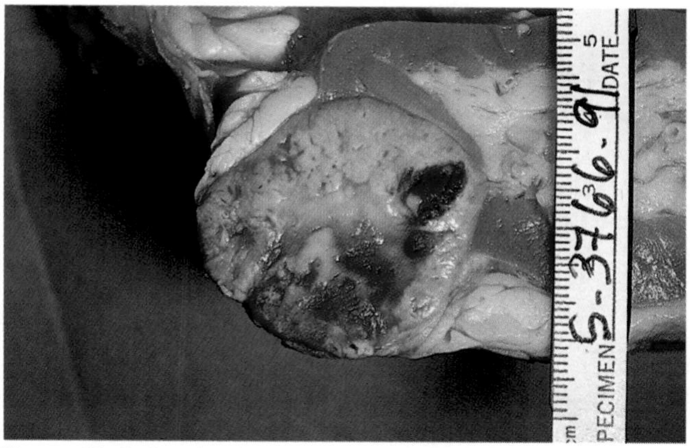

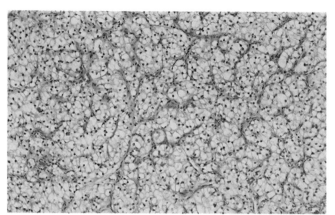

Figure 23–2. Renal cell carcinoma, clear cell type. This relatively small, well-circumscribed tumor has characteristic tan-yellow areas interspersed with hemorrhage and central pale gray hyalinization. The tumor bulges into perinephric fat but would be staged as confined to the kidney unless histologic sections showed infiltrative growth into perinephric fat.

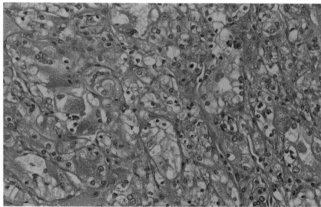

Figure 23–5. Renal cell carcinoma, clear cell type. Tumor cells with clear cytoplasm are invested by sparse stroma with prominent thin-walled blood vessels, creating a compact alveolar architecture. This characteristic histologic appearance is one of the most common of many patterns that can be found in any individual tumor.

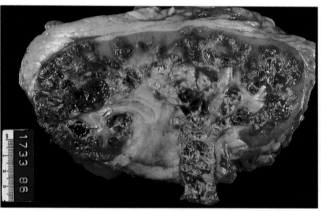

Figure 23–3. Renal cell carcinoma, clear cell type. This large tumor has characteristic variegated tan-yellow to brown areas with extensive hemorrhage and necrosis. The tumor largely replaces renal parenchyma and invades the renal vein.

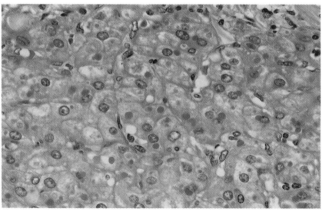

Figure 23–6. Renal cell carcinoma (RCC), clear cell type with eosinophilia. Many of the tumor cells have fine eosinophilic or slightly granular eosinophilic cytoplasm and are admixed with cells having the characteristic lucent cytoplasm. These tumors were previously classified as RCC of mixed clear and granular cell type.

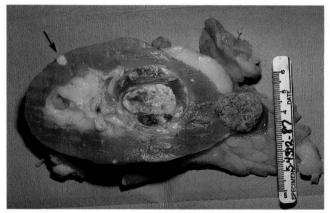

Figure 23–4. Multicentric renal cell carcinoma. Two separate renal cell carcinomas are associated with a small subcapsular tumor nodule *(small arrow).*

Figure 23–7. Renal cell carcinoma, clear cell type with eosinophilia and hyaline globules. An admixture of cells with cytoplasmic eosinophilia and clear cytoplasm have fairly numerous eosinophilic hyaline globules.

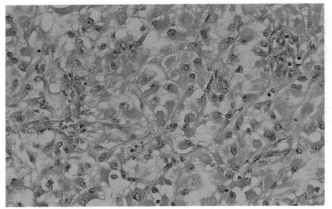

Figure 23–8. Renal cell carcinoma (RCC), clear cell type with eosinophilia. This tumor consists of cells with optically lucent cytoplasm and prominent cytoplasmic eosinophilia and has "rhabdoid features" that may mimic rhabdomyoblastic differentiation. These features may occasionally be seen in high-grade clear cell RCCs and should not be confused with rhabdoid tumor.

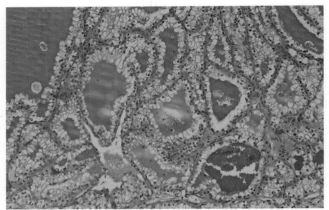

Figure 23–9. Renal cell carcinoma, clear cell type. A tubular and microcystic architecture is created by spaces, some of which are cystically dilated and filled with proteinaceous fluid or blood.

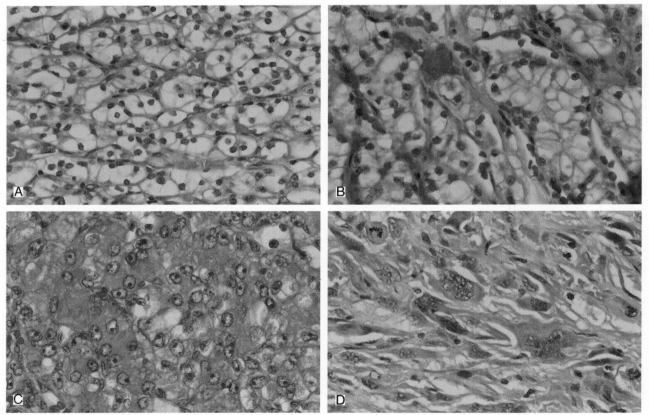

Figure 23–10. Nuclear grading of renal cell carcinoma (RCC). This composite photograph shows the four nuclear grades of RCC in the Fuhrman system. *A,* Fuhrman nuclear grade 1 with uniform round tumor nuclei and absent to inconspicuous nucleoli. *B,* Fuhrman nuclear grade 2 with slightly larger tumor cells with small nucleoli. *C,* Fuhrman nuclear grade 3 with more nuclear and nucleolar enlargement. *D,* Fuhrman nuclear grade 4 with bizarre multilobated and spindled nuclei.

PAPILLARY (CHROMOPHIL) RENAL CELL CARCINOMA

General Features

- Papillary RCCs have been described under the designation of chromophil RCC in the Mainz (Thoenes et al) classification and have also been called tubulopapillary. Papillary RCC was originally defined as a histologic subtype of RCC in which at least 50% of the tumor is composed of true papillae. A papillary or tubulopapillary architecture predominates in the vast majority and is present, at least focally, in almost all cases; compact (solid) and cystic patterns may also be seen. Papillary (chromophil) RCC may encompass some of the so-called granular cell tumors of other classification schemes.
- Papillary RCCs account for about 10% to 15% of surgically resected adult renal epithelial tumors.
- Multifocality and bilaterality are more common than in classic clear cell carcinoma.
- Papillary RCCs are also more often associated with adenomas and dysplastic changes within renal tubules.
- Angiographically, the majority of these tumors are hypovascular, a reflection of the hemorrhage and necrosis, which is extensive in many cases.
- An additional unique clinical feature is the tendency of papillary tumors to occur in patients with end-stage renal disease, especially after prolonged dialysis.

Gross Pathology

- Tumors are usually well circumscribed, often surrounded by a thick pseudocapsule, and appear red-brown to tan-yellow.
- The cut surface most often appears friable secondary to extensive necrosis; hemorrhage and cystic change may be conspicuous; crumbling tissue may have a crystalline sheen.
- Sizes range widely, and many tumors are large.

Microscopic Pathology

- Most tumors have a predominant papillary or tubulopapillary growth pattern; solid or trabecular components may be seen in areas of more compact tumor growth (compact packing of papillae may impart a solid architecture whereas parallel arrays of papillae may produce a trabecular pattern); hyalinization of papillary cores may produce a sclerotic appearance.
- Foamy macrophages are often present within fibrovascular stalks.
- Psammoma bodies may be present.
- Papillary (chromophil) tumors are subclassified as basophilic, eosinophilic, or mixed (duophilic) on the basis of cell type:
  - Basophilic cells have small round nuclei with dense chromatin and inconspicuous nucleoli, small volume of cytoplasm, and a high nuclear-cytoplasmic ratio, and the nuclear staining enhances the impression of basophilia in hematoxylin and eosin–stained sections.
  - Eosinophilic cells are characterized by more abundant granular cytoplasm that ultrastructurally contains numerous organelles; chromatin pattern is more open than in the basophilic cell type, and nucleoli are often prominent.
  - Mixed (duophilic) types consist of a mixture of basophilic and eosinophilic cell types.
- Papillary RCCs of basophilic type are predominantly low nuclear grade while eosinophilic variants are often high grade.
- Solid variants of papillary RCC composed of solid growth patterns lacking true papillae have been estimated to represent fewer than 3% of all papillary RRCs.
- High-grade papillary RRCs, although predominantly papillary, often exhibit tubular and solid growth patterns, show intratubular spread, and may elicit a prominent desmoplastic stromal response.
- Cases with clear cells can be included if the clear cells are a minor component of the tumor.

Special Studies

- Periodic acid–Schiff with and without diastase shows scant glycogen; these tumors do not stain with Hale's colloidal iron (except for hemosiderin).
- Like the clear cell carcinomas, papillary RCCs express low-molecular-weight cytokeratins 8/18, 19, and 7; in contrast to clear cell RCCs, vimentin expression is often very weak to negative but can be pronounced at the basal pole in basophilic cell types.
- Ultrastructurally, papillary-basophil RCCs contain only a few organelles, mainly endoplasmic reticulum, whereas the eosinophilic type contains more abundant mitochondria.
- Papillary RCCs are characterized by polysomies involving chromosomes 7 and 17 and loss of Y plus a number of other abnormalities including trisomies of chromosomes 16, 20, and 12 (see Table 23–4).

Differential Diagnosis

- *Clear cell RCC with cytoplasmic eosinophilia:* Papillary (chromophil) tumors must be distinguished from clear cell RCCs in which the majority of cells have eosinophilic cytoplasm. A predominant papillary or tubulopapillary architecture is characteristic of papillary RCCs. Clear cell RCCs usually show multiple architectural patterns in any single tumor; a tubulopapillary component may be present, but usually as a focal (not a predominant) pattern.
- *Collecting duct carcinoma (CDC):* These tumors have a papillary architecture and an infiltrating tubular component with prominent desmoplasia and may occasionally be difficult to distinguish from high-grade papillary RCCs (see discussion of CDCs later).
- *Metanephric adenoma:* Low-grade papillary RCCs with a tubular or solid (vague tubular) architecture may resemble metanephric adenoma. Papillary RCCs usually have more abundant cytoplasm, greater nuclear atypia, and at least occasional nucleoli in contrast to the scant

cytoplasm, more uniform nuclei, and lack of nucleoli characteristic of metanephric adenoma.

Clinical Course

■ Past studies have variably reported the prognosis of papillary RCC to be better than or similar to the prog-

nosis of clear cell RCC. Recent literature suggests that papillary RCC tends to present at a lower stage and has a better overall 5-year survival rate than clear cell RCC. Papillary RCCs do, however, have the potential for aggressive behavior. Stratification of papillary RCCs according to cell type, nuclear grade, and stage appears to provide useful prognostic information.

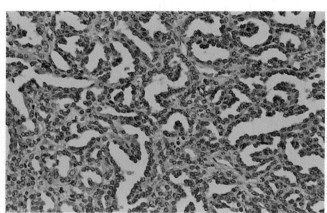

Figure 23–13. Papillary renal cell carcinoma, chromophil-basophilic cell type. The papillary chromophil-basophilic cell type has tumor cells with scant amphophilic cytoplasm and a high nuclear-to-cytoplasmic ratio that on hematoxylin and eosin stain imparts a basophilic appearance.

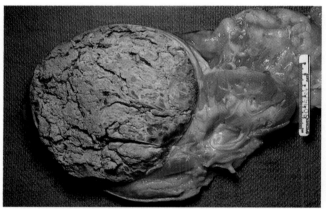

Figure 23–11. Renal cell carcinoma, papillary (chromophilic) type. A well-circumscribed tumor is surrounded by a pseudocapsule composed of compressed renal parenchyma. The tumor has extensive necrosis and a friable crumbling appearance.

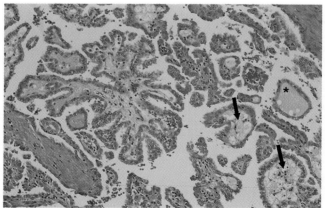

Figure 23–12. Papillary (chromophil) renal cell carcinoma. The prominent papillary architecture is created by neoplastic cells lining central fibrovascular cores that focally contain foamy macrophages *(arrows)* and edema *(asterisk)*.

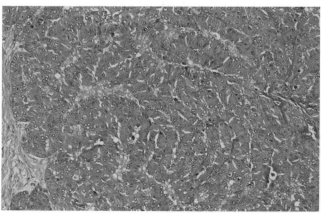

Figure 23–14. Papillary renal cell carcinoma, chromophil-eosinophilic cell type. The eosinophilic variant of papillary tumors is characterized by columnar tumor cells with eosinophilic granular cytoplasm and nuclei with prominent nucleoli. In this example the papillary architecture is more compacted and mimics a trabecular pattern.

CHROMOPHOBE RENAL CELL CARCINOMA

General and Clinical Features

- Chromophobe RCC is a variant that was first described as a distinctive clinicopathologic entity by Thoenes and colleagues in 1985.
- This tumor is believed to arise from intercalated cells in the renal collecting ducts and may be the malignant counterpart of renal oncocytoma.
- Chromophobe RCCs account for approximately 5% of surgically resected adult renal epithelial tumors.
- They occur predominantly in middle-aged patients and show no sex predilection.

Gross Pathology

- Tumors are well circumscribed, homogeneous, and tan-brown.
- In contrast to oncocytoma, these tumors frequently show hemorrhage and necrosis but lack a central scar; cystic change is uncommon.

Microscopic Pathology

- Classic and eosinophilic variants have been described.
  - The classic type is characterized by cells with abundant pale, finely reticular cytoplasm, often with perinuclear clearing and a more dense peripheral zone of cytoplasmic condensation adjacent to the cell membrane (producing a halo around the nucleus). Nuclei tend to be central but may have an eccentric location and have coarse chromatin with variable nucleoli. Scattered large pleomorphic tumor cells are often concentrated along small blood vessels.
  - The eosinophilic variant contains cells with cytoplasmic eosinophilia, often with perinuclear clearing; in most cases classic areas can be identified focally. The eosinophilic variant may also contain areas that closely resemble oncocytoma.
  - Solid architecture is most common without the prominent vascular network characteristic of clear cell RCCs.

- Nuclear grading has not been validated for chromophobe RCCs, but most are grade 2.
- Sarcomatoid transformation has been reported.

Special Studies

- The histochemical hallmark of chromophobe RCC is diffuse and strong reticular cytoplasmic staining with Hale's colloidal iron.
- Immunohistochemically, the tumors express low-molecular-weight cytokeratin but not vimentin.
- Ultrastructurally, numerous cytoplasmic microvesicles are characteristic and distinctive; some evidence suggests that these vesicles are derived from the mitochondrial membrane.
- Cytogenetic studies demonstrate distinctive karyotypic abnormalities, including multiple monosomies involving chromosomes 1, 2, 6, 10, 13, 17, and 21 (in decreasing order of frequency) and hypodiploidy; rearrangement of mitochondrial DNA has also been reported (see Table 23-4).
- DNA flow cytometry shows a mixed population of hyperdiploid and hypodiploid cells.

Differential Diagnosis

- *Clear cell RCC with cytoplasmic eosinophilia, papillary RCC (eosinophilic type), and oncocytoma:* Chromophobe carcinoma, especially the eosinophilic variant, must be differentiated from other RCCs with eosinophilic cytoplasm. Oncocytoma may closely mimic the eosinophilic variant of chromophobe carcinoma, grossly and histologically. Generous tissue sampling and close attention to cytologic features are crucial. Special stains (Hale's colloidal iron) or electron microscopy may be required for resolving this sometimes difficult differential diagnosis.

Clinical Course

- Current data suggest that this tumor has a better prognosis than the usual clear cell RCC of similar grade and stage.

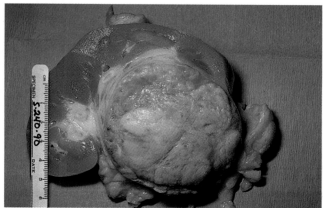

Figure 23-15. Chromophobe renal cell carcinoma. This renal cell carcinoma is well circumscribed, homogeneous, and tan-pink and has an appearance often seen in tumors of the chromophobe cell type.

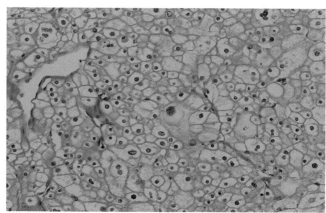

Figure 23-16. Chromophobe renal cell carcinoma. The classic type is characterized by polygonal tumor cells with pale-staining, finely reticular cytoplasm, perinuclear clearing, and a peripheral zone of cytoplasmic condensation. Scattered, large pleomorphic tumor cells are an additional characteristic feature.

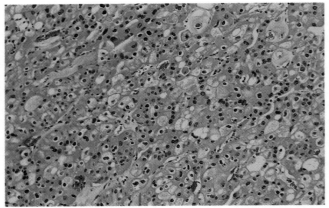

Figure 23–17. Chromophobe renal cell carcinoma. Hale's colloidal iron stain colors the cytoplasm of chromophobe cells blue; this strong diffuse staining pattern is a characteristic histochemical feature. (Hale's colloidal iron stained section courtesy of Dr. Mahul Amin, Detroit.)

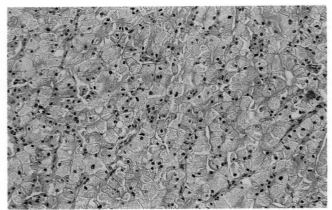

Figure 23–18. Chromophobe renal cell carcinoma, eosinophilic variant. Most tumor cells have eosinophilic cytoplasm, often with perinuclear clearing, and are intermingled with pale-staining cells that retain the cytologic features characteristic of classic chromophobe carcinoma.

COLLECTING DUCT CARCINOMA

Synonym: Bellini duct carcinoma.

General and Clinical Features

- Collecting duct carcinoma (CDC) is a recently described variant of RCC that accounts for fewer than 1% of all surgically resected renal epithelial neoplasms. Current morphologic, immunohistochemical, and lectin-binding studies suggest histogenesis and differentiation toward terminal medullary collecting (Bellini's) ducts.
- The current literature suggests that these tumors tend to occur in a similar or slightly younger age group than usual RCCs and have an aggressive clinical course. Metastases are common at diagnosis.
- Davis and associates recently described a tumor termed *renal medullary carcinoma,* also of purported collecting duct origin, that is seen in young black patients with sickle cell trait. This tumor shares many histologic similarities with CDC but may also display some unusual histologic patterns, including yolk sac carcinoma–like and adenoid cystic carcinoma–like areas. The reported cases of renal medullary carcinoma have been aggressive; the majority of patients had metastases, and all died within 1 year of diagnosis.
- On the less aggressive end of the spectrum, there are several reports of low-grade carcinomas of putative collecting duct origin that have behaved in a more indolent fashion than typical CDC.
- Additional morphologic, cytogenetic, and molecular studies will be necessary for determining whether renal medullary carcinoma and the putative low-grade CDC are part of a continuum in the spectrum of collecting duct neoplasia or whether they are distinct clinicopathologic entities.

Gross Pathology

- The main tumor mass has a central or medullary location and often impinges on and distorts the pelvicalyceal system.
- Tumors are gray-white with infiltrative borders; variegation with areas of necrosis is common.
- Extensive renal, extrarenal (especially hilar), and vascular (intrarenal and hilar) infiltration is characteristic.

Microscopic Pathology

- Collecting duct carcinomas have a complex tubular and tubulopapillary architecture often admixed with solid, cribriform, and microcystic patterns. Irregular infiltrating tubules associated with marked desmoplasia are characteristic and have a tendency to entrap intact glomeruli and benign renal tubules in the midst of tumor.
- Tumor cells characteristically have abundant pale eosinophilic cytoplasm but may be admixed with focal clear cell components. Cells with a hobnail appearance may be seen lining tubules and microcysts.
- Typical CDCs are characteristically of high nuclear grade (Fuhrman grades 3 and 4).
- The absence of urothelial carcinoma (a papillary or carcinoma in situ component) within the renal pelvis is an additional major diagnostic criterion.
- Dysplastic changes bordering on carcinoma in situ within collecting ducts adjacent to the tumor and a prominent neutrophilic infiltrate are helpful secondary features present in some cases.
- Sarcomatoid dedifferentiation has been reported.

Special Studies

- Mucin stains (periodic acid–Schiff with diastase, mucicarmine, alcian blue pH 2.5) may demonstrate focal cytoplasmic mucin.
- Immunohistochemically, tumors may coexpress cytokeratins 8/18 and vimentin. Reactivity for cytokeratin 19, high-molecular-weight cytokeratin (34βE12), *Ulex europaeus* agglutinin, and *Arachis hypogaea* peanut lectin support differentiation toward inner medullary collecting ducts.
- No consistent pattern of cytogenetic abnormalities has been established for CDC; a few reported cases have shown loss of chromosomes 1, 6, 14, 15, and 22 (see Table 23–4).

Differential Diagnosis

- *Papillary RCC:* High-grade papillary and tubulopapillary RCCs are sources of potential misdiagnosis. Tubulopapillary architecture associated with an infiltrative tubular component, striking desmoplasia, and expression of high-molecular-weight cytokeratin and *Ulex europaeus* agglutinin are quite distinctive to CDC.
- *Transitional cell carcinoma and adenocarcinoma of the renal pelvis:* Pelvic urothelial carcinoma can spread into collecting ducts, infiltrate the kidney, and mimic CDC; the presence of a papillary or an in situ component in the renal pelvis favors urothelial origin. Cases of urothelial carcinoma with glandular differentiation and adenocarcinoma of the renal pelvis also enter the differential diagnosis.
- *Metastatic adenocarcinoma:* Metastasis (especially from a primary adenocarcinoma in the lung or gastrointestinal tract) should be excluded.

Clinical Course

- A limited number of cases reported to date suggest that typical CDCs are often of advanced stage with metastases common at diagnosis; these tumors usually pursue an aggressive clinical course, and most patients die of disease within 2 years of diagnosis.

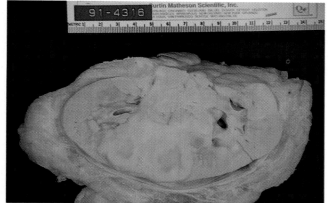

Figure 23–19. Collecting duct carcinoma. Grossly, this large tumor has a central location, distorts the pelvicalyceal system, and irregularly infiltrates the cortex and hilar connective tissue.

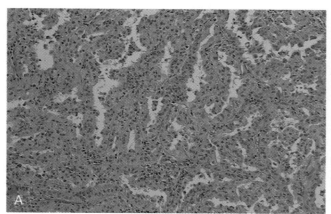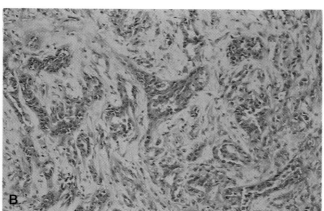

Figure 23–20. Collecting duct carcinoma. *A,* Histologically, the tumor is characterized by a tubulopapillary growth pattern. *B,* Irregular infiltrating angulated tubules associated with marked desmoplasia are a characteristic histologic feature.

SARCOMATOID RENAL CELL CARCINOMA

General and Clinical Features

- Sarcomatoid or spindle cell change may occur in all types of RCC. Sarcomatoid RCCs do not represent a distinct entity in regard to their genetic features and are probably a manifestation of tumor dedifferentiation from an antecedent RCC. Their distinctive features warrant further discussion because they include true sarcomas within the differential diagnosis and are usually associated with a poor prognosis.
- Sarcomatoid change occurs in about 1% to 6% of RCCs. When the antecedent carcinoma can be recognized (as is usual when ample tissue sections are reviewed), the various components and their relative proportion of the tumor composition should be noted. When the sarcomatoid component predominates and the antecedent carcinoma cannot be recognized, these tumors may be appropriately assigned to the unclassified RCC category.
- Clinical features of sarcomatoid RCC are similar to those of conventional clear cell RCC.

Gross and Microscopic Pathology

- The sarcomatoid component is characterized by a fleshy, pale tan-white appearance with infiltrative margins.
- The sarcomatoid component may predominate or may be focal.
- The sarcomatoid component is composed of cells with markedly enlarged pleomorphic or multilobated nuclei

or spindle cells and is by definition high nuclear grade (Fuhrman nuclear grade 4, see Table 23–4).
- Sarcomatoid carcinomas are seen most often in association with classic clear cell RCC, but they may also occur in association with papillary (chromophil), chromophobe, and collecting duct carcinoma.

Special Studies

- The epithelial nature of these neoplasms can usually be recognized by identification of a more classic renal epithelial component on hematoxylin and eosin–stained sections. Immunohistochemical or electron microscopic studies for identification of cells immunoreactive for pan-cytokeratin (using broad-spectrum antibody cocktails) or ultrastructural identification of desmosomes and microvilli may occasionally be necessary.

Differential Diagnosis

- *Primary renal sarcomas:* Renal sarcomas are very uncommon, and malignant spindle cell tumors of the kidney in adults most often represent sarcomatoid RCC. Generous tumor sampling (at least one block per centimeter of tumor) may be required to identify a focal epithelial component in sarcomatoid RCCs.

Clinical Course

- Tumors with sarcomatoid change are often advanced in stage at diagnosis and highly aggressive (median survival is 6.8 months and the 3-year survival rate is only about 19% in some series).

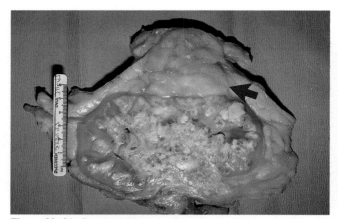

Figure 23–21. Sarcomatoid renal cell carcinoma. This large tumor with extrarenal invasion has peripheral pale tan-gray, solid areas *(arrow)* that corresponded histologically to a sarcomatoid component. Centrally, the tumor has mottled hemorrhagic areas with necrosis that histologically represented classic renal cell carcinoma of the clear cell type.

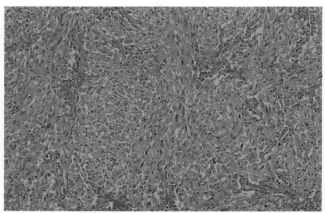

Figure 23–22. Sarcomatoid renal cell carcinoma. Tumors with sarcomatoid change may be composed of spindle cells that create histologic patterns easily confused with primary renal or metastatic sarcomas.

CYSTIC RENAL CELL CARCINOMA

- Focal cystic change is common in RCCs and, when extensive, may dominate the gross and microscopic features of the tumor. Cystic RCCs do not represent a homogeneous group of tumors in regard to their gross, histologic, or genetic features, but they warrant separate discussion because correct diagnosis of them may often be problematic.
- Renal cell carcinomas with extensive cystic degeneration may be deceptive on radiologic, gross, and histologic examination inasmuch as they may mimic benign unilocular or multilocular cysts.
- Cystic renal masses containing necrotic or hemorrhagic material should be suspected to be malignant; extensive tissue sampling may be necessary to identify viable areas of diagnostic tumor.
- In a review of cases from the Armed Forces Institute of Pathology, Hartman and colleagues classified cystic RCCs into four subtypes:

  i. Those resulting from an intrinsic multilocular pattern of growth (the most common type)
  ii. Those resulting from an intrinsic unilocular pattern of growth
  iii. Those resulting from cystic degeneration of a previously solid tumor
  iv. Those originating in a benign cyst

- Multilocular cystic RCCs are composed of variably sized, noncommunicating cysts separated by irregular, fibrous septa of variable thickness.
  - The septa may show marked hyalinization and focal calcification or ossification.
  - The cysts may be lined by a single layer of uniform cells, which may be markedly attenuated or absent.
  - Multiple sections will often reveal solid nests of clear tumor cells within the cyst wall.
  - These tumors are usually of low nuclear grade, are confined to the kidney, and have an excellent prognosis.
- Unilocular cystic RCCs usually have thick irregular walls and are generally lined by clear cells; papillae lined by clear cells may also be seen.
- Cystic tumors originating from previously solid tumors are characterized by central tumor necrosis and areas of old and recent hemorrhage.
  - Papillary (chromophil) RCCs often show extensive central cystic degeneration resulting from necrosis of a previously solid tumor.
  - Clear cell RCCs may also undergo massive central cystic degeneration.
- Renal cell carcinomas may rarely arise in benign cysts in the kidney (see discussion in Chapter 20 regarding adult polycystic and acquired cystic disease).

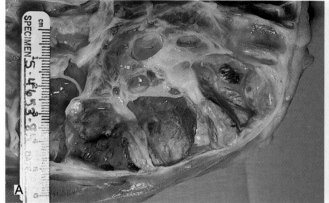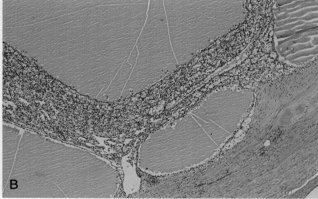

Figure 23–23. Multilocular cystic renal cell carcinoma (RCC). *A,* This RCC has extensive cystic change and can be confused grossly with cystic nephroma (multilocular renal cyst). *B,* Histologic sections reveal variably sized cysts lined by single to multiple layers of clear cells that form a solid component diagnostic of RCC. The clear cells have low-grade nuclear features.

RENAL CELL CARCINOMA, UNCLASSIFIED

- The diagnostic category of unclassified RCC includes renal epithelial malignancies that do not fit any of the established categories; it does not represent a homogeneous morphologic or genetic entity.

- This group accounts for less than 1% of cases in most large surgical series.
- Features that might prompt assignment of a carcinoma to this category include apparent composites of recognized types, sarcomatoid tumors without recognizable epithelial elements, mixtures of epithelial and stromal components, mucin production, and unrecognizable cell types.

■ Other differential diagnostic possibilities should be considered before assigning a neoplasm to this category. In particular, metastatic carcinoma and epithelioid angiomyolipoma should be considered when an intrarenal neoplasm of unusual morphology is encountered.

RENAL EPITHELIAL HYPERPLASIA AND CORTICAL ADENOMA

General Features

■ Microscopic, compact clusters of uniform epithelial cells arranged in a tubular or papillary pattern may be seen as multiple, unilateral, or bilateral lesions in the renal cortex. Such foci of tubular hyperplasia are often not visible grossly.
■ Cortical adenomas are small, grossly recognizable, asymptomatic cortical nodules found commonly as incidental autopsy findings (in between 4% and 37% of autopsy patients, depending on the autopsy population and study methods).
■ Focal tubular epithelial hyperplasia may be associated with adenomas and small cortical cysts. Adenomas are found in increasing frequency with advancing age, renal scars, and arterial nephrosclerosis; they develop frequently in patients maintained on long-term dialysis and have been reported in up to one third of patients with acquired cystic disease.
■ Adenomas are reported to be more common in kidneys containing RCCs.
■ Although all classification schemes recognize adenomas as an entity, no absolute criteria are currently known that can distinguish papillary adenoma from small papillary carcinomas.

Gross and Microscopic Pathology

■ Adenomas are usually pale yellow to gray well-circumscribed nodules located in the cortex (most commonly subcapsular with slight protrusion above the cortical surface). Adenomas under 1 mm may be visible; the upper size limit is not well defined.
■ Bell (1950) proposed criteria, based on size, for differentiating adenomas from malignant epithelial tumors. In his review of renal epithelial tumors having a diameter less than 3 cm, metastases developed in only 3 of 65 patients (about 5%). Bell therefore arbitrarily classified adenomas as including all asymptomatic renal epithelial tumors smaller than 3 cm. But definitions based arbitrarily on size are problematic, in that they include small renal epithelial neoplasms with malignant potential. Size is not an absolute criterion, since tumors as small as 0.8 cm have been reported to metastasize.
  • Farrow (1989) developed a definition of adenoma based on histologic features. He defined adenomas as small cortical nodules composed of small cells with uniform nuclei lacking nuclear atypia that are arranged in a tubular or papillary architecture. This definition corresponds to papillary adenomas of the chromophil-basophil cell type and excludes tumors with a predominantly clear cell composition or a solid pattern. Cortical nodules composed of compact nests of clear cells are regarded as potentially malignant regardless of size.
■ Grignon and Eble (1998) proposed that diagnostic criteria for a papillary adenoma should include the following: (1) papillary, tubular, or tubulopapillary architecture; (2) diameter less than or equal to 5 mm; and (3) no histologic resemblance to clear cell, chromophobe, or collecting duct RCCs. This recommendation acknowledges that papillary adenomas closely resemble low-grade papillary RCCs histologically and that no absolute morphologic criteria allow their distinction from small low-grade papillary cancers. These criteria are believed to define a large group of incidental tumors with little or no potential for growth or metastasis.

Special Studies

■ Papillary adenomas exhibit polysomies of chromosomes 7 and 17 and loss of Y (+7, +17, −Y), genetic abnormalities that are similar to but less extensive than those found in papillary RCCs. Kovacs believes that cytogenetic analysis can distinguish benign from malignant papillary tumors because the latter have additional chromosome abnormalities (including +12, +16, +20, and −14). Additional studies will be needed to validate this concept.

Additional Note

■ *Small renal epithelial neoplasms of low malignant potential:* Small renal epithelial neoplasms are a matter of practical concern for the surgical pathologist inasmuch as radiologic studies have increased the discovery of small renal lesions. The term *small renal epithelial neoplasm of low malignant potential* has been suggested by Epstein as a diagnostic term for "histologically benign" tumors smaller than 3 cm. In this approach, all neoplasms (including clear cell tumors) that are less than 3 cm and lack cytologic atypia, infiltrative growth, necrosis, and vascular invasion are placed in a subset of tumors with probable low metastatic potential.

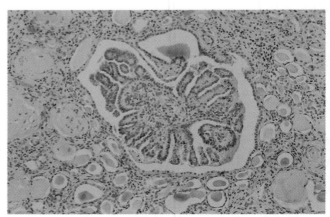

Figure 23–24. Renal epithelial hyperplasia. Papillary projections extend into a cystically dilated tubular space.

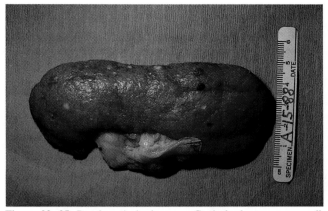

Figure 23–25. Renal cortical adenomas. Cortical adenomas are small, grossly recognizable yellow nodules that are common incidental autopsy findings. They are often associated with small renal cysts and renal scarring most often caused by vascular nephrosclerosis.

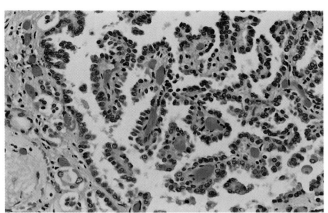

Figure 23–26. Papillary renal cortical adenoma. A small tubulopapillary epithelial proliferation composed exclusively of small round cells with scant amphophilic cytoplasm is present within the cortex; the tumor lacks cytologic atypia, a clear cell component, and an infiltrative growth pattern.

ONCOCYTOMA

General and Clinical Features

■ Oncocytomas are a clinicopathologically distinct group of renal neoplasms that were only recently separated from the spectrum of RCC (Klein and Valensi, 1976); when defined by strict morphologic criteria, they behave as benign neoplasms. Variation in the application of diagnostic criteria has resulted in controversial terms such as atypical oncocytoma and grade 2 oncocytoma.

■ Patients are usually asymptomatic (66% in published cases); initial symptoms may include a flank or abdominal mass (19%), pain (18%), or microscopic or gross hematuria (30%).

■ Patients with oncocytomas are slightly older than those with RCC (median age, 62 years; range, 10 to 94 years); men are affected twice as often as women (2.1:1).

■ Oncocytomas are usually detected during radiologic studies performed to evaluate an unrelated symptom. Clinically detected lesions are usually large (median, 6 cm; the largest reported is 26 cm); tumors identified incidentally at autopsy are small (median, 2 cm).

■ Radiologically, the tumor classically appears solid and may show a central stellate scar corresponding to a relatively avascular region. Four characteristic angiographic features have been reported:
  • The "lucent rim" sign created by the sharp smooth tumor margin and capsule.
  • A homogeneous capillary pattern with a density similar to that of normal renal parenchyma.

  • Absence of marked vascular disarray producing no pooling of contrast material or arteriovenous shunting in neoplastic vessels.
  • A spoke-wheel appearance of the feeding arteries.
■ Tumor differentiation toward the intercalated cell of the collecting duct has been demonstrated in some studies.
■ Oncocytoma may rarely coexist with RCC or angiomyolipoma and may coexist with adenomas as incidental autopsy findings.

Gross and Microscopic Pathology

■ Adequate tissue sampling and adherence to strict morphologic criteria are essential to make the correct diagnosis.
■ Characteristic gross features are a well-circumscribed, roughly spherical, homogeneous, tan to mahogany-brown mass, often with a cental stellate hyaline-fibrous scar; tumors lack the prominent necrosis and cystic change often seen in RCCs and do not invade the renal vein.
■ Tumors may grossly involve perinephric fat.
■ Most tumors are solitary; multicentric or bilateral tumors have been reported in 3% to 5% of cases. Rarely, numerous lesions are present in cases of so-called oncocytomatosis.
■ Microscopically, the tumor is composed exclusively or predominantly of cells with markedly eosinophilic, abundant, coarsely granular (oncocytic) cytoplasm. The cytoplasmic granularity correlates ultrastructurally to an increased number of mitochondria. Tumor cells are nested or arranged in tubular, trabecular, and more compact "solid" patterns. Cellular formations are em-

bedded within characteristically poorly cellular edematous, myxoid, or hyalinized stroma. Microcysts may be present.

■ The nuclei are generally round with smooth nuclear contours; nucleoli may range from invisible or inconspicuous to prominent (equivalent to Fuhrman's nuclear grade 3 or 4). Mitoses are absent to vanishingly rare.

■ The focal presence of cells with pleomorphic, hyperchromatic nuclei, occasional multinucleation, and monstrocellular elements is acceptable and is believed to represent degenerative-ischemic changes.

■ Features that exclude the diagnosis of oncocytoma and support a diagnosis of RCC include
  • The presence of clear cells or spindle cells.
  • Prominent papillary architecture.
  • Gross or conspicuous microscopic necrosis.
  • The presence of more than a rare mitotic figure.

■ Permissible "atypical features" for the diagnosis of oncocytoma include
  • Gross or microscopic infiltration of perinephric fat or focal extension into adjacent renal parenchyma.
  • Hemorrhage.
  • Rare foci of microscopic necrosis.
  • Rare mitosis without atypia.
  • Very focal papillary arrangement.
  • Microvascular invasion.

■ Because oncocytomas are benign neoplasms, nuclear grading and pathologic staging are not applicable.

Special Studies

■ Ultrastructurally, very numerous abnormal, swollen mitochondria and a decreased prominence of other organelles are the defining features.

■ Tumor cells stain negative or show focal weak positive staining for Hale's colloidal iron.

■ Immunohistochemically, oncocytomas express low-molecular-weight cytokeratins and epithelial membrane antigen and do not express vimentin.

■ The lectin-binding pattern supports differentiation toward collecting ducts.

■ Oncocytomas lack the 3p deletion or polysomies characteristic of clear cell and papillary RCCs, respectively. Cytogenetically, two groups of karyotypic abnormalities have been identified.
  • One cytogenetic pattern shows loss of chromosomes Y and 1 and the other has translocations involving breakpoint 11q13 (see Table 23–2).
  • Unique mitochondrial DNA alterations have also been reported.

■ Flow cytometric studies have shown diploid (50% of tumors), polyploid (39%), and aneuploid (11%) DNA content.

Differential Diagnosis

■ *Chromophobe RCC* (particularly the *eosinophilic* variant) shares overlapping morphologic features with oncocytoma and is the major diagnostic pitfall. Chromophobe RCCs grossly are often homogeneous, solid, beige to light brown tumors that rarely show a central scar. Chromophobe RCCs grow in solid masses, broad trabeculae, or alveolar patterns, unlike the compact

nested or tubular pattern of oncocytoma. Chromophobe RCCs are usually composed of an intimate admixture of cells with pale cytoplasm (which differ from clear cells) and eosinophilic cells that have perinuclear clearing and peripheral cytoplasmic condensation. Immunohistochemically, both tumors are immunoreactive for pan-cytokeratin and lack immunoreactivity for vimentin. Diffuse staining for Hale's colloidal iron indicating the presence of acid mucopolysaccharides and the presence ultrastructurally of unique cytoplasmic vesicles are additional differentiating features of chromophobe carcinoma.

■ *So-called RCC with oncocytic features, papillary (chromophil) RCC, and clear cell RCCs with cytoplasmic eosinophilia:* Renal cell carcinomas composed of cells with eosinophilic or oncocytic cytoplasm may mimic the gross and cytoarchitectural features of oncocytoma and need to be excluded. These tumors often show nuclear pleomorphism with irregular nuclear contours, mitoses, and a characteristic supporting fibrovascular framework. Although papillary (chromophil) carcinoma may have tumor cells with granular or oncocytic cytoplasm, the presence of a prominent papillary or tubulo-papillary architecture excludes oncocytoma.

Treatment and Clinical Course

■ Surgical resection is usually the treatment of choice. Partial nephrectomy may be recommended in patients with solitary kidneys or compromised renal function.

■ When strict diagnostic criteria are applied, oncocytoma is a benign neoplasm; there have been no well-documented cases of metastases. Reports of "metastatic oncocytoma" may represent misdiagnosed cases of chromophobe carcinoma (particularly the eosinophilic variant), cases with concurrent clear cell carcinoma, or tumors subject to inadequate sampling or nonstringent diagnostic criteria.

■ Core needle biopsy, fine-needle aspiration, and frozen section evaluation may suggest a differential that includes oncocytoma; they play a limited role in the definitive diagnosis of this renal neoplasm in that oncocytoma is a diagnosis of exclusion that can only be made after adequate tissue sampling.

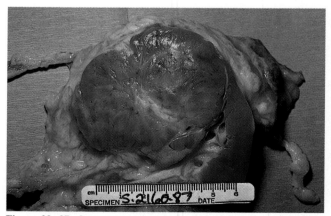

Figure 23–27. Oncocytoma. Grossly, the tumor is well circumscribed, dark tan–mahogany brown, with a central pale scar.

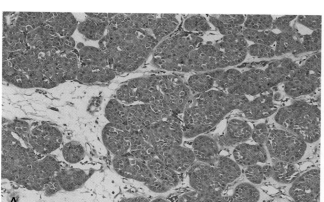
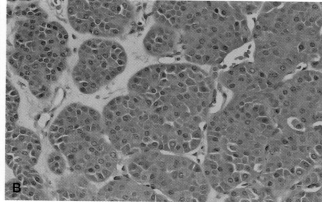

Figure 23–28. Oncocytoma. Nests of tumors cells are embedded within a characteristically edematous and poorly cellular stroma. The tumor cells have abundant granular (oncocytic) cytoplasm, lack cytologic atypia, and do not show mitoses.

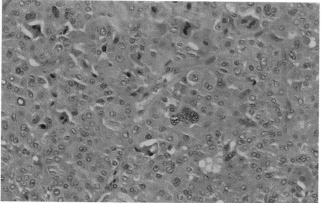

Figure 23–29. Oncocytoma with focal cytologic atypia. Oncocytomas may contain foci with pleomorphic nuclei and monstrocellular elements, which may arise through ischemic-degenerative changes.

METANEPHRIC ADENOMA

General and Clinical Features

- Metanephric adenoma is a rare lesion of uncertain histogenesis that has only recently been recognized and described in detail.
- These tumors are most common in middle age (age range, 38 to 64) and predominate in females by well over 2:1.
- Patients are usually asymptomatic, and 50% of reported cases are incidental findings.
- Some patients have polycythemia, abdominal or flank pain, a mass, or hematuria.
- Metanephric adenoma shares some clinicopathologic features with the lesion recently described as metanephric (nephrogenic) adenofibroma by Hennigar and Beckwith (see Chapter 22). Metanephric adenoma and meta-

nephric adenofibroma may form a spectrum encompassing epithelial proliferation with or without accompanying mesenchymal proliferation.

Gross and Microscopic Pathology

- Tumors are well circumscribed, solid or lobulated, and gray-white and range from 0.3 to 15.0 cm.
- Cyst formation, focal hemorrhage, and calcification may be present.
- The tumor consists of small, rounded uniform acini and tubules admixed with more solid areas. Tumor cells have scant cytoplasm, bland dark-staining nuclei, and absent or inconspicuous nucleoli. Stroma is usually minimal and acellular but can be edematous or hyalinized.
- Short papillae reminiscent of the "glomeruloid" bodies of nephroblastoma may be present.

- Hemorrhage, necrosis, and calcifications with psammoma bodies are common; microcystic growth patterns occur less commonly.

Special Studies

- Tumor cells lack glycogen and mucin (periodic acid–Schiff with and without diastase).
- Immunohistochemical and lectin studies have shown varied results; reactivity for keratin, vimentin, and *Arachis hypogaea* (peanut) lectin has been variably present or absent. One study showed expression of the *WT1* gene protein that is commonly expressed in Wilms tumors.
- Ultrastructural studies have shown the presence of cilia on the luminal surface of tumor cells and apical secretory granules.
- A few tumors studied cytogenetically had normal karyotypes; other studies have found frequent gain of chromosomes 7 and 17 and loss of the Y chromosome (similar to papillary neoplasms).
- Flow cytometric analysis has shown diploid DNA content in four analyzed cases.

Differential Diagnosis

- *Adult nephroblastoma, nephrogenic rest, papillary adenoma, papillary RCC, and metanephric adenofibroma* enter the differential diagnosis. Adult nephroblastoma, particularly the monophasic epithelial type, is the most likely source of potential misdiagnosis. Metanephric adenoma lacks a proliferatively active blastema component and has a uniformly bland cytologic appearance. Metanephric adenoma can also be confused with low-grade papillary neoplasms (basophilic type) that have a tubular architecture and psammoma bodies.

Treatment and Clinical Course

- Reported cases have been treated with total nephrectomy. No recurrence or metastasis has been reported; however, some cases have had relatively short follow-up. Nephron-conserving surgery may be a clinical consideration in the future if additional cases with long-term follow-up support a benign outcome.

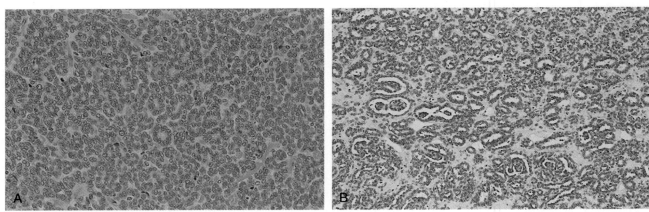

Figure 23–30. Metanephric adenoma. *A,* The tumor is composed of solid nests of cells and small tubules. Tumor cells have cytologically bland nuclei and scant cytoplasm and are embedded within minimal acellular stroma. *B,* In other areas, the tumor has well-formed tubules and short papillae resembling immature glomeruli.

MISCELLANEOUS TUMORS WITH EPITHELIAL OR RENAL PARENCHYMAL DIFFERENTIATION

NEUROENDOCRINE TUMORS

General and Clinical Features

- Renal neuroendocrine neoplasms are rare, and the spectrum includes carcinoid tumors, atypical carcinoids, and small cell carcinomas.

- Intrarenal pheochromocytoma and neuroblastoma have been reported rarely; neuroblastoma occurs rarely in adult kidneys and may be better classified within the group of primitive neuroectodermal tumors.
- Neuroendocrine tumors usually occur in older patients (age range from adolescence to the ninth decade).
- Patients typically have tumors of advanced stage when seeking medical attention for hematuria and abdominal pain.
- Endocrine manifestations, including carcinoid syndrome and excessive secretion of glucagon and vasoactive intestinal polypeptides, have been reported.

Gross and Microscopic Pathology

- Neuroendocrine tumors are often large and show invasion of adjacent structures; hemorrhage, necrosis, and cystic change are variable.
- Renal neuroendocrine tumors appear identical to their counterparts arising in other organs.
  - In two cases of renal carcinoid tumors, the tumor was associated with teratoma.
  - Small cell carcinomas may show classic oat cell or intermediate cell morphology (a subclassification that holds no significance in terms of prognosis or therapy); tumor cells characteristically have inconspicuous to scant cytoplasm, prominent nuclear molding, frequent mitoses, and prominent necrosis.

Special Studies

- Tumors generally stain with silver stains (e.g., Grimelius).
- Immunohistochemically, carcinoid tumors are cytokeratin positive; small cell carcinomas may be cytokeratin negative or show a paranuclear dot-like reactivity for keratin characteristic of neuroendocrine carcinoma; neuroendocrine markers such as chromogranin, synaptophysin, neuron-specific enolase, and Leu-7 are much more frequently positive in carcinoid tumors than in small cell carcinomas.
- Electron microscopy reveals membrane-bound neurosecretory granules with dense cores ranging from 150 to 400 nm in diameter. Granules are sparse in small cell carcinomas and numerous in carcinoid tumors.

Differential Diagnosis

- Other "small cell tumors," including metastatic small cell carcinoma, malignant lymphoma, and adult nephroblastoma: Clinical information is necessary to exclude metastatic small cell carcinoma; the latter rarely involves the kidney in the absence of a known lung primary and systemic disease. Malignant lymphoma infiltrates the renal parenchyma, spares normal structures, and immunohistochemically stains for leukocyte common antigen. Adult nephroblastoma, although usually triphasic, may in a biopsy sample appear as a pure blastema component; immunohistochemically, blastema is cytokeratin negative and usually vimentin positive. Neuroblastoma is recognized by the presence of neuropil and the formation of Homer-Wright rosettes.

Treatment and Clinical Course

- Renal carcinoids and small cell carcinomas have behaved as aggressive neoplasms in the few reported cases. The majority of patients have metastases or metastases develop, and these patients have a poor prognosis.

PRIMITIVE NEUROECTODERMAL TUMOR (PNET)

Synonym: Peripheral neuroepithelioma.

General and Clinical Features

- Peripheral primitive neuroectodermal tumors (PNETs) are members of the Ewing family of tumors, including osseous and extraosseous Ewing's sarcoma and Askin's tumor of the thorax. These tumors typically arise in the soft tissues of the chest wall and paraspinal region. PNETs occasionally occur in an internal organ, and the kidney may represent the most frequent site of organ-based PNET.
- There have been less than a dozen published reports of PNET in the literature; additional cases seen at the Pathology Center of the National Wilms Tumor Study (reported in abstract form) suggest that this neoplasm may be more common than would be judged by published accounts.
- The peak prevalence of renal PNET is during the second and third decades (reported age range 17 to 62 years).
- Histogenesis and putative neural crest derivation of PNET and Ewing's sarcoma remain controversial.

Gross and Microscopic Pathology

- Grossly, the tumors are multinodular and tan-white and often show extrarenal extension. Areas of hemorrhage and extensive necrosis are common.
- Microscopically, small, round, uniform cells with overlapping nuclei, heterogeneous chromatin patterns, prominent nucleoli, and scanty cytoplasm form solid areas of tumor with a vague lobular pattern; focal rosette formation is seen. Mitotic figures and individual necrotic cells are often numerous.

Special Studies

- Renal PNETs show immunoreactivity for vimentin, cytokeratin, neuron-specific enolase, and the MIC2 gene product 013 (CD99).
- The translocation t(11,22), that is considered specific to PNET and Ewing's sarcoma, has been detected in several cases by polymerase chain reaction, tissue culture cytogenetics, and fluorescence in situ hybridization.

Differential Diagnosis

- Blastemal predominant nephroblastoma, small cell neuroendocrine carcinoma, and lymphoma (small non-cleaved cell type): PNETs may be more common than Wilms tumor in individuals between the ages of 15 to 30 years. PNET should be a diagnostic consideration whenever an unusual small cell tumor is encountered in an adolescent or a young adult. Immunohistochemistry and molecular studies, as detailed earlier, can aid in the differential diagnosis.

Treatment and Clinical Course

- Treatment includes nephrectomy and chemotherapy with or without radiation therapy.
- The number of reported cases with follow-up is small, but patients often died of tumor within months to 5 years.

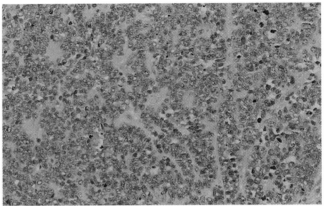

Figure 23–31. Primitive neuroectodermal tumor. Small round cells with scanty cytoplasm, overlapping nuclei, and prominent nucleoli form a vague lobular pattern. There are numerous individually necrotic cells.

JUXTAGLOMERULAR CELL TUMOR

Synonym: "Reninoma."

General and Clinical Features

- Juxtaglomerular cell tumor is a rare tumor originating from the renal-juxtaglomerular cells and is usually characterized by hypertension from excess renin production. Cases reported in the literature to date number over 50.
  - Measurement of plasma renin by selective vein catheterization may be important in the diagnosis and resection of small tumors.
- These tumors occur in young adults and adolescents (average age, 27 years at the time of resection) and show a 2:1 female preponderance.
- No cases of metastasis, recurrence, multifocality, or bilaterality have been reported.

Gross and Microscopic Pathology

- Tumors are small (usually < 3 cm), well circumscribed, and rubbery gray-white and may contain small cystic cavities.
- Histologic features are quite variable:
  - The tumor most often consists of trabeculae of small polygonal cells within a myxoid stroma.
  - The tumor may also form solid islands, tubules, cysts, and broad papillae.
  - Prominent vascularity may lead to an appearance reminiscent of hemangiopericytoma.

Special Studies

- Tumor cells have cytoplasmic granules staining with modified Bowie's stain and periodic acid–Schiff.
- Immunohistochemically, granules stain for renin.
- Electron microscopy reveals characteristic rhomboid crystals.

Differential Diagnosis

- The clinical, gross, and histologic features are usually distinctive.

Note: Renin secretion is associated with other renal and extrarenal tumors, including RCC, nephroblastoma, and pancreatic adenocarcinoma. Theoretically, any strategically located tumor can compress the renal artery and lead to increased renin production and hypertension.

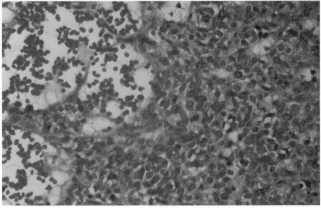

Figure 23–32. Juxtaglomerular cell tumor. Polygonal tumor cells are associated with a prominent vascular component.

CYSTIC NEPHROMA AND CYSTIC PARTIALLY DIFFERENTIATED NEPHROBLASTOMA

Synonyms: Multilocular renal cyst and multilocular cystic nephroma are synonyms for cystic nephroma.

General and Clinical Features

- The clinicopathologic spectrum of cystic nephroma (CN) and cystic partially differentiated nephroblastoma (CPDN) in the pediatric population has been previously outlined in Chapter 22. As discussed earlier, CN and CPDN are multilocular cystic lesions that are distinguished histologically by the presence (CPDN) or absence (CN) of intraseptal blastema and other immature elements.
- Most cases of CPDN occur in children within the first 36 months of age, with a slight predominance in boys. Among adults, CN affects primarily individuals older than the age of 30 years and has a striking female predominance (women predominate over men by approximately 8:1). Reports of CPDN in adults are rare.
- Diagnostic criteria for CN and CPDN have varied among different authors and have been recently reviewed and refined by Eble and Bonsib. Based on published accounts and differences in age distribution and gender predominance, Eble et al. conclude that (1) CN and CPDN are unrelated entities, (2) CN is unrelated to nephroblastoma, and (3) tumors in children should be classified as CPDN, while all but exceptional cases in adults should be classified as CN.
- In adults, many cases are asymptomatic and are found incidentally by radiologic examination; abdominal pain and hematuria are the most common initial symptoms.

Gross Pathology

- CN is indistinguishable from CPDN on gross inspection. Multiple fluid-filled cysts form a bulging, well-demarcated mass (usually unilateral and solitary), surrounded by a thick, fibrous pseudocapsule that compresses adjacent renal tissue.
- The interior is composed of cysts and septa with no expansile solid nodules.
- Tumors vary widely in size (average 9 cm in one large series). Location within the kidney is also variable. CN commonly herniates into the renal pelvis or renal sinus or may bulge from the convexity of the renal cortex.
- Cysts vary in size from microscopic to greater than 5 cm and contain clear or hemorrhagic fluid. Septa are typically thin (less than 5 mm).

Microscopic Pathology

- Septa in CN consist predominantly of fibrous tissue that varies from myxoid to collagenous but may at times be more cellular, with a resemblance to ovarian stroma; the septa may contain small cysts and mature renal tubules.
- Foci of blastema, immature stromal or epithelial elements, and skeletal muscle, smooth muscle, or fat are not present within septa in CN.
- Fibrous septa are partially lined by a single layer of flattened, cuboidal, or hobnail epithelial cells that usually have eosinophilic cytoplasm; occasional lining epithelial cells may show cytologic atypia, including hyperchromatism and nuclear enlargement.
- The presence of clear cells is allowed if they are restricted to the single layer of lining epithelium and do not form nests.

Special Studies

- The cyst lining epithelium is immunoreactive for cytokeratin; lectin histochemical and immunohistochemical studies show variable expression of proximal and distal tubular and collecting duct markers.

Differential Diagnosis

- *Multilocular cystic renal cell carcinoma* is the major differential diagnosis in adults. Adequate tissue sampling of the cyst walls is essential to exclude the presence of nests of clear cells indicating RCC.

Treatment and Clinical Course

- CN and CPDN are cured by surgical excision. They require complete excision because of preoperative diagnostic uncertainty based on imaging studies or tissue biopsy and the potential for recurrence with incomplete excision. Excision is also required because continued growth of these lesions may compromise renal function.
- Cystic RCCs and sarcomas have rarely been reported to occur in adult CN, but it is unclear whether these malignant tumors arose in preexisting cystic lesions or whether they represent cystic degeneration of a primary malignant neoplasm.

NEPHROBLASTOMA (WILMS TUMOR)

- Adult nephroblastomas are rare.
- Nephroblastomas can be confused with other mixed malignant tumors; acceptable cases should contain diagnostic areas of blastema.
- Prognosis is poor; metastases are present in 13% of patients at diagnosis. Despite multimodal therapy, only 50% of patients have a 5-year disease-free survival.

TERATOMA

- Teratoma rarely occurs as a primary renal tumor.
- Two of the reported cases contained areas of carcinoid; one tumor occurred in a dysplastic kidney.

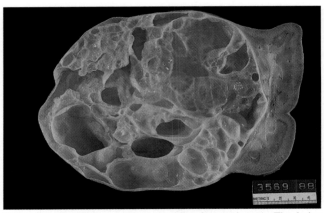

Figure 23–33. Cystic nephroma (multilocular renal cyst). The lesion consists of multiple smooth-walled noncommunicating locules formed by septa that lack solid expansile tumor nodules.

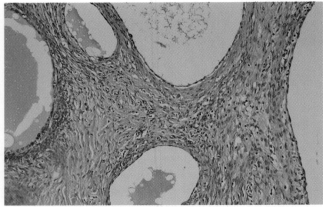

Figure 23–34. Cystic nephroma. Histologically, variably sized cysts are lined in part by a single layer of flattened epithelium.

BENIGN RENAL MESENCHYMAL NEOPLASMS

ANGIOMYOLIPOMA

General and Clinical Features

- Angiomyolipomas are benign lesions composed of thick-walled blood vessels and variable amounts of mature adipose and smooth muscle tissue.
- The true nature and pathogenesis of these lesions remain controversial; once thought to represent hamartomas or choristomas (disordered arrangement of mature tissue present in an abnormal location), new evidence suggests that they represent neoplasms of perivascular epithelioid cells with the potential to differentiate toward smooth muscle, fat, and blood vessels.
- With the advent of CT, most angiomyolipomas are diagnosed preoperatively on the basis of their characteristic fat density; fine-needle aspiration may be used to confirm the diagnosis.
- Angiomyolipomas occur both sporadically and in association with several hereditary disorders, including von Recklinghausen's disease, von Hippel–Lindau disease, and autosomal dominant (adult) polycystic kidney disease. The association is particularly strong with the tuberous sclerosis complex, an autosomal dominant disorder with variable penetrance characterized by mental retardation, epilepsy, central nervous system neoplasms, and cutaneous hamartomas.
  - The literature on renal angiomyolipoma is confusing because authors have variably defined their criteria for the tuberous sclerosis complex and have incom-

pletely reported the clinical investigations used to detect the lesions of tuberous sclerosis.
  - Most large surgical series report that about 80% of angiomyolipomas occur sporadically while most of the remaining cases are associated with tuberous sclerosis.
  - Angiomyolipomas occur in 50% to 80% of patients with tuberous sclerosis.
  - The hereditary syndrome may be partially expressed, so patients with multiple renal angiomyolipomas should be evaluated for tuberous sclerosis.
- Affected patients are predominantly female (ratio of 4:1); the average age at diagnosis is 41 years, but children have been affected.
- Among symptomatic patients, flank pain caused by intratumoral hemorrhage is the most common manifestation. Life-threatening complications include massive retroperitoneal hemorrhage and progressive renal failure from replacement and compression of renal parenchyma.
- According to Steiner et al., patients with tuberous sclerosis and renal angiomyolipoma are seen at a younger age, are more often symptomatic, more often have bilateral tumors, and more often require surgery.
- Large angiomyolipomas are more common in women than men, and tumors often show rapid growth during pregnancy. Recent studies have shown frequent progesterone receptor immunoreactivity in tuberous sclerosis–associated renal angiomyolipomas and suggest that hormones may play a role in stimulating their growth.
- Multiple or bilateral lesions and extrarenal involvement of retroperitoneal tissue, regional lymph nodes, renal vein and inferior vena cava, spleen, liver, or other organs may occur and are generally interpreted as multi-

centric lesions and local spread rather than metastatic disease.
- Lymphangioleiomyomatosis of the lung can be associated with the tuberous sclerosis complex in females.
- Renal cell carcinoma has rarely been reported in the ipsilateral or contralateral kidney of patients with angiomyolipoma. Simultaneous occurrence of oncocytoma in the same kidney has also been reported.

Gross and Microscopic Pathology

- Angiomyolipoma is usually a circumscribed (not encapsulated) intrarenal tumor that replaces renal parenchyma. Tumors may also arise from the renal capsule.
- Lesions may range from small (usually a few millimeters) capsular nodules to large 20-cm tumors located within renal or perirenal tissues. Tumors may increase in size through replacement of renal parenchyma and entrap isolated islands of renal tissue; entrapped tubules may form cysts and rarely produce a polycystic appearance. Tumors seldom extend into the renal vein, vena cava, or collecting system.
- Most angiomyolipomas are solitary; multiple tumors have been observed in as many as 20% of cases.
- Tumors are usually yellow and have a fatty appearance when adipose tissue predominates. Tumors composed predominantly of smooth muscle are firm and pale gray. Hemorrhage is common, and degenerative changes may result in a mottled, friable appearance.
- Histologically, adipose tissue, thick-walled blood vessels, and smooth muscle are usually haphazardly admixed.
  - Mature adipose tissue, often with focal fat necrosis, lipophages, and giant cells, usually predominates.
  - Blood vessels typically have thickened and abnormally formed walls in which muscle tissue is partially replaced by dense fibrous tissue. These vessels may resemble the arterialized veins seen in arteriovenous malformations. Internal elastic laminae are often absent or fragmented, and tortuous vessels with focally thinned and dilated walls may form small aneurysms.
  - The smooth muscle component is usually associated with the outer muscular walls of blood vessels, and the elongated nuclei of muscle cells typically radiate out perpendicular to the vessels walls. The smooth muscle component often forms interlacing fascicles interrupted by islands of adipose tissue and vessels but may produce broad fields composed exclusively of smooth muscle. Nuclear enlargement, hyperchromatism, and mitoses may be present. The smooth muscle usually consists of both spindle and epithelioid cells.
- Epithelioid angiomyolipoma is a recently recognized variant in which there is a large component of polygonal smooth muscle cells with abundant eosinophilic cytoplasm and an epithelioid or oncocytoma-like appearance. The epithelioid cells vary from polygonal with mild nuclear atypia to markedly atypical and variably sized, including multinucleate giant cells. Spindle

cells and large mononuclear cells with eccentric nuclei and large nucleoli that superficially resemble ganglion cells may be present. Mitotic activity, hemorrhage, and necrosis may be prominent. Fat cells and thick-walled blood vessels diagnostic of angiomyolipoma may be inconspicuous or absent.

Special Studies

- The smooth muscle cells react with antibodies to smooth muscle actin, and to a lesser extent desmin. Reactivity for melanoma-associated antigen HMB-45 is commonly seen in the smooth muscle and epithelioid cell component. Epithelial markers, such as cytokeratins and epithelial membrane antigens, are negative.
- Electron microscopy has shown the presence of a spectrum of granules and typical premelanosomes in a few cases.

Differential Diagnosis

- *Renal cell carcinoma with cytoplasmic eosinophilia:* Angiomyolipomas in which the smooth muscle component consists predominantly of spindled or epithelioid cells with mitotic activity, necrosis, and nuclear pleomorphism may lead to a mistaken diagnosis of sarcomatoid RCC or clear cell RCC with cytoplasmic eosinophilia. Thorough tissue sampling usually demonstrates areas with more characteristic triphasic composition in angiomyolipoma. Immunohistochemistry is helpful in that angiomyolipomas do not react with antibodies to pancytokeratin or epithelial membrane antigen and do react with antibodies to smooth muscle actin and HMB-45.
- *Leiomyoma* and *leiomyosarcoma*: A predominance of smooth muscle cells with spindle cell morphology may mimic leiomyoma or leiomyosarcoma (in cases with high cellularity and nuclear atypia). Reactivity for HMB-45 can be useful in differentiating monotypic leiomyoma-like angiomyolipomas from smooth muscle neoplasms.
- *Lipoma and well-differentiated liposarcoma:* Angiomyolipomas composed predominantly of adipose tissue may be misdiagnosed as lipoma or well-differentiated (lipoma-like) liposarcoma.

Treatment and Clinical Course

- Typical angiomyolipomas are benign regardless of size.
- Recommendations regarding treatment are based on size, clinical symptoms, association with tuberous sclerosis, and detectable tumor growth on periodic radiographic follow-up.
  - Rupture and hemorrhage are uncommon in tumors smaller than 4 cm. Patients with tumors smaller than 4.0 cm are more likely to be asymptomatic; they may be monitored conservatively with periodic CT or ultrasound and rarely require surgical intervention.
  - Patients with tumors larger than 4.0 cm who have symptoms of bleeding or uncontrollable pain gener-

ally undergo renal-sparing surgery (i.e., partial nephrectomy) or renal arterial embolization.

• Patients with tumors larger than 4 cm who are
asymptomatic or have mild symptoms may be monitored conservatively with periodic CT or ultrasound
or may be treated prophylactically with tumor embolization or renal-sparing surgery. They should be
warned of possible future complications, including
spontaneous rupture and hemorrhage. Tumors shown
to grow during follow-up may be treated with tumor
embolization or renal-sparing surgery.

■ Sarcomatous transformation of angiomyolipoma is exceedingly rare; there are two case reports of high-grade
leiomyosarcoma arising from angiomyolipoma, including one report of sarcomatous transformation with bi-
opsy-proven pulmonary metastases. Although most
cases of the recently recognized epithelioid variant of
angiomyolipoma behave in a benign fashion, a minority
recur locally and may have malignant potential.

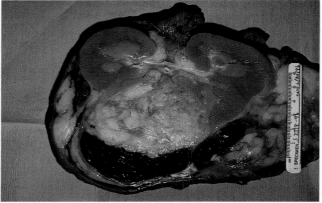

Figure 23–35. Angiomyolipoma. The tumor is yellow and lobulated
and has a fatty appearance. Extensive subcapsular hemorrhage prompted
surgical resection.

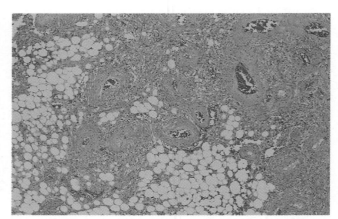

Figure 23–36. Angiomyolipoma. The tumor has a characteristic triphasic composition of smooth muscle, fat, and thick-walled vessels.

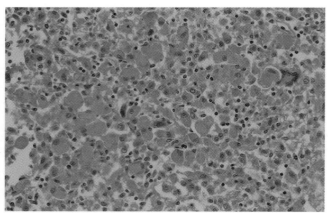

Figure 23–37. Epithelioid angiomyolipoma. The smooth muscle cells
predominate and have an epithelioid appearance with abundant cytoplasm, atypical enlarged nuclei, and visible nucleoli; occasionally, a
multinucleate cell is present; these features may create diagnostic confusion with renal cell carcinomas or sarcomas.

RENOMEDULLARY INTERSTITIAL CELL TUMOR

Synonyms: Medullary fibroma; medullary harmartoma.

General and Clinical Features

- Renomedullary interstitial cell tumors are small nodules that are common asymptomatic and incidental findings at autopsy.
- Controversy persists about whether these represent neoplasms or hyperplastic nodules that form secondary to hypertension.
- Renomedullary interstitial cell tumors occur rarely in patients less than 20 years of age but have been reported to occur in almost half of patients over 20 years of age in one large autopsy series.
- Rare symptomatic tumors are usually manifested as pedunculated masses in the proximal ureter or renal pelvis and have been reported as renal pelvic polyps (fibromas) (see Chapter 24).

Gross and Microscopic Pathology

- Nodules are well circumscribed, usually spherical, slightly bulging, pale white-gray, and firm and are generally located within the midportion of the renal medulla; nodules are usually 2 to 3 mm and very rarely larger than 5 mm.

- The nodules are sparsely to moderately cellular and composed of small spindle or stellate cells embedded in a stroma closely resembling that of the renal medulla. Some thick and interlacing bundles of loose fibers are often present, and amyloid may be deposited in irregular clumps.
- Medullary tubules are often entrapped at the periphery of the nodules.

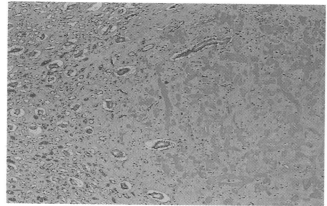

Figure 23–38. Renomedullary interstitial cell tumor. This small circumscribed nodule is poorly cellular and composed of mesenchymal cells embedded in a loose matrix with thick eosinophilic bundles of collagen; medullary tubules are entrapped at the periphery.

ADULT MESOBLASTIC NEPHROMA

Synonym: Cystic hamartoma of the renal pelvis.

General and Clinical Features

- This rare but distinctive biphasic (stromal and epithelial) lesion of the adult kidney has been described under several names in the literature, including cystic hamartoma of the renal pelvis (see review by Truong et al, 1998). The descriptive term *solid and cystic biphasic tumor of the kidney* has been used to refer to a series of seven similar adult lesions published in abstract form (Adsay et al, 1998).
- The concept of adult mesoblastic nephroma is challenged by some experts who believe that mesoblastic nephroma is an entity restricted to infants usually within the first 12 months of age. These experts argue that adult cases have no known histogenetic relationship to congenital mesoblastic nephroma and show significant morphologic differences. The stromal component appears similar in infantile and adult cases. However, in adult mesoblastic nephroma, epithelial-lined tubules and cysts are an integral component dispersed throughout the tumor, whereas in infantile cases

entrapped non-neoplastic nephron elements are present predominantly at the peripheral tumor-kidney interface.
- There are 22 published cases of adult mesoblastic nephroma; adults range from 19 to 78 years (mean 42 years) and are predominantly women (20 cases).
- Initial symptoms may include abdominal mass, flank pain, or hematuria; asymptomatic cases are detected by radiologic imaging.
- Additional molecular and cytogenetic studies are needed to refine our understanding of this entity and its relationship (or probable lack thereof) with congenital mesoblastic nephroma.

Gross and Microscopic Pathology

- Tumors are solitary and solid but often have cystic spaces; in contrast to infantile cases, adult cases are well circumscribed. The reported size ranges from 2 to 24 cm (mean 8 cm). Tumors frequently involve the renal sinus but do not extend beyond the renal capsule.
- Histologically, the tumor consists of epithelial and stromal components in various combinations.
  - Tubules and variably sized cysts are lined by a single layer of cuboidal, flattened, or hobnail cells that may

form intracystic papillary proliferations; the epithelial cells lack significant cytologic atypia or mitoses. Tubules and cysts are dispersed throughout the tumor.

- The stroma consists of spindle cells (fibroblastic and myofibroblastic) with scattered bundles of smooth muscle cells. Adult cases typically show low stromal cellularity and mitotic activity (the classic variant), but rare cases may show higher stromal cellularity, moderate nuclear atypia, and brisk mitotic activity (the cellular variant).
- Occasionally, tumors may be almost purely cystic.

Special Studies

- Tumors show immunoreactivity for vimentin, desmin, and smooth muscle actin in the spindle cell component and reactivity for keratin and epithelial membrane antigen in the epithelial component. Immunohistochemical and lectin studies show that the cysts and tubules typically display the phenotype of collecting ducts.

Differential Diagnosis

- *Cystic nephroma:* Cystic nephroma lacks a significant solid component, and the fibrous stromal component lacks smooth muscle differentiation.
- *Sarcomatoid RCC:* Prominent cytologic atypia, numerous mitotic figures, and epithelial differentiation within the spindle cell component (which may be confirmed by immunohistochemistry or electron microscopy) are the major features that differentiate sarcomatoid RCC from adult mesoblastic nephroma.

Treatment and Clinical Course

- Nephrectomy or partial nephrectomy has been standard treatment.

- Metastases do not develop; tumor recurrence has been documented in only one patient (reported 21 years after the initial resection).

OTHER BENIGN MESENCHYMAL NEOPLASMS

- A wide variety of soft tissue lesions have been described within the kidney.
- The terms *capsuloma* or *capsular leiomyoma* have been used to describe a variety of lesions that may be found incidentally in autopsies or nephrectomy specimens. Grossly they appear as small (0.1 to 0.3 cm) gray-white nodules attached to the capsule. Histologically they are composed of variable amounts of fibrous, smooth muscle, and adipose tissue and less commonly contain epithelial elements. Whether these lesions are true neoplasms or choristomas remains controversial.

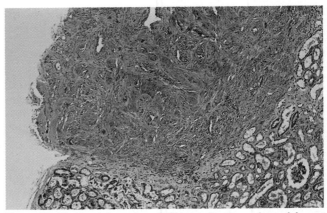

Figure 23–39. Renal "capsuloma." This small subcapsular nodule was an incidental autopsy finding. Trichrome stain colors the smooth muscle tissue red and the fibrous component blue. This tumor was not immunoreactive for HMB-45.

LEIOMYOMA

- Clinically significant or symptomatic benign smooth muscle tumors are rare in the kidney.
- The peak frequency is in the fourth to fifth decades, but cases in neonates and children have been reported.
- Grossly, tumors are solid, well circumscribed and pale tan with a whorled, bulging cut surface.
- Microscopically, tumors consist of bundles of smooth muscle fibers that may show focal calcification and other degenerative changes.
- Criteria for differentiation of benign from malignant smooth muscle tumors are uncertain. Tumor necrosis, nuclear pleomorphism, or mitotic activity (one or more mitoses per 10 high-power fields) favor a diagnosis of leiomyosarcoma.

- Some tumors recognized as capsular leiomyoma may represent a monotypic variant of angiomyolipoma (leiomyoma-like angiomyolipoma) composed of smooth muscle. Immunohistochemically, these tumors coexpress smooth muscle and melanogenesis (HMB-45) markers and represent tumors of perivascular epithelioid cells.

HEMANGIOMA

- Most renal hemangiomas occur in young and middle-aged adults.
- Lesions are usually single, small, asymptomatic, and possibly congenital.
- Multifocal and a few bilateral lesions also occur.

- Multifocal cases may be associated with syndromes such as Klippel-Trénaunay and Sturge-Weber.
- Hematuria is the most common symptom; massive bleeding may occur, especially in large lesions that involve the renal pelvis.
- Most renal angiomas are cavernous rather than capillary.

LYMPHANGIOMA

- Lymphangiomas are less frequent than hemangiomas.
- Lymphangiomas typically occur in young adults or children.
- Most cases are peripelvic or pericalyceal and may actually represent lymphangiectasia secondary to pelvic inflammation and lymphatic obstruction.
- Rare intrarenal lymphangiomas have a multicystic gross appearance.
- Histologically, cavernous spaces of variable size are lined by flattened endothelial cells and filled with lymphatic fluid; the septa may contain smooth muscle.

LIPOMA

- Renal lipomas are extremely rare and occur in much fewer than 1% of kidneys at autopsy.
- Most tumors are intrarenal and occur in middle-aged women.
- Most lipomas are found incidentally; very few are symptomatic.
- Most appear to arise from the renal capsule or the hilar fat.
- Gross and microscopic features are those of benign adipose tumors in other sites.

Differential Diagnosis

- *Angiomyolipomas:* The presence of thick-walled blood vessels and a smooth muscle component are differentiating features.
- *Peripelvic lipomatosis:* This condition frequently follows renal atrophy, most commonly in nephrosclerosis and hydronephrosis.

SOLITARY FIBROUS TUMOR

- Solitary (or localized) fibrous tumors (SFTs) are relatively rare neoplasms that were originally described and are most commonly encountered as a pleural mass. Solitary fibrous tumors have subsequently been described in many other anatomic locations, including rare reports involving the renal parenchyma and capsule.
- Most SFTs occur in patients in the fourth decade of life or older, with a female predilection. They are often asymptomatic and incidentally discovered during radiologic evaluation for unrelated clinical symptoms. Patients with SFTs in the kidney may have gross painless hematuria.
- Histologically, the tumor is composed of spindled (occasionally ovoid, rarely epithelioid) cells interspersed among varying amounts of collagen. Tumor cells usually have bland nuclei with inconspicuous nucleoli and

a low mitotic rate. Cellularity usually varies from low to moderate, and variation in the degree of cellularity in different areas of the neoplasm is a characteristic feature. Tumors are often quite vascular and feature vessels with a zone of hyalinization around the walls; hemangiopericytoma-like areas may be seen.
- Immunohistochemically, strong diffuse staining of tumor cells for vimentin and CD34 is characteristic; keratin, S-100 protein, and HMB-45 are negative; actin and desmin are usually negative.
- Most SFTs behave in a benign fashion. Complete resection is the most important prognostic factor. Although follow-up is short, the few SFTs of the kidney reported to date have behaved in a benign fashion following nephrectomy.
- The differential diagnosis for SFT in the kidney includes a wide variety of lesions, including *sarcomatoid RCC, mesoblastic nephroma, angiomyolipoma, medullary fibroma,* and other *spindle cell neoplasms.*

MALIGNANT MESENCHYMAL TUMORS

LEIOMYOSARCOMA

General and Clinical Features

- Leiomyosarcoma is the most common primary sarcoma of the kidney and represents 40% to 60% of reported sarcomas.

Gross Pathology

- Tumors are usually located peripherally and appear to arise from the renal capsule or from smooth muscle in the renal pelvis or large renal blood vessels; approximately one third of cases are intrarenal.
- Tumors are pale gray, firm, and fleshy with a nodular or bosselated cut surface.

Microscopic Pathology

- Histologic features are similar to those of leiomyosarcomas at other sites (intersecting fascicles of elongated tumor cells with blunt-ended or "cigar-shaped" nuclei and eosinophilic fibrillary cytoplasm); various subtypes have been reported.
- No established criteria can reliably distinguish benign from malignant lesions.
- The most important features separating benign from malignant smooth muscle tumors include size, the presence of necrosis, nuclear pleomorphism, or one or more mitoses per 10 high-power fields.

Special Studies

- Immunohistochemistry is positive for smooth muscle markers (actin and desmin).

Differential Diagnosis

- A primary leiomyosarcoma of the kidney must be differentiated from retroperitoneal soft tissue sarcomas (leiomyosarcomas, dedifferentiated liposarcomas, and others) that may secondarily invade or compress the kidney. With large tumors, the site of origin (kidney versus retroperitoneal soft tissue) may be difficult or impossible to establish.

■ *Angiomyolipoma* and *sarcomatoid RCC* must be distinguished from leiomyosarcoma. Generous tissue sampling is crucial, and the use of immunohistochemical stains and/or electron microscopy may aid in establishing the correct diagnosis.

Treatment and Clinical Course

■ Most patients die of disease within 2 years of diagnosis.
■ Local recurrence and metastases to bone and lung are common.

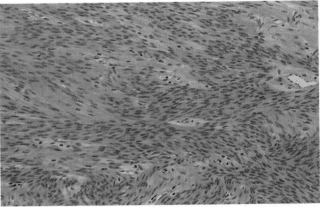

Figure 23–40. Renal leiomyosarcoma. This primary smooth muscle neoplasm is composed of fascicles of spindle cells with moderate cellularity.

LIPOSARCOMA

■ Most retroperitoneal liposarcomas arise in soft tissue and may secondarily involve the kidney, but when tumors are large, the precise site of origin may be indeterminate.
■ Liposarcomas limited to the kidney are exceptionally rare. Some of the reported cases of renal liposarcoma have, in retrospect, been large solitary angiomyolipomas.
■ Various histologic patterns have been observed; the myxoid type is the most common.
■ Complete surgical excision is difficult; recurrence and tumor-related death are expected.

HEMANGIOPERICYTOMA

■ Hemangiopericytomas may occur as primary renal neoplasms; about 50% actually represent tumors arising in perirenal tissue or the renal capsule.
■ Renal tumors are usually large, circumscribed, and fibrous.
■ Microscopically, oval to spindle cells are arranged around variably sized blood vessels, many of which are branching and exhibit a characteristic "staghorn" configuration.
■ Criteria for malignancy in an intrararenal location are not well established.
■ Three reported cases were associated with paraneoplastic syndromes, including hypoglycemia.
■ The prognosis for malignant lesions is better than for most other renal sarcomas.

FIBROSARCOMA AND MALIGNANT FIBROUS HISTIOCYTOMA

■ These tumors may be less common than the literature suggests because some reported cases may actually represent sarcomatoid RCC.
■ Most tumors are large and involve perirenal structures; the primary site of involvement is often impossible to determine.
■ Both tumors are characteristically solid and fleshy with variable hemorrhage and necrosis.
■ The clinical course is aggressive and the prognosis is poor.

OTHER RENAL SARCOMAS

■ Osteosarcoma, rhabdomyosarcoma, and angiosarcoma have also been reported rarely as primary renal neoplasms; the prognosis and survival are poor.
■ A variety of other, even more rare sarcomas, including malignant mesenchymoma, angiomyoliposarcoma, malignant schwannoma, and undifferentiated spindle and round cell sarcoma, have been reported as primary renal malignancies.

METASTATIC NEOPLASMS INVOLVING THE KIDNEY

■ The kidneys are involved by metastasis from extrarenal primaries in about 2% to more than 10% of autopsy studies of patients dying of malignant diseases. At autopsy the most common primary malignancies metastasizing to the kidney include melanoma (skin) and tumors primary in the lung, contralateral kidney, gastrointestinal tract, breast, ovary, and testis.

■ Extrarenal tumors may infrequently occur with renal metastasis as the primary manifestation and are not often encountered in surgical pathology. Primary neoplasms giving rise to clinically diagnosed renal metastases include carcinomas of the lung, thyroid, breast, esophagus, larynx, and anus and liposarcoma of the leg.

■ Metastases can be single or multiple, and their clinical features may mimic those of RCC by producing hematuria or a palpable mass. Some metastases may closely simulate primary renal tumors grossly and even histologically. Knowledge of the patient's clinical history and review of tissues obtained from previous resections are often necessary for correct interpretation.

■ Widespread microscopic metastases to glomeruli, some associated with the clinical picture of proteinuria or acute renal failure, have been reported.

■ Renal cell carcinoma is the most common recipient tumor involved in cancer-to-cancer metastasis; lung carcinoma is the most common donor neoplasm in such instances. Immunohistochemical and ultrastructural studies may be helpful in correctly interpreting the resulting microscopic appearance.

■ Renal involvement by lymphoreticular and hematopoietic tumors is discussed in Chapter 18.

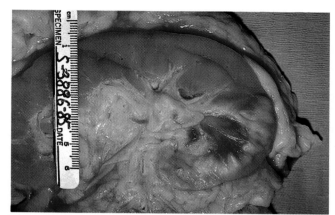

Figure 23–41. Metastatic squamous cell carcinoma involving the kidney. This metastatic tumor is characteristically located within the renal cortex. The primary squamous cell carcinoma originated in a previously resected lung.

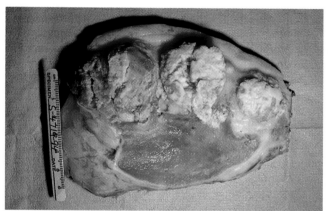

Figure 23–42. Metastatic adenocarcinoma involving the kidney. This metastatic tumor clinically and grossly mimicked a primary renal malignancy. The primary adenocarcinoma originated in a previously resected colon.

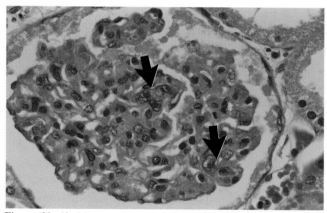

Figure 23–43. Microscopic metastasis to the kidney. A microscopic metastasis of lung adenocarcinoma is present within a renal glomerulus *(arrows)*.

References

Introduction

Association of Directors of Anatomic and Surgical Pathology: Recommendations for the reporting of resected neoplasms of the kidney. Hum Pathol 20:1005, 1996.
Eble JN: Recommendations for examining and reporting tumor-bearing kidney specimens from adults. Semin Diagn Pathol 15:77, 1998.
Guinan P, Sobin LH, Algaba F, et al: TNM staging of renal cell carcinoma. Cancer 80:992, 1997.
Rosai J: Ackerman's Surgical Pathology, 8th ed. St Louis, Mosby, 1996.

Classification

Kovacs G: Molecular differential pathology of renal cell tumors. Histopathology 22:1, 1993.
Kovacs G, Akhtar M, Beckwith B, et al: The Heidelberg classification of renal cell tumours. J Pathol 183:131, 1997.
Mostofi FK, Sesterhenn IA, Sobin LH: Histological Typing of Kidney Tumours: International Histological Classification of Tumours, No. 25. World Health Organization, Geneva, 1981.
Steiner G, Sidransky D: Commentary: Molecular differential diagnosis of renal carcinoma: From microscopes to microsatellites. Am J Pathol 149:1791, 1996.
Störkel S, Eble JN, Adlakha K, et al: Classification of renal cell carcinoma. Cancer 80:987, 1997.

Thoenes W, Störkel S, Rumpelt HJ: Histopathology and classification of renal cell tumors (adenomas, oncocytomas and carcinomas). The basic cytological and histomorphological elements and their use for diagnostics. Pathol Res Pract 181:125, 1986.

Thoenes W, Störkel ST, Rumpelt HJ, et al: Cytomorphological typing of renal cell carcinoma—a new approach. Eur Urol 18:6, 1990.

Renal Cell Carcinoma (General and Clear Cell Type)

Bjornsson J, Short MP, Kwiatkowski, et al: Tuberous sclerosis–associated renal cell carcinoma: Clinical, pathological, and genetic features. Am J Pathol 149:1201, 1996.

Eble JN: Neoplasms of the kidney. In: Bostwick DG, Eble JN (eds): Urologic Surgical Pathology. St. Louis, Mosby, 1997, p 82.

Fuhrman SA, Lasky LC, Limas C: Prognostic significance of morphologic parameters in renal cell carcinoma. Am J Surg Pathol 6:655, 1982.

Goldstein NS: The current state of renal cell carcinoma grading. Cancer 80:977, 1997.

Grignon DJ, Staerkel GA: Surgical diseases of the kidney. In: Silverberg SG, DeLellis RA, Frable WJ (eds): Principles and Practice of Surgical Pathology and Cytopathology, 1st ed. New York, Churchill Livingstone, 1997, p 2147.

Guinan P, Sobin LH, Algaba F: TNM staging of renal cell carcinoma. Cancer 80:992, 1997.

Motzer RJ, Bander NH, Manus DM: Medical progress, renal-cell carcinoma. N Engl J Med 335:865, 1996.

Murphy WM, Beckwith JB, Farrow GM: Tumors of the Kidney, Bladder, and Related Urinary Structures, 3rd series. Washington, DC, Armed Forces Institute of Pathology, 1994, p 92.

Nappi O, Mills SE, Swanson PE, et al: Clear cell tumors of unknown nature and origin: A systematic approach to diagnosis. Semin Diagn Pathol 14:164, 1997.

Weiss LM, Gelb AB, Medeiros LJ: Adult renal epithelial neoplasms. Am J Clin Pathol 103:624, 1995.

Papillary (Chromophil) Renal Cell Carcinoma

Amin MB, Corless CL, Renshaw AA, et al: Papillary (chromophil) renal cell carcinoma: Histomorphologic characteristics and evaluation of conventional pathologic prognostic parameters in 62 cases. Am J Surg Pathol 21:621, 1997.

Delahunt B, Eble JN: Papillary renal cell carcinoma: A clinicopathologic and immunohistochemical study of 105 tumors. Mod Pathol 10:537, 1997.

Lager DJ, Huston BJ, Timmerman TG, et al: Papillary renal tumors, morphologic, cytochemical, and genotypic features. Cancer 76:669, 1995.

Mancilla-Jimenez R, Stanley RJ, Blath RA: Papillary renal cell carcinoma. A clinical, radiologic and pathologic study of 34 cases. Cancer 38:2469, 1976.

Renshaw AA, Corless CL: Papillary renal cell carcinoma, histology and immunohistochemistry. Am J Surg Pathol 19:842, 1995.

Renshaw AA, Zhang H, Corless CL, et al: Solid variants of papillary (chromophil) renal cell carcinoma: Clinicopathologic and genetic features. Am J Surg Pathol 21:1203, 1997.

Chromophobe Renal Cell Carcinoma

Akhtar M, Tulbah A, Kardar AH, et al: Sarcomatoid renal cell carcinoma: The chromophobe connection. Am J Surg Pathol 21:1188, 1997.

Bonsib SM: Renal chromophobe cell carcinoma: The relationship between cytoplasmic vesicles and colloidal iron stain. J Urol Pathol 4:9, 1996.

Bugert P, Gaul C, Wever K, et al: Specific genetic changes of diagnostic importance in chromophobe renal cell carcinomas. Lab Invest 76:203, 1997.

Crotty TB, Farrow GM, Lieber MM: Chromophobe renal cell carcinoma: Clinicopathologic features of 50 cases. J Urol 154:356, 1995.

Durham JR, Keohane M, Amin MB: Chromophobe renal cell carcinoma. Adv Anat Pathol 3:336, 1996.

Speicher MR, du Manoir S, Schoell B, et al: Specific loss of chromosomes 1, 2, 6, 10, 13, 17, and 21 in chromophobe renal cell carcinomas revealed by comparative genomic hybridization. Am J Pathol 145:356, 1995.

Störkel S, Steart PV, Drenckhahn D, et al: The human chromophobe cell renal carcinoma: Its probable relation to intercalated cells of the collecting duct. Virchows Arch 56:237, 1989.

Thoenes W, Störkel S, Rumpelt HJ, et al: Chromophobe cell renal cell carcinoma and its variants. A report of 32 cases. J Pathol 155:1277, 1988.

Tickoo SK, Amin MB, Zarbo RJ: Colloidal iron staining in renal epithelial neoplasms, including chromophobe renal cell carcinoma: Emphasis on technique and patterns of staining. Am J Surg Pathol 22:419, 1998.

Collecting Duct and Renal Medullary Carcinoma

Amin Mahul B, Varma MD, Tickoo SK, et al: Collecting duct carcinoma of the kidney. Adv Anat Pathol 4:85, 1997.

Baer SC, Ro JY, Ordonez NG, et al: Sarcomatoid collecting duct carcinoma: A clinicopatholgic and immunohistochemical study of five cases. Hum Pathol 24:1017, 1993.

Davis CJ, Mostofi FK, Sesterhenn IA: Renal medullary carcinoma—the seventh sickle cell nephropathy. Am J Surg Pathol 19:1, 1995.

Dimopoulos MA, Logothetis CJ, Markowitz A, et al: Collecting duct carcinoma of the kidney. Br J Urol 71:388, 1993.

Fleming S, Lewi HJE: Collecting duct carcinoma of the kidney. Histopathology 10:1131, 1986.

Kennedy SM, Merino MJ, Linehan WM, et al: Collecting duct carcinoma of the kidney. Hum Pathol 21:449, 1990.

Rumpelt J-H, Storkel S, Moll R, et al: Bellini duct carcinoma: Further evidence for this rare variant of renal cell carcinoma. Histopathology 18:115, 1991.

Srigley JR, Eble JN: Collecting duct carcinoma of the kidney. Semin Diagn Pathol 15:54, 1998.

Sarcomatoid Renal Cell Carcinoma

Baer SC, Ro JY, Ordonez NG, et al: Sarcomatoid collecting duct carcinoma: A clinicopathologic and immunohistocheical study of five cases. Hum Pathol 24:1017, 1992.

Farrow GM, Harrison EG Jr, Utz DC: Sarcomas and sarcomatoid and mixed malignant tumors of the kidney in adults—part III. Cancer 22:556, 1968.

Ro JY, Ayala AG, Sella, et al: Sarcomatoid renal cell carcinoma: A clinicopathologic study of 42 cases. Cancer 59:516, 1987.

Cystic Renal Cell Carcinoma

Eble JN, Bonsib SM: Extensively cystic renal neoplasms: Cystic nephrons, cystic partially differentiated nephroblastoma, multilocular renal cell carcinoma, and cystic hamartoma of the renal pelvis. Semin Diagn Pathol 15:2, 1998.

Hartman DS, Davis CJ Jr, Johns T, et al: Cystic renal cell carcinoma. Urology 28:145, 1986.

Murad T, Komako W, Oyasu R, et al: Multilocular cystic renal cell carcinoma. Am J Clin Pathol 95:633, 1991

Cortical Adenoma

Aizawa S, Suzuki M, Kikuch Y, et al: Clinicopathological study on small renal cell carcinoma with metastasis. Acta Pathol Jpn 37:947, 1987.

Bell E: Renal Disease. Philadelphia, Lea & Febiger, 1950.

Budin RE: Renal cell neoplasms: Their relationship to arteriolonephrosclerosis. Arch Pathol Lab Med 108:138, 1984.

Cristol DS, McDonald JR, Emmett JL: Renal adenomas in hypernephromatous kidney: A study of their incidence, nature and relationship. J Urol 55:507, 1946.

Epstein JI: Differential Diagnosis in Pathology: Urologic Disorders. New York, Igaku-Shoin, 1992.

Farrow GM: Diseases of the kidney. In: Murphy WM (ed): Urological Pathology. Philadelphia, WB Saunders, 1989, p 409.

Grignon DJ, Eble JN: Papillary and metanephric adenomas of the kidney. Semin Diagn Pathol 15:41, 1998.

Reese AJM, Winstanley DP: The small tumor-like lesions of the kidney. Br J Cancer 12:507, 1958.

Trinkle AJ: The origin and development of renal adenomas and their relation to carcinoma of the renal cortex (hypernephroma). Am J Cancer 27:676, 1936.

Oncocytoma

Ambos MA, Bosniak MA, Valensi QJ, et al: Angiographic patterns in renal oncocytomas. Radiology 129:615, 1978.

Amin MB, Crotty TB, Tickoo SK, et al: Renal oncocytoma, a reappraisal of morphologic features with clinicopathologic findings in 80 cases. Am J Surg Pathol 21:1, 1997.

Davis CJ Jr, Mostofi FJ, Sesterhenn IA, et al: Renal oncocytoma, clinicopathological study of 166 patients. J Urogenital Pathol 1:41, 1991.

Klein MJ, Valensi QJ: Proximal tubular adenomas of kidney with so-called oncocytic features. Cancer 38:906, 1976.

Merino MJ, LiVolsi VA: Oncocytomas of the kidney. Cancer 50:1852, 1982.

Morra NM, Das S: Renal oncocytoma: A review of histogenesis, histopathology, diagnosis and treatment. J Urol 1:295, 1993.

Morell-Quadreny L, Gregori-Romero MA, Carda-Batalla C, et al: Renal oncocytomas (typical and atypical variants). Int J Surg Pathol 3:210, 1996.

Rainwater LM, Farrow GM, Lievber MM: Flow cytometry of renal oncocytoma: Common occurrence of deoxyribonucleic acid polyploidy and aneuploidy. J Urol 135:1167, 1986.

Metanephric Adenoma

Davis CJ Jr, Barton JH, Sesterhenn IA, et al: Metanephric adenoma: Clinicopathological study of fifty patients. Am J Surg Pathol 19:1101, 1995.

Gatalica A, Grujic S, Kovatich A, et al: Metanephric adenoma: Histology, immunophenotype, cytogenetics, ultrastructure. Mod Pathol 9:329, 1996.

Jones EC, Pins M, Dickersin RD, et al: Metanephric adenoma of the kidney: A clinicopathological, immunohistochemical, flow cytometric, cytogenetic and electron microscopic study of seven cases. Am J Surg Pathol 19:615, 1995.

Strong JW, Ro JY: Metanephric adenoma of the kidney: A newly characterized entity. Adv Anat Pathol 3:172, 1996.

Neuroendocrine Tumors

Cauley JE, Almagro UA, Jacobs SC: Primary renal carcinoid tumor. Urology 32:564, 1988.

Fetissof F, Benatre A, Dubois MP, et al: Carcinoid tumor occurring in a teratoid malformation of the kidney: An immunohistochemical study. Cancer 54:2305, 1984.

Gohji K, Nakanishi T, Hara I, et al: Two cases of primary neuroblastoma of the kidney in adults. J Urol 137:966, 1987.

Kojiro M, Ohishi H, Isobe H: Carcinoid tumor occurring in a cystic teratoma of the kidney, a case report. Cancer 38:1636, 1976.

Raslin WF, Ro JY, Ordonez NJ, et al: Primary carcinoid of the kidney. Immunohistochemical and ultrastructural study of 5 patients. Cancer 72:2660, 1993.

Rothwell DL, Vorstman B, Patton I, et al: Intrarenal pheochromocytoma. Urology 31:175, 1988.

Tetu B, Ro JY, Ayala AG, et al: Small cell carcinoma of the kidney: A clinicopathologic, immunohistochemical, and ultrastructural study. Cancer 60:1809, 1987.

Primitive Neuroectodermal Tumor (PNET)

Marley EF, Liapis H, Humprey PA, et al: Primitive neuroectodermal tumor of the kidney—another enigma: A pathologic, immunohistochemical, and molecular diagnostic study. Am J Surg Pathol 21:354, 1997.

Roloson GJ, Beckwith JB: Primary neuroepithelial tumors of the kidney in children and adults: A report from the NWTS Pathology Center (abstract). Mod Pathol 6:67A, 1993.

Sheaff M, McManus A, Scheimberg I, et al: Primitive neuroectodermal tumor of the kidney confirmed by fluorescence in situ hybridization Am J Surg Pathol 21:461, 1997.

Takeuchi T, Iwasaki H, Ohjimi J, et al: Renal primitive neuroectodermal tumor: An immunohistochemical and cytogenetic analysis. Pathol Int 46:292, 1996.

Juxtaglomerular Cell Tumor

Kihara I, Kitamura S, Hoshino T, et al: A hitherto unreported vascular tumor of the kidney: A proposal of "juxtaglomerular cell tumor." Acta Pathol Jpn 18:197, 1967.

Kodet R, Taylor M, Vachalova H, et al: Juxtaglomerular cell tumor. An immunohistochemical, electron-microscopic and in situ hybridization study. Am J Surg Pathol 18:837, 1994.

Robertson PW, Klidjian A, Harding LK, et al: Hypertension due to a renin-secreting renal tumor. Am J Med 43:963, 1967.

Tetu B, Vaillancourt L, Camilleri J-P, et al: Juxtaglomerular cell tumor of the kidney. Report of two cases with a papillary pattern. Hum Pathol 24:1168, 1993.

Cystic Nephroma (Multilocular Cyst) and Cystic Partially Differentiated Nephroblastoma

Castillo OA, Boyle ET Jr: Multilocular cysts of kidney, a study of 29 patients and review of the literature. Urology 37:156, 1991.

Eble JN, Bonsib SM: Extensively cystic renal neoplasms: Cystic nephroma, cystic partially differentiated nephroblastoma, multilocular renal cell carcinoma, and cystic hamartoma of the renal pelvis. Semin Diagn Pathol 15:2, 1998.

Joshi VV, Beckwith JB: Multilocular cyst of the kidney (cystic nephroma) and cystic, partially differentiated nephroblastoma. Cancer 64:466, 1989.

Kajani N, Rosenberg BF, Bernstein JL: Multilocular cystic nephroma. J Urol Pathol 1:33, 1993.

Madewell JE, Goldman SM, Davis CJ, et al: Multilocular cystic nephroma: A radiographic-pathologic correlation of 58 patients. Radiology 146:309, 1983.

Powell T, Shackman R, Johnson HD: Multilocular cysts of the kidney. Br J Urol 23:142, 1951.

Taxy JB, Marshall FF: Multilocular renal cysts in adults: Possible relationship to renal adenocarcinoma. Arch Pathol Lab Med 107:633, 1983.

Adult Nephroblastoma

Byrd RL, Evans AE, A'Angio GJ: Adult Wilms' tumor: Effect of combined therapy on survival. J Urol 127:648, 1982.

Huser J, Grignon DJ, Ro JY, et al: Adult Wilm's tumor: A clinicopathological study of 11 cases. Mod Pathol 3:321, 1990.

Teratoma

Aaronson IA, Sinclair-Smith C: Multiple cystic teratomas of the kidney (letter). Arch Pathol lab Med 104:614, 1980.

Fetissof F, Benatre A, DuBois MP, et al: Carcinoid tumor occurring in a teratoid malformation of the kidney: An immunohistochemical study. Cancer 54:2305, 1984.

Kojiro M, Ohishi H, Isobe H: Carcinoid tumor occurring in a cystic teratoma of the kidney: A case report. Cancer 38:1636, 1976.

Angiomyolipoma

Ashfaq R, Weinberg AG, Albores-Saavedra J: Renal angiomyolipoma and HMB-45 reactivity. Cancer 71:3091, 1993.

Bernstein J, Robbbins TO, Kissane JM: The renal lesions of tuberous sclerosis. Semin Diagn Pathol 3:97, 1996.

Bonetti F, Pea M, Martignoni G, et al: The perivascular epithelioid cell and related lesions. Adv Anat Pathol 4:343, 1997.

Eble JN: Angiomyolipoma of kidney. Semin Diagn Pathol 15:21, 1998.

Eble JN: Epithelioid angiomyolipoma of the kidney: A report of five cases with a prominent and diagnostically confusing epithelioid smooth muscle component. Am J Surg Pathol 21:1123, 1997.

Farrow GM, Harrison EG Jr, Uta DC, et al: Renal angiomyolipoma: A clinicopathologic study of 32 cases. Cancer 22:564, 1968.

Ferry JA, Malt RA, Young RH: Renal angiomyolipoma with sarcomatous transformation and pulmonary metastases. Am J Surg Pathol 15:1083, 1991.

Henske EP, Xiang H, Short P, et al: Frequent progesterone receptor immunoreactivity in tuberous sclerosis–associated renal angiomyolipomas. Mod Pathol 11:665, 1998.

Kaiserling E, Krober S, Xiao JC, et al: Angiomyolipoma of the kidney. Immunoreactivity with HMB-45. Light and electron-microscopic findings. Histopathology 25:41, 1994.

Steiner MS, Goldman SM, Fishman EK, et al: The natural history of renal angiomyolipoma. J Urol 150:1782, 1993.

Renal Medullary Interstitial Cell Tumors

Eble JN: Unusual renal tumor and tumor-like conditions. In: Eble JN (ed): Tumors and Tumor-like Conditions of the Kidneys and Ureters. New York, Churchill Livingstone, 1990, p 145.

Warfel KA, Eble JN: Renomedullary interstitial cell tumors. Am J Clin Pathol 83:262, 1985.

Zimmermann A, Lusciti P, Flury B, et al: Amyloid-containing renal interstitial cell nodules (RICNs) associated with chronic arterial hypertension in older age groups. Am J Pathol 105:288, 1981.

Mesoblastic Nephroma

Adsay V, Grignon D, Eble J, et al: Solid and cystic biphasic tumor of the adult kidney. Mod Pathol 11:74A, 1998.

Durham JR, Bostwick DG, Farrow GM, et al: Mesoblastic nephroma of adulthood. Report of three cases. Am J Surg Pathol 10:1029, 1993.

Levin NP, Damjanov I, Depillis VJ: Mesoblastic nephroma in an adult patient. Recurrence 21 years after removal of the primary lesion. Cancer 49:573, 1982.

Pawade J, Soosay GN, Delprado W, et al: Cystic hamartoma of the renal pelvis. Am J Surg Pathol 17:1169, 1993.

Truong LD, Williams R, Ngo T, et al: Adult mesoblastic nephroma: Expansion of the morphologic spectrum and review of literature. Am J Surg Pathol 22:827, 1998.

Other Benign Mesenchymal Neoplasms

Bonsib SM: HMB-45 reactivity in renal leiomyomas and leiomyosarcomas. Mod Pathol 9:664, 1996.

Colvin SH Jr: Certain capsular and subcapsular mixed tumors of the kidney herein called "capsuloma." J Urol 48:585, 1942.

Grignon DJ, Ro JY, Ayala AG: Mesenchymal tumors of the kidneys. In: Eble JN (ed): Tumors and Tumor-like Conditions of the Kidney and Ureters. New York, Churchill Livingstone, 1990, p 123.

Palmer FJ, Tynan AP: Leiomyoma of the kidney. J Urol 112:22, 1974.

Solitary Fibrous Tumor

Gelb A, Simmons ML, Weidner N: Solitary fibrous tumor involving the renal capsule. Am J Surg Pathol 20:1288, 1996.

Fain JS, Eble J, Nascimento AF, et al: Solitary fibrous tumor of the kidney: Report of three cases. J Urol Pathol 4:227, 1996.

Nascimento AG: Solitary fibrous tumor: A ubiquitous neoplasm of mesenchymal differentiation. Adv Anat Pathol 3:388, 1996.

Sarcomas

Grignon DJ, Ayala AG, Ro JY, et al: Primary sarcomas of the kidney: A clinicopathologic and DNA flow cytometric study of 17 cases. Cancer 65:1611, 1990.

Farrow GM, Harrison EG, Utz DC, et al: Sarcomas and sarcomatoid and mixed malignant tumors of the kidney in adults—part I. Cancer 22:545, 1968.

Mayes DC, Fechner RE, Gillenwater JY: Renal liposarcoma. Am J Surg Pathol 14:268, 1990.

Murphy WM, Beckwith JB, Farrow GM: Tumors of the Kidney, Urinary Bladder, and Related Structures, 3rd series. Washington, DC, Armed Forces Institute of Pathology, 1994, p 158.

Metastatic Neoplasms Involving the Kidney

Petersen RO: Kidney. In: Petersen RO (ed): Urologic Pathology, 2nd ed. Philadelphia, JB Lippincott, 1992, p 132.

Toth T: Extracapillary tumorous metastatic crescents in glomeruli of the kidney. Pathol Res Pract 182:240, 1987.

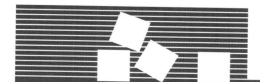

CHAPTER 24

Tumors and Tumor-Like Conditions of the Renal Pelvis

INTRODUCTION

- Embryologically, the renal pelvis and major and minor calyces form through branching and expansion of the ureteral bud and are lined by urothelium (transitional epithelium) that is continuous with that of the ureter and urinary bladder.
- The urothelium lining the upper and lower urinary tract is specialized to protect subepithelial tissue from harmful substances. It is of variable thickness (dependent in part on the degree of organ distention). Normally, the urothelium ranges from three to seven cell layers (three to five layers in the renal pelvis) and is composed of basal and intermediate cells covered by a protective layer of large, frequently multinucleated umbrella cells. The urothelium rests on a basement membrane overlying lamina propria that consists of loose connective tissue. In the renal pelvis, an outer layer of smooth muscle forms a spiral that is continuous with the muscularis of the ureter.
- Lesions involving the renal pelvis are similar to those of the urinary bladder and ureter. Approximately 5% to 10% of primary renal tumors occur in the renal pelvis and arise from the pelvic urothelium.
- The majority of these tumors are transitional cell (urothelial) carcinomas (TCCs). Squamous cell carcinoma and adenocarcinoma of the renal pelvis are much less common.
- Tumor stage (Table 24–1) and grade are the most important predictors of prognosis in patients with renal pelvic carcinomas.

- Benign epithelial neoplasms, including transitional cell papilloma and inverted papilloma, are rare.

Table 24–1
TNM STAGING OF RENAL PELVIC CARCINOMA

Primary Tumor (T)

TX	Primary tumor cannot be assessed
T0	No evidence of primary tumor
Ta	Papillary noninvasive carcinoma
Tis	Carcinoma in situ
T1	Tumor invades subepithelial connective tissue
T2	Tumor invades the muscularis
T3	Tumor invades peripelvic fat or the renal parenchyma
T4	Tumor invades adjacent organs or through the kidney into the perirenal fat

Regional Lymph Nodes (N)

NX	Regional lymph nodes cannot be assessed
N0	No regional lymph node metastasis
N1	Metastasis in a single lymph node, 2 cm or less in maximum dimension
N2	Metastasis in a single lymph node >2 cm but <5 cm in maximum dimension; or multiple lymph nodes none >5 cm in greatest dimension
N3	Metastasis in a lymph node >5 cm in maximum dimension

Distant Metastasis (M)

MX	Distant metastasis cannot be assessed
M0	No distant metastasis
M1	Distant metastasis

Adapted from AJCC Cancer Staging Manual, 5th ed. American Joint Committee on Cancer, Philadelphia, Lippincott–Raven, 1997.

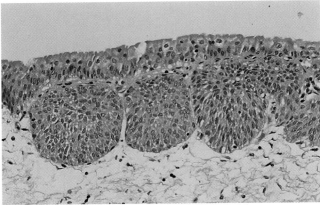

Figure 24-1. Urothelium of the renal pelvis. The epithelium consists of basal and intermediate cell layers with a surface layer of umbrella cells. Invaginations of urothelium (von Brunn's nests) are seen within the subepithelial connective tissue (lamina propria).

MALIGNANT EPITHELIAL NEOPLASMS

TRANSITIONAL CELL CARCINOMA

Synonym: Urothelial carcinoma.

Note: Some authors prefer the term *urothelial carcinoma* to *transitional cell carcinoma*. These terms are used interchangeably in this text.

General and Clinical Features

- Transitional cell carcinoma (TCC) is the most common renal pelvic neoplasm and accounts for about 90% of these tumors.
- Peak incidence occurs in the sixth and seventh decades of life; children are rarely affected.
- There is a male preponderance (3:1) except for analgesic-associated cancers, which do not show sex predilection.
- Epidemiologic risk factors include tobacco use, occupational exposure to azo dyes and pigments, chronic inflammation, and calculi (similar to those for the urinary bladder and ureter).
- Analgesic abuse (long-term ingestion of phenacetin-containing drugs) is an important risk factor for the development of renal pelvic cancers (up to 25% of cases) in some populations. Balkan nephropathy (a form of chronic tubulointerstitial nephritis of uncertain etiology) has a strong association with renal pelvic TCC in some Balkan nations.
- Thorotrast-associated renal pelvic carcinomas have been reported rarely, have often shown squamous differentiation, and have been reported 16 to 40 years after the administration of thorium-containing radiologic contrast material.

- Painless gross hematuria is the most common initial symptom (70% to 80% of patients); flank pain and/or mass are additional symptoms.
- Radiologic studies, including intravenous and/or retrograde pyelography, ultrasonography, and computed tomography, urine cytology, and renal pelvic brush/wash cytology aid in the diagnostic evaluation.
- Renal pelvic TCCs are commonly associated with multifocal urothelial neoplasia; synchronous or metachronous urothelial carcinomas involving the ipsilateral or contralateral ureter, renal pelvis, or urinary bladder are identified in about 40% to 50% of patients.
- Renal cell carcinoma has been reported rarely as a coexisting primary tumor.

Gross Pathology

- Pelvic urothelial tumors most commonly form exophytic papillary masses with frond-like growth on the mucosal surface.
- Invasive solid (nonpapillary/sessile) tumors often with surface necrosis and ulceration also occur (some of these tumors may arise from high-grade urothelial dysplasia-carcinoma in situ).
- Depending on their location relative to the ureteropelvic junction, large tumors may cause urinary outflow obstruction and hydronephrosis.
- Tumors may be localized or diffusely involve the renal pelvis, extend down the ureter, or invade the renal medulla and cortex with extension through the renal capsule and penetration into perinephric fat.

Microscopic Pathology

- Renal pelvic TCCs have the same histologic spectrum as urothelial carcinomas of the urinary bladder and ureter (see references for a detailed review).

- Most tumors have a papillary growth pattern with central, thin, and often branching fibrovascular cores lined by urothelium of variable thickness with varying degrees of cytologic abnormalities. Papillary tumors may be invasive or noninvasive. Infiltrative urothelial carcinomas that lack a papillary component are also seen.
- Papillary and invasive urothelial carcinomas may be associated with high-grade urothelial dysplasia–transitional cell carcinoma in situ (CIS). CIS is defined as a full-thickness proliferation of malignant urothelial cells confined to the epithelium. CIS is rarely observed in the renal pelvis in the absence of an accompanying papillary or invasive TCC.
- Specimens should be evaluated for the presence of multifocal tumors or high-grade urothelial dysplasia-CIS. In a majority of cases, the mucosa adjacent to invasive renal pelvic TCCs shows dysplasia or CIS (this finding identifies patients at increased risk for metachronous urothelial tumors).
- The presence (and depth) or absence of stromal and smooth muscle invasion and lymphatic or vascular invasion should be documented.
- Tumors are graded in terms of cytologic features. Several systems have been developed for the grading of urothelial carcinoma. Although some systems have had four grades, the system proposed by the World Health Organization (WHO) has been widely accepted. This system divides urothelial carcinomas into three grades (1–3), corresponding to well, moderately, and poorly differentiated, on the basis of nuclear pleomorphism, mitotic activity, prominence of nucleoli, loss of polarity, and nuclear crowding.
  - Grade 1 tumors are almost always papillary and noninvasive. They are lined by more than seven cell layers that resemble normal urothelium, but have slight nuclear enlargement without significant nuclear pleomorphism or mitotic activity.
  - Grade 2 tumors are often papillary and show a greater degree of nuclear pleomorphism, more prominent nucleoli, and more readily identified mitoses. The number of cell layers may be increased, normal, or decreased.
  - Grade 3 tumors are usually sessile and invasive but occasionally have a papillary architecture. They are composed of markedly pleomorphic cells with marked nuclear enlargement, prominent nucleoli, and frequent mitoses.
- Tumor grade usually correlates with stage. Low-grade (grades 1 and 2) tumors may show minimal or absent invasion, whereas high-grade (grade 3) tumors are often of advanced stage at diagnosis.
- Carcinomas arising from urothelium have a great potential for divergent differentiation and may show squamous, glandular, and occasionally neuroendocrine (small cell) differentiation.
  - Squamous differentiation (defined by the presence of intercellular bridges or keratinization) is common. The proportion of the squamous component varies but is most frequently observed as focal squamous differentiation in a high-grade TCC.
  - Glandular (adenocarcinomatous) differentiation (defined as the presence of true glandular spaces) is less common than squamous differentiation. Focal glandular differentiation in a high-grade TCC must be distinguished from pseudoglandular spaces created by artifact or tumor necrosis.
  - Mucin-containing (alcian blue-positive) cells occur and are more common in high-grade TCCs. Their presence is not classified as glandular differentiation unless accompanied by unequivocal gland formation.
- Sarcomatoid transformation and rare variants with trophoblastic or hepatoid differentiation and osteoclast-type giant cells have been reported.
  - Sarcomatoid urothelial carcinoma may have a partial or complete spindle cell pattern of growth that may mimic true sarcomas. Immunohistochemical and electron microscopic studies may be useful in identifying carcinomatous elements obscured by the sarcomatoid spindle cell component (see later).

Special Studies

- Immunohistochemically, TCCs express both high- and low-molecular-weight cytokeratins. In low-grade TCCs, cytokeratins 7, 8, 13, and 19 predominate. Higher grade urothelial carcinomas preferentially express cytokeratin 18. TCCs also express other epithelial markers, including epithelial membrane antigen, Leu-M1, and carcinoembryonic antigen. Vimentin is not expressed in low-grade urothelial carcinoma but is commonly coexpressed with cytokeratin in poorly differentiated tumors.
- Ultrastructural studies reveal desmosomes and tonofilaments (features of epithelial differentiation) that decrease in number with increasing tumor grade. High-grade urothelial carcinomas may show focal presence of glandular differentiation with microlumen formation and microvillous projections.

Differential Diagnosis

- *Renal cell carcinoma:* Renal pelvic TCCs with renal medullary and cortical extension may be difficult to distinguish from renal cell carcinoma, both grossly and histologically. Renal cell carcinomas that are characteristically centered on the renal medulla (e.g., collecting duct carcinoma and renal medullary carcinoma) may pose particular problems in the differential diagnosis. The identification of a papillary or in situ urothelial component within the renal pelvis favors TCC.
- *Squamous cell carcinoma and adenocarcinoma of the renal pelvis:* Urothelial carcinomas may show focal or extensive squamous or glandular differentiation. Tumors with any identifiable urothelial component (including CIS) are classified as urothelial carcinomas with squamous or glandular differentiation.
- *Sarcoma:* Primary sarcomas of the renal pelvis are very rare and must be differentiated from sarcomatoid renal pelvic carcinomas, in which the malignant spindle cell component predominates. Electron microscopy or immunohistochemical techniques (employing antibodies to cytokeratin) may be useful in demonstrating epithelial differentiation in sarcomatoid carcinomas.

Treatment and Clinical Course

- Nephroureterectomy (with bladder cuff) is the standard therapy for pyeloureteral TCC; radical resection is usually chosen owing to the high incidence of renal and perirenal invasion, multicentric tumor, and recurrence in the ureteral/bladder stump.
- Retroperitoneal lymphadenectomy is advocated by some. Adjuvant chemotherapy and radiation therapy may be used in the treatment of advanced disease.
- More conservative resection may be considered in select cases in which the risk of renal and perirenal invasion and multicentricity is low or in the setting of compromised renal function.

- Approximately 75% of renal pelvic TCCs are low-grade and low-stage.
- Muscle invasion is a critical prognostic factor that adversely affects survival.
- Regional metastasis to para-aortic lymph nodes is a poor prognostic finding.
- Distant metastases to lung, liver, bone, and peritoneum are most common.
- Patients with high-grade/high-stage lesions usually die within 2 years of diagnosis; overall 5-year survival rate after radical surgery ranges from 20% to 45%.
- Endoscopic and cytologic follow-up is essential because of the high rate of recurrence and the risk of metachronous tumors.

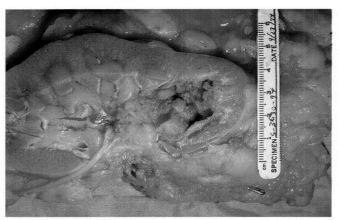

Figure 24–2. Papillary transitional cell carcinoma of the renal pelvis. An exophytic papillary urothelial tumor extensively involves the renal pelvis and calyces.

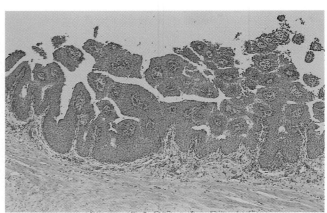

Figure 24–4. Papillary transitional cell carcinoma of the renal pelvis. Branching frond-like stalks lined by neoplastic cells are seen on the renal pelvic surface. The tumor has a broad pushing base that invades the lamina propria and extends near the muscular layer.

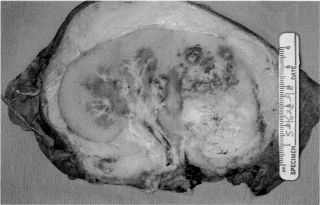

Figure 24–3. Transitional cell carcinoma of the renal pelvis. A solid sessile neoplasm involves the calyceal system and extensively invades the kidney and hilar tissue.

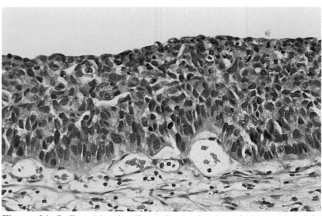

Figure 24–5. Transitional cell carcinoma in situ of the renal pelvis. Large pleomorphic cells with hyperchromatic nuclei and high nuclear-cytoplasmic ratios show loss of polarity and no evidence of maturation. The dysplastic changes involve the full thickness of the urothelium. The basement membrane is intact.

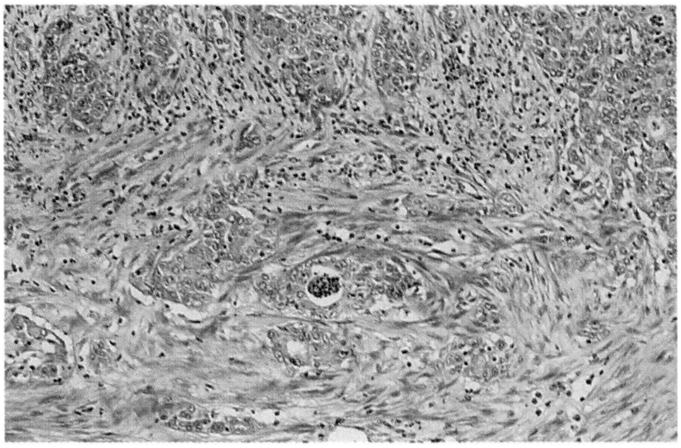

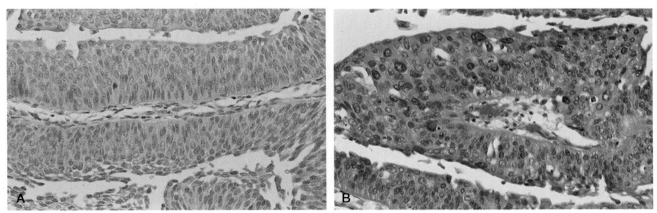

Figure 24-6. Transitional cell carcinoma with myoinvasion. Irregular nests of urothelial carcinoma invade smooth muscle.

Figure 24-7. Papillary transitional cell carcinoma. *A,* Low-grade (well-differentiated) papillary TCC has slight nuclear enlargement without significant nuclear pleomorphism. *B,* Pleomorphic cells with marked nuclear enlargement are seen in this example of a high-grade (poorly differentiated) papillary TCC.

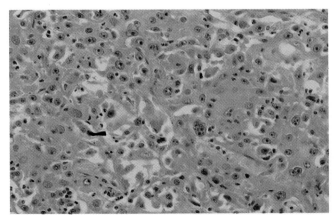

Figure 24-8. Invasive transitional cell carcinoma. This poorly differentiated urothelial carcinoma is characterized by marked nuclear pleomorphism and has focal squamous differentiation (a feature commonly seen in high-grade urothelial neoplasms).

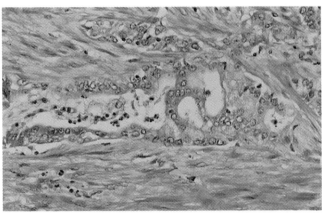

Figure 24-9. Transitional cell carcinoma with glandular differentiation. Invasive urothelial carcinomas may form true glandular spaces (glandular differentiation) and have mucin-containing cells.

SQUAMOUS CELL CARCINOMA

General and Clinical Features

- Squamous cell carcinoma of the renal pelvis accounts for about 5% to 10% of renal pelvic malignancies.
- These tumors have a strong association with renal pelvic calculi and chronic infection and may be associated with squamous metaplasia involving the renal pelvis and calyces.
- This neoplasm occurs most frequently in men during the sixth and seventh decades, but rare pediatric cases have been reported.
- Patients usually have gross painless hematuria; a palpable mass is common (75% of patients).

Gross and Microscopic Pathology

- Grossly, squamous cell carcinomas are poorly circumscribed, infiltrating, friable to firm, and gray-white and often show ulceration and necrosis. With most tumors, there is invasion of the pelvic wall and adjacent peripelvic adipose tissue at the time of diagnosis.
- Histologically, squamous differentiation, typically with prominent keratinization and intercellular bridges, is seen throughout the tumor. The diagnosis of squamous cell carcinoma is reserved for pure tumors without identifiable urothelial components, including transitional cell carcinoma in situ. (*Note:* Renal pelvic carcinomas with identifiable urothelial and squamous components are classified as TCC with squamous differentiation.)
- Squamous cell carcinomas range from well differentiated (abundant keratinization, prominent intercellular bridges, and minimal nuclear pleormorphism) to poorly differentiated with marked nuclear pleomorphism.
- Renal pelvic urothelium adjacent to tumor may show squamous metaplasia.

Differential Diagnosis

- *Metastatic squamous cell carcinoma* should be excluded. Knowledge of the clinical history usually enables the correct diagnosis to be made.
- *Transitional cell carcinoma with squamous differentiation* should be excluded by generous tissue sampling that fails to disclose a urothelial component.

Treatment and Clinical Course

- Invasion of retroperitoneal soft tissue and lymph node metastases are commonly present at the time of diagnosis.
- Renal pelvic squamous cell carcinomas are more aggressive and have a worse prognosis than renal pelvic TCCs; most patients die within 2 years of diagnosis.

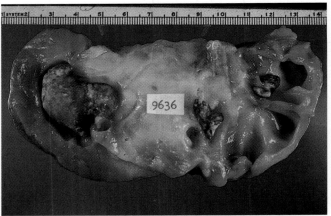

Figure 24–10. Squamous cell carcinoma of the renal pelvis. This carcinoma is associated with a large staghorn renal calculus.

ADENOCARCINOMA

General and Clinical Features

- Primary adenocarcinoma of the renal pelvis is rare and accounts for fewer than 1% of renal pelvic malignancies. Reports consist of single cases or small series.
- Factors predisposing to the development of pelvic adenocarcinoma include glandular (intestinal) metaplasia (pyelitis glandularis of the intestinal type) with a frequent history of lithiasis, chronic pyelonephritis, and hydronephrosis.

- The peak frequency is in the sixth and seventh decades, but rare pediatric cases have been reported. There is no sex predilection.

Gross and Microscopic Pathology

- Most tumors have invasion of the pelvic wall and adjacent peripelvic adipose tissue.
- Papillary and glandular architecture and resemblance to mucinous adenocarcinoma of the colon are common. Mucin production is variable, and signet-ring cell features may be seen.

- Most tumors will be associated with pyelitis glandularis of the intestinal type involving the adjacent mucosa.

Differential Diagnosis

- *Metastatic adenocarcinoma* should be excluded before accepting a diagnosis of primary adenocarcinoma of the renal pelvis.

Treatment and Clinical Course

- Most patients have advanced disease at diagnosis and a poor prognosis.

SMALL CELL CARCINOMA

- Small cell neuroendocrine carcinoma has been reported very rarely in the renal pelvis (see references for a few case reports).
- Histologic, immunohistochemical, and ultrastructural features of small cell carcinoma of the renal pelvis are similar to those that occur more commonly in the lungs and other sites (see Chapter 23).
- Histologically, nests and sheets of undifferentiated small to intermediate-sized tumor cells have been admixed with invasive urothelial carcinoma and carcinoma in situ in the few reported cases of small cell carcinoma of the renal pelvis. Unlike urothelial carcinoma with squamous or glandular differentiation, such mixed tumors are reported as small cell carcinoma with other histologic components. This difference in terminology relates to therapy and the potential response of small cell carcinoma to combined surgery and adjuvant multiagent chemotherapy.
- These tumors pursue the typically aggressive course of small cell carcinomas in other body sites, with metastasis and death often within less than 1 year following diagnosis and nephrectomy.

BENIGN EPITHELIAL NEOPLASMS

Transitional Cell Papilloma

- The diagnostic criteria for transitional cell (urothelial) papilloma and its frequency within the urinary tract remain controversial (see references for a detailed discussion of these issues). Most authorities currently accept the existence of urothelial papilloma based on restrictive diagnostic criteria.
- The World Health Organization classification defines papilloma as a usually solitary papillary tumor covered by normal-appearing urothelium consisting of no more than six or seven layers of cells that generally lack mitotic figures.
- Urothelial papilloma occurs in a younger age group (usually younger than age 50 years) than most urothelial cancers.
- Transitional cell papilloma of the renal pelvis is rare.
- Grossly, transitional cell papilloma is usually small (several millimeters or less).
- Microscopically, delicate fibrovascular stalks are covered by cytologically and architecturally normal urothelium.

Inverted Papilloma

Synonym: Brunnian adenoma.

- Inverted papilloma occurs less commonly in the renal pelvis than in the urinary bladder and ureter.
- Its etiology remains uncertain, and it is variably viewed as a benign neoplasm or a reactive proliferative lesion (possibly related to pyelitis glandularis and pyelitis cystica).
- Hematuria and flank pain are common presenting symptoms.
- Grossly and endoscopically, it may form a domed mass that mimics TCC.
- Microscopically, anastomosing islands and trabeculae of urothelium proliferate downward into the lamina propria. The surface urothelium is normal or attenuated, and an exophytic papillary component should not be present. There is usually little or no cytologic atypia, and mitotic figures are rare or absent.
- The major differential diagnosis is TCC with an inverted growth pattern mimicking inverted papilloma. TCC shows more significant cytologic atypia and mitotic figures.
- Inverted papillomas are curable with surgical resection and have a low rate of recurrence. They may, however, be associated with synchronous or metachronous TCCs in the urinary tract.

NON-NEOPLASTIC PROLIFERATIVE AND METAPLASTIC LESIONS

Von Brunn's Nests and Pyelitis Cystica and Glandularis

- Von Brunn's nests and pyelitis cystica and glandularis are non-neoplastic urothelial proliferative lesions that are regarded as normal or reactive in nature.
- Von Brunn's nests are invaginations of urothelium present within the lamina propria of the urinary tract; they are more common in the urinary bladder than in the ureter or renal pelvis.
- When von Brunn's nests within the renal pelvis acquire central cystic lumens lined by urothelium or columnar cells, they are referred to as pyelitis cystica and pyelitis glandularis, respectively. In pyelitis cystica, the lumina are lined by cuboidal or flattened urothelium; the lumina may become dilated and filled with eosinophilic fluid. In the typical type of pyelitis glandularis, the lumina of von Brunn's nests are lined by nonmucinous columnar cells that are surrounded by one or more layers of urothelial cells. Similar epithelium may be present on the mucosal surface.
- Pyelitis cystica and glandularis is usually an incidental microscopic finding, but may rarely produce grossly visible nodular elevations or fluid-filled cysts that protrude into the renal pelvis.

Squamous and Intestinal Metaplasia

■ Squamous and intestinal metaplasia involving the renal pelvis usually arises in a background of chronic inflammation, chronic infection, calculi, or chronic irritation (e.g., indwelling catheters).

■ Squamous metaplasia is the most common form of urothelial metaplasia and may be nonkeratinizing or keratinizing. Keratinizing squamous metaplasia may result in abundant keratin accumulation, which may form renal pelvic masses.

■ In the intestinal type of pyelitis glandularis, colonic-type mucinous epithelium, often containing goblet cells (and rarely enterochromaffin cells), replaces urothelium. Intestinal metaplasia of the renal pelvis is rare and has been associated with adenocarcinoma.

Nephrogenic Metaplasia (Adenoma)

■ Nephrogenic metaplasia (nephrogenic adenoma) is more commonly encountered in the urinary bladder and ureter but has been reported rarely in the renal pelvis.

■ It may appear as an exophytic lesion that grossly and histologically mimics carcinoma. It is usually associated with chronic inflammation and is currently recognized as a metaplastic process.

■ Microscopically, papillary and tubular proliferations (resembling renal tubules) and cystically dilated tubules are lined by cytologically bland cuboidal, low columnar, or hobnail cells. Tubules and cysts often contain eosinophilic or basophilic secretions.

■ Familiarity with this tumor-like lesion is important in distinguishing it from adenocarcinoma or urothelial carcinoma.

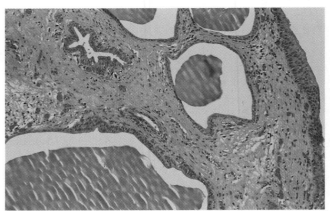

Figure 24–11. Pyelitis cystica and glandularis (typical type). Von Brunn's nests have central lumina, most of which are cystically dilated, lined by cuboidal to flattened urothelium, and filled with eosinophilic secretions (pyelitis cystica). In a few nests, the lining cells are columnar (nonmucinous) and represent glandular metaplasia (pyelitis glandularis) of the typical type.

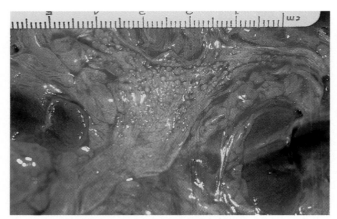

Figure 24–12. Pyelitis cystica. The renal pelvis has numerous thin-walled mucosal cysts that corresponded histologically to the cystic change of Von Brunn's nests.

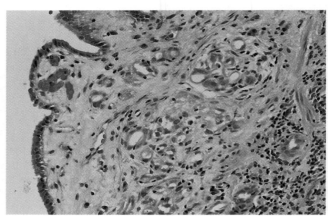

Figure 24–13. Nephrogenic metaplasia (adenoma). A proliferation of small tubules lined by cuboidal to flattened epithelium resembling renal tubules is present within the lamina propria. The surface is lined by metaplastic cuboidal to low columnar epithelium. (Note: This example of nephrogenic metaplasia involving the urinary bladder shows histologic features identical to rare reported cases of this entity in the renal pelvis).

MESENCHYMAL NEOPLASMS

Fibroepithelial Polyp

- Renal pelvic fibroepithelial polyps are benign mesenchymal lesions that are considered by some to be hamartomatous, rather than neoplastic.
- Both adults and children are affected.
- The ureteropelvic junction is a common site of involvement, and the polyp may cause obstruction.
- Flank pain and hematuria are the most common symptoms.
- Grossly, a fibroepithelial polyp consists of single or multiple slender, vermiform projections that usually arise from a common base.
- Histologically, polyps consist of edematous and mildly inflamed fibrovascular cores covered by benign urothelium that may be focally eroded; the stalks may undergo hyalinization or contain smooth muscle.

OTHER UNCOMMON NEOPLASMS

- Other benign and malignant mesenchymal neoplasms are exceedingly rare in the renal pelvis. Hemangioma, leiomyoma, leiomyosarcoma, choriocarcinoma, malignant melanoma, lymphoma, carcinosarcoma, and other rare sarcomas have been reported. Wilms tumor and mesonephric adenosarcoma, an aggressive entity that may be linked histogenetically to nephroblastoma, have been reported.
- Metastatic tumors involving the renal pelvis are rare.

References

Transitional Cell Carcinoma

Bonsib SM, Eble JN: Renal pelvis and ureter. In: Bostwick DG, Eble JN (eds): Urologic Surgical Pathology. St. Louis, Mosby, 1997, p 150.

Eble JN, Young RH: Carcinoma of the urinary bladder: A review of its diverse morphology. Semin Diagn Pathol 14:98, 1997.

Melamed MR, Reuter VE: Pathology and staging of urothelial tumors of the kidney and ureter. Urol Clin North Am 20:333, 1993.

Mostofi FK, Sobin LH, Torloni H: Histological typing of urinary bladder tumors. In: International Classification of Tumors. vol 10. Geneva, Switzerland, World Health Organization, 1973.

Murphy WM, Beckwith JB, Farrow GM: Tumors of the Kidney, Bladder and Related Structures, 3rd series. Washington, DC, Armed Forces Institute of Pathology, 1994.

Wick MR, Perrone TL, Burke BA: Sarcomatoid transitional cell carcinoma of the renal pelvis. Arch Pathol Lab Med 109:55, 1985.

Wick MR, Zarbo RJ, Hitchcock CL: Special techniques for the pathologic analysis of lesions of the urinary bladder. In: Young RH (ed): Pathology of the Urinary Bladder. New York, Churchill Livingstone, 1989, p 285.

Squamous Cell Carcinoma

Blacher EJ, Johnson DE, Abdul-Karim FW, et al: Squamous cell carcinoma of renal pelvis. Urol 25:124, 1985.

Li MK, Cheung WL: Squamous cell carcinoma of the renal pelvis. J Urol 138:269, 1987.

Adenocarcinoma

Ackerman LV: Mucinous adenocarcinoma of the pelvis of the kidney. J Urol 55:35, 1946.

Mirone V, Prezioso D, Palombini S, et al: Mucinous adenocarcinoma of the renal pelvis. Eur Urol 10:284, 1984.

Petersen RO: Renal Pelvis. In: Petersen RO (ed): Urologic Pathology. Philadelphia, JB Lippincott Co, 1992, p 170.

Shibahara N, Okada S, Onishi S, et al: Primary mucinous carcinoma of the renal pelvis. Pathol Res Pract 189:946, 1993.

Small Cell Carcinoma

Essenfeld H, Manivel JC, Benedetto P, et al: Small cell carcinoma of the renal pelvis: A clinicopathological, morphological and immunohistochemical study of 2 cases. J Urol 144:344, 1990.

Mills SE, Weiss MA, Swanson PE, et al: Small cell undifferentiated carcinoma of the renal pelvis. A light microscopic, immunocytochemical and ultrastructural study. Surg Pathol 1:83, 1988.

Ordonez NG, Horsand J, Ayala AG, et al: Oat cell carcinoma of the urinary tract: An immunohistochemical and electron microscopic study. Cancer 58:2519, 1986.

Benign Epithelial Neoplasms

Amin MB, Murphy WM, Reuter VE, et al: A symposium on controversies in the pathology of transitional cell carcinomas of the urinary bladder, part I. Anat Pathol 1:1, 1996.

Eble JN, Young RH: Benign and low-grade papillary lesions of the urinary bladder: A review of the papilloma–papillary carcinoma controversy and a report of 5 typical papillomas. Semin Diagn Pathol 6: 351, 1989.

Kyriakos M, Royce RJ: Multiple simultaneous inverted papillomas of the upper urinary tract. Cancer 63:368, 1989.

Non-Neoplastic Proliferative and Metaplastic Lesions

Bullock PS, Thoni DE, Murphy WM: The significance of colonic mucosa (intestinal metaplasia) involving the urinary tract. Cancer 59: 2086, 1987.

Hertle L, Androulakakis P: Keratinizing desquamative squamous metaplasia of the upper urinary tract: Leukoplakia-cholesteatoma. J Urol 114:165, 1987.

Mostofi FK: Potentialities of bladder epithelium. J Urol 71:705, 1954.

Murphy WM, Beckwith JB, Farrow GM: Tumors of the Kidney, Bladder, and Related Urinary Structures, 3rd Series. Washington, DC, Armed Forces Institute of Pathology, 1994, p 275.

Oliva E, Young RH: Nephrogenic adenoma of the urinary tract: A review of the microscopic appearance of 80 cases with emphasis on unusual features. Mod Pathol 8:722, 1995.

Young RH, Eble JN: Non-neoplastic Disorders of the Urinary Bladder. In: Bostwick DG, Eble JN (eds): Urologic Surgical Pathology. St. Louis, Mosby, 1997, p 166.

Mesenchymal and Other Uncommon Neoplasms

Bonsib SM, Eble JN: Renal pelvis and ureter. In: Bostwick DG, Eble JN (eds): Urologic Surgical Pathology. St. Louis, Mosby, 1997, p 150.

Murphy WM, Beckwith JB, Farrow GM: Tumors of the Kidney, Bladder, and Related Urinary Structures, 3rd Series. Washington, DC, Armed Forces Institute of Pathology, 1994, p 313.

Wolgel CD, Parris AC, Mitty HA, et al: Fibroepithelial polyp of renal pelvis. Urology 19:436, 1982.

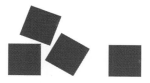

INDEX

Note: Page numbers in *italics* refer to illustrations; page numbers followed by t refer to tables.

    focal segmental, 39t, 45–50. See also Focal
        segmental glomerulosclerosis.
Glomerulus(i), anatomy of, gross, 2, 3
    microscopic, 4–6
    in acute diffuse intracapillary proliferative
        glomerulonephritis, 17, 18
    in Alport's syndrome, 119
    in amyloidosis, 223, 225
    in C1q nephropathy, 202
    in chronic pyelonephritis, 145, 149
    in Churg-Strauss syndrome, 180
    in collagen Type III glomerulopathy, 204
    in diabetic nephropathy, 98–99, 101–103
    in diffuse extracapillary proliferative
        (crescentic) glomerulonephritis, 29,
        31–32
    in end-stage renal disease, 114–115, 115–
        116
    in essential mixed cryoglobulinemia, 12–13,
        182
    in fibrillary glomerulonephritis, 229, 232
    in fibronectin glomerulopathy, 206
    in focal glomerulonephritis, 35, 35–36
    in focal segmental glomerulosclerosis, 45–
        46, 47
    in HBV-associated membranous glomerulo-
        nephropathy, 196
    in hemolytic-uremic syndrome and throm-
        botic thrombocytopenic purpura, 70,
        72
    in Henoch-Schönlein purpura, 64–65
    in heroin-associated nephropathy, 192
    in HIV-associated nephropathy, 187, 189
        activity and chronicity indices in, 80t
        WHO classification of, 80, 81t
    in IgA nephropathy, 59, 61–62
    in interstitial nephritis, 138
    in ischemic acute tubular nephropathy, 127
    in lupus nephritis, 80–82, 84–86
    in membranoproliferative (mesangiocapil-
        lary) glomerulonephritis, Type I, 22,
        24–25
        Type II, 23, 26
    in membranous glomerulonephropathy, 51,
        52
    in minimal change nephrotic syndrome, 40,
        41–42
    in obstructive nephropathy, 154
    in polyarteritis nodosa, 173
    in progressive systemic sclerosis, 94
    in sickle cell anemia, 200, 201
    in Wegener's granulomatosis, 178, 179
    normal, 4–6
Glycogen deposits, in diabetic nephropathy, 99
Goldblatt kidney, 160
Goodpasture's syndrome, 28
Gouty nephropathy, 107–108, 108
Grading, Fuhrman, of renal cell carcinoma,
    278, 278t
    nuclear, of renal cell carcinoma, 278, 278t,
        282
    WHO, of renal pelvic transitional cell carci-
        noma, 311
Granulomatosis, allergic, 180–181
    Wegener's. See Wegener's granulomatosis.
Granulomatous interstitial nephritis, 139, 141
Grawitz's tumor. See Renal cell carcinoma.

H
HBc antigen, 195
HBe antigen, 195
HBsAg antigen, 195
HBV. See Hepatitis B virus (HBV).
Heidelberg classification, of renal epithelial tu-
    mors, 275, 276t
Hemangioma, 302–303
Hemangiopericytoma, 304
Hematopoietic tumors, 273
Hematoxylin bodies, in lupus nephritis, 81, 83
Hematuria, benign familial, 124, 125
    condition(s) with, 57–58, 58t
        Henoch-Schönlein purpura as, 64–65, 65
        IgA nephropathy as, 58–63. See also IgA
            nephropathy (Berger's disease).
        loin pain–hematuria syndrome as, 66–67
    in sickle cell anemia, 199
    microscopic or gross, 57
Hemodialysis, long-term, acquired cystic kid-
    ney disease associated with, 242
Hemodialysis-associated amyloidosis, 222
Hemodynamic factors, in glomerular injury,
    10
Hemolytic-uremic syndrome, 68–76
    biology of disease in, 68–69
    diarrhea-negative (atypical form of), 69
    diarrhea-positive (classic form of), 69
    electron microscopy of, 71, 74–76
    immunofluorescent microscopy of, 71, 73–
        74
    laboratory findings for, 69
    light microscopy of, 70–71, 72–73
    treatment and clinical course of, 69–70
Hemorrhage, interstitial, in renal transplants,
    252
Hemosiderin, in renal tubular epithelium, 130,
    132
Henoch-Schönlein purpura, 64–65, 65
Hepatic cirrhosis, effect of, on kidneys, 197,
    197–198
Hepatic cysts, in autosomal dominant polycys-
    tic kidney disease, 236–237
Hepatitis, chronic, renal disease associated
    with, 197
Hepatitis B virus (HBV), 194–197
    antigens associated with, 195
    biology of disease and, 194–195
    glomerular lesions associated with, 196–197
    IgA nephropathy associated with, 196
    membranous glomerulonephropathy associ-
        ated with, 195–196
    polyarteritis nodosa associated with, 195
Hepatorenal system, 194
Heroin-associated nephropathy, 46, 192–193,
    193
    vs. HIV-associated nephropathy, 188
Hippel-Lindau disease, renal cell carcinoma
    associated with, 276
Histiocytoma, malignant fibrous, 304
HIV-associated nephropathy, 47, 187–191
    biology of disease in, 187
    clinical features of, 187
    differential diagnosis of, 188
    electron microscopy of, 188, 190–191
    immunofluorescent microscopy of, 188, 190
    laboratory values for, 187

Tubulitis, in acute interstitial allograft rejection, 249, *250*
Tubulovenous reflux, *156*
Tumor(s), extrarenal, 209–211. See also *Extrarenal neoplasm(s).*
  metastatic, involving kidney, 304–305, *305*
  neuroendocrine, 294–295
  renal. See also specific tumor, e.g., *Oncocytoma.*
    classification of, 275, 276t
    mesenchymal, benign, 298–303
      malignant, 303–305
    pediatric, 261–273. See also specific type, e.g., *Nephroblastoma (Wilms tumor).*
      differential diagnosis and frequency of, 264t
      ossifying, 273
    renal pelvic, 309–317. See also under *Renal pelvis.*
      benign epithelial, 315
      malignant epithelial, 310–315
      mesenchymal, 317
      proliferative, metaplastic, and inflammatory, 315–316
      TNM staging of, 309t
Tumor lysis syndrome, acute, extrarenal neoplasms and, 210

U

Urate nephropathy, 107–108, *108*
Urate tophus, *108*
Urinary tract, obstruction of, 153. See also *Obstructive nephropathy.*
  causes of, 154t
Uropontin, 111
Urothelial carcinoma. See *Transitional cell carcinoma.*
Urothelium, of renal pelvis, 309, *310*
Uveitis, interstitial nephritis with, 139–140

V

Vascular abnormalities, in loin pain–hematuria syndrome, 66

Vasculitis, renal, 172–186. See also specific type, e.g., *Polyarteritis nodosa.*
  conditions associated with, 173t
VHL gene, 280
Viral infections, interstitial nephritis associated with, 137t, 139, *141*
Von Brunn's nests, within renal pelvis, 315

W

WAGR syndrome, nephroblastoma and, 262
Waldenström's macroglobulinemia, 221, *221*
Wegener's granulomatosis, 177–179
  biology of disease in, 177
  clinical features of, 177–178
  differential diagnosis of, 179
  electron microscopy of, 179
  gross appearance of kidney in, 178
  immunofluorescent microscopy of, 179
  laboratory values for, 178
  light microscopy of, 178–179, *179*
  treatment and clinical course of, 179
  vs. polyarteritis nodosa, 174
WHO. See *World Health Organization (WHO).*
Wilms tumor. See *Nephroblastoma (Wilms tumor).*
"Wire loop" lesion, of lupus nephritis, 81, 82, *85*
World Health Organization (WHO) classification, of lupus glomerulonephritis, 80, 81t
  of renal epithelial tumors, 275, 276t
World Health Organization (WHO) definition, of focal glomerulonephritis, 34
  of hypercellularity, 9
  of mesangial proliferative glomerulonephritis, 15
World Health Organization (WHO) grading, of renal pelvic transitional cell carcinoma, 311
WT1 gene, 262
WT2 gene, 262

X

Xanthogranulomatous pyelonephritis, 146, *150*
  vs. clear cell renal cell carcinoma, 280